F. Schmitt · M. K. Stehling · R. Turner

Echo-Planar Imaging

Springer

Berlin
Heidelberg
New York
Barcelona
Budapest
Hong Kong
London
Milan
Paris
Santa Clara
Singapore
Tokyo

F. Schmitt · M. K. Stehling · R. Turner

Echo-Planar Imaging

Theory, Technique and Application

Foreword by Sir Peter Mansfield, FRS

With Contributions by

P. A. Bandettini, R. Bowtell, R. Brüning,
M. S. Cohen, A. J. S. de Crespigny, J. C. Duerk,
D. A. Feinberg, D. N. Firmin, H. Fischer, J. Hennig,
W. Irnich, B. Kiefer, K. Kwong, R. Ladebeck,
C. H. Meyer, M. F. Müller, B. Poncelet, P. V. Prasad,
P. Reimer, B. R. Rosen, F. Schmitt, B. Siewert,
O. P. Simonetti, M. K. Stehling, R. Turner, S. Warach,
P. A. Wielopolski, and E. C. Wong

With 386 Figures and 10 Tables

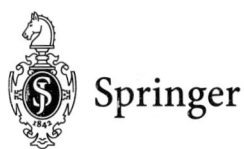 Springer

Franz Schmitt
Siemens Medical Systems
Department MRG
Henkestraße 127
91052 Erlangen, Germany

Michael K. Stehling, PhD, MD
Heinrich-Heine-Straße 4
63303 Dreieich, Germany

Robert Turner, PhD
Wellcome Department of Cognitive Neurology
Institute of Neurology, University College London
12 Queen Square
London WCIN 3BG, UK

The cover illustrations were kindly provided by Dr. Alistair Howseman (Wellcome Department of Cognitive Neurology, London), Dr. Betina Siewert and Dr. Stephen Warach (Beth Israel Hospital, Boston), and Dr. Piotr Wielopolski (Dr. Daniel Den Hoed Kliniek, Rotterdam, Holland).

ISBN 3-540-63194-1 Springer-Verlag Berlin Heidelberg New York

Library of Congress Cataloging-in-Publication Data

Echo-planar imaging : theory, technique, and application / [edited by] F. Schmitt, M. K. Stehling, R. Turner ; with contributions by P. A. Bandettini ... [et al.]. p. cm. Includes bibliographical references and index.
ISBN 3-540-63194-1
1. Magnetic resonance imaging. I. Schmitt, F. (Franz), 1953-. II. Stehling, M. K. (Michael K.), 1961-. III. Turner, R. (Robert), 1944-. IV. Bandettini, P. A. (Peter A.) [DNLM: 1. Echo-Planar Imaging. WN 185E18 1998] RC78.7.N83E24 1998 616.07'548-dc21

© Springer-Verlag Berlin Heidelberg 1998
Printed in Germany

The use of general descriptive names, registered names, trademarks, etc. in this publication does not imply, even in the absence of a specific statement, that such names are exempt from the relevant protective laws and regulations and therefore free for general use.

Product liability: The publishers cannot guarantee the accuracy of any information about the application of operative techniques and medications contained in this book. In every individual case the user must check such information by consulting the relevant literature.

Production: ProEdit GmbH, 69126 Heidelberg, Germany
Cover design: Erich Kirchner, 69126 Heidelberg, Germany
Typesetting: Hagedorn Kommunikation, 68519 Viernheim, Germany
SPIN 10104822   21/3135-5 4 3 2 1 0 - Printed on acid-free paper

Preface

*"Dost thou love life?
Then do not squander time,
for that's the stuff
life is made of".*

Benjamin Franklin

This book describes the technical principles and applications of echo-planar imaging (EPI) which, as much as any other technique, has shaped the development of modern magnetic resonance imaging (MRI). The principle of EPI, namely, the acquisition of multiple nuclear magnetic resonance echoes from a single spin excitation, has made it possible to shorten the previously time-consuming MRI data acquisition from minutes to much less than a second. Interestingly, EPI is one of the oldest MRI techniques, conceived in 1976 by Sir Peter Mansfield only 4 years after the initial description of the principles of MRI. One of the inventors of MRI himself, Mansfield realized that fast data acquisition would be paramount in bringing medical applications of MRI to full fruition. The technological challenges in implementing EPI, however, were formidable. Until the end of the 1980s few people believed that EPI would be clinically useful, since its complexity was far greater than that of "conventional" MRI methods. Many fundamental improvements in hardware, such as high performance gradient coil systems, magnetic screening of gradient and RF coils, improved gradient amplifiers, as well as more sophisticated and faster image formation algorithms, had to be developed to make EPI work, In turn, these technological improvements laid the foundation for most modern MRI techniques. Fast spin-echo (FSE) imaging, which is ubiquitously used in modern MRI, snap-shot FSE, used for abdominal and cardiac imaging, BOLD (blood oxygen level dependent) and diffusion techniques, used in neurofunctional and stroke research, as well as fast gradient echo techniques employed for 3D musculoskeletal imaging and gadolinium-enhanced MR-angiography have all profited directly or indirectly from EPI.

The idea to write this book first emerged during the final year of my PhD studies at the University of Nottingham in 1989 when I realized the profound impact EPI would have on the further development of MRI. Two years later, while working at the Siemens MR-research and development laboratory, Franz Schmitt enthusiastically supported my idea and, 1 year later, after we had both moved to Boston's Beth Israel Hospital to join Siemen's EPI prototype project headed by Robert Edelman, we signed the contract with Springer to get the book underway. Some time later Robert Turner joined us and provided crucial support in guiding the project through a difficult phase of its genesis. The book in its final form, however, would not exist without the enormous enthusiasm and discipline and the skills of Franz Schmitt in leading all the contributors to the finish line.

Our book endeavors to provide the first comprehensive treatment of the physics and technology of EPI and its applications in research and medicine. The editors were fortunate to have obtained the support of many pioneers and international experts in the field of EPI and related subjects whose contributions to this book give profound insights into the current development of EPI and its applications. Since the book is aimed at both scientists and medical doctors, it covers the range from profound mathematical treatments to illustrative medical examples, both of which can be studied independently.

On behalf of my coauthors Franz Schmitt and Robert Turner I would like to express gratitude to everybody who has contributed to this book, including the many unnamed supporters.

Dreieich   Michael K. Stehling
London   Robert Turner
Erlangen   Franz Schmitt
April 1998

Foreword

Some 23 years have passed since the idea of echo-planar imaging was conceived. In its original form it was called "Multi-planar Image Formation using NMR Spin-Echoes", but as time evolved it seemed necessary to follow the then current vogue of using catchy acronyms to encapsulate the technique. The nomenclature became reduced to echo-planar imaging (EPI), which is now the accepted term for this high-speed, one-shot imaging modality.

I well remember a symposium of experts convened at the University of Nottingham in 1977. I was asked to speak on a topic and chose to unveil the EPI method. The audience of about 20–25 people included Richard Ernst, Paul Lauterbur and others, and I recollect the look of disbelief and incredulity that greeted my presentation. There were no questions and it was as if I had never spoken. To put things in perspective, one has to remember that imaging times were typically of the order of 1 h and there was I proposing a method which would produce images in milliseconds. The response was not entirely surprising.

A lot of water has passed under the bridge from those heady and exciting days until today. From conception, EPI took a year or two before implementation of the crudest kind, and following those early 18-ms images there was a long struggle to raise funds and convince people by example that EPI could eventually work and compete in clinical imaging. Countless numbers of students, postdocs and visitors passed through Nottingham and made their contribution to the development of EPI, but it was not until a superconductive magnet had been acquired in the late 1970s, and not without the enthusiasm and dedication of a group of people at Nottingham and two of my former students, Ian Pykett and Richard Rzedzian, who went to the United States to set up their own company to make EPI machines, that the topic took off in a way which convinced far-sighted radiologists that there was something to the method. Once clinical interest was aroused, the various major companies in MRI took an interest in the technique and with that came final acceptance of the method.

The many aspects of this developmental process are encapsulated in the different chapters of this book, which also include EPI variants such as spiral scan EPI. The three authors are themselves pioneers in the subsequent development of EPI and especially its application, in the clinical radiological sense, the functional imaging research sense and the industrial sense. Two of the authors, I am proud to say, are ex-Nottingham researchers.

The editors of this book have, in my view, succeeded in producing a fine balance between the basics of EPI, the hardware aspects, safety issues and the clinical and radiological application.

This book, which is long overdue, certainly has my imprimatur. Aspects of EPI have been mentioned in other texts and in other reviews, but this is the first major book dedicated entirely to EPI and its hybrid variants. I have found the book generally very informative and stimulating. It is a book that will be of considerable value to MRI experts as well as to new students in the topic. Its appearance signals the coming of age of EPI.

Nottingham, April 1998   Peter Mansfield

Contents

List of Contributors

Bandettini, Peter A., PhD
Biophysics Research Institute
Medical College of Wisconsin
8701 W. Watertown Plank Rd.
Milwaukee, WI 53226, USA

Bowtell, Richard, PhD
Magnetic Resonance Centre
Department of Physics, Science Park
University of Nottingham
Nottingham, NG7 2RD, UK

Brüning, Roland, MD
Magnetic Resonance Imaging Unit
Clinic for Diagnostic Radiology
Klinikum Großhadern
Marchioninistr. 15
81377 München, Germany

Cohen, Mark S., PhD
Brain Mapping Division
School of Medicine
University of California Los Angeles
RNRC 3256, 710 Westwood Plaza
Los Angeles, CA 90024, USA

de Crespigny, Alexander, J. S., PhD
Department of Radiology
Stanford University Medical Center
Lucas MRS Building
Stanford, CA 94305-5488, USA

Duerk, Jeffrey C., PhD
Department of Radiology
University Hospitals
11100 Euclid Avenue
Cleveland, OH 44106, USA

Feinberg, David A., PhD, MD
Neuro Radiology Section
Mallinckrodt Institute
510 South Kingshighway Blvd.
St. Louis, MO 63110, USA

Firmin, David N., PhD
Royal Brompton Hospital Magnetic Resonance Unit
Sydney Street
London SW3 6NP, UK

Fischer, Hubertus, PhD
Siemens Medical Systems
Department MRO
Henkestr. 127
91052 Erlangen, Germany

Hennig, Jürgen, MD
Department of Diagnostic Radiology
Radiological University Hospital
Albert Ludwigs University of Freiburg
Hugstetter Str. 55
79106 Freiburg, Germany

Irnich, Werner, Professor Dr. Dipl.-Ing.
Institute of Medical Technics
University of Gießen
Aulweg 123
35392 Gießen, Germany

Kiefer, Berthold, PhD
Siemens Medical Systems
Department MRIS
Henkestr. 127
91052 Erlangen, Germany

Kwong, Kenneth, PhD
Massachusetts General Hospital
NMR Center
Building 149, 13th Street
Charlestown, MA 02129, USA

Ladebeck, Ralph, Dipl.-Phys.
Siemens Medical Systems
Department MRIS
Henkestr. 127
91052 Erlangen, Germany

Meyer, Craig H., PhD
Information Systems Laboratory
Department of Electrical Engineering
Stanford University
120 Durand Street
Stanford, CA 94305, USA

Müller, Markus, F., MD
Department of Diagnostic Radiology
Inselspital, University of Berne
Freiburgstrasse 4
3010 Bern, Switzerland

Poncelet, Brigitte, MD
Department of Radiology
NMR Center Massachusetts General Hospital
Building 149, 13th Street
Charlestown, MA 02129, USA

Prasad, Pottumarthi Vara, PhD
Department of Radiology
Beth Israel Hospital
330 Brookline Avenue, AN-242
Boston, MA 02215, USA

Reimer, Peter, MD
Institute of Clinical Radiology
Westfälische Wilhelms University
Albert-Schweitzer-Str. 33
48129 Münster, Germany

Rosen, Bruce R., PhD, MD
MRI
Massachusetts General Hospital
2nd Floor, Building 149, 13th Street
Charlestown, MA 02129, USA

Schmitt, Franz
Siemens Medical Systems
Department MRG
Henkestr. 127
91052 Erlangen, Germany

Siewert, Betina, MD
915 Tenth Street
Hermosa Beach, CA 90254, USA

Simonetti, Orlando P., PhD
Siemens Medical Systems
MR Research & Development
448 East Ontario, Suite 700
Chicago, IL 60611, USA

Stehling, Michael K., PhD, MD
Heinrich-Heine-Str. 4
63303 Dreieich, Germany

Turner, Robert, PhD
Wellcome Department of Cognitive Neurology
Institute of Neurology
University College London
12 Queen Square
London WCIN 3BG, UK

Warach, Steve, PhD, MD
Department of Neurology
Beth Israel Hospital
Harvard Medical School
330 Brookline Avenue
Boston, MA 02215, USA

Wielopolski, Piotr A., PhD
Department of Radiology
University Hospital Rotterdam
P.O. Box 5201
Rotterdam 3008 AE, The Netherlands

Wong, Eric C., PhD, MD
Departments of Radiology and Psychiatry
University of San Diego MRI
410 Dickinson Street
San Diego, CA 92103-8749, USA

CHAPTER 1

The Historical Development
of Echo-Planar Magnetic Resonance Imaging

R. Turner, F. Schmitt, and M. K. Stehling

Historical Introduction

During 1972 Paul Lauterbur at the State University of New York at Stonybrook in the United States and Peter Mansfield at Nottingham University in the United Kingdom stumbled their way [1, 2] to the common realization that the phenomenon of nuclear magnetic resonance (NMR) could be used to create a two-dimensional map of the density of nuclear spins within a sample of material. The crucial insight, arising from the earlier work of Gabillard [3], was that when a magnetic field gradient is established across an object containing NMR-sensitive nuclear spins, for each position in space there corresponds a different frequency at which the spins resonate. Thus frequency analysis of the NMR signal could provide an indication of how many spins are to be found at any particular plane in space, corresponding to a given contour of the magnetic field; in short, a *profile* of the spin density in the object.

Although initial progress was slow, since few scientists believed that the very low sensitivity technique of NMR could possibly be useful outside the physics or chemistry laboratory, by 1980 several practical magnetic resonance imaging (MRI) scanners had been developed [4–6], and commercial interest was mounting rapidly. As was natural, simplicity was sought in these early implementations, both in the new equipment that had to be manufactured and in the imaging technique decided upon. Thus one of the earliest practical ideas for forming an image with NMR [7], termed echo planar imaging (EPI) by its discoverer in 1977, Sir Peter Mansfield, was deemed by manufacturers to be too complicated for further development. Since EPI can produce images about 1000 times more rapidly than the method opted for by manufacturers in the early 1980s – spin-warp imaging [6] – this might be seen in hindsight to be a decision lacking in vision. It was not until 1987 that a handful of researchers, based mainly at the University of Nottingham and at a small research and development company, Advanced NMR Systems Inc., in Woburn, Massachusetts, were able to solve the practical difficulties surrounding EPI and to produce images of comparable quality to those available with the now burgeoning "conventional" MRI equipment [8, 9].

The historical development of EPI began, as noted, with the early realization that NMR can provide images of the density of nuclear spins in a piece of matter. To understand how this can be achieved we must first introduce the phenomenon of NMR. For a more detailed treatment of the basics of NMR see [10, 11] and Chap. 2 of this volume.

Nuclear Magnetic Resonance

Neutrons and protons, which each have a spin of 1/2, arrange themselves in atomic nuclei in such a way that in many cases the nucleus has a nonzero net spin. Associated with this spin is a small but well-defined magnetic moment, which means that a very large applied magnetic field tends to align the nucleus in a preferred direction. Putting this in another way, there is an energy difference between the state in which the nuclear spin is aligned with the magnetic field, and that in which the spin is in the opposite direction to the field. The Larmor equation states that this energy is proportional to the strength of the magnetic field and to the size of the magnetic moment of the nucleus:

$$\Delta E = h\nu = h\gamma B_o/2\pi \tag{1}$$

where ΔE is the energy difference between the parallel and antiparallel spin orientations, expressed here as a frequency ν using Planck's constant h, γ is the magnetogyric ratio describing the size of the nuclear magnetic moment, and B_o is the applied magnetic field. Exposing the sample to an additional radio-frequency (RF) magnetic field, varying in time at the Larmor frequency, results in a transfer of energy to the nuclear spins. This phenomenon is known as NMR. The angular frequency $2\pi\nu$ is usually written as ω.

In the language of classical physics, spins in a steady magnetic field precess about B_o at the Larmor frequency, with a mean magnetization vector directed along the static magnetic field. Application of the RF field causes the mean magnetization to nutate away from B_o, at a rate depending on the amplitude B_1 of the RF field. If this field is switched off when the nuclear magnetization is not parallel to B_o, the magnetization vector, continuing to precess in space, induces a current in a loop of wire with its plane parallel to the direction of B_o, just as the operation of a dynamo. The signal decays over time as the nuclear spins in different parts of the sample gradually lose their phase coherence and become realigned with B_o. This decaying signal is called the free induction decay (FID). The characteristic time for loss of phase coherence is called the transverse relaxation time, T2, and realignment with B_o takes place over the longitudinal relaxation time, T1.

The most abundant nuclear species having a nonzero magnetic moment is the hydrogen nucleus, consisting of a single proton. This has a Larmor frequency of 42.6 MHz at a field of 1.0 T. It also happens that protons have the largest magnetogyric ratio of any nucleus, giving them the greatest NMR sensitivity. Water protons in biological soft tissue at this field have a transverse relaxation time of about 30–100 ms and a longitudinal relaxation time of about 200–1500 ms, depending on tissue type. MRI is possible in human and animal subjects because biological tissue is mostly water, and because the relaxation times are long enough that state-of-the-art data acquisition techniques can collect enough useful data before the NMR signal decays to nothing.

Consider an extended sample, containing water (say), placed inside an RF coil, within a uniform magnetic field. If an RF pulse with a magnetic field component oscillating at the Larmor frequency is applied to the sample, and subsequently the frequency content of the induced free induction decay is analyzed, a single spectral line at the Larmor frequency is observed. The line width corresponds to the inverse of the transverse relaxation time, T2.

Now consider the effect of an additional static magnetic field, varying in space. By convention, the direction of the main field B_o is taken to be the z direction in a cartesian coordinate system. The RF pulse is applied in a direction perpendicular to this, and the magnetic field gradients necessary for imaging are dB_z/dx, dB_z/dy, and dB_z/dz. Suppose we have imposed a gradient $dB_z/dx = G_x$ (for details on gradient coils see Chap. 3). The Larmor frequency is now:

$$\omega = \gamma(B_o + G_x x) \tag{2}$$

and varies spatially in the x direction. If the sample extends a distance d in this direction, the FID contains frequency components over a range $\Delta\omega$, where:

$$\Delta\omega = \gamma G_x d \tag{3}$$

Frequency analysis (Fourier transform) of the FID shows a broadened line which contains some indication of the water distribution in the sample – in fact, it represents a profile of the sample in the x direction. If a series of data sets of this kind is acquired, with a range of angles at which the applied gradient is oriented to the sample, enough information is available to deduce the internal water distribution in the sample, by means of the so-called "back projection" algorithm [1], a method which was already employed in computed tomography (CT) [12]. This is the basis of the earliest method of magnetic resonance imaging of liquid samples, devised by Lauterbur in 1972 [1], and given the name projection reconstruction (PR).

While PR requires only modest additions of hardware to typical NMR instruments, the reconstruction algorithm is complex, and the time over which data are acquired is not used very efficiently. It retains a place on commercial MRI scanners because it performs well with tissues, such as lung, which have a very short transverse relaxation time [13]. However, for most purposes techniques which allow simple two- and three-dimensional Fourier transforms for image reconstruction have come to dominate MRI.

The earliest of these methods, Fourier zeugmatography [14] was itself foreshadowed by the insight of Mansfield and Grannell in 1973 [2] that the FID, when plotted in a space corresponding to the time integral of the magnetic field gradients applied to the object during acquisition, can be regarded as the diffraction pattern of the object.

If the time integral of the magnetic field gradients applied after the initial RF excitation pulse is written:

$$k = \gamma \int_0^t G(t') dt' \tag{4}$$

then the amplitude of the FID, S(t), can be expressed [2]:

$$S(t) = C \int_V \rho(\underline{r}) \exp(i\underline{k}\cdot\underline{r}) d^3\underline{r} \tag{5}$$

where C is a constant and $\rho(r)$ is the density of nuclear spins in the object of volume V. The quantity k has units of inverse distance, and corresponds precisely to the "reciprocal space" used in X-ray crystallography. Commonly, by using an RF excitation pulse containing a limited range of frequencies in the presence of a magnetic field gradient (the "slice select gradient") only a slice of spins in the object is excited, and the integral in Eq. 5 reduces to:

$$S(t) = Cd \int_A \rho(\underline{r})\exp(i\underline{k}\cdot\underline{r})\underline{d}^2\underline{r} \qquad (6)$$

where d is the slice thickness and A is the area of the section of the sample.

In either case the FID is revealed as the Fourier transform, or diffraction pattern, of the spin density. If the FID is sampled at a sufficiently large number of points in k space, the resulting data set may be inverse-Fourier transformed to provide an image of the selected section of the object. All gradient-based MRI methods can be regarded as differing ways of sampling FID data in k space, by means of various strategies for varying the gradients. Once gradients are switched on, the variable k traces out a trajectory [15] in k space, while FID data are continuously sampled. The earlier MRI methods to be commercially developed sampled only a small proportion of k space after each RF excitation, tracing a different trajectory each time, and building up a complete picture of the diffraction pattern only after (say) 128 excitations. EPI, by using larger and more rapidly switched magnetic field gradients which causes the trajectory to make a raster scan, is able to sample the whole of k space (for a given spatial resolution) after one excitation. This is discussed in much greater detail in other chapters.

Historical Development of EPI

As mentioned above, EPI was first conceived in 1977 by Mansfield [7]. The scanning of k space was performed with the use of two consecutive RF pulses, each followed by gradient switching and signal acquisition, the entire process taking less than 40 ms. Ordidge [16] provided the crucial insight that for correct image reconstruction it is vital to reverse the temporal order of data points obtained during gradient reversals. In the early years of its development EPI was viewed primarily as a means of forming acceptable images of rapidly moving parts of the body, such as the heart. The first in vivo dynamic study was of a rabbit heart [17], which was followed by a series of papers characterizing congenital heart defects in neonates [18]. The images shown in the earliest studies had a pixel matrix of 32×32 and were obtained at a field strength of only 0.1 T. It is remarkable how clearly the pediatric heart was delineated in these images, which had acquisition times of 35 ms, considering the poor signal-to-noise ratio inevitably associated with MRI at this low static field. By 1985 the MRI hardware at Nottingham had been developed sufficiently to allow the formation of images with pixel matrices [19] of 64×128 [20], and later improvements have resulted in single-shot images with 128×128 and 128×256 resolution [21].

In the meantime, important EPI developments were taking place in other establishments. In 1982 two of Mansfield's former research students, Rzedzian and Pykett set up a venture-capital research and development company in Massachusetts (Advanced NMR Systems, Inc.) to implement EPI at the much higher field of 2 T, with a view to creating a commercial product. In this they had the far-sighted support of radiological researchers at the Massachusetts General Hospital, notably Tom Brady. By 1986 most of the hardware problems had been solved [8], and diagnostic-quality images of the chest were shown, with pixel resolution of 64×128 and good single-shot signal-to-noise ration. A special feature of this implementation was the use of sinusoidally switched imaging gradients, in contrast with the original EPI method using a trapezoidal read-gradient waveform. The relative advantages and disadvantages of this method are discussed elsewhere in this book. While both the groups in Nottingham and Boston were able to obtain impressive real-time movies of cardiac function and other new applications, lack of clinical evaluation and medical conservatism led to slow commercial uptake of the now-marketable product, until the early 1990s (see below).

Elsewhere, Johnston [22] and Edelstein (personal communication), at the University of Aberdeen, in the United Kingdom, realized that a modification to the original EPI sequence, the so-called "blipped" technique, would allow a genuinely single-shot acquisition, at the expense of the potential formation of a spurious "ghost" image, half-way across the field of view from the correct image (commonly referred to as N/2 ghost; for details see Chap. 8). The advantages of this approach, however, were so obvious that most EPI developments since 1985 have been made with this type of sequence, referred to as blipped echo-planar single-pulse technique (BEST) [23]. A variety of methods for removing or avoiding the ghost artifact have been devised [24]; these are discussed in Chaps. 4 and 8. The tenacity of this problem has led to the implementation of many variants of EPI, such as asymmetric BEST (ABEST) [25].

Further pioneering studies were made at the University of California at San Francisco, by Crooks and coworkers. Again, working at low field (0.35 T), they implemented the blipped version of the EPI sequence and showed images of reasonable quality in 1986, using a small gradient coil insert designed initially for pediatric studies but suitable for head imaging. With this equipment they produced the first diffusion-weighted EPI image of human brain [26]. Parallel to this, two other laboratories in California [27–30] worked on a variant of the original EPI version. Following the suggestion by Ljunggren [15] that the demands on gradient switching can be reduced if a spiral trajectory through k space can be utilized, these researchers succeeded in developing image reconstruction algorithms which allowed images to be forned from data spliced from several spiral passes through k space, using a series of RF pulses. This research culminated in excellent quality cardiac images allowing visualization of proximal coronary arteries [30].

Simultaneously with these developments in the United Kingdom and the United States, initial EPI images were acquired on a 2.0-T experimental scanner at the Siemens research laboratory in Erlangen, Germany, at the end of 1987, initially with a head gradient insert [31]. In 1989 the first experimental whole-body

EPI scanner was set up, and initial experiments with whole-body gradient coils showed that fast switching gradients can cause peripheral stimulations [32] (for details see Chap. 6).

After the difficulties had been realized of obtaining good-quality EP images at field strength of 2.0 T and over organs other than the brain, the subsequent development of a whole-body prototype was continued successfully at 1.0 T [33, 34]. Studies of brain activation and oxygenation changes were carried out [35] in the same laboratory in 1993.

Among the other companies that embarked on the development of EPI, General Electric as early as 1989 established a collaboration with Advanced NMR Systems, but simultaneously developed their own version of nonsinusoidal EPI in 1991 [36]. Phillips and other companies such as Picker and Toshiba followed in the early 1990s.

EPI diffusion imaging was conceived by Turner at a NATO Advanced Scientific Institute in 1986 [37]. By 1989 Turner and Le Bihan [38] had developed this technique to the point that it could be used to evaluate variations in tissue water mobility in brain tumors and stroke, paving the way for the diffusion studies of McKinstry and collaborators [39], and those described in Chap. 20 of this book.

Many of the research and clinical applications of EPI were first pioneered at Massachusetts General Hospital [40] and later at Beth Israel Hospital in Boston [41] in the early 1990s. At Massachusetts General Hospital the group around Brady and Rosen carried out fundamental work on human brain perfusion [42] and functional MRI of the brain [43] on a 1.5-T General Electric system with an Advanced NMR Systems EPI add-on. The group of Edelman at Beth Israel Hospital, using a 1.5-T Siemens prototype scanner, focused on the clinical application of diffusion-weighted EPI for the early detection of stroke [44] and the development of segmented EPI techniques [45]. At the same institution the use of the high-performance EPI gradient system was demonstrated for magnetic resonance angiography with very short echo times [46].

EPI at higher field strength was demonstrated to be feasible [47], where the technique was implemented on commercial 2.0-T [48] and 4.7-T [49, 50] horizontal bore systems for animal studies. This led to EPI of small plant specimens at 7 T by Sukumar et al. in 1990 and at 11.4 T by Bowtell et al. (personal communication). Due to image artifacts – distortion and signal drop-out – associated with magnetic susceptibility variations in the object, which become very severe at high magnetic fields, it is unlikely that EPI in humans will be pursued at fields higher than 4 T. The first such results at 4 T were obtained at the National Institues of Health in Bethesda, Maryland [51]. EPI of human brain at 3 and 4 T has now been demonstrated in several laboratories, for instance, Nottingham [52], Milwaukee, Wisconsin, and Hershey, Pennsylvania. Many laboratories have now conducted studies in animals on 2-T systems.

A major obstacle in the development of EPI were the technical demands, especially on gradient coil and amplifier performance. These problems were overcome by the use of more powerful gradient current amplifiers [53, 54] and by fundamental changes in gradient coil design. Early gradient coils had extensive fringe fields inductively coupled with conducting structures in the magnet assembly, resulting in slow switching and troublesome eddy currents. Addition of a set of appropriately designed [55–58] shielding coils around the primary gradient coils removed the fringe fields almost entirely, allowing much cleaner gradient switching to be achieved.

Interest was quickened still further by the discovery of methods for imaging brain activity, known collectively as magnetic resonance functional neuroimaging, or functional MRI, in the early 1990s [43, 59–63]. The excellent time resolution and freedom from motion artifact of EPI made it the method of choice for the new and expanding field of MRI studies of brain functional anatomy, and several research hospitals with interests in neuroscience are in the process of installing the commercial EPI equipment that has recently become available. Top-of-the-line MRI systems produced by the largest MRI manufacturers since 1995 feature EPI capability.

A Guide to This Book

To provide a text that is useful to a wide range of readers we include introductory and advanced descriptions of EPI techniques and a broad variety of applications. The book begins with an overview of the fundamental concepts of EPI, stressing the idea of reciprocal or "k space" (Chap. 2, Cohen). This is followed by a description of the hardware requirements for MRI equipment for performing good-quality EPI imaging (Chap. 3; Bowtell and Schmitt). Chapter 4 (Wielopolski, Schmitt, and Stehling) and Chap. 5 (Schmitt and Wielopolski) discuss the methods of EPI image formation, including advanced EPI pulse sequences and sources of image artifacts. Image artifacts are then the subject of Chap. 6 (Fischer and Ladebeck). Chapter 7 (Schmitt, Irnich, and Fischer) considers the limitations of EPI imposed by interaction of rapidly switched magnetic fields with tissue, and the effects of flow on EPI images are examined in Chap. 8 (Wielopolski, Simonetti, and Duerk), including the potential of this technique for rapid and precise measurement of flow.

The next nine chapters cover most of the most important applications of EPI in recent years. A major advantage of EPI is freedom from motion artifacts when images are sensitized to microscopic diffusive motion of water molecules, and Chap. 9 describes the application of this technique to imaging of diffusion in the brain, which shows great promise in the early evaluation of stroke, a recurrent theme in this book by reason of its great clinical potential. Chapter 10 (Reimer and Ladebeck) describes EPI abdominal imaging and Chap. 11 (Müller, Pottumarthi, and Prasad) diffusion imaging of the kidney. Major progress has been made in using the unequaled speed of EPI to image the beating heart, and Chap. 12 (Firmin and Poncelet) provides a comprehensive summary of achievements and prospects in this area. EPI enables the monitoring of contrast agents passing through tissue in real time and can thus provide well-localized maps of relative blood volume. Chapter 13 (Stehling, Bruning, and Rosen) describes progress made in this application, with special reference to assessments of tumor vascularity.

Other important clinical applications of neuroimaging are described in Chap. 14 (Siewert and Warach). Perhaps the most remarkable use of EPI so far has been in the field of functional neuroimaging. The paramagnetic properties of hemoglobin allow EPI to depict local changes in blood flow arising from functional brain activity. Contributions from pioneers in the field (Chap. 15, Bandettini and Wong; Chap. 16, Kwong) describe the theoretical basis of functional contrast and the value of EPI methods in this area, and provides examples of the ground-breaking applications that are currently transforming the field of cognitive neuroscience. EPI also lends itself to well-characterized experimental studies in animals using specialized smaller MRI systems, and some of the technical issues and applications are described by de Crespigny in Chap. 17.

Chapters 18–20 deal with closely related methods for obtaining very rapid MRI images, which share with EPI the collection of data from two- or three-dimensional portions of k space after each RF spin excitation. The first (Chap. 18, Hennig) is a description of single-shot rapid spin-echo imaging (RARE), by Hennig. This is followed by a discussion of "segmented" versions of this method using several excitation pulses (Chap. 19, Kiefer), and a detailed description of the highly efficient sequence which in which a train of refocused spin echoes is further subdivided into groups of gradient echoes, known as gradient and spin echo (GRASE (Chap. 20, Feinberg). A final chapter (Chap. 21, Meyer) examines on techniques closely related to EPI, dealing with curvilinear, or spiral, acquisition trajectories in k space.

References

1. Lauterbur PC (1973) Image formation by induced local interaction: examples employing nuclear magnetic resonance. Nature 243:190–191
2. Mansfield P, Grannell PK (1973) NMR 'diffraction' in solids? J Phys C 6:L422–426
3. Gabillard R (1952) A steady state transient technique in nuclear magnetic resonance. Physiol Rev 85:694–705
4. Mansfield P, Pykett IL (1978) Biological and medical imaging by NMR. J Magn Reson 29:355–372
5. Bottomley PA (1982) NMR imaging techniques and applications: a review. Rev Sci Instr 53:1319–1334
6. Edelstein WA, Hutchison JMS, Johnson G, Redpath T (1980) Spin warp NMR imaging and applications to human whole body imaging. Phys Med Biol 25:751–756
7. Mansfield P (1977) Multi-planar image formation using NMR spin echoes. J Phys C 10:L55–L58
8. Rzedzian RR, Pykett IL (1987) Instant images of the human heart using a new, whole-body MR imaging system. Am J Roentgenol 149:245–250
9. Ordidge RJ, Coxon R, Howseman A, Chapman B, Turner R, Stehling M, Mansfield P (1988) Snapshot head imaging at 0.5T using the echo planar technique. Magn Reson Med 8:110–115
10. Wehrli F (1992) Principles of magnetic resonance. In: Stark DD, Bradley WG (eds) Magnetic resonance imaging. Mosby–Year Book, St Louis
11. Edelman RR, Messelink JR, Zlatkin MB (1996) Clinical Magnetic Resonance Imaging. Second Edition. W.B. Saunders Company. A division of Harcourt Brace and Company, Philadelphia
12. Cormack AM (1964) Representation of a function by 1st line integrals, with some radiological applications. II J Appl Phys 35:2908–2913
13. Castagno AA, Shuman WP (1987) MR imaging in clinically suspected brachioplexus tumor. AJR 149:1219–1230
14. Kumar A, Welti D, Ernst R (1975) NMR Fourier zeugmatography. J Magn Reson 18:69–83

15. Ljunggren S (1983) A simple graphical representation of Fourier based imaging methods. J Magn Reson 54:338–343
16. Ordidge RJ, Mansfield P (1985) NMR methods. United States patent 4509015
17. Ordidge RJ, Mansfield P, Doyle M, Coupland RE (1981) Real-time movie images of NMR. Br J Radiol 55:729–733
18. Rzedzian RR, Mansfield P, Doyle M, Guilfoyle D, Chapman B, Coupland RE, Chrispin A (1983) Real time NMR clinical imaging in paediatrics. Lancet II:1281–1282
19. Howseman Am, Stehling MK, Chapman B, Coxon R, Turner R, Ordidge RJ, Crawley MG, Glover P, Mansfield P, Coupland RE (1988) Improvements in snapshot nuclear magnetic resonance imaging. Br J Radiol 61:822–828
20. Stehling MK, Evans DS,Lamont G, Ordidge RJ, Howseman AM, Chapman B, Coxon R, Mansfield P, Hardcastle JD, Coupland RE (1989) Gastrointestinal tract: dynamic MR studies with echo-planar imaging. Radiology 171:41–46
21. Stehling MK (1989) Echo-planar proton magnetic resonance imaging. PHD Thesis, University of Nottingham, UK.
22. Johnson G, Hutchinson JMS (1985) The limitations of NMR recalled echo imaging techniques. J Magn Reson 63:14–30
23. Doyle M, Turner R, Cawley M, Glover P, Morris GK, Chapman B, Ordidge RJ, Coxon R, Coupland RE, Worthington BS, Mansfield P (1986) Real-time cardiac imaging of adults at video frame rates by magnetic resonance imaging. Lancet II:682–683
24. Bruder H, Fischer H, Reinfelder HE, Schmitt F (1992) Image reconstruction for echo planar imaging with nonequidistant k-space sampling. Magn Reson Med 23:311–323
25. Feinberg D, Turner R, Jakab P, von Kienlin M (1990) Echo-planar imaging with asymmetric gradient modulation and inner volume excitation. Magn Reson Med 13:162–169
26. Avram HE, Crooks LE (1988) Effect of self-diffusion on echo-planar imaging. Proc Soc Magn Reson Med:980–980
27. Ahn CB, Kim JH, Cho ZH (1986) High speed spiral-scan echo planar NMR imaging. IEEE Trans Med Imag MI-5:2
28. Macovski A, Meyer CH (1986) A novel fast-scanning system. Proc Soc Magn Reson Med, 5th annual meeting, WIP, p 156
29. Meyer CH, Macovski A, Nishimura DG (1989) Square-spiral fast imaging. Proc Soc Magn Reson Med, 8th annual meeting, p 362
30. Meyer CH, Hu BS, Nishimura DG, Macovski A (1992) Fast spiral coronary artery imaging. Magn Reson Med 28:202–213
31. Schmitt F, Fischer H, Ladebeck R (1988) Double acquisition echo planar imaging. Proceedings of the 2nd European Congress of NMR in Medicine and Biology, Berlin
32. Fischer H (1989) Physiological effects by fast oscillating magnetic field gradients. Radiology:382–382
33. Schmitt F, Stehling MK, Ladebeck R, Fang M, Quaiyumi A, Bärschneider E, Huk W (1992) Echo-planar imaging of the central nervous system at 1.0 T. J Magn Reson Imaging 2:473–478
34. Reimer P, Schmitt F, Ladebeck R, Graessner J, Schaffer B, Galinski M (1993) Experimental evaluation of potential bowel contrast agents for echo planar MR imaging. Eur Radiol 3:487–492
35. Stehling MK, Schmitt F, Ladebeck R (1993) Echo-planar imaging of human brain oxygenation changes. J Magn Reson Imaging 3:471–474
36. Souza SP, Roemer PB, StPeter RL, Mueller OM, Rohling KW, Dumoulin CL, Hardy CJ (1991) Echo Planar Imaging with a non-resonant gradient power system. In: Book of abstracts: Society of Magnetic Resonance in Medicine, p 217
37. Turner R (1988) Perfusion studies and fast imaging. In: Rescigno A, Boicelli A (eds) Cerebral blood flow. Plenum, New York, pp 245–258
38. Turner R, Le Bihan D, Maier J, Vavrek R, Hedges LK, Pekar J (1990) Echo-planar imaging of intra-voxel incoherent motion. Radiology 177:407–414
39. McKinstry RC, Belliveau JW, Buchbinder BR, Cohen MS, Weisskoff RM et al (1990) Instant NMR diffusion and susceptibility-contrast CBV imaging of patients with increased blood-brain-barrier permeability. Proc Soc Magn Reson Med, 9th annual meeting, p 1139
40. Cohen MS, Weisskoff RM (1991) Ultra-fast imaging. Magn Reson Imaging 9(1):1–37
41. Edelman RR, Wielopolski PA, Schmitt F (1994) Echo-planar MR imaging. Radiology 192:600–612
42. Rosen B, Belliveau JW, Chien D (1989) Perfusion imaging by nuclear magnetic resonance. Magn Reson Q 5:263–281

43. Belliveau JW, Kennedy DN, McKinstry RC et al (1991) Functional mapping of the human visual cortex by magnetic resonance imaging. Science 254:716–719
44. Warach S, Gaa J, Sievert B, Wielopolski PA, Edelman RR (1995) Acute human stroke studied by whole brain echo planar diffusion weighted MRI. Ann Neurol 37:231–241
45. Wielopolski PA, Manning JW, Edelman RR (1995) Single breath-hold volumentric imaging of the heart using magnetization-prepared 3-dimensional segmented echo-planar imaging. J Magn Reson Imaging 4:403–409
46. Wielopolski PA, Zisk J, Patel M, Edelman RR (1993) Evaluation of ultra-short echo time MR angiography with a whole body echo planar imager. In: Book of abstracts: Society of Magnetic Resonance in Medicine, 93:384
46. Pykett IL, Rzedzian RR (1987) Instant imaging of the body by magnetic resonance. Magn Reson 5:563–571
48. Turner R, Le Bihan D (1990) Single-shot diffusion imaging at 2.0 Tesla. J Magn Reson 86:445–452
49. Turner R (1989) Single shot imaging at 4.7 tesla. Relaxation times, GE NMR Instrum Newslett 6:4–6
50. Turner R, von Kienlin M, Moonen CTW, van Zijl PCM (1990) Single shot localized echo-planar imaging (STEAM-EPI) at 4.7 tesla. Magn Reson Med 14:401–408
51. Turner R, Jezzard P, Wen H, Kwong KK, Le Bihan D, Zeffiro T, Balaban RS (1993) Functional mapping of the human visual cortex at 4 tesla and 1.5 tesla using deoxygenation contrast EPI. Magn Reson Med 29:281–283
52. Mansfield P, Coxon R, Glover P (1994) Echo-planar imaging of the brain at 3.0T: first normal volunteer results. J Comput Assist Tomogr 18:339–343
53. Mueller OM, Roemer PB, Park JN, Souza SP (1991) A general purpose non-resonant gradient power system. In: Book of abstracts: Society of Magnetic Resonance in Medicine, p 130
54. Ideler KH, Nowak S, Borth G, Hausmann R, Schmitt F (1992) A resonant multipurpose gradient power switch for high performance imaging. In: Book of abstracts: Society of Magnetic Resonance in Medicine, p 4044
55. Turner R, Bowley RM (1986) Passive screening of switched magnetic field gradients. J Phys E Sci Instr 19:876–879
56. Turner R (1993) Gradient coil design: a review of methods. Magn Reson Imaging 11:903–920
57. Mansfield P, Chapman BLW (1986) Active magnetic screening of gradient coils in NMR imaging. J Magn Reson 66:573–576
58. Roemer PB, Hickey JS (1986) Self-shielded gradient coils for nuclear magnetic resonance imaging. European patent application 87101198
59. Ogawa S, Tank DW, Menon R et al (1992) Intrinsic signal changes accompanying sensory stimulation–functional brain mapping with magnetic resonance imaging. Proc Natl Acad Sci USA 89:5951–5955
60. Kwong KK, Belliveau JW, Chesler DA et al (1992) Dynamic magnetic resonance imaging of human brain activity during primary sensory stimulation. Proc Natl Acad Sci USA 89:5675–5679
61. Bandettini PA, Wong EC, Hinks RS, Tikofsky RS, Hyde JS (1992) Time course EPI of human brain function during task activation. Magn Reson Med 25:390–397
62. Stehling MK, Fang M, Ladebeck R, Schmitt F (1992) Functional magnetic resonance imaging with echo planar imaging at 1 T. Proceedings of the Society of Magnetic Resonance Imaging, New York
63. Stehling MK, Turner R, Mansfield P (1991) Echo-planar imaging: magnetic resonance imaging in a fraction of a second. Science 254:43–50

CHAPTER 2

Theory of Echo-Planar Imaging

M. Cohen

Generalized Overview

Magnetic resonance (MR) imaging always involves a complex balance of final signal-to-noise ratio (SNR) against a host of user-specified parameters such as resolution, contrast, scan time, and field of view. The total available nuclear MR signal in biological tissues is extremely small, a problem aggravated by the typical needs of the researcher or clinician for contrast and resolution. Improvements in spatial resolution, for example, necessitate dividing that limited quantity of signal into ever smaller chunks or voxels; improvements in contrast ordinarily are made by selectively *diminishing* the signal from some tissues while attempting to retain signal from others.

In MR imaging as currently practiced [we call this "conventional" as distinct from "echo-planar" imaging (EPI)] this challenge is addressed by sampling the signal repeatedly and building up an image data set gradually from these repeated samples. Simply stated, EPI demands the formation of a complete image following a single excitatory pulse, collecting the complete data set in the short time that the free induction nuclear MR signal is still detectable, for example, in a time limited by T2*.

In practice, EPI places enormous demands on the imaging hardware and on the creativity of the physicist and engineers constructing system hardware and software, and the specific technologies used to answer to these demands form much of the text of this chapter. Here we consider some of the principles of MR imaging with field gradients and try to place EPI in this context.

Capsule Review of Magnetic Resonance Imaging

The nuclei of many atoms, most typically hydrogen, behave as though they are spinning about an axis. The motion of these positively charged particles results in the creation of a magnetic field. When such a particle is placed into a static magnetic field (usually known as "B_o") its *angular momentum* results in *precession* of the nuclear spin about the B_o field. The precessional frequency (f) is a simple function of the magnitude of B_o:

$$f = \gamma B_o \tag{1}$$

where, for proton, $\gamma \approx 42.58$ MHz/T. In other words, in a 1-T magnetic field the hydrogen nuclei (protons) precess about the axis of the applied field at a rate of about 42 million cycles per second. The precessional motion of these tiny nuclear magnets can be observed by the current they induce in any nearby conductor or antenna. It is this set of fundamental principles that forms the physical basis of both nuclear MR spectroscopy and imaging.

Spatial Encoding

Once the MR signal has been created, it is necessary to spatially encode it in order to form an image: one must develop a means to determine the strength of the signal as a function of position. The method for this is based upon the realization that creating a spatially variant (inhomogeneous) magnetic field causes the signal frequency to vary with position (as in Eq. 1). In the simplest case the magnetic field (and therefore the MR frequency) is a linear function of position:

$$B_o = Gx + K = f/\gamma \tag{2}$$

where G is the magnitude of a "gradient" field, x is the position in space, and K is a constant field onto which that gradient is imposed (Fig. 1). When a gradient is applied, the strength of the MR signal at each frequency gives a measure of the signal strength at each position.

With larger gradient field amplitudes the frequency differences between adjacent spins are increased; it is thus possible to resolve smaller differences in position and thereby to improve the spatial resolution of the images. The key to observing the frequency differences is to sample the MR signal during the time that the gradients are applied.

What is needed, then, is a means for determining the signal strength as a function of frequency. Fortunately, this tool was provided us some 170 years ago and is known as the Fourier transform (FT) after its creator, Joseph Fourier. He showed that any signal can be generated by combining a possibly infinite series of sine waves at different frequencies, and showed further how to determine these frequencies and their amplitudes. While this chapter does not attempt to deal analytically with FT, we refer to it and its properties from time to time.

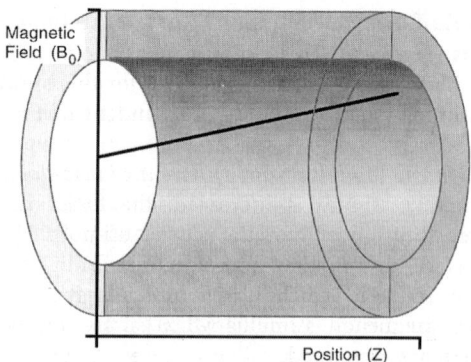

Fig. 1. Electromagnetic gradient coils are used to impose a spatially variant magnetic field within a large homogeneous magnetic field. The graph (*black*) shows the resulting magnetic field as a function of position within the static magnet (*gray*)

Magnetic Field (B_0)

Position (Z)

For a more complete picture the reader is directed to any of a number of texts on the topic, such as that of Bracewell [1].

Generally, we must localize the MR signal in three dimensions. Currently for most MR imaging one dimension of localization is performed using slice selective excitation [2]; the remaining two-dimensional localization is performed using field gradients as described above. To explain how the latter is carried out we first explore the manner in which the MR signal evolves while a gradient is turned on, and then introduce the concept of "k space" as a description of the MR raw data. With this background it is a relatively straightforward task to understand the many variants of EPI.

Magnetic Resonance Signals in the Presence of Gradients

After the initial radiofrequency (RF) excitation, or during the spin echo, the magnetization from protons everywhere throughout the sample is precessing in-phase and, to the extent that the magnetic field is homogeneous and uniform, these protons are precessing at the same frequency. In imaging, as mentioned above, gradients are used to convert position to frequency. Once such gradients are turned on, the protons along the gradient axis begin to precess at different frequencies and thus begin to dephase. (Along axes perpendicular to the gradients the spins are at the same frequency. A collection of spins at the same frequency is referred to as a *spin isochromat*.) Therefore one effect of the gradients is to cause a position-dependent phase shift.

Clearly, since frequency is a temporal phenomenon, it is not possible to detect it instantaneously. Less obvious is the fact that the so-called "discrete Fourier transform" (the digital version of the FT) can differentiate the locations of isochromats with one-full cycle (360°) of phase difference. This has a direct impact upon the achievable spatial resolution.

Consider the following example. Suppose that we are able to produce a magnetic field gradient of 10^{-3} T/m (1 G/cm). This causes spins 1 cm apart to differ in frequency by about 4258 Hz (from Eq. 1). If this gradient is left on for 1/4258 s (about 0.25 ms), spins 1 cm apart differ in phase by 360° and can thus be detected as different in position by FT. To achieve millimeter resolution the gradients must be left on for ten times as long (2.5 ms) or run at ten times the amplitude (10 G/cm). It is the product of the gradient amplitude and its duration that determines the final resolution. It also follows that if the gradients are left on for only a very brief period, there is very little net spatial encoding; the resulting images have very poor spatial resolution and differentiate only the largest features of the images. In general then, as the gradient-time product increases, the phase difference between spins in different positions increases, and we are able to detect smaller differences in position through FT.

Recognizing that the gradient-time product determines the spatial resolution, we are ready to introduce the concept of "k space." Note that the MR signals are collected in the presence of field gradients. If we were to plot the received MR signal starting at the moment when the gradients are switched on, we would see that the data accumulate features about smaller and smaller features of the images (as the gradient-time product increases). This would be a graph of k space where the horizontal, or "k" axis is the cumulative gradient-time product. Clearly the larger k values refer to finer image details (i.e., higher spatial frequency).

Because the gradient amplitudes may vary with time, we generally look at the integral of the gradient-time product to obtain a sense of the amount of spatial encoding that has occurred:

$$k_i = gG_i(t)dt \tag{3}$$

where the subscript i indicates that the gradient is applied along the i axis.

To develop intuition about the two-dimensional case consider that:

- In the *absence* of gradients all spins precess at the same rate, regardless of their position. Thus their relative phase does not change.

Fig. 2. Spin isochromats. A spin isochromat refers to a collection of nuclear spins precessing at the same frequency. In the presence of magnetic field gradients, spins along a line perpendicular to the gradients are arranged in isochromats. Continued application of the gradients results in a phase dispersion between isochromats. The phase differences increase as long as the gradients are applied. *Top,* the phase dispersion after a brief period of t seconds; *bottom,* the accumulated phase difference after $2t$ seconds

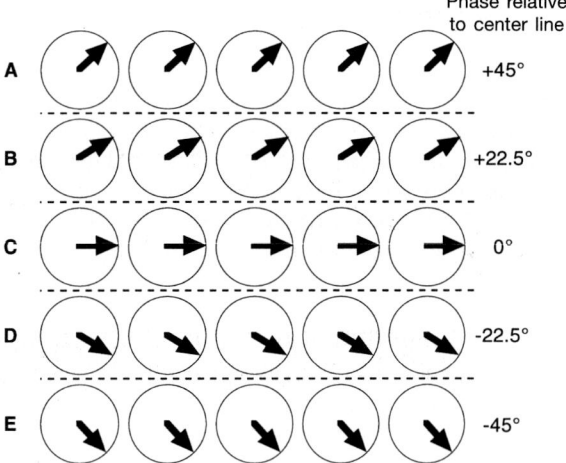

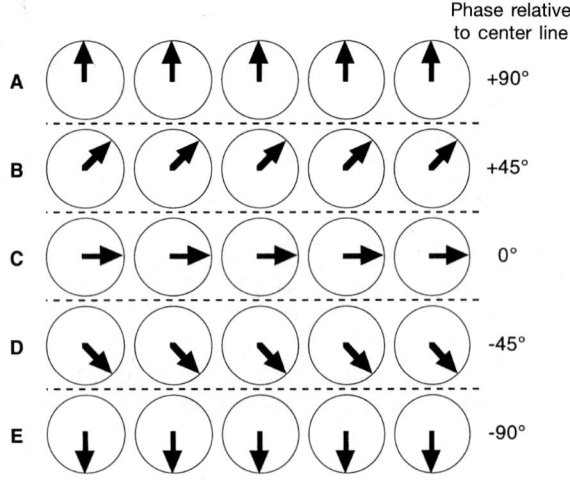

- A brief, high amplitude gradient pulse produces the same phase dispersion (as long as the spins do not move, i.e., the same phase difference with position) as a low amplitude gradient of longer duration.
- Since the data are sampled (digitized) at discrete intervals, there is no way to distinguish between the briefly pulsed gradients and the longer duration gradients.
- By reversing the polarity of the gradient (i.e., by changing which end of the magnet is in the higher field) the direction that the signal traverses in k space is reversed (i.e., referring to Fig. 2, the signs of the accumulated phase differences are reversed).

Figure 3 shows presents the concepts in (1) and (2) graphically. As the data are sampled at discrete points in time (in the process of analog to digital conversion) the phase evolution of the signal depends on the history of the signal prior

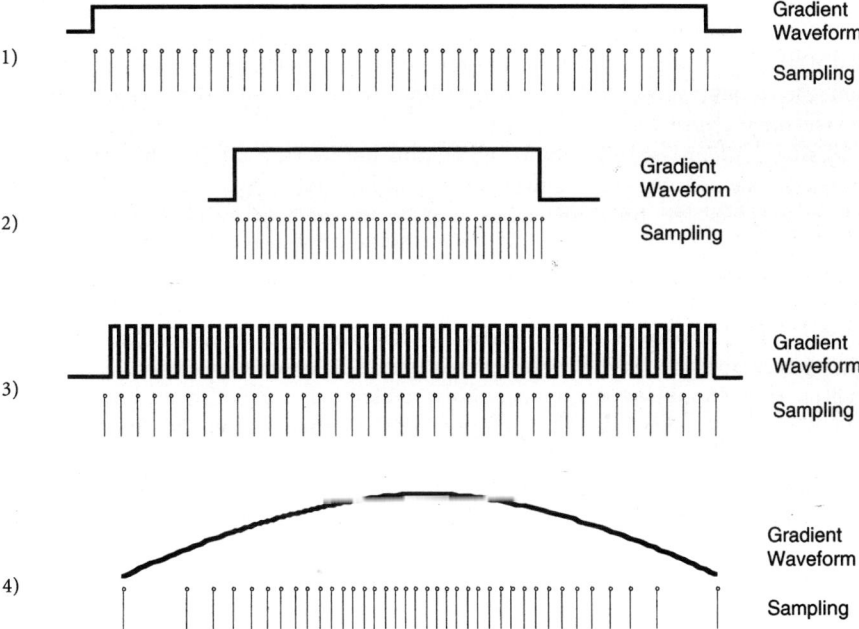

Fig. 3. The MR signal is sampled digitally in the presence of magnetic field gradients that cause the precessional frequency of the protons to vary as a function of position. Each digital sample represents a single data point in the raw data (k) space As the signal is sampled discretely, rather than continuously, the spatial encoding depends only on the integral of the gradient waveform, rather than its shape. Thus the four spatial encoding schemes sketched above all perform identical spatial encoding. In the first, a modest gradient amplitude is used with regularly spaced samples in time to produce equally spaced samples in k space. In the second scheme, application of a larger gradient amplitude allows the use of more rapid sampling. In the third scheme, the gradients are pulsed at high amplitude between successive points. This is analogous to the approach used for "phase" encoding in conventional imaging. The final scheme shows the use of a time-varying gradient waveform. By appropriately adjusting the sample points in time it becomes possible to space the data samples evenly in k space in the final data. The amplitude of the gradient determines the rate at which k space is traversed

to each sample point. To the extent that the gradients alter the signal, small gradient amplitudes for long durations are equivalent to large gradient amplitudes for short durations. When the gradients are turned off, and the field is everywhere uniform, the signal (or at least its spatial encoding) remains constant.

In conventional imaging we take advantage of this by applying a gradient along one axis (the "readout" or "frequency-encoding" axis) during signal acquisition, which in typical clinical instruments lasts for 5–10 ms (see Figs. 4 and 5). The gradient along the second axis (the "phase-encoding" axis) is applied briefly, immediately prior to readout. Adjacent points along each of the two axes are ordinarily separated by the same "k" distance. However, the time that passes between collection of adjacent points in the two directions can differ substantially. For the conventional imaging schemes the time between adjacent points along the phase-encode axis is equal to "TR," because the signal, whose T2 is often only slightly longer than the nominal 5- to 10-ms readout period, must be reformed in the time between the collection of each readout line.

At this point the phase-encoding gradient is pulsed briefly, displacing the signal in the k phase direction, and the readout process is repeated. The excitation–phase-encode–readout cycle is repeated until the desired net displacement in the phase-encode direction is achieved.

Using standard gradient and digitization hardware it ordinarily takes about 3 ms to encode the MR signal, in one dimension, to 1 mm resolution. In order to form the final image we require the data at every combination of phase and frequency encoding, and we thus must repeat the readout encoding once for each k step in the phase direction. To acquire 64 such readout lines, each at a different displacement along the k phase direction, would therefore require at least 64×3 ms, or nearly 200 ms. Since this is far longer than the T2 of typical body tissues, this is not a practical readout period. It is for this reason that the pulsed phase-encoding gradient scheme outlined above is used since it ensures adequate MR signal during the entire data encoding and collection period.

Consider how this might appear in a map of k space. During the time that gradients are applied the signal makes a trajectory to a new position, corresponding to a new gradient-time product, in a direction determined by the magnitude of the gradients (the vector sum of any applied gradients). Starting from $k = 0$, the origin of k space, when a readout gradient is applied, the signal advances in the k readout direction. When a phase-encoding gradient is applied, the path is advanced along the phase-encoding axis. Thus the scheme outlined in Fig. 4 can be plotted as shown in Fig. 5. Here one line at a time is acquired in the k readout direction. After waiting for TR and reforming the signal, the readout is repeated at a new phase-encode displacement.

Because the central point in k space is acquired with zero net gradient encoding, it contains no spatial information about the signal (or, more precisely, it represents the component of the signal that is of uniform intensity throughout the image. Points that are displaced from the k space origin represent information about smaller features of the image. This relationship between k space location and spatial resolution (spatial frequency) is demonstrated in Fig. 6, showing

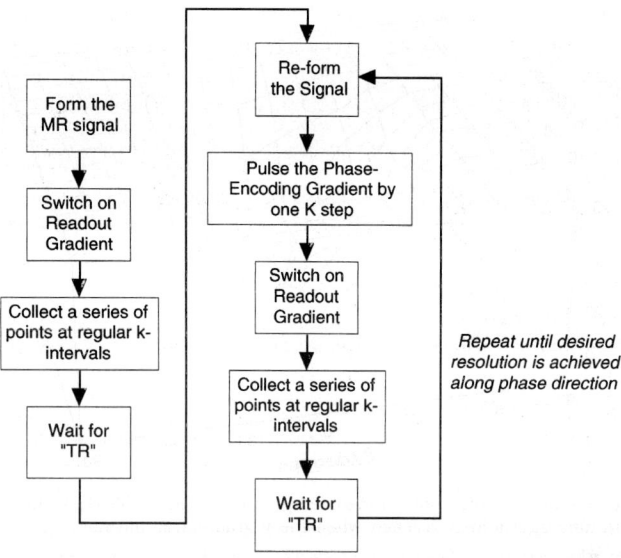

Fig. 4. Flow chart of the gradient encoding scheme for conventional imaging. After the initial formation of the MR signal a readout gradient is turned on, causing it to be encoded in the readout direction, that, is to move along the k readout direction. Each time the gradient-time product has reached a desired increment, the data are sampled, until a sufficient total displacement has occurred to achieve the desired spatial resolution along that axis. By this time the MR signal has generally decayed to the point that it needs to be reformed, either through another excitation or, in the case of RARE or fast spin-echo imaging, by an additional echo forming 180° pulse

Fig. 5. Conventional k encoding. In the conventional approach, raw data lines are acquired one at a time, separated by a "TR" period – typically from 10 to 3000 ms. Prior to the collection of each data line a gradient is applied along the phase-encoding and readout directions, causing the MR signal to be displaced in the k space plane (*gray*). After this preencoding the data are collected in the presence of the frequency-encoding or "readout" gradient. Following each data collection the signal is reformed in the TR period, usually by the application of one or more additional RF pulses. The encoding process is then repeated with a different k phase and k frequency displacement, until a sufficient number of data lines are collected

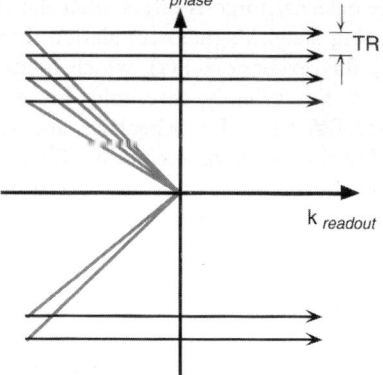

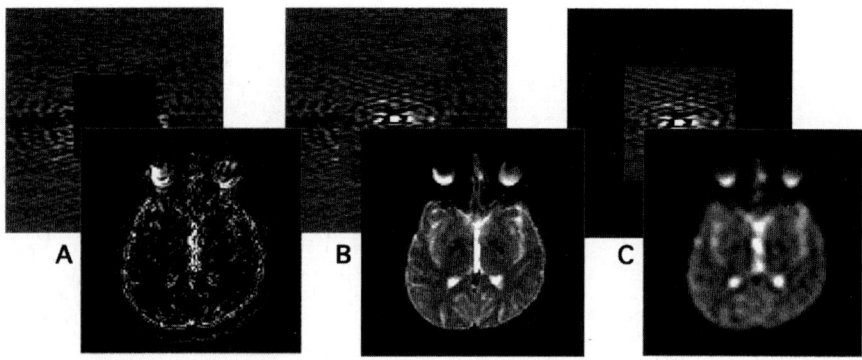

Fig. 6A–C. Data acquired near the origin of k space contain low spatial frequency information about the image, that acquired towards the k space periphery represents high spatial frequencies. **B** *Above*, the k space raw data (from an EPI scan) and resulting image for a normal EPI scan. If the k space data are zeroed, as in **A**, only the high spatial frequencies remain, and the resulting image contains mostly thin lines. When only the low spatial frequency data are used (**C**), a low-resolution image is produced. Note that the broad image contrast features are reasonably well represented in **C**. Many strategies for increased conventional imaging speed, such as "fast spin-echo [3]" and "keyhole imaging [4]" take advantage of this in controlling image contrast

that the points near the center of k space form a low-resolution map of the signal, and points near the periphery encode the image details [4].

A few added notes about k space (stated without proof):

- The spacing between points in k space determines the image field of view (FOV). The smaller the k displacement between adjacent points the wider the FOV. Expanding the FOV is thus accomplished simply by sampling the signal more rapidly (in time) in the presence of the gradient.
- To form an image using the Fourier transform it is necessary to have data from all four quadrants of k space, symmetrically about the origin along positive and negative k axes. (As shown below, in many cases the MR data have an intrinsic symmetry such that only half of the data need be explicitly acquired. This can be used in "partial-Fourier" or "half-NEX" imaging to reduce total acquisition time).

The flow chart for true EPI (Fig. 7A) is much simpler than that for conventional encoding (we use the term "true EPI" to refer to scan techniques using a single excitation pulse) in that all data are acquired following a single excitation pulse, so that the signal need not be repeatedly reformed. The key in this case is to use higher gradient amplitudes and faster sampling (both requiring more advanced hardware) so that the total spatial encoding process is completed in a shorter time short than T2, in other words, before the MR signal has decayed away. The path shown is for a particular k space traversal known as MBEST [5] or Instascan [6], though others are discussed below.

For completeness, we note that the so-called rapid spin-echo (RARE) [7] or fast spin-echo technique [3] is somewhere in the middle. In RARE, rather than use a new excitation pulse with each readout line, an additional 180° echo-form-

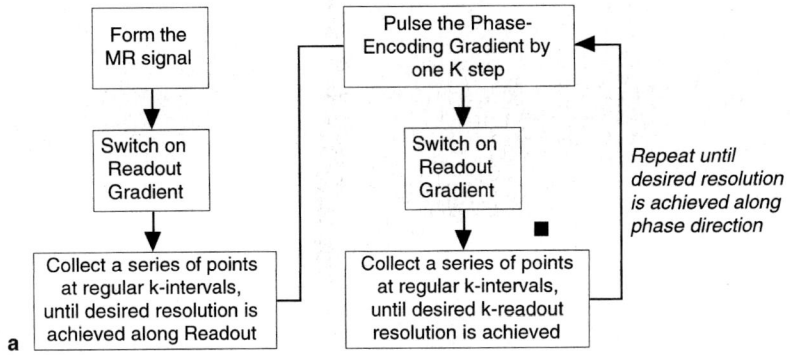

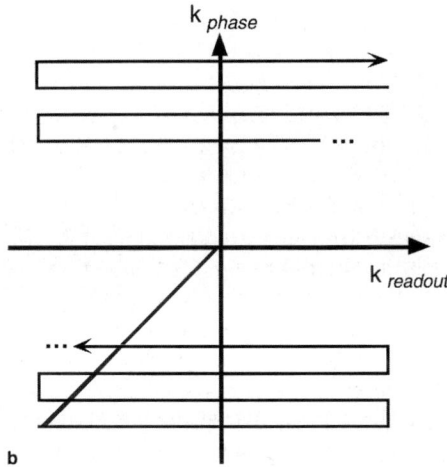

Fig. 7. a Similar to the flow chart shown for conventional imaging in Fig. 4, in the scheme for the most common form of EPI, each line of data collection on the readout axis is separated by a brief pulse of the phase-encoding gradient. The key, in true EPI, is to acquire each readout line fast enough that *all* can be acquired in the short time that the MR signal is present. **b** The k space trajectory for this form of EPI forms a rasterlike path. Note that the direction of traversal for alternate lines of readout must be reversed by switching the polarity of the readout gradients

ing pulse is used to re-form the signal. With RARE the number of lines acquired per RF excitation may be increased easily (and the scan time correspondingly decreased) as much as 16-fold that of conventional imaging. Likewise, the gradient- and spin-echo (GRASE) technique [8] acquires a few readout lines following each of several RF spin echoes, finding a further spot in the middle ground between conventional and EPI approaches.

The EPI Pulse Sequence

Having determined the desired method of collecting the raw data, and given our simple knowledge of k space, it is a relatively simple matter to write out the MR pulsing sequence needed for EPI. Figure 8 shows a straightforward version, using only a single excitation pulse. The RF pulse is made slice selective by simulta-

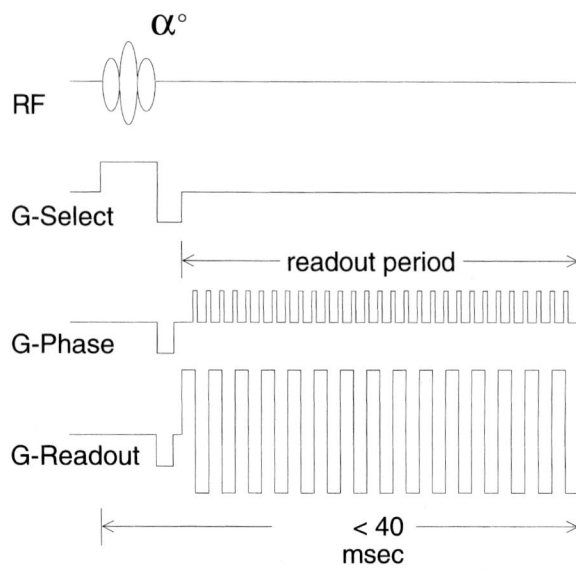

Fig. 8. EPI pulse sequence used to create the k space trajectory of Fig. 5. G select, G phase, and G readout refer to gradients on the slice selection, phase encoding, and readout axes, respectively. Excitation is limited to a single slice by transmitting the RF pulse in the presence of G select. Thereafter, brief negative pulses of G phase and G readout displace the signal to the lower left corner of k space. Rapidly oscillating the readout gradient causes the signal trajectory to alternate in the positive and negative directions in the readout axis. The brief pulses or "blips" of G phase cause the trajectory to move up one line at a time along k phase. A typical EPI scan time of 40 ms is shown to scale

neously turning on a gradient along the slice selection axis. The phase and readout gradients (G phase and G readout, respectively) give the k space trajectory of Fig. 5. Note that the positive-negative alternation of the readout gradient gives the alternating positive and negative velocities in k readout, while the brief pulses, or "blips" [5] of the phase-encoding gradient move the data from line to line along that axis.

Note the burden placed on the gradient system to perform such a sequence. For example, let us assume that we desire 2-mm pixels with a 0.5-ms readout period per line (a 32-ms readout for 64 phase-encode lines). We more or less invert the discussion on resolution above and calculate that 2-mm resolution implies one cycle per 2 mm, and that this must take place in 0.5 ms. The spin isochromats must therefore differ by 2 kHz in 2 mm, or 10 kHz/cm, which is a rather large gradient amplitude of (10 kHz/cm)/(4258 Hz/gauss), or 2.35 G/cm. Furthermore, this assumes that the gradients can be switched on to that value instantaneously – an unlikely feat.

All of the data points that make up the scan matrix along the readout axis must be acquired during the readout of each line. Thus for a 128 point readout resolution 128 points must be sampled during the gradient pulse. With readout periods of only 0.5 ms, the points must be sampled at 256 kHz, typically with 16 bits of precision, again assuming that the gradients have instantaneous rise times. This is quite close to today's (1998) practical limit for analog to digital conversion.

Sufficient Sampling Points

Just how many points need actually to be acquired depends upon the final image resolution and FOV needed. Where the maximum displacement along the k axis determines the image resolution, the FOV is determined by the number of points along that line, that is, the number of data samples acquired between $k = 0$ and k_{max}. For example, 128 pixels of 2 mm width give a 25.6 cm FOV. Acquiring additional lines in the k phase direction is performed easily by simply extending the pulse sequence for a longer period. Unfortunately, this can result in some image distortion [9], as the T2* values of the sample may not be long enough to yield signal for the extended readout duration. With today's imagers matrix sizes of 128 lines (in the phase-encode direction) are common, with readout periods as short as 60 ms.

As mentioned above, there is an important redundancy in the k space raw data. The raw data can be decomposed into two components. One is symmetrical about the origin (as a cosine wave), and the other is antisymmetric (as a sine wave). Knowing this, as long as one knows the precise location of that point of symmetry it is possible to make a full image from only half of the data [1, 10] since the symmetrical and antisymmetrical parts of the data are easily constructed. Figure 9 shows the time evolution of the MR signal in the presence of gradients as the gradient-time integral approaches and passes through zero (k goes from negative to positive values). The magnetization of the sample is a

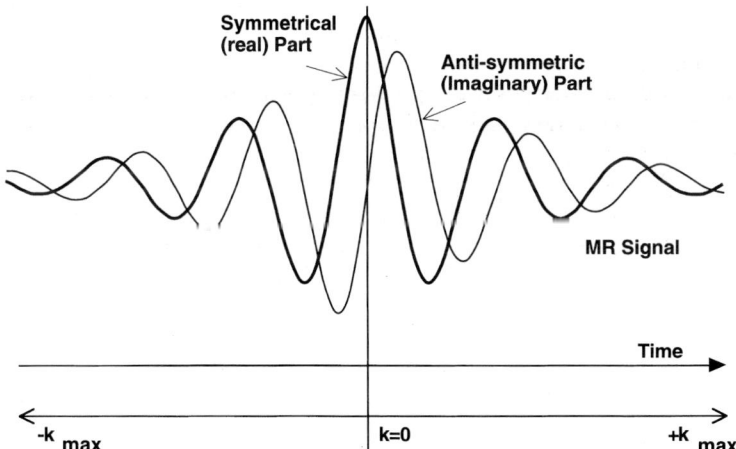

Fig. 9. The MR signal during gradient encoding. The MR signal is a rotating magnetic vector. Receivers 90° of rotation apart detect the waveforms shown above, one of which is symmetric about $k = 0$, and one of which is antisymmetric. The technique of conjugate synthesis is frequently used in both conventional and echo-planar MR imaging to "synthesize" half of the data when the other half is explicitly collected. For example, if only the data in the positive portion of k space are collected, it is a simple task to reconstruct the data for negative k values. In practice, the symmetry is not perfect, due to such effects as T2 decay, motion and magnetic field inhomogeneity. It is usually therefore necessary to collect more than half of the data to form a satisfactory estimate of the other half

rotating signal. If one imagines detecting the signal from two receivers rotated 90° with respect to one another, one would obtain the signals shown. One portion of the signal is symmetric about the k = 0 point, and the other is *anti*symmetric – its amplitude at time = –t is equal and opposite that at time = t. Clearly for waveforms of this kind it would not be necessary to explicitly acquire the data at positive and negative k values.

One way to understand this is the following. The Fourier transform in general operates between functions of complex variables. Even if the input function contains only real components, its transform generally contains an imaginary part, usually represented as a separate data set. Thus for a single real input signal (from a real patient or phantom) two raw data sets are produced – real and imaginary. This implies that the transformed MR data are over-specified, giving two transform points for every input point. This over specification is manifest as a symmetry in the MR raw data: if the value of the signal at k(m, n) is A+iB, the value at k(–m, n) is A–iB, the complex conjugate. Knowing this, it is a trivial matter to calculate k(–m, n), if k(m, n) is known.

This so-called "conjugate symmetry" of the MR raw data for real objects affords great savings in EPI and in conventional imaging because only half of the raw data points need be acquired to form a complete image. Therefore only half of the readout time is needed. In practice, however, determining the point of symmetry in the MR raw data requires collecting just slightly more than half of the data. Conjugate symmetry may be used in a variety of important ways in EPI, either to reduce the total scan time (relaxing somewhat the gradient requirements) or to improve the spatial resolution with a constant total readout.

Let us suppose, for example, that we have a gradient set capable of achieving a desired FOV (say 20×40 cm) in a readout period of 32 ms, sweeping out the area of k space shown in Fig. 10. One important use of conjugate symmetry is in echo time reduction. Because the overall readout periods in EPI are rather long, the echo time (usually coincident with the collection of the central region of

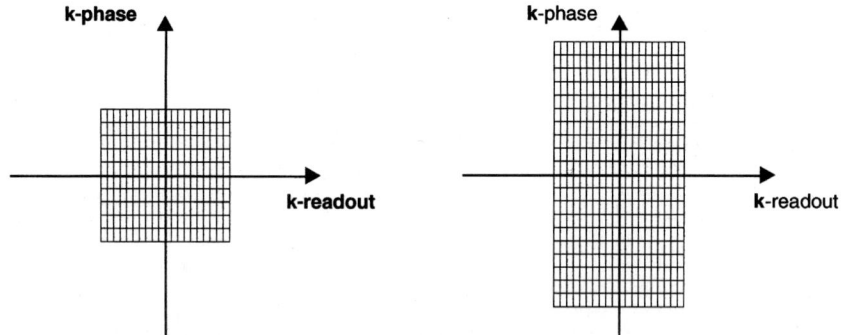

Fig. 10. During a single encoding cycle with EPI a sufficient region of k space is covered to produce a single image of moderate resolution, as indicated by the sampling grid (*above*). Extending the overall readout duration (*below*) results in increased coverage of the k phase axis, and thus improved resolution in that dimension

Fig. 11. Conjugate synthesis may be used for echo time reduction in EPI. The raw data are collected starting near the origin, closely following the RF excitation pulse, and slightly more than half of k space is covered. Conjugate symmetry is then exploited to complete the raw data set, and a complete image is reconstructed. Using this approach, it is practical to achieve effective echo times of only a few milliseconds

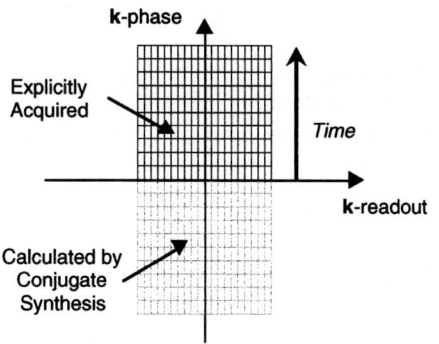

k space) tends to be long as well. By explicitly collecting only half k space, and starting near the origin, it is possible to dramatically reduce the effective TE. The data are then reconstructed by calculating the symmetrical half of the raw data space. Figure 11 outlines this scheme.

It is also common to use conjugate synthesis to enhance spatial resolution. As suggested in Fig. 12, one can acquire for a long readout period (as in Fig. 10, right) offset to one side of the k readout axis. The other half of the raw data is then formed as before by conjugate synthesis. Using this approach, it is straightforward to acquire single-shot images of 128×256 resolution, with pixel sizes of 1.5×3 mm.

Near the origin of k space there is very little net spatial encoding, implying that these points represent the signal intensities of large areas in the image. As a result, these data points dominate the overall contrast features. Figure 6 (above) shows the contributions of the central and peripheral data points in k space to the final image contrast.

Fig 12 The conjugate symmetry of k space may be used for resolution-enhancement as shown above. Here half of the data are explicitly collected along the k readout axis, and the remaining half of the data are calculated. In combination with an extended readout duration as diagrammed in Fig. 11 (*right*), useful matrix sizes of 128×256 points may be collected in about 60 ms

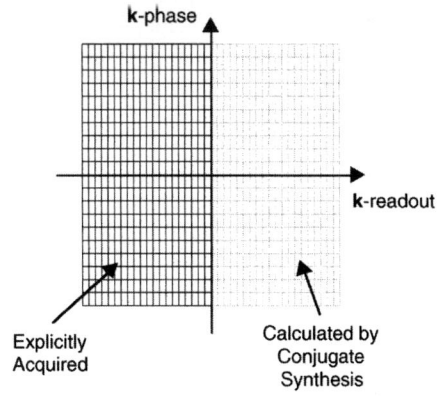

Number of Data Points and Bandwidth

For many applications it is convenient to express the bandwidth of MR images as the frequency difference from one pixel to the next; this in turn is determined by the time that elapses between collection of adjacent pixels: with longer times resulting in lower effective bandwidths. The bandwidth is an extremely important parameter for the final image quality as it determines the distortion in the final image from chemical shift and magnetic susceptibilities. Differences in susceptibility or chemical shift result in small differences in the proton resonant frequency. Since the positions of the signal are mapped onto the image by frequency, this can result in positional shifts and distortion. For typical conventional images the frequency difference between pixels is generally set to about 125 Hz. Fat and water have a relative chemical shift of about 3.5 parts per million (ppm), meaning that their resonant frequencies differ by $3.5 \times 10^{-6} \times 42.6$ MHz/T, or about 150 Hz/T. Thus in a 1-T field fat and water would differ in position by about 1 pixel. In addition to the more familiar chemical shift, biological samples (such as people) typically exhibit susceptibility gradients on the order of 1–2 ppm between body tissues.

With the bandwidths used in conventional MR imaging, these susceptibility variations seldom exert much influence on the scans. In EPI, however, the effective bandwidth can be quite low, as the time between adjacent points on the k phase axis can be quite long (0.5–1 ms), and there is no intervening RF pulse to rephase the MR signal. With a resulting bandwidth of 15–30 Hz/pixel, displacements of 8–10 pixels between water and fat, or in magnetically inhomogeneous regions such as the sella, are not uncommon. This problem is particularly serious in very high field imaging, as is being explored currently   , because the frequency difference is proportional to the main magnetic field strength. As a consequence the EPI readout must be faster at higher fields to maintain the same degree of image distortion.

Bandwidth is also related to SNR. Lower image bandwidths incorporate less noise in the final images, as the higher frequencies are not sampled, and therefore high frequency noise does not contaminate the data set. The longer readout periods used for EPI at lower magnetic fields thus mitigate somewhat the reduction in signal strength in those instruments.

In the vast majority of applications the EPI scans are acquired with lipid suppression to minimize the image degradation of prominent chemical shift artifacts. The most common scheme is to apply a saturating pulse to the fat resonance prior to data acquisition [11, 12], although other methods are viable. One promising approach is to use combined chemical shift and slice selective excitation (the so-called spatial-spectral pulse) [13], or short TI inversion recovery (STIR) [11, 14].

Encoding Order (BEST, Zig-Zag, Spiral, Square Spiral)

The rasterlike k space traversal shown above is only one of several that have been used for EPI. What is most important is that the raw data space be adequately covered by whatever traversal is used, regardless of the order in which the points are collected. One attractive approach is to cover the raw data space in a spiral pattern from the center of k space outward (Fig. 13). Using this scheme, the echo time (defined as the time from the RF pulse to acquisition of the center of k space) can be kept to an absolute minimum. (Note that the overall contrast behavior of the image is largely dominated by the data acquired at or near the center of k space, as mentioned above). Interestingly, the spiral acquisition pattern is self-refocusing for motion, so that velocity-dependent phase changes are minimized. This may become an advantage in vascular applications where velocities can be high even by comparison to the short overall readout used in EPI. Furthermore, the power requirements for the gradient sets are somewhat less severe, as the high amplitude gradient waveforms need not be reached instantaneously, as suggested in the raster EPI scheme described above.

The "square spiral" traversal shown in Fig. 13 on the left (as proposed and used by [15]), similarly to the MBEST/Instascan patterns in Fig. 7, has the advantage that the data are acquired on a regularly spaced grid. When acquired in this way, the data must only be sorted before using a two-dimensional FT for image reconstruction. When nonsquare (e.g., circular) spirals are used, as in Fig. 13 on the middle and right, the data cannot be acquired on such a grid. It therefore becomes necessary to adjust for the spacing of the data points, either by interpolation (which results in some loss of resolution and SNR) or by non-Fourier reconstruction. On the other hand, while the gradient switching cycle for the square spiral is extremely demanding. That for the circular spiral (Fig. 14) is much less so, being essentially a sinusoidal modulation of the form: $G_x = ktsin(\omega t)$, $G_y = ktcos(\omega t)$.

The most challenging aspect of the spiral acquisitions, however, is the propagation of chemical shift and susceptibility artifacts. The raster scans of Fig. 7B

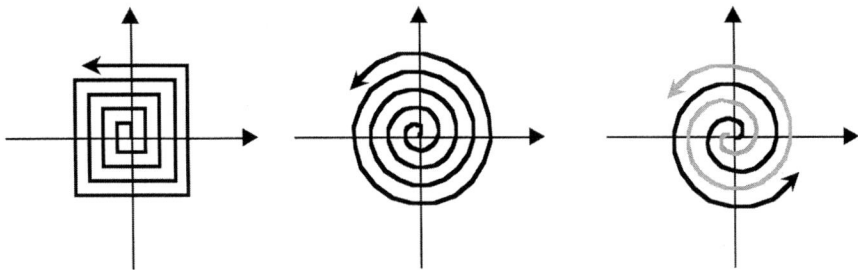

Fig. 13. As long as a sufficient number of points are acquired throughout the k space plane, it is possible to form a complete MR image. A variety of different traversal patterns have been proposed and used. The "square spiral" scan (*left*) has the advantage (as does the raster pattern shown in Fig. 7B *above*) that the data are acquired on a regular grid, so that a simple fast FT reconstructs the image. For the circular spiral and interleaved circular spiral trajectories on the middle and right; the gradient switching burden is minimized

Fig. 14. Gradient switching pattern required for the implementation of a circular spiral traversal of k space, as sketched in Fig. 13. The gradient waveform can be drawn directly from the k space traversal. Note that this is essentially a sinusoid of constantly increasing amplitude

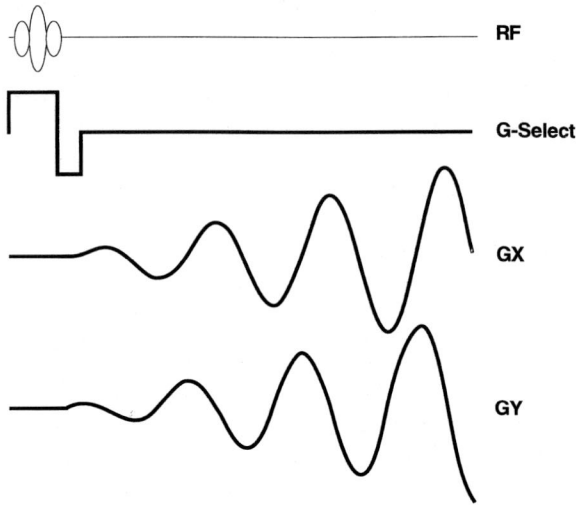

result in the data along the phase (or frequency) encoding axis being sampled uniformly in time and therefore have a consistent effective bandwidth in either direction: chemical shift and susceptibility result in uniform positional shifts. In the spiral scans the data points are sampled irregularly in time along these axes and thus result in blurring. The correction currently in practice for this problem is to reconstruct the raw data repeatedly at a variety of frequency offsets and then to "focus" the image data from the various reconstructions [16]. This method is somewhat complex and computation-intensive, although nevertheless effective.

Encoding Accuracy

Gradient Waveforms

Errors in the amplitude of the gradient waveforms (or, more accurately, errors in positioning the sampling points with respect to the integral of the gradient) can result in improper location of the data points in k space. The SNR of single short EPI experiments can be surprisingly high, on the order of several hundred to one in head images at 1.5 T when surface coils are used. Thus such artifacts frequently become visible. In order to use simple Fourier methods to reconstruct the EPI scans it is desirable that the data points be spaced on a regular two-dimensional grid. As suggested in Fig. 3, this may be accomplished either by sampling at a constant rate in the presence of a constant gradient amplitude or by sampling at an irregular rate in the presence of a nonconstant gradient, as long as the integral of the gradient, with respect to time, is kept constant between successive data points. Many current practical implementations of gradient power systems utilize sinusoidal gradient waveforms as they can be made quite power efficient through the use of resonant controllers [17]. Such an approach to sampling requires high resolution in the sampling control system, as small timing errors in each data point may result in noticeable artifacts.

The most common, and ultimately most challenging, source of such sampling errors is through the introduction of magnetic eddy currents in the conducting surfaces of the magnet due to the relatively high switching fields from the gradients. Such eddy currents results in time-dependent distortions of the magnetic field and thus in variations in the precessional frequency of the protons. The spatial distribution of the eddy current fields depends upon their conduction paths; in some cases they may result primarily in an overall field shift (when, for example, the conducting path forms a loop around the magnet's imaging bore) or in gradient fields. Either of these introduces distortion into the spatial encoding of the signal.

Eddy currents in EPI are so serious that in practice some sort of gradient shielding is generally required (unless local gradient coils are used that are at a considerable distance from the conducting surfaces of the magnet). The most commonly used approach to gradient shielding is to use a concentric, counter-wound gradient set that cancels the gradient fields outside of the coil [18]. Of course, this also attenuates the gradients on the *inside* of the coil so that the overall efficiency of the gradient may be reduced.

The timing of the samples must also be quite accurate to minimize artifacts. Collecting 256 data samples during a 500-µs gradient pulse requires sampling at an average of 500 kHz. In most practical applications of EPI the actual sampling rate is much higher, as the gradient waveshape is sinusoidal or trapezoidal (rather than square). Since the gradient is not on at full strength for the entire 500-µs readout, the peak amplitudes, and thus sampling rate, must be higher. Roughly speaking, the amplitude of the artifacts increases linearly with the errors in sampling rate. Thus, to keep such artifacts below the 200:1 SNR, the sampling must be accurate to within 0.5 parts per hundred, or 1×10^{-8} s with the 2-µs samples described above.

Once common form of sampling error is for the entire sampling train to be offset by a few microseconds from the gradient waveform. This can happen

Fig. 15. So-called "N/2" ghost artifact that appears when alternating lines of k space are not sampled in proper phase coherence, as can happen when sampling time points are shifted slightly with respect to gradient switching

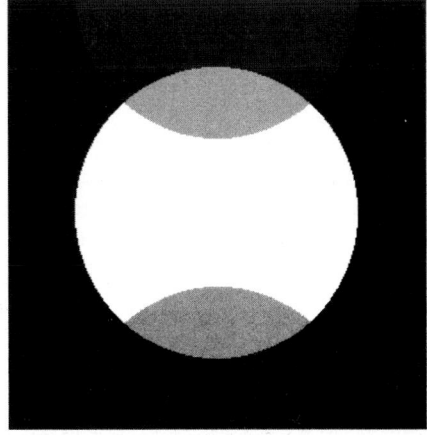

when, for example, eddy currents are conducted in the RF coils, introducing a coil-specific phase lag. Because the data in ordinary EPI are acquired in a back-and-forth trajectory in k space, alternate data lines must be reversed in time prior to Fourier reconstruction. A small lag in the sampling therefore results in a line to line k space discrepancy, with alternate lines being properly phased. This results in the introduction of ghost artifacts into the image, as schematized in Fig. 15.

Multi-Shot Experiments

In much the same way that individual raw data lines may be concatenated across excitations to form a complete conventional image, it is reasonable, and practical, to concatenate one or more EPI data acquisitions traversing different regions of k space to form a higher resolution image. This is the principal behind both the "Mosaic" and "MESH" methods proposed by Rzedzian [14, 19]. In the Mosaic scan, two-dimensional tiles of k space data are acquired and concatenated prior to image reconstruction. In the MESH scans, the EPI data collections are interleaved along the phase-encoding axis.

Another multiple excitation ("multi-shot") EPI approach is to provide phase-encoding along the slice selection axis between each EPI data collection. A three-dimensional FT of this data set results in a multi-slice, volume data set [20]. Because each of the resulting images is formed from the entire data set, a net improvement in SNR is achieved. As a result it is possible to form very high-resolution contiguous data sets in an extremely short period. Cohen [28], for example, has demonstrated 4-mm contiguous sections of the heart in total scan times of only 400 ms, easily fast enough to minimize artifacts from cardiac motion. Volume acquisitions, however, place a significant burden on the analog to digital conversion system in the scanner, as achieving the predicted high SNR requires high digitization depth (on the order of 16 bits) while maintaining the high EPI sampling rate. Fortunately, this is now becoming economically feasible.

dB/dt: A Nagging Issue of Safety

As shown by Ampére, time-varying magnetic fields (dB/dt) results in the development of an electromotive force and thus a current in nearby conductors. The switching rate of gradients used in EPI systems can readily reach amplitudes of more than 100 T/s that can produce significant electrical currents in the body of the subject being imaged [21–24] which can, under certain circumstances, be perceived and can even become quite noxious. The current magnitude depends on such factors as the orientation of the time-varying fields with respect to the conducting paths of the body, the local electrical conductivity etc. The sensory effects depend, in addition, on the direction of the nerve fiber bundles with respect to the induce electric fields. In humans, in body gradient sets, the threshold for delectability of the gradients seems to be about 60 T/s rms with gradients operating near 1 kHz [24, 25]. On theoretical grounds the use of trapezoidal as opposed to sinusoidal gradient waveforms may result in slightly greater total gradient areas and thus higher spatial resolution before stimulation can be detected. Safety of the EPI system is thus of significant concern to both the system designers and to regulatory agencies.

The available evidence on safety is presently very limited, as there are no reports of practical imaging designs that are able to cross safety thresholds. One group has studied the effects of extremely high magnetic field switching rates (3000 T/s) applied locally to the myocardium of laboratory animals. At these dB/dt values they were able to produce extra-systoles [26]. Such data suggest a considerable safety margin between the detection of gradient induced currents in the body and their possible harmful effects. Prudent gradient designs, however, ordinarily minimize the dB/dt where possible.

To π or Not To π?

It is sometimes convenient to consider EPI as a sort of stand-alone imaging block in a pulse sequence, where the RF pulse sequence determines the image contrast and an EPI encoding step forms an image from the MR signal at any time point. For example, performing EPI spatial encoding following a single excitation pulse results in an image whose contrast is T2* dominated (i.e., its signal intensity depends strongly on local magnetic field variations). Using a two-pulse series, typically a 90° pulse followed by a 180° pulse (a Hahn spin-echo series [27]), with a subsequent EPI data collection results in an image where the T2* contrast is minimized. The typical readout periods of 30–128 ms in EPI are rather longer than those in conventional imaging, and T2* losses are considerable during the readout period. Hahn echoes are commonly required for reasonably image quality.

Current State of The Art

As practiced at the time of this writing, EPI is a rapidly emerging approach to MR imaging. Compared to conventional scanning it offers tremendous speed advantages (of several hundred-fold for comparable contrast) and a greatly expanded range of applications. Because the sampling duration is considerable shorter, the SNR may be limited; therefore EPI is predominantly a high-field (1.5 T or more) technique. The engineering difficulties in high speed, high amplitude gradient, and analog to digital conversion designs have been largely overcome, so that readout gradient oscillation rates of 800–1400 Hz are now practical, enabling 256×256 images to be collected in as little as 90 ms (using conjugate synthesis). EPI imaging speed is thus facing other practical limits, such as the threshold of sensation from the large dB/dt and the SNR loss that can result from extremely short readouts (and large bandwidths). The gradient hardware, in particular, remains quite costly. EPI is therefore not yet widely available, but costs are showing a definite trend downwards. The ultimate acceptance of EPI will now depend primarily on the value of the new applications as compared to the cost of the technology conversions.

References

1. Bracewell R (1978) The Fourier transform and its applications. II. McGraw-Hill, New York
2. Mansfield P, Morris PG (1982) NMR Imaging in biomedicine. In: Waugh JS (ed) Advances in magnetic resonance. Academic, New York
3. Mulkern RV, Wong ST, Winalski C, Jolesz FA (1990) Contrast manipulation and artifact assessment of 2D and 3D RARE sequences. Magn Reson Imaging 8(5):557–566
4. van Vaals JJ, Brummer ME, Dixon WT, Tuithof HH, Engels H et al (1993) "Keyhole" method for accelerating imaging of contrast agent uptake. J Magn Reson Imaging 3(4):671–675
5. Howseman AM, Stehling MK, Chapman B, Coxon R, Turner R et al (1988) Improvements in snap-shot nuclear magnetic resonance imaging. Br J Radiol 61(729):822–888
6. Pykett I, Rzedzian R (1987) Instant images of the body by magnetic resonance. Magn Reson Med 5:563–571
7. Hennig J, Nauerth A, Friedburg H (1986) RARE imaging: a fast method for clinical MR. Magn Reson Med 3:823–833
8. Oshio K, Feinberg DA (1991) GRASE (gradient- and spin-echo) imaging: a novel fast MRI technique. Magn Reson Med 20(2):344–349
9. Farzaneh F, Riederer SJ, Pelc NJ (1990) Analysis of T2 limitations and off-resonance effects on spatial resolution and artifacts in echo-planar imaging. Magn Reson Med. 14(1):123–139
10. Margosian P (1985) Faster MR imaging – imaging with half the data. In: Book of abstracts: Society of Magnetic Resonance in Medicine, 1024
11. Weisskoff R, Cohen M, Rzedzian R (1989) Fat suppression techniques: a comparison of results in instant imaging. In: Book of abstracts: Society of Magnetic Resonance in Medicine, 836
12. Weisskoff R (1990) Improved hard-pulse sequences for frequency-selective presaturation in magnetic resonance. J Magn Reson 86:170–175
13. Meyer C, Pauly J, Macovski A, Nishimura D (1990) Simultaneous spatial and spectral selective excitation. Magn Reson Med 15(2):287–304
14. Cohen MS, Weisskoff RM (1991) Ultra-fast imaging. Magn Reson Imaging 9(1):1–37
15. Meyer C, Macovski A (1987) Square spiral fast imaging: interleaving and off-resonance effects. In: Book of abstracts: Society of Magnetic Resonance in Medicine, 230
16. Noll DC, Pauly JM, Meyer CH, Nishimura DG, Macovski A (1992) Deblurring for non-2D Fourier transform magnetic resonance imaging. Magn Reson Med 25(2):319–333
17. Rzedzian R (1987) A method for instant whole-body MR imaging at 2.0 tesla and system design considerations in its implementation. In: Book of abstracts: Society of Magnetic Resonance in Medicine, 229
18. Turner R, Bowley RM (1986) Passive screening of switched magnetic field gradients. J Phys E (Sci Instr) 19 (10):876–879
19. Rzedzian R (1987) High speed, high resolution, spin echo imaging by Mosaic scan and MESH. In: Book of abstracts: Society of Magnetic Resonance in Medicine, 51
20. Cohen M, Rohan M (1989) 3D volume imaging with instant scan. In: Book of abstracts: Society of Magnetic Resonance in Medicine, 831
21. Reilly J (1989) Peripheral nerve stimulation by induced electric currents: exposure to time-varying magnetic fields. Med Biol Eng Comput 27:101–110
22. Reilly J (1990) Peripheral nerve stimulation and cardiac excitation by time-varying magnetic fields: a comparison of thresholds. Office of Science and Technology Center for Devices and Radiological Health. United States Food and Drug Administration
23. Cohen MS, Weisskoff RM, Rzedzian RR, Kantor HL (1990) Sensory stimulation by time-varying magnetic fields. Magn Reson Med 14(2):409–414
24. Budinger TF, Fischer H, Hentschel D, Reinfelder HE, Schmitt F (1991) Physiological effects of fast oscillating magnetic field gradients. J Comput Assist Tomogr 15(6):909–914
25. Cohen M, Weisskoff R, Kantor H (1989) Evidence of peripheral stimulation by time-varying magnetic fields. Radiological Society of North America, abstract 382
26. Bourland J, Mouchawar G, Nyehuis J, Geddes L, Foster K et al (1990) Transchest magnetic (eddy-current) stimulation of the dog heart. Med and Biol Eng Comput 28:196–198
27. Hahn E (1990) Spin echoes. Phys Rev 80(4):580–594
28. Cohen MS, Weisskoff R, Rohan M, Brady T (1991) 400 msec volume imaging of the heart. In: Tenth Annual Meeting of the Society of Magnetic Resonance in Medicine. San Francisco, CA, pp. 840

CHAPTER 3

Echo-Planar Imaging Hardware

R. Bowtell and F. Schmitt

Introduction

The extremely short image acquisition times afforded by the echo-planar imaging (EPI) technique [1] can only be achieved by imposing heavy demands on magnetic resonance (MR) scanner hardware. The high performance required, particularly in the generation of large rapidly switched magnetic field gradients, meant that in the past it was generally not possible to implement EPI on standard clinical imaging systems, and consequently much of the development of the technique has taken place on dedicated, research-oriented systems with modified hardware. Over recent years, however, a number of technical developments have made the fulfilment of EPI's technical requirements more straightforward, and the new generation of commercial MR scanners incorporate hardware improvements which will allow the routine implementation of EPI.

In EPI an image is generated from a train of gradient-recalled echoes which are usually acquired after a single radio-frequency (RF) excitation. EPI's rigorous demands on scanner hardware result mainly from the need to acquire these echoes before they decay through T_2^* relaxation. Generation of an echo-planar image consisting of $N \times N$ pixels requires the acquisition of N echoes, giving an approximate time per echo of $\tau \approx T_2^*/N$. Usually this time must be less than 1 ms, which is considerably shorter than in most other MRI techniques. Since the spatial resolution in an MR image is proportional to $(G \times \tau)^{-1}$, where G is the strength of the magnetic field gradient, it can be seen that the reduction in τ required by EPI necessitates a compensating increase in gradient strength if the resolution is not to be compromised. Unfortunately, not only does the applied magnetic field gradient have to be large, but it also must be rapidly reversed so as to produce a train of gradient echoes. The generation of large, rapidly switched magnetic field gradients requires the use of highly efficient gradient coils, of low inductance in conjunction with powerful amplifiers and often special gradient switching circuitry. The design and implementation of such hardware, which is most crucial in the implementation of EPI, is discussed in detail below (see 'Gradient Coil Requirements for EPI' and 'Gradient Coil Design').

Because of the small amount of time available per echo in EPI the dwell time between sample points is generally very short (<10 μs), and consequently the bandwidth which must be used in signal acquisition is large. The spectrometer used in an EPI system must therefore be capable of high digitisation rates and be able to accommodate signals with large bandwidths. Analogue to digital converter (ADC) units which are able to sample 16-bit complex data at rates in excess of 1 MHz are currently available, giving a minimum time per echo in 128×128 imaging of just over 100 μs in the case of linear sampling. Although EPI is actually very efficient in terms of the image signal to noise ratio (SNR) achievable per unit time, the large bandwidths which this technique requires inevitably mean that the SNR in a single-shot image is low compared to that achieved with other, slower techniques. It is consequently important to ensure when implementing EPI that the RF coil design is optimised to give maximum sensitivity in detection of the MR signal. The particular technical requirements of EPI in this area are, however, not significantly different from those of any MRI technique in which SNR is at a premium. Consequently the RF coil designs used in conventional applications are generally well suited to use in EPI, with bird-cage coils [2] most widely used as volume resonators for whole-body and head imaging and surface coils employed in the imaging of localised anatomical regions [3]. Two points which may be of some importance in the construction of RF coils for use in EPI are that (a) at very low magnetic fields the wide bandwidth required by EPI may not be compatible with the use of an RF coil with a high Q factor, and (b) it is important to ensure that any conducting sheet acting as an RF screen does not sustain eddy currents at the gradient switching frequencies used in EPI. This is best accomplished by slotting the RF screen and building it out of very thin copper which is thicker than the skin depth at RF but much thinner than the skin depth at the audio frequencies used in gradient switching.

With a data acquisition period which is generally less than 100 ms in duration, EPI clearly offers the possibility of 'real-time' imaging, with the associated benefits of interactive patient positioning and interactive optimisation of image contrast [4]. Implementation of this technique also requires that images can be reconstructed and displayed at a similar rate to that of data acquisition. Echoplanar image reconstruction requires a significant amount of data re-ordering, as well as application of a two-dimensional Fourier transformation. 'Real-time' imaging therefore poses heavy demands on computer hardware. The increasing power of high-speed parallel processing technology, however, now means that it is routinely possible to process and display 128×128 images at rates of more than ten frames per second. When images are acquired at this speed, data accumulate at a rate of more than 0.6 Mbyte per second (assuming 16-bit digitisation of the MR signal). Clearly the high speed of EPI can therefore pose some data archiving problems, and efficient implementation of the technique requires the use of computing systems with large data storage areas which can be accessed at high speed.

The need to acquire a train of echoes generally means that the MR signal is sampled longer in EPI than in other techniques. The long duration of the sampling window, Nτ, translates into a low-frequency separation between pixels in the direction of the blipped gradient in the resulting image. This makes the echoplanar technique sensitive to image distortion resulting from inhomogeneities in the magnetic field. For example, in an experiment in which τ is 0.5 ms and 128 echoes are gathered, the frequency separation of pixels is only 16 Hz, which corresponds to a variation in the MR frequency of only 0.25 ppm at

1.5 T. EPI therefore requires the use of superconducting magnets which produce highly homogeneous magnetic fields.

Gradient Coils

Gradient Coil Characteristics

The magnetic field gradients used in MR imaging (MRI) are almost always generated by passing currents through specially arranged conductors, known as gradient coils. Three independent coils are employed, each of which generates a linear variation of the z component of the magnetic field, B_z, along one of the Cartesian axes, x, y or z, i.e. $B_z = G \times x$, $G \times y$ or $G \times z$, where G is the gradient strength. By convention the z direction is defined as that of the main magnetic field. A linear variation of the field with x or y position is known as a transverse gradient, whilst a longitudinal gradient corresponds to a linear field variation with z position. The strength of the magnetic field gradient produced by a gradient coil is always directly proportional to the current which it carries, so that:

$$G = \eta \times I \tag{1}$$

where, η is known as the gradient coil efficiency. Ideally a gradient coil should have as high an efficiency as possible, so that the largest gradient can be generated per unit current. The efficiency of a coil is proportional to the number of turns, n, that it carries, so that it might be thought that ever-increasing efficiency could be achieved by increasing n. This route to improved efficiency might be acceptable if a continuously applied gradient were required, but usually in MRI it is necessary to be able rapidly to switch magnetic field gradients on and off. In this context the coil inductance, L, is also an important parameter since it determines the minimum achievable gradient switching time. The larger the inductance, the more energy is required to establish a given current through the coil and consequently the slower the gradient rise time. Unfortunately, L scales as the square of the number of turns on a coil, and increasing the gradient efficiency by adding more turns therefore rapidly leads to excessive coil inductance and consequently long gradient rise times. As a result of the respective variations in the inductance and efficiency with the number of coil turns, the ratio η^2/L is independent of n and consequently is a good measure of the intrinsic performance of a gradient coil design.

Two other gradient coil attributes are also very important: the size of the region over which the coil produces a homogeneous gradient and the coil resistance. The power dissipated by a coil of resistance, R, carrying current, I, is I^2R. Significant power dissipation in the gradient coils is undesirable since it leads to heating of the coil wires and consequently of the environment inside the magnet's room temperature bore. Excessive heating can lead to coil failure. Low resistance is therefore a desirable characteristic in gradient coil design, which is best achieved by ensuring that there is an adequate current-carrying cross section in all parts of the coil.

An ideal gradient coil produces a magnetic field gradient that is perfectly linear in its variation with either x, y or z position over the whole region from which the MR signal is to be detected. In reality, apart from certain impractical exceptions, it is not possible to design a gradient coil which produces a perfectly linear field variation over large regions of space. Usually the spatial variation of the field produced by a gradient coil is most linear at the centre of the coil and shows increasing deviations from linearity as the distance from the coil centre increases. Since the process of image formation in MRI relies on a linear relationship between magnetic field strength and position, departure from gradient linearity leads to image distortion. Although some degree of image deformation can be corrected by image processing, it is desirable to minimise the amount of distortion. This is accomplished by limiting the maximum deviation from linearity in the magnetic field produced by the gradient coil over a specified region of interest. The specified region should of course be large enough to encompass all of the body anatomy which is to be simultaneously imaged. Increasing the size of the linear field region inside a coil usually leads to a reduction in coil efficiency at fixed inductance. The process of designing a gradient coil therefore requires compromises to be made between the gradient coil's efficiency, inductance, homogeneity and resistance. Other attributes which must also be considered are the size of the coil and the ease of coil fabrication. The particular trade-offs which are made depend to a large extent on the region of the body to be imaged and on the imaging sequence to be employed. Generally the smaller a gradient coil is made, the better its performance. This is because the ratio of η^2/L scales as the inverse fifth power of the coil size. It is consequently very important to use as small a coil as is allowed by the constraints of: (a) achieving adequate gradient linearity over the region of interest and (b) allowing straightforward access of the subject to the imaging area.

Gradient Coil Requirements for EPI

The use of a large rapidly switched magnetic field gradient in EPI means that low coil inductance and high gradient coil efficiency are both particularly important for this technique. Figure 1 shows the two types of switched gradient waveform (trapezoidal and sinusoidal) commonly used in EPI. The spatial resolution which can be achieved in the switched gradient direction depends on the area under one-half cycle of the gradient waveform. For the same peak gradient strength, G, in each waveform the resolution is given by:

$$\Delta x_{trap} = \frac{4\pi f}{\gamma G(1-\frac{\Delta}{\tau})} \qquad \Delta x_{sin} = \frac{2\pi^2 f}{\gamma G} \tag{2}$$

where $f = (2\tau)^{-1}$ is the gradient switching frequency, and it is assumed that the MR signal is sampled on the trapezoidal gradient ramps. Clearly in the case of a trapezoidal gradient the shortest possible ramp time, Δ, is advantageous, but this time is limited by the maximum rate at which the amplifier can slew the current through the coil. The slew rate is usually set by the coil inductance and the

Fig. 1. Sinusoidal and trapezoidal gradient waveforms

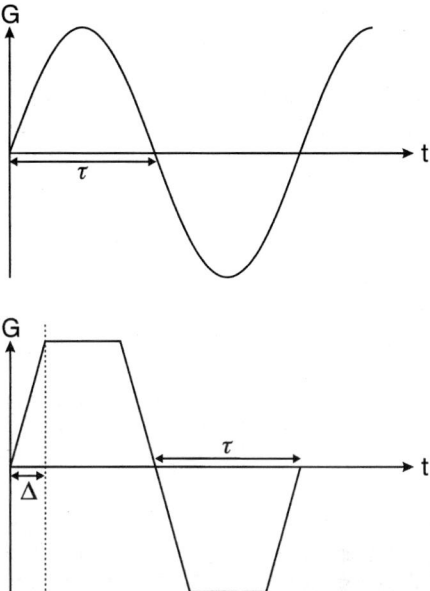

Fig. 1. Sinusoidal and trapezoidal gradient waveforms

maximum voltage which the amplifier can generate, since linearly ramping up to a gradient of strength G in a time Δ requires a voltage:

$$V = \frac{G \times L}{\eta \times \Delta} \qquad (3)$$

When the ramp time is small ($\Delta < 0.363\tau$) a trapezoidal gradient waveform always yields better resolution than a sinusoidal gradient for the same frequency and peak gradient strength. However, sinusoidal gradients are more straightforward to generate using simple resonant gradient coil drivers. Since these usually allow larger peak gradient amplitudes to be attained than do non-resonant circuits (as described under 'Gradient Coil Drivers), sinusoidal gradients are quite commonly employed in EPI. Figure 2 shows the variation in spatial resolution with gradient strength at three different switching frequencies for the two types of waveform. For the trapezoidal waveform a gradient slew rate of $200 \text{ Tm}^{-1}\text{s}^{-1}$ has been assumed. The current required to generate these gradients has been indicated for a well-designed body gradient coil with an inner diameter of 64 cm, an efficiency of $0.045 \text{ mTm}^{-1} \text{ A}^{-1}$ and an inductance of 130 μH.

As can be seen in Fig. 2, large currents are required in EPI, even when high-performance gradient coils are used. Gradient coil resistance must therefore be made as low as possible to limit coil heating and the power demanded from the gradient coil driving circuitry. The problems of power dissipation in the gradient coils can be alleviated by water-cooling the coils. This usually involves passing water through pipes placed in close proximity to the coil conductors. Unfortunately, gradient coil resistance usually increases with frequency, because of local eddy current effects and electro-mechanical coupling [5]. Problems asso-

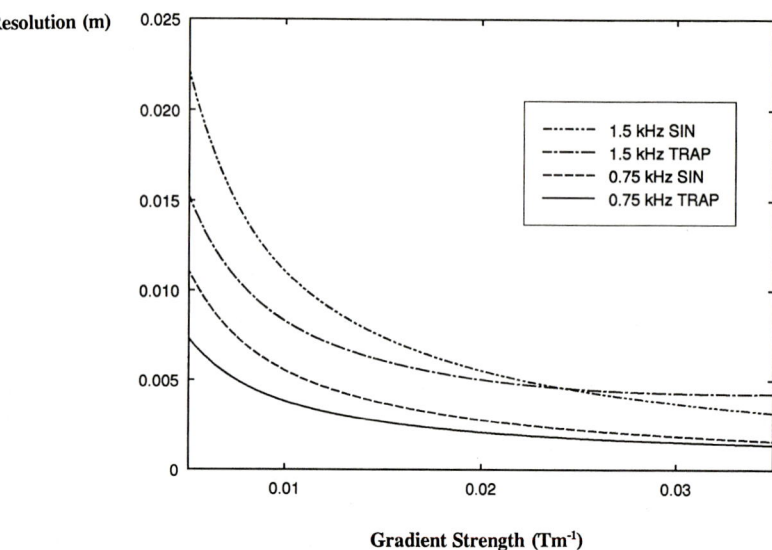

Fig. 2. Variation of the achievable resolution as a function of gradient strength for trapezoidal and sinusoidal gradient waveforms of frequency 0.75 and 1.5 kHz

ciated with gradient coil resistance are thus intensified when high gradient switching frequencies are used.

Several other coil attributes assume increased importance when implementing EPI. The first is the degree of interaction of the gradient coils with any proximal conducting structures. In addition to the magnetic field gradient produced internally, a gradient coil also generates some magnetic field in the surrounding volume. In MRI this volume usually contains electrical conductors, such as the magnet heat shields. If the current through the gradient coil is changed, eddy currents are induced in the conductors so as to oppose any change in flux. Once generated, these eddy currents decay exponentially with time, but with time constants that may be hundreds of milliseconds long. The decaying eddy currents generate magnetic fields inside the imaging region, which vary with time and spatial position, thus potentially causing image distortion and variation in the phase of the MR signal. The low frequency separation of pixels in EP images, which results from the relatively long time for which the MR signal must be sampled, makes the EPI sequence quite sensitive to the small magnetic fields which are generated by eddy currents. The rapidly switched gradient used to form the echo train, which might be expected to cause the most eddy current problems, actually generates little effect because of its repetitive nature and its short period compared with typical eddy current time constants. Problems may, however, arise as a result of switched gradients used in other parts of the imaging sequence. The method of active magnetic screening [6] which is commonly used to ameliorate eddy currents problems is described below.

The level of acoustic noise produced by a gradient coil when it is generating the large switched gradient is also of some importance. In MRI the conducting elements of the gradient coil are immersed in the large static magnetic field, B_o, and consequently they experience a Lorentz force, $\underline{F}$, which for an element of length, $\underline{l}$, carrying a current, I, is given by:

$$\underline{F} = IB_o\underline{l} \times \underline{k} \tag{4}$$

where $\underline{k}$ is a unit vector in the z-direction.

Consider a typical situation: a 50-cm-long wire arranged at 90° to a magnetic field of 1.5 T and carrying a current of 300 A experiences a force of 225 N, equivalent to a weight of 23 kg. This force inevitably leads to some small displacement of the gradient coil wires. When the current is switched on or off, the resulting wire movements lead to the production of acoustic noise. The situation is particularly awkward in EPI because a large current oscillating at audio frequency has to be passed through the gradient coil. The resulting acoustic noise can cause some discomfort to the subject and those operating the system. A number of steps can be taken to reduce the noise produced by a gradient coil. These include making the coil very heavy so that it cannot easily vibrate at the frequency of the switched gradient waveform [7], using active noise cancellation to null the sound from the gradient coil at the subject's ears, and designing coils in which the forces are locally cancelled so that the coil vibration is reduced at source [8]. The latter approach is described in more detail in the next section.

Finally, the peak magnetic fields generated in the body of the subject being imaged must be very carefully considered in EPI. As is described in Chap. 7, the flux changes resulting from the application of a rapidly switched magnetic field gradient induce electric fields in body tissues. These can lead to undesirable nerve stimulation. The size of the induced electric field depends on the rate of change in flux inside the body. This is largest in regions where the magnetic field generated by the gradient coil is largest. With a linear field variation with position, the maximum field generally increases with the extent of the region of homogeneity. The size of this region must therefore be subjected to prudent restriction when designing coils for use in EPI.

Gradient Coil Design

Cylindrical Geometry

Most gradient coils consist of conducting elements arranged on a cylindrical surface. Cylindrical geometry is the natural choice for gradient coil design because of the cylindrical nature of most of the magnets used in MRI and because of the ease of access to the imaging area which this geometry offers. However, in some situations better gradient coil performance can be achieved by adopting alternative geometries, as described below.

Discrete Wire Coils

The simplest cylindrical gradient coils consist of simple wire units, such as saddles and hoops. These are arranged with appropriate symmetry on a cylindrical surface so as to produce a magnetic field which varies linearly with one of the three Cartesian co-ordinates. The magnetic field produced by any coil can be described by the superposition of an appropriate family of functions, each having a different spatial variation. In coil design the functions used to describe the field variation with position are often the spherical harmonics, which have the property of orthogonality in spherical geometry. The positions of the units which make up the simple coils described above are chosen so as to eliminate as many undesired terms in the spherical harmonic expansion of the field variation as is possible, thus leaving the low-order harmonic corresponding to the desired gradient as the dominant term [9]. Simple application of this process leads to the Maxwell coil, which generates a z gradient, and the Golay coil [10], which can be used to produce an x or y gradient.

A Maxwell coil consists of two circular wire loops of radius, a, which are spaced by a distance of $\sqrt{3}$ a, and which carry currents circulating in opposite senses, as shown in Fig. 3. These produce a pure linear gradient ($B_z = 8.06 \times 10^{-7}$ a^{-2} z) [11] at the coil centre. The loop spacing is chosen so as to eliminate the spherical harmonic terms which produce fields varying as z^3 and $\rho^2 z$ (in cylindrical co-ordinates). The first undesired terms in the spherical harmonic expansion, which vary as z^5, $z^3\rho^2$ and $z\rho^4$, have an increasingly strong perturbative effect on the linearity of the field variation as the distance from the coil centre increases, and their presence means that the Maxwell coil produces a gradient with less than 5% deviation from uniformity only inside a sphere of radius 0.5 a.

Figure 4 shows a Golay coil which generates an x gradient. It consists of four saddle units arranged symmetrically about the planes z = 0 and x = 0, on a cylinder of radius, a. The angle subtended by each of the arcuate segments is 120°, chosen so as to eliminate spherical harmonic terms varying as cos(3φ). The arc positions along the z axis are fixed so as to null other high order terms. A y gradient coil is generated by a simple rotation of all the saddle units by 90°

Fig. 3. A Maxwell coil, consisting of two counter-rotating current loops, of radius a. The loop separation is $\sqrt{3}$ a

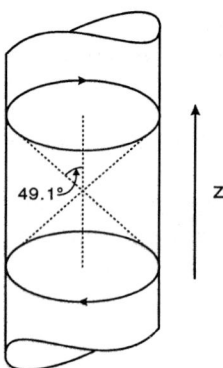

49.1°

z

Fig. 4. A Golay coil consisting
of four saddle units

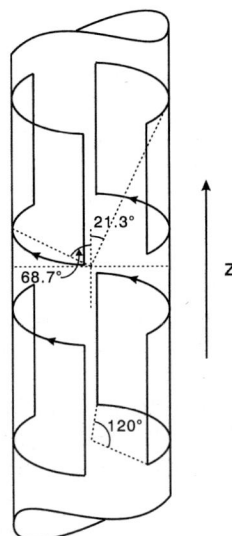

about the z axis. The field produced at the origin by the Golay coil is
$B_z = 9.18 \times 10^{-7} \, a^{-2}x$, and the field variation deviates from linearity by less
than 5% inside a sphere of radius 0.6 a [11].

For both of these coils the volume of the region within which a sufficiently
pure field gradient obtains is a relatively small fraction of the volume enclosed
by the coil and the coil efficiency is also quite low for a reasonable inductance.
Although some improvement in the size of the homogeneous volume can be
achieved by adding more units so as to null further, undesired harmonic
terms [12], better performance can be achieved by using coils consisting of distributed rather than discrete wire paths. In this type of coil multiple conducting
paths are placed on a cylindrical surface in order to approximate a continuous
current distribution. Such coils can produce pure field gradients over large relative volumes and also tend to have better η^2/L values because there is less flux
concentration close to the coil windings than in coils with discrete wire paths.

The design of gradient coils composed of distributed wire paths may be
accomplished using two classes of method, those based on the use of finite element analysis and those based on the use of analytic expressions.

Analytic Design of Coils with Distributed Wirepaths

The analytic methods start from the Green's function expansion of the vector
potential resulting from a current distribution:

$$\underline{J}(\phi,z) = J_z(\phi,z)\underline{\hat{z}} + J_z(\phi,z)\underline{\hat{\phi}} \tag{5}$$

confined to the surface of a cylinder of radius, a. Using this expression, Turner and Bowley were able to derive the following equation for the variation of the magnetic field, $B_z(r,f,z)$ in the region where $\rho < a$ [13]:

$$B_z = -\frac{\mu_o}{2\pi} \sum_{m=-\infty}^{m=\infty} \int_{-\infty}^{\infty} dk\, e^{ikz} e^{im\phi}\, J_\phi^m(k)\, ka\, I_m(k\rho)\, K_m'(ka) \qquad (6)$$

Here $J_\phi^m(k)$ is the Fourier transform with respect to z and ϕ, of the azimuthal component of the current distribution:

$$J_\phi^m(k) = \frac{1}{2\pi} \int_{-\pi}^{\pi} d\phi e^{-im\phi} \int_{-\infty}^{\infty} dz\, e^{-ikz}\, J_\phi(\phi,z) \qquad (7)$$

and $I_m(x)$, $K_m(x)$ are the modified Bessel functions.

By defining a similar Fourier transform of the magnetic field variation at radius, $c < a$, $(B_z^m(c,k) = FT[B_z(c,\phi,z)])$ Eq. 6 can be inverted to give:

$$J_\phi^m(k) = -\frac{B_z^m(c,k)}{\mu_o ka\, K_m'(ka) I_m(kc)} \qquad (8)$$

This equation can be used to implement the target field approach to coil design, which was developed by Turner [14]. Here a desired or target field variation is first specified over a cylindrical surface inside the coil cylinder. The target field is Fourier transformed and substituted into Eq. 8 to yield the Fourier transform of the current distribution, $J_\phi^m(k)$, which generates this field variation. Inverse Fourier transformation then gives the actual current distribution. Finally, wire paths which mimic the calculated current distribution are determined. This is accomplished by placing wires at contours of the integrated current density or 'stream function'. Implementation of the target field approach requires the use of an appropriate target field. For a longitudinal gradient coil a sensible field variation is:

$$B_z = \frac{z}{1 + (\frac{z}{d})^6} \qquad (9)$$

whilst for a transverse coil:

$$B_z = \frac{Gx}{d_2 - d_1} \left(\frac{d_2}{1 + (\frac{z}{d_1})^6} - \frac{d_1}{1 + (\frac{z}{d_2})^6} \right) \qquad (10)$$

is appropriate [15]. The size of the volume within which a linear field variation is generated, depends on the target field parameters (d or d_1 and d_2) and the target radius. Designing a particular coil with this method, involves choosing these parameters so as to produce an appropriate region of gradient homogeneity. In assessing the resulting coil design, it is also useful to be able to evaluate the coil's inductance and the power which it dissipates. This is straightforward since using the formalism described above, relatively simple expressions can be derived for the inductance:

$$L = -\frac{\mu_0 a^2}{I^2} \sum_{m=-\infty}^{\infty} \int_{-\infty}^{\infty} dk |J_\phi^m(k)|^2 I_m'(ka) K_m'(ka) \tag{11}$$

and for the power dissipation:

$$P = \frac{\rho a}{t} \sum_{m=-\infty}^{\infty} \int_{-\infty}^{\infty} dk |J_\phi^m(k)|^2 \left(1 + \frac{m^2}{k^2 a^2}\right) \tag{12}$$

of a coil in which a current, I, flows in a conducting cylinder of thickness, t, and resistivity, ρ [11]. As well as being useful in evaluating coil performance, these expressions can be directly minimised in the process of coil design. In the minimum inductance approach [16] Lagrange's undetermined multipliers are used to minimise the coil inductance subject to the constraint that the field produced by the coil corresponds to specified values at n target points. By appropriately choosing the position of these target points a coil of minimum inductance, which generates a pure field gradient over a particular region of interest can be designed. By a similar process coils with the lowest possible power dissipation can also be designed [17].

When designing a cylindrical gradient coil, it is often necessary to constrain the length of the coil. Such length constraints can be added into the minimisation techniques described above, but it is often more straightforward automatically to incorporate the finite coil length into the current density. This can be accomplished by writing the z variation of the current density as a Fourier series:

$$j(z) = \sum_{n=1}^{N} a_n \sin\left(\frac{n\pi z}{L}\right) + b_n \cos\left(\frac{n\pi z}{L}\right) \tag{13}$$

truncated to length 2L [18]. The process of coil design then becomes one of setting the values of the coefficients, a_n and b_n.

Active Magnetic Screening

The method of active magnetic screening, which can be used to eliminate the detrimental effects of eddy currents induced in structures surrounding a gradient coil, follows naturally from the ideas used in the analytic design of coils with distributed wirepaths. Eddy currents are generated by the time varying fringe fields produced when a gradient coil is switched on or off. Once produced, eddy currents decay slowly, producing spatial and temporal variation in the magnetic field. One way of ameliorating the problems associated with eddy currents is to alter the form of the gradient waveform so as to cancel the magnetic field generated by the eddy currents in the region enclosed by the gradient coil [19]. Unfortunately, the spatial variation of the magnetic field generated by the eddy currents is usually not the same as that produced by the gradient coil, so full cancellation of the eddy current fields cannot be achieved everywhere within the region of interest for imaging. A better solution to the eddy current problem is to exclude the fringe fields from surrounding areas, thus preventing the formation of any eddy currents. In active magnetic screening introduced by Mansfield and Chapman [6] and by Roemer *et al.* [20] flux exclusion is realised by surrounding the gradient coil, with a second coil wound on a concentric cylinder of greater radius. This coil, known as the active screen or active shield, is designed so that the field which it generates exactly cancels that from the inner or primary gradient coil at all points outside the cylinder on which it is wound. If the screening coil is described by a current distribution $j(\phi,z)$ on a cylinder of radius, b, then using the cylindrical harmonic expansion of the magnetic field it can be shown that the screening condition is given by:

$$j_\phi^m(k) = -\frac{aI_m'(ka)}{bI_m'(kb)} J_\phi^m(k) \tag{14}$$

This expression was first derived by Turner and Bowley [13]. From this equation it is straightforward to calculate the screen for a previously designed gradient coil. For production of useful coils this approach is usually inadequate, since as well as generating the required nulling field externally the screening coil produces a field internally which generally upsets the required gradient linearity. It is better therefore to integrate the screen into the process of coil design by incorporating its presence in the expressions for the magnetic field, inductance, power dissipation, etc. The analytic methods of coil design may then be applied to the production of naturally screened gradient coils [21].

Addition of a screen inevitably lowers the gradient coil efficiency and inductance, since the screening coil produces a field of opposite sign to that of the primary coil. As might be expected the reduction in efficiency always dominates, and the price paid for magnetic screening is therefore a reduced coil efficiency

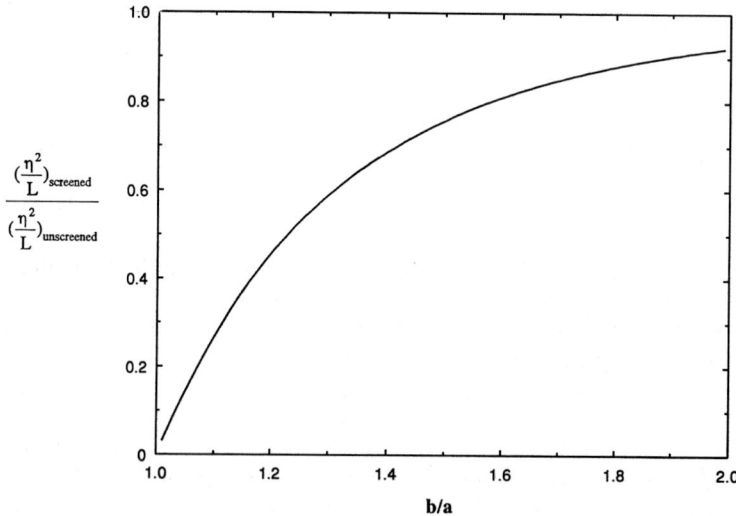

Fig. 5. Variation of the ratio of η^2/L of an actively screened x gradient coil to that of an unscreened coil, which generates the same internal field variation, for varying values of b/a. To generate these curves, b, the screen radius is varied at fixed inner coil radius, a

at fixed inductance. As indicated in Fig. 5, this reduction becomes more pronounced as the ratio of screen to primary coil radius decreases. This behaviour, which also occurs for longitudinal gradient coils, means that it is advantageous to have as large a separation between the screen and inner coil as is allowed by the magnet geometry. The current required in the screening coil to give external field cancellation depends on the number of turns it carries. A large number of turns on the screen is desirable since the larger this number is, the better the screen mimics the required continuous current distribution, and hence the better the field cancellation close to the screening cylinder is. However, it is very important that the screen and primary currents show exactly the same temporal variation so that screening obtains at all times whilst a gradient waveform is being played out. The best way of achieving this requirement is to connect the screen and primary coil in series. Use of this arrangement fixes the number of turns in the screen and, as it turns out, always requires that screen has fewer turns than the primary. If the degree of screening achieved with this number of turns is insufficient, an alternative arrangement may be used in which symmetry units of the screen are connected in parallel with one another and then in series with the primary coil. This can allow the number of turns in the screen to be doubled, but does require careful setting up [22]. It is interesting to note that the screening coil links no flux, and therefore increasing the number of turns on the screen does not significantly change the coil inductance [23].

Figure 6 shows the wirepaths of an actively screened transverse gradient coil which was designed via the target field approach for use in whole-body EPI. The diameter of the inner and outer coils are 64 and 88 cm, respectively, and the coil has an efficiency of 0.062 mTm^{-1} A^{-1} at an inductance of 420 μH, whilst producing a field which is homogeneous to greater than 5 % within a cylinder of diameter 50 cm and length 35 cm. It is designed so that the ratio of currents in inner and outer coils is 2:1, allowing the two halves of the screen to be connected in parallel with one another and then in series with the primary. The degree of magnetic screening which has been achieved is indicated in Fig. 7, which shows the how the magnetic field generated by the inner coil and screen, divided by that generated by the inner coil alone, varies along axial lines close to the surface of the screen. The field variation was calculated by applying the Biot-Savart law to small elements of the individual wirepaths. At a radius of 46 cm, only 2 cm from the screen surface, the degree of screening shows some fluctuation with axial position. This results from using discrete wires to mimic the required continuous screening current distribution. As the distance from the screen is increased this fluctuation is reduced. It is usually unimportant at distances from the screen which are greater than the local wire spacings in the screen.

An actively screened z gradient coil which was designed to operate on similar diameter coil cylinders and to produce a pure gradient over the same region of interest is shown in Fig. 8. It has an inductance of 520 μH and produces a gradient strength per unit current of 0.094 mTm^{-1} A^{-1} efficiency. As is usually the case, the longitudinal coil has a significantly higher η^2/L value than its transverse counterpart.

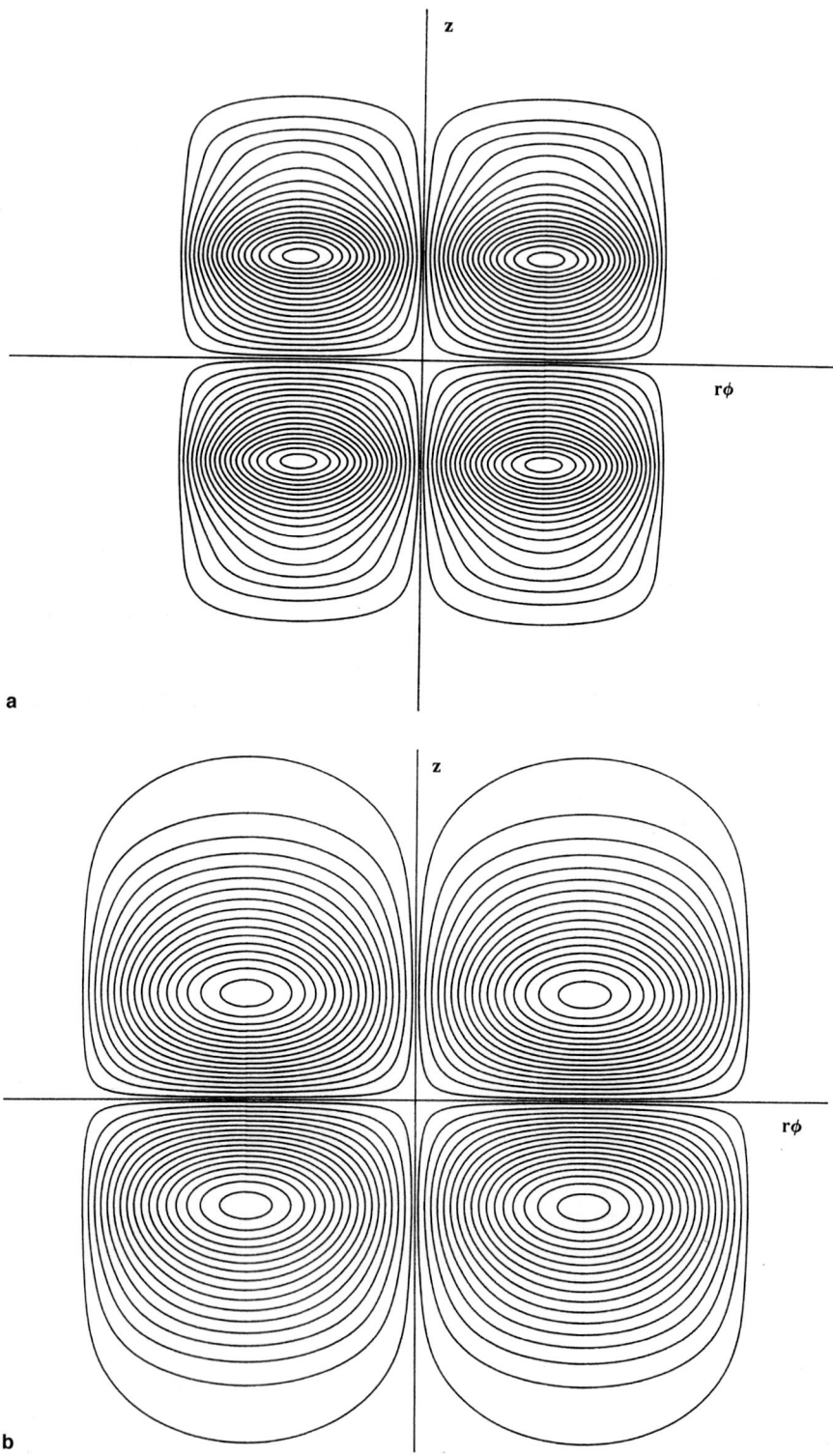

Fig. 6a,b. Wirepaths for a screened x gradient coil. **a** Inner coil. **b** Screen. In each case the coil is shown with the coil cylinder rolled out flat. b/a = 1.375 in this coil design

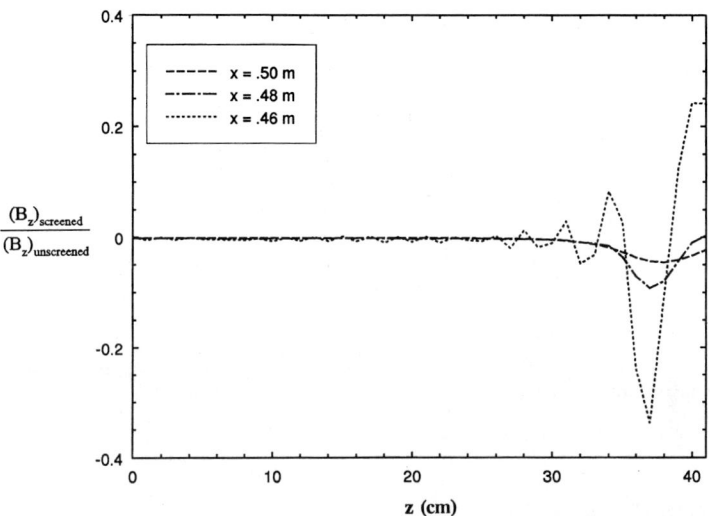

Fig. 7. Variation of the ratio of the field from the screened coil of Fig. 6 to that from the inner coil alone. The field is calculated along axial lines at y = 0, x = 46, 48 and 50 cm

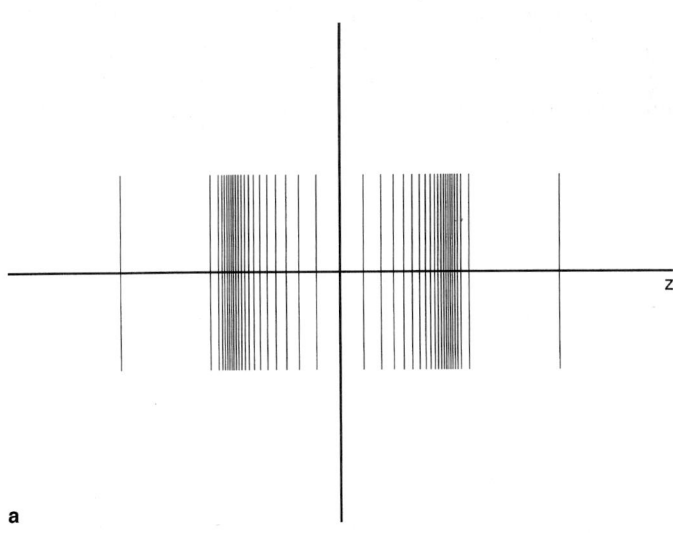

Fig. 8a,b. Wire positions for an actively screened z gradient coil. **a** Inner coil

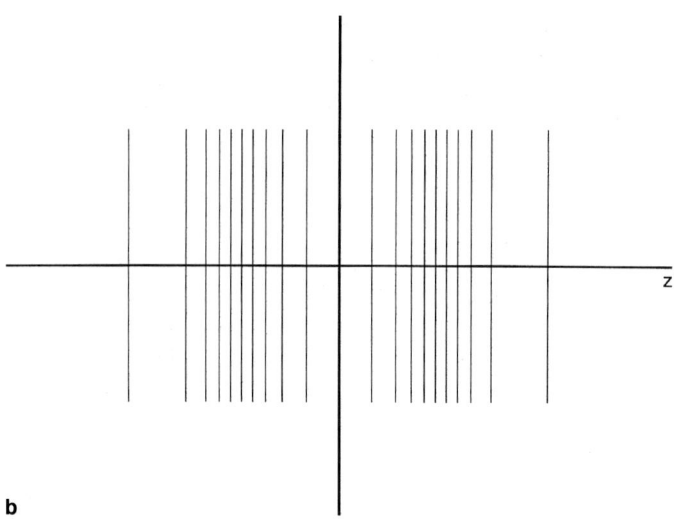

Fig. 8a,b. (continued) **b** Screen. The lines indicating the wire positions are drawn with a length equivalent to the coil diameter

Finite Element Methods in Coil Design

A number of gradient coil design techniques which are based on some form of finite element analysis have been developed. In one of the earliest approaches [24] the surface of the cylinder on which the coil is to be wound is divided up into small elements. The current flow required in each element so as to produce the minimum deviation from a pure gradient over a set of points defining the region of interest is then calculated by matrix inversion. Wire paths which mimic this distribution of currents may then be calculated in the manner described previously. In this way Compton was able to design high-quality transverse and longitudinal gradient coils in the early 1980's. More recently Pissanetzky [25] has extended this approach by including the coil inductance in a least-squares optimisation procedure based on a similar division of the current carrying surface into small elements.

An alternative finite element method involves optimising the position of a number of conducting elements so as to minimise an error function which may contain contributions from the inductance and power dissipation as well as the deviation of the magnetic field from the required value at a number of specified points. In this sort of approach the relationship between the error function and wire positions is generally not a straightforward quadratic, which means that some sort of non-linear minimisation technique must be used. Wong and colleagues [26] have used the method of conjugate gradient descent to minimise an appropriate error function, whilst more recently Crozier and Doddrell have employed the method of simulated annealing [27]. The use of the actual conducting element positions in the minimisation process is advantageous since it means that there is no stage of approximation in going from a continuous current distribution to discrete elements. The effect of such an approximation is usually small, however, when a reasonable number of turns are used to mimic the current distribution [11].

In the simple geometries, which can be handled by the analytic approach, the two methods of coil design produce very similar coil designs when reasonable numbers of turns can be used. Since the methods of coil design based on finite element analysis are generally computationally more intensive than the analytic methods, there is little need for their use in this sort of situation. The finite element methods can, however, be used to design coils with less straightforward geometries [28] for which it is not possible to develop analytic expressions, and it is here and in the analysis of time-dependent effects that finite element analysis may have most significant application in gradient coil design.

Head Gradient Coils

The strong dependence of η^2/L on coil diameter means that there is considerable advantage in using a dedicated, small-diameter head gradient coil set for EPI of the brain and spinal cord. The problem in designing such coils is that they must be truncated at the shoulders to allow access for the head. This truncation does not pose serious problems in the design of longitudinal coils, but does relatively compromise the performance of transverse coils, so that the expected increase in η^2/L due to small diameter is eroded. Thus for example, with a coil of inner diameter 38 cm and length 38 cm, with a region of 5 % homogeneity corresponding to a central cylinder of 20 cm diameter and 20 cm radius, it is possible to design a z gradient coil with an efficiency of 0.34 mTm^{-1} A^{-1} at about 260 µH inductance whilst the best transverse coil would produce a gradient per unit current of only 0.062 mTm^{-1} A^{-1} at the same inductance. This loss of performance results from the fact that truncation forces the transverse coil's return arcs to be positioned too close to the coil centre. A number of ways around this problem have been suggested. One way of ameliorating the loss of performance caused by truncation is to truncate the coil asymmetrically so that the region of interest is no longer centrally located within the coil. This is possible because there is of course no need to truncate the coil in the z direction superior to the head. A simple way of implementing this idea is to use half of a conventional non-truncated design [29]. Unfortunately, the positioning of the wirepaths in this sort of coil means that it experiences a strong torque when energised inside the magnet. This makes clinical use of such a coil system difficult. This difficulty can, however, be eliminated by incorporating the requirement that the asymmetric coil is torque balanced into the process of coil design [30, 31].

An alternative solution to the problem of truncation is to use a long coil but to exclude the wirepaths from a sufficiently large region to allow slots to be cut in the former to permit access for the shoulders [11]. This solution is feasible, however, only for the y gradient coil, whose symmetry allows shoulder slots to be formed naturally.

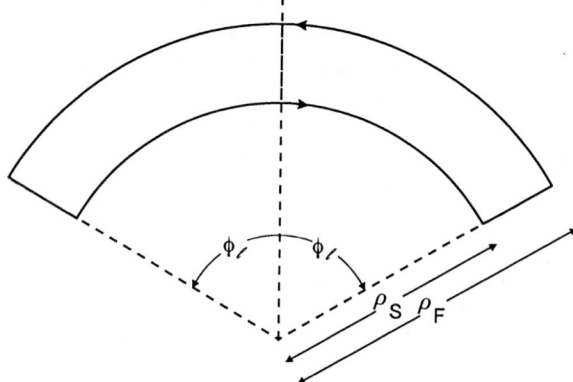

Fig. 9. Closed current loop consisting of two azimuthal and two radial sections. This construction can be used as the basis of heavily truncated gradient coils

A final option is to displace the return arcs radially so that they do not get in the way of the shoulders. In one approach the return arcs are placed on conical surfaces placed at either end of a truncated cylinder [32]. Alternatively, the return arcs can be formed on a concentric cylinder of larger radius [28]. A good way of achieving this sort of design is to compose the coil of units such as those shown in Fig. 9 [33, 34]. These units have a number of good features: they are easy to manufacture, there is no net force or torque on a single unit, and it is possible to derive an analytic expression for the field for an array of such units [35]. Coils composed of these units provide some gain in efficiency at fixed inductance compared with conventional cylindrical coils in the case of significant truncation. The design of head gradient coils is currently an active area of research, with improved designs still appearing and as yet no clear consensus on the best approach to the amelioration of truncation effects.

Other Geometries

Although cylindrical geometry is often the natural choice for gradient coil design, there are situations in which alternative geometries offer advantages. For imaging of the abdomen the use of planar or bi-planar coils can be advantageous since the shape of the human torso allows the coil wires to be brought into closer proximity to the body than in cylindrical coils. This proximity is translated into higher efficiency at fixed inductance by the a^{-5} dependence of η^2/L. Coils consisting of wires confined to a single plane can be made arbitrarily small since their size is not fixed by any constraint of subject access. Size reduction obviously limits the region over which a homogeneous gradient can be generated, and a particular problem in the design of uni-planar coils is that it is difficult to control the field variation in the direction normal to the coil plane. Such coils may be usefully employed as surface gradient coils [36], however, and the field variation which they produce may be matched to the drop-off in sensitivity of a surface RF coil, so that after image post-processing a uniform SNR is achieved within the image [37]. A larger region of gradient homogeneity can be generated using a bi-planar coil design [17, 38, 39], and although the plane separation must be large enough to maintain an adequate subject access, gains in η^2/L over whole-body cylindrical coils can be achieved.

Planar coil design can be performed using the analytic or finite element methods. The former relies on the use of 'Fourier-space' expressions for the magnetic field produced by, and the inductance or power dissipation of, a current distribution confined to a plane. Active screening can be implemented in planar geometry through the use of screening coils wound on outer planes, which sandwich the inner coil, or on a surrounding cylinder [40]. The natural planar geometry to use in designing coils for whole-body imaging is one in which the current carrying elements are confined to x-z planes since this allows the smallest plane spacing. This geometry allows highly efficient y and z gradient coils of low inductance to be designed, but the symmetry means that an x gradient coil inevitably has poorer performance. Figure 10 shows the wirepaths on one

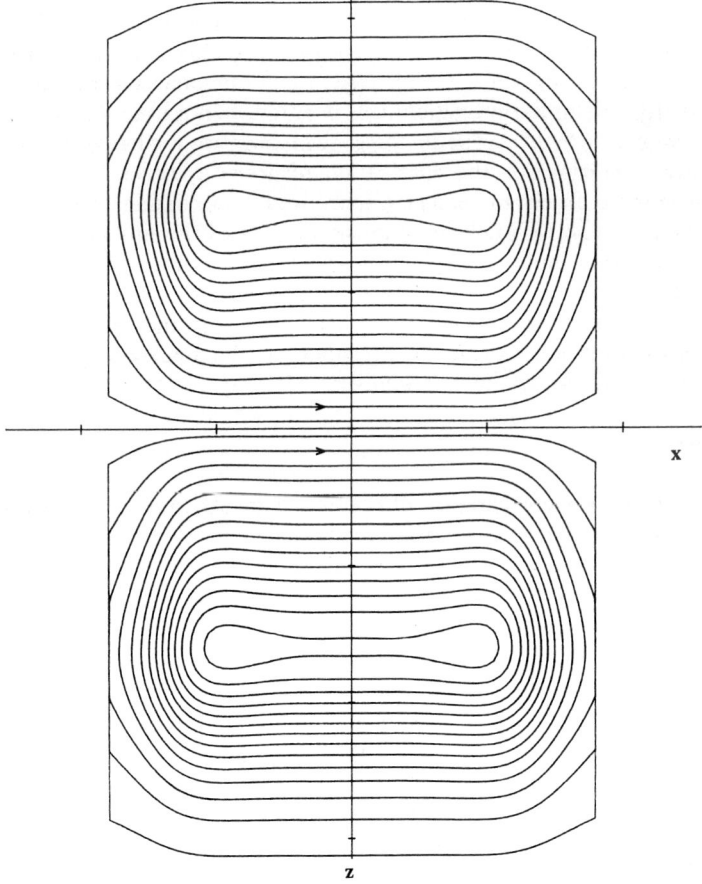

Fig. 10. Wire paths on one plane of a bi-planar y gradient coil. The distance between ticks on the axes is one half of the plane spacing. The wirepaths on the opposite plane carry current in the same sense

plane of a y gradient coil, which was designed for cardiac imaging [41]. The plane spacing is 30 cm and this coil has an efficiency of 0.22 mTm^{-1} A^{-1} at 310 µH inductance, whilst generating a field gradient which is uniform to better than 5 % within a cube of side 18 cm. A z gradient coil with similar attributes has also been designed.

Whole-body gradient coils with elliptical cross section may well offer further improvements in performance [42]. The mathematics required in the analytic approach to the design of elliptical coils is complicated and consequently finite element analysis may be a more sensible approach to the design of this type of coil.

Active Acoustic Screening

The acoustic noise generated by gradient coils results from small movements of the gradient coil wires and former which occur in sympathy with the oscillating Lorentz forces experienced by the current carrying elements. A powerful way of eliminating the acoustic noise is therefore to null the forces on the current carrying elements. A symmetric gradient coil positioned in a homogeneous magnetic field experiences no net torque or force when carrying a current, but this is not a sufficient condition for the elimination of acoustic noise. To move towards this goal it is necessary to achieve a more local cancellation of the forces. One way of doing this is to build the gradient coil out of the units shown in Fig. 9. These form closed loops in a plane perpendicular to the static magnetic field and therefore experience no net force or torque. If the segments are coupled together tightly by filling the loop with a medium in which the speed of sound, v, is large, reasonable local force cancellation can be achieved. This yields good noise cancellation for gradient waveforms with frequencies, f, such that:

$$f \ll \frac{v}{2\Delta} \tag{15}$$

where $\Delta = \rho_f - \rho_s$ is the separation of the arc segments [34]. As described above, coils composed of these units are also naturally well suited to use in head gradient coils, where significant truncation is required. An alternative method of producing local force cancellation is to surround the gradient coil with an active acoustic screen. This is a second coil wound on an outer cylinder, tightly bonded to the first, and arranged so that the force produced by the second coil locally cancels that on the inner coil [43]. It is also possible to incorporate active magnetic screening into this approach, by adding further coils.

Nerve Stimulation

The application of a rapidly switched magnetic field gradients can lead to nerve stimulation in patients. This stimulation results from the electric field induced in tissues when the flux linked by the body changes. Full modelling of the process of stimulation is difficult because of the heterogeneity of the body's electrical conductivity, but stimulation is obviously more likely the larger the peak magnetic field generated inside the body. Consequently it is sensible to limit this peak field in the process of coil design. To evaluate the magnitude of the peak field it is necessary to consider all the components of the magnetic field generated by a gradient coil. Although gradient coils are designed to generate a linear variation of the z component of the magnetic field, Maxwell's equations imply that field components directed along the x and y axes must also be present. Simple analysis [44] indicates that for example in a region where $B_z = G_z$, the magnitude of the field is:

$$|B| = G\sqrt{\frac{(x^2 + y^2)}{4} + z^2}$$
(16)

whilst for an x or y gradient it is:

$$|B| = G\sqrt{x^2 + z^2}$$
(17)

or:

$$|B| = G\sqrt{y^2 + z^2}$$
(18)

It is clear from these expressions that the largest magnetic field is generated at large values of x, y or z, so that restricting the extent of the region over which a pure gradient is produced tends to limit the peak magnetic field induced in the body. Outside the region of homogeneity the magnitude of the field may well show further increase in size, and it is likely that regions of very high field intensity occurs close to the coil windings. Some steps have been taken to incorporate the elimination of regions of high field intensity in the process of coil design [44], but it is likely that there will be further developments in this area in the near future.

Gradient Coil Construction

The current carrying elements of a gradient coil are usually formed from copper wires or from slotted copper sheet. Most commonly these elements are fixed to a fibre glass coil former. Accurate positioning of the conducting elements is important and in constructing a wire wound coil this can be facilitated by cutting a groove into the surface of the coil former using a computer controlled milling machine or lathe. The wire may then be wound into the groove and fixed in place with epoxy resin or by over-wrapping with a fibre glass layer so as to produce a robust coil. In cylindrical whole-body coils a large-scale computer-controlled machine tool is required to cut grooves into the cylindrical surface. In the absence of access to such a machine the wires can be wound on a flat surface which carries grooves defining the wire paths and then bent and wrapped onto a cylindrical surface. Coils made from slotted copper sheet may be formed in a number of ways. The simplest is to using etching techniques in which the wire-paths are defined by chemically cutting away a spiral track of copper. Unfortunately, etching methods can be used only with relatively thin copper sheet, which may make it difficult to achieve an adequate current carrying cross section. Computer-controlled machine tools allow thicker copper sheet to be cut and therefore obviate this problem.

Wire wound coils are generally easier to construct, but the use of copper sheet confers a number of advantages on the constructed coil. These mainly result from the fact that in such coils the current is spread over a much larger fraction of the coil former's surface. Consequently the coil provides a better approximation of a continuous current distribution and in addition has a lower resistance than a wire wound coil which produces an equivalent radial build up of the coil former surface. This means that better active shielding and lower power dissipation can often be achieved with this sort of coil construction.

Gradient Coil Drivers

Non-resonant Drive and Simple Resonant Circuits

The simplest way of driving a gradient coil is to directly connect the coil to a powerful amplifier. This amplifier operates in 'current mode' so that the large current that it generates through the gradient coil follows a voltage waveform input from the waveform controller. In this mode of operation the amplifier must generate enough voltage to overcome the inductive impedance of the coil when the waveform controller demands a changing coil current and enough voltage to overcome the coil resistance when a constant current is necessary. When large rapidly switched gradients are produced by reasonably well-designed gradient coils, it is the inductive impedance which requires the largest voltages. For example, in the whole-body z gradient coil described above (see 'Gradient Coil Requirements for EPI') which has a resistance of 0.05 Ω a linear ramp from zero up to a gradient strength of 20 mTm^{-1} in 200 μs requires more than 550 V, whilst maintaining a constant gradient at this level requires only 11 V. The high-power delivery required from the amplifier is therefore a result of the voltage needed to establish the current through the coil. The energy used to establish this current is stored rather than dissipated, and a considerable reduction in the average power demanded from the gradient coil amplifiers can therefore be achieved if steps are taken to recover the stored energy and to then re-use it. Periodic waveforms such as the switched gradient used in EPI lend themselves naturally to a scheme whereby energy recycling can be utilised.

The simplest such scheme is to use the resonant circuit shown in Fig. 11, in which a capacitor is connected in series with the gradient coil. For a sinusoidal

Fig. 11. A simple resonant circuit produced by connecting a capacitor, C, in series with the gradient coil

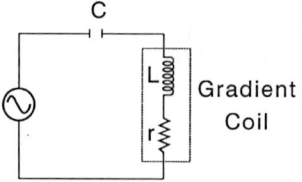

waveform at frequency, $f = \omega/2\pi$, the impedance of this arrangement is of course:

$$Z = r + j(\omega L - \frac{1}{\omega C})$$ (19)

which means that the circuit is resonant at frequency:

$$f = \frac{1}{2\pi\sqrt{LC}}$$ (20)

At this frequency the impedance of the circuit is just equal to the coil resistance. It is therefore possible to generate a high-current waveform through the gradient coil with a relatively low voltage. A significant amount of energy is still needed to establish the current in the gradient coil, but subsequently this energy oscillates between being stored as current through the inductor and as charge on the capacitor, with the amplifier only having to top-up the energy dissipated by the coil resistance.

Multi-Mode Resonant Gradient Coil Drivers

The simple circuit of Fig. 11 significantly reduces the power demanded from the gradient coil amplifier, but can be used to generate only a sinusoidal waveform. This is a drawback since as described above (see 'Gradient Coil Requirements for EPI') a trapezoidal waveform with reasonably short ramp times always yields better spatial resolution. To overcome this problem Mansfield and colleagues [45] developed a multi-mode resonant gradient coil driver which can be used in the resonant generation of trapezoidal gradient waveforms. The multi-mode resonant circuit is based on the realisation that it is possible to represent a trapezoidal waveform as a quite rapidly converging Fourier series composed of sinusoids oscillating at the fundamental gradient switching frequency, f, and at odd harmonics of this frequency. A trapezoidal waveform can therefore be synthesised from a small number of sinusoidal oscillations. By using a multi-mode resonant circuit which is designed to be resonant at all of the discrete frequencies, the circuit exhibits the same low resistance to each sinusoid allowing resonant generation of the trapezoidal waveform. Figure 12 shows a tri-modal resonant circuit [45] which can be used to generate a trapezoid composed of three different frequency sinusoids. The capacitance values C_3 and C_5 are chosen so that the two simple parallel LCR arrangements are resonant at frequencies, 3f and 5f. This means that the upper arms of the circuit pass no current at these frequencies. Using this feature it is straightforward to choose the other component values to give identical resonances at the three different frequencies. This circuit, which relies only on passive components has been constructed and used to generate trapezoidal waveforms with peak currents of over 500 A.

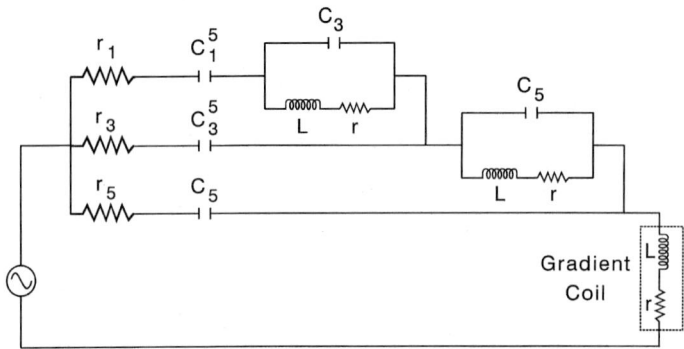

Fig. 12. A tri-modal resonant circuit, used in the resonant generation of trapezoidal gradient waveforms

Resonant Booster

Another way to provide the voltage needed to drive the coil rapidly is to combine a resonant circuit with high power semiconductor switches [58, 59]. This combination is called a resonant booster because it allows the voltage at the coil to be boosted. The most commonly used semiconductor switches are thyristors, gate turn-off thyristors and insulated gated bipolar transistors (IGBT). Thyristors are used in the circuit shown in Fig. 13, which represents a simple version of a resonant booster [46]. We introduce this simple booster version because it explains the basics of switchable resonant circuits. The resonance frequency is a function of the capacitance and the inductance used in the circuit as described in Eq. 20. Using this circuit any combination of fast sinusoidal and slower trapezoidal gradient pulses is possible. In this context 'fast' refers to the gradient rise time set by the voltage, U_c, of the booster and slow means with the time given by the voltage U_{PSU} of the standard gradient power supply unit (G-PSU). This allows much more flexibility in gradient pulse sequence programming, that for example, the multi-mode resonant gradient driver described above (see 'Multi-Mode Resonant Gradient Coil Drivers').

Fig. 13. Resonant circuit controlled by semiconductor switches. Switch S_1 is used to bypass the capacitor which enables non-resonant pulses. When switch S_0 is closed, the circuit is driven in resonance

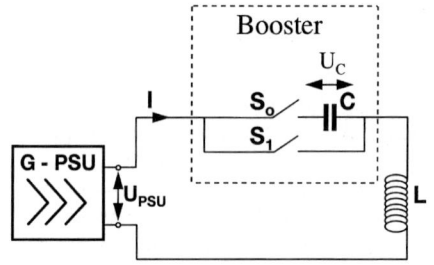

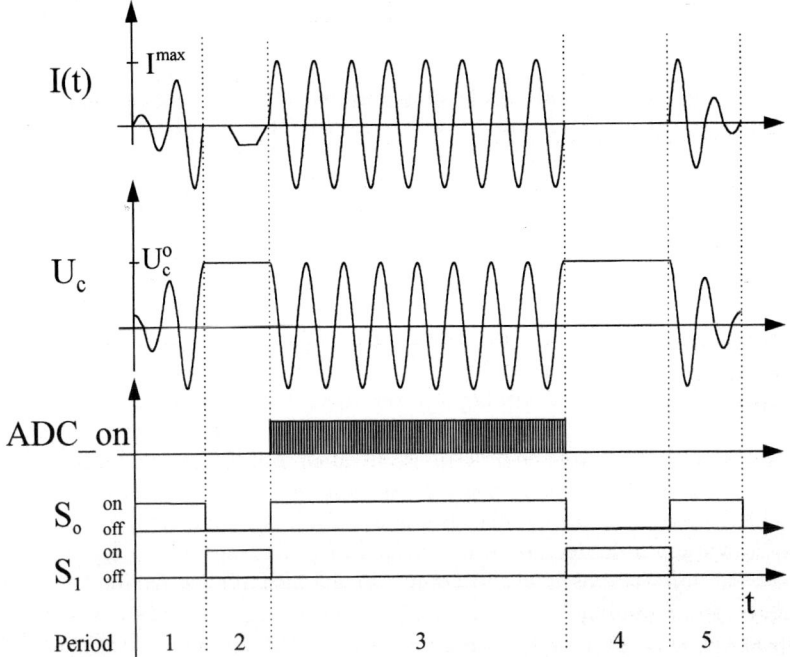

Fig. 14. Switching diagram for resonant circuit of Fig. 13. S_0 *on*, switch is closed. A typical EPI readout train is shown. *ADC on*, MR data acquisition time

Figure 14 shows an example of the way in which the switches S_0 and S_1 are triggered for an EPI readout gradient pulse train [I(t) in upper row of Fig. 14]. Period 2 represents the pre-phasing and period 3 the readout period. Before driving the coil with the maximum possible speed the capacitor must be charged to the voltage required. Periods 1 and 5 represent the charging and discharging of the capacitor, respectively.

In order to charge the capacitor, switch S_0 is closed in period 1. The circuit is driven in resonant mode because the coil and capacitor are in series. The capacitor is charged by cycling the current through the circuit with the resonant frequency [47]. The envelope of the current can be linear or exponential. The amplitude of the last half wave must be the same as the readout gradient amplitude of period 3. At the end of period 1 switch S_0 is opened. This yields a capacitor voltage, U_c^o, of:

$$U_c^o = \frac{1}{\omega C} I^{max} \tag{21}$$

When switch S_1 (period 2) is closed, capacitor C is bypassed and consequently any type of gradient pulse can be produced. The rate of change of current, dI/dt, is now defined by the G-PSU output voltage, U_{PSU}:

$$\left|\frac{dI}{dt}\right| = \frac{U_{PSU}}{L} \tag{22}$$

The sinusoidal periodic pulse train shown in period 3 can be generated by opening switch S_1 and closing switch S_0 simultaneously. This pulse train is usually applied in the acquisition of EPI MR signal data as indicated by the ADC-on trace. When data acquisition is completed, switch S_0 is opened exactly at the zero crossing of the current wave form, and the capacitor is charged again to the voltage U_c^o as calculated in Eq. 21. In order to discharge the capacitor the switch S_0 is closed again at the start of period 4. When the current is zero, with the same envelope and time as during charging period 1, the capacitor is discharged to a voltage $U_c = 0$ V. The main disadvantage of thyristor switches is that they can be switched only when the current is equal to zero.

During the past 5–10 years high-power IGBTs which overcome this problem have become available. These semiconductors allow switching of high currents and voltages at any time. IGBTs in a so-called full-bridge configuration [48, 49], as shown in Fig. 15, comprise the best solution. As well as resonant sinusoidal and conventional trapezoidal gradient pulses, this booster provides the so called 'catch and hold' feature, which means that fast sinusoidal ramps combined with a flat top are possible and results in a much higher flexibility in pulse sequence programming.

Figure 16 explains how the booster circuit of Fig. 15 is switched in order to supply high voltage to the coil. In period 1 the current is slowly ramped up to $I = I^{max}$. dI/dt in this pulse is set by the output voltage U_{PSU} of the standard gradient PSU, as described in Eq. 22. Switches S_1 and S_3 are closed to bypass the capacitor. This means that the coil is driven by the G-PSU only. When all switches are opened, and simultanously a sinusoidal ramp down current is driven through the coil (period 2), the current passes through the 'free wheel' diodes D_1, the capacitor C and the 'free wheel' diode D_4. In this state the coil and capacitor form a resonant circuit and therefore oscillate for a quarter sine wave with the resonance frequency f. At the end of period 2 the capacitor is charged to the voltage U_c^o, as can be calculated with Eq. 21. In period 3 (switches S_1 and S_3

Fig. 15. A full-bridge config-uration resonant booster. The coil (L) is switched in series to the capacitor when diagonals S_1S_4 or S_2S_3 are closed. The coil is driven by the gradient amplifier (G-PSU) when switches S_1 and S_3 are closed

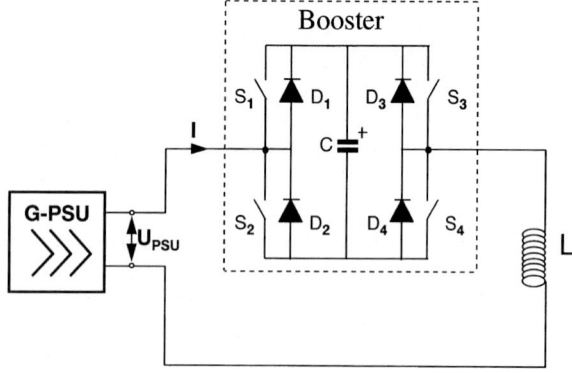

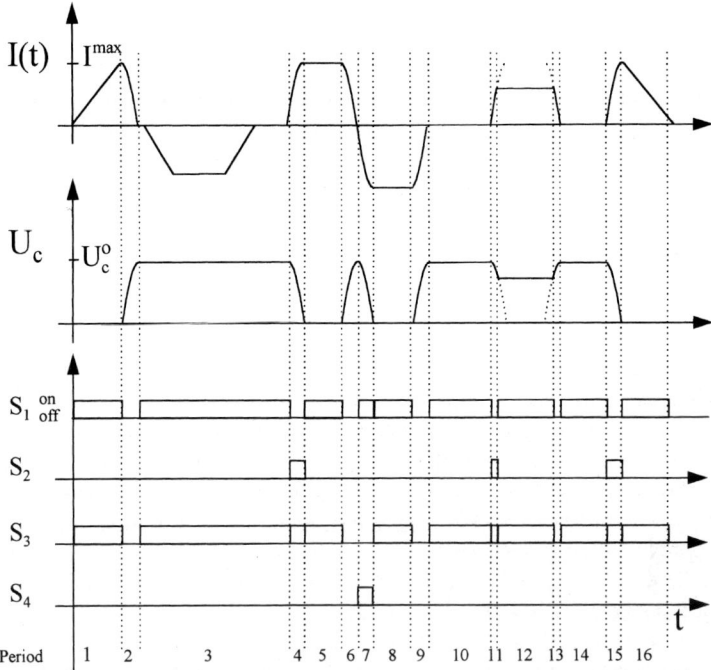

Fig. 16. Switching diagram for resonant booster of Fig. 15. The capacitor is charged to voltage U_c^o in period 2 and discharged to zero in period 15. For further explanation see text

closed) any type of gradient pulse can be performed with the dI/dt value described in Eq. 22. Period 4 shows a positive sinusoidal current ramp up to $I = I^{max}$. In order to achive this switches S_2 and S_3 are closed causing a discharge of the capacitor at the end of period 4. A flat top current is produced by bypassing the capacitor C (switches S_1 and S_3 closed). Period 6 shows the same switching diagram as shown in period 2, yielding a recharge of the capacitor. A negative sinusoidal ramp down to $I = -I^{max}$ is achieved when switches S_1 and S_4 are closed. The constant negative current in period 8 is produced by bypassing capacitor C (switches S_1 and S_3 closed). Opening all the switches in period 9 again results in a recharging of the capacitor (the current returns through the 'free wheel' diodes D_2 and D_3).

Segments of quarter sinusoidal ramps can be generated when the capacitor is only partially discharged (period 11). Recharge of capacitor C to the orginal voltage, U_c^o, is achieved when periods 11 and 13 have the same duration. Finally, the capacitor is discharged in period 15 (same switching scheme as in period 4), and the current is ramped down slowly in period 16.

The booster shown in Fig. 15 can generate a variety of arbitrary pulse shapes [50] depending on the output voltage U_{PSU} of the standard G-PSU. In order to understand how this works G-PSU and the booster (when charged) can be considered as voltage sources. The standard G-PSU delivers any voltage between

+U_{PSU} and -U_{PSU} at any time on demand. The booster itself can be considered as a voltage supply which loses its voltage when pulses are ramped to positive or negative currents (for example, periods 4, 7 or 11) and regains the voltage when the gradient pulses are ramped down to zero (for example, periods 6, 9, 13). The polarity of the booster voltage is determined by the switch diagonals S_1 and S_4 (negative current) and S_2 and S_3 (positive current). When S_1 and S_4 are closed, the negative pole of the capacitor is connected to the coil. On the other hand, when S_2 and S_3 are closed, the positive pole is connected to the coil. When both voltage sources are switched in series, the circuit can generate a maximum voltages of:

$$|U^{max}| = |U_{PSU}| + |U_c^o| \tag{23}$$

Figure 17 shows a simulation for a trapezoidal current pulse (square box markers). As an example, a coil inductance of L = 1200 µH, DC resistance of R = 200 mW, capacitance of C = 43 µF and maximum current of I^{max} = 250 A were chosen. We assume that the capacitor was charged to U_c^o = 2000 V before the beginning of the trapezoidal pulse. The voltage U_{PSU} at the terminals of the G-PSU can be calculated by the differential equation of a damped harmonic oscillator [51]:

$$U_{PSU} = I(t) \cdot R - L \cdot \frac{dI(t)}{dt} + U_c^o - \frac{1}{C} \int_t I(t') dt' \tag{24}$$

During period 1 the coil needs a constant voltage of U_L = -2000 V in order to produce a linear current ramp with a duration of T_{Rise} = 150 µs, while the voltage

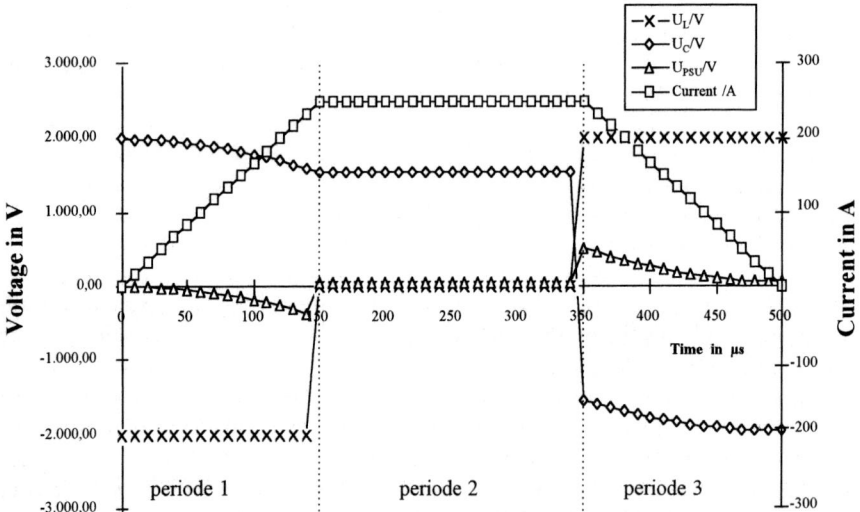

Fig. 17. The booster of Fig. 15. allows a manifold of gradient pulses beside the sinusoidal shapes. For example, a trapezoidal current pulse (*squares*) with a rise time of 150 µs can be generated requiring a voltages of 2000 V at coil U_L (*X*). The gradient amplifier must provide the voltage U_{PSU} (*triangles*) to compensate the voltage drop U_C (*rhombi*) of the capacitor. For more explanation see text

of the capacitor U_c drops from +2000 to about +1600 V. Capacitor and coil voltages have opposite polarity at the terminal of the G-PSU. Therefore a net voltage of about 400 V results at the end of period 1. During the flat top the capacitor is bypassed (S_1 and S_3 on). The coil is driven by the G-PSU only. In period 3 the polarity of the capacitance is changed (all switches off: current flow through D_1 and D_4). (The reader should not be confused by the U_c voltage train of Fig. 17. Here the polarity of the capacitance voltage changes. We introduce this reversal to better explain the net voltage at the G-PSU terminal. In Fig. 16 the voltage on the capacitance is shown in a monopolar format.) This causes a recharge of the capacitor at the end of period 3. At the terminals the G-PSU consequently drops from about 500 V to 0V.

The ability to generate waveforms which are not pure sinusoidal waves with a 'resonant' booster is strongly dependent on the output voltage of the G-PSU. Keeping in mind that the standard G-PSU can supply any voltage up to some maximum value at any time on demand, trapezoidal pulses can be generated as long as the capacitance voltage drop during the ramps (periods 1 and 3) is smaller than the output voltage, U_{PSU}, minus the resistive losses, $U_R = I^{max} \cdot R$, as demonstrated in Fig. 17. As long as this holds true the standard G-PSU compensates the voltage loss of the capacitance. This capability can be used for oblique and double-oblique imaging [52] and for driving offset currents as may be required for shimming [53].

From this fact it is also obvious that the minimum rise time produced with this type of booster is a function of the resonant frequency f (see Eq. 20):

$$T_{Rise} < \frac{1}{4 \cdot f} \tag{25}$$

This means that when this booster is used to produce trapezoidal pulses, the achievable rise time is always shorter than the duration of a quarter sine wave of corresponding frequency, f.

Non-resonant Booster

In contrast to resonant boosters, which provide a changing capacitance voltage to the coil, non-resonant boosters supply a constant voltage. An example of a non-resonant booster, shown in Fig. 18, was introduced by Mueller et al. [54, 55] and appied to single-shot EPI [56] in 1991. The low voltage (LV) and the high voltage (HV) G-PSU can be switched in series by means of the switches (S_1, S_2, S_3 and S_4), forming a double-stage booster. For constant or slowly varying gradient pulses the LV G-PSU provides any voltage between $+U_{LV}$ and $-U_{LV}$ at any time on demand. For very short linear gradient rise times the HV G-PSU is used. The HV power stage is used to boost the voltage at the coil, while the LV power stage is used accurately to regulate the current at the coil to achieve the precision needed for MRI. The capacitance, C_1, at the output of the HV G-PSU is needed to stabilize the output voltage U_{HV} and consequently plays a completely different role to the resonance capacitor described in the previous section on resonant boosters. This capacitance (C_1) is typically of the order of millifarads (mF)

Fig. 18. A nonresonant booster with a double power stage LV and HV is shown. Constant or slowly varying currents are driven by the low voltage amplifier LV G-PSU. Rapidly changing current pulses are generated by means of the high voltage amplifier HV G-PSU

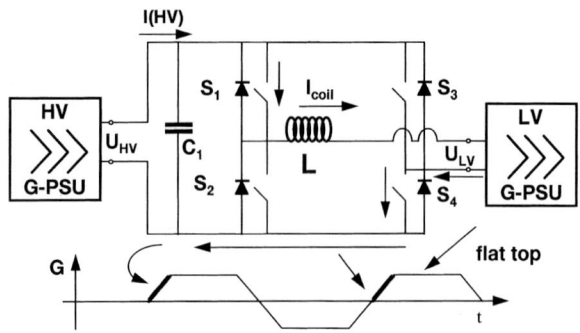

while the resonant booster capacitance is of the order of microfarads (μF) only. The major difference in the circuit of Fig. 18 when compared to a resonant booster is that the coil is be connected inside the full bridge. Figure 18 shows a double-stage booster. The first stage is represented by the conventional LV G-PSU and the second by the HV G-PSU. In general the two power stages can have different output voltages. When both power stages are switched in series, the achievable rise time can be calculated from Eq. 22 as:

$$T_{Rise} = \frac{I^{max} \cdot L}{U_{LV} + U_{HV}} \tag{26}$$

The concept of non-resonant boosters can be expanded to multi-stage boosters [57]. Both linear and binary staging are possible. A variant of linear power staging is explained in the left portion of Fig. 19. In this case the voltage of the booster stages is equal to the LV-GPSU voltage U_{LV} so that:

$$U_{HV} = U_{LV} \tag{27}$$

In general, with N such power stages a total voltage U_{Tot} at the coil of:

$$|U_{Tot}| = U_{LV} \sum_{n=1}^{N} (n+1) \tag{28}$$

is achieved. When, for example, $N = 3$ power stages are used, the total voltage gained is four times U_{LV}. Linear power staging of this type has the advantage that only one booster stage type is used, and this is used several times. This offers some advantage in terms of cost because of component commonality. The disadvantage is that the total voltage is rather small compared with binary staging.

With binary staging the voltage of the HV power stages differ, as described in Eq. 2.29:

$$U_{HV}^{n} = U_{LV} \cdot 2^{n} \tag{29}$$

When N power stages are combined a total output voltage of:

$$|U_{Tot}| = |U_{LV}| \cdot (2^{N} + 1) \tag{30}$$

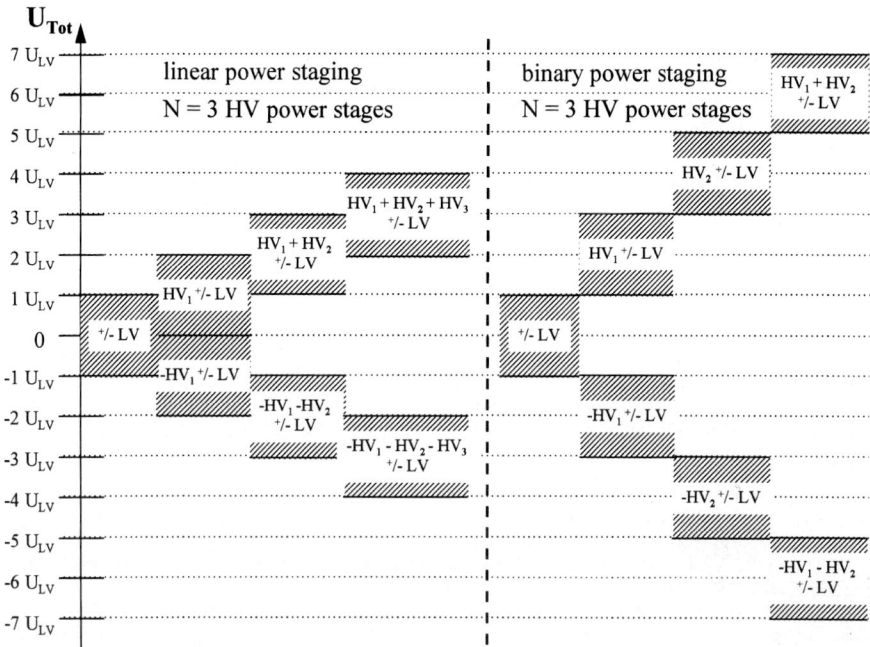

Fig. 19. Linear (*left*) and binary (*right*) power staging for non-resonant boosters is shown. Binary staging is more effective in terms of attainable total voltage per power stage. For further explanation see text

can be achieved. Figure 19 (right) shows an example with $N = 2$ HV power stages. The total output voltage gained is 5 times U_{LV}. The advantage of this type of power staging is the high voltage gained. However, it has some technical drawbacks, and because of the different output voltages it cannot benefit from component commonality, as is possible with linear power staging.

Conclusions

This chapter describes the demands which EPI makes on scanner hardware and the technical developments which now allow these demands to be properly fulfilled. A heavy emphasis is placed here on the methods for generating large, rapidly switched gradients because the need to generate such gradients routinely in EPI probably posed the main obstacle to the clinical implementation of the technique. The development of methods for designing highly efficient, low-inductance gradient coils and of techniques for producing large, rapidly changing electric currents has largely removed this obstacle. The clinical potential of EPI, conceived by Mansfield nearly 20 years ago, can now be fully realised.

References

1. Mansfield P (1977) Multi-planar image formation using NMR spin echoes. J Phys C 10:L55–L58
2. Hayes CE, Edelstein WA, Schenck JF, Mueller OM, Eash M (1985) An efficient, highly homogeneous radiofrequency coil for whole-body NMR imaging at 1.5 T. J Magn Reson 63:622–628
3. Ackerman JJH, Grove TH, Wong GG, Gadian DG, Radda GK (1980) Nature 283:167–170
4. Stehling MK, Turner R, Mansfield P (1991) Echo planar imaging: magnetic resonance imaging in a fraction of a second. Science 254:43–50
5. Rohan M (1995) Electro-mechanical coupling at high fields: increased gradient resistance. Proceedings of the 3rd Annual Meeting of the SMR, Nice, p 937
6. Mansfield P, Chapman B (1986) Active magnetic screening of gradient coils in NMR imaging. J Phys E15:235–239
7. Rzedzian R, Martin C (1991) Shielded gradient coil for nuclear magnetic resonance imaging. International patent WO 91/19209, 12 December
8. Mansfield P, Glover P, Bowtell R (1994) Active acoustic screening: design principles for quiet gradient coils in MRI. Meas Sci Technol 5:1021–1025
9. Romeo F, Hoult DI (1984) Magnetic field profiling: analysis and correcting coil design. Magn Reson Med 1:44–65
10. Golay MJE (1957) Magnetic field control apparatus. U.S. patent 3,515,979, 4 November
11. Turner R (1993) Gradient coil design: a review of methods. Magn Reson Imaging 11:903–920
12. Siebold H (1990) Gradient field coils for MR imaging with high spectral purity. IEEE Trans Magn 26:897–900
13. Turner R, Bowley RM (1986) Passive screening of switched magnetic field gradients. J Phys E 19:876–879
14. Turner R (1986) A target field approach to optimal coil design. J Phys D 19:L147–151
15. Turner R, Mansfield P, Chapman BLW (1986) Magnetic field coils. U.K. patent GB 2193322B, 28 June
16. Turner R (1988) Minimum inductance coils. J Phys E 21:948–952
17. Bowtell R, Mansfield P (1989) Minimum power flat gradient pairs for NMR microscopy. Proceedings of the 8th Annual Meeting of the SMRM, Amsterdam, p 977
18. Carlson JW, Derby KA, Hawrysko KC, Weidemann M (1992) Design and evaluation of shielded gradient coils. Magn Reson Med 26:191–206
19. Morich MA, Lampman DA, Daniels WR, Goldie FT (1988) Exact temporal eddy current compensation in magnetic resonance imaging systems. IEEE Trans Med Imaging 7:247–254
20. Roemer P, Edelstein WA, Hickey J (1986) Self shielded gradient coils. Proceedings of the 5th Annual Meeting of the SMRM, Montreal, p 1067
21. Mansfield P, Chapman BLW (1987) Multishield active magnetic screening of coil structures in NMR. J Magn Reson 72:211–223
22. Freeman A, Bowtell R, Glover P, Paterson-Stephens I, Issa B, Mansfield P (1995) A potential problem with operating gradient coils in parallel mode. Proceedings of the 3rd Annual Meeting of the SMR, Nice, p 949
23. Bowtell RW, Mansfield P (1990) Screened coil designs for NMR imaging in magnets with transverse field geometry. Meas Sci Technol 1:431–439
24. Compton RC (1982) Gradient coil apparatus for a magnetic resonance system. U.S. patent 4,456,881, 18 January
25. Pissanetzky S (1992) Minimum energy MRI gradient coils of general geometry. Meas Sci Technol 3:667–673
26. Wong EC, Jesmanowicz A, Hyde JS (1991) Coil optimization for MRI by conjugate gradient descent. Magn Reson Med 21:39–48
27. Crozier S, Doddrell DM (1993) Gradient-coil design by simulated annealing. J Magn Reson A 103:354–357
28. Wong EC, Hyde JS (1992) Short cylindrical transverse gradient coils using remote current return. Proceedings of the 11th Annual Meeting of the SMRM, Berlin, p 583
29. Myers CC, Roemer PB (1991) Highly linear asymmetric transverse gradient coil design for head imaging. Proceedings of the 10th Annual Meeting of the SMRM, San Francisco, p 711
30. Alsop DC (1993) A torque-balanced asymmetric gradient coil for imaging of the brain. Proceedings 12th Annual Meeting of the SMRM, New York, p 359
31. Abduljalil AM, Aletras AH, Robitaille P-ML (1994) Torque free asymmetric gradient coils for echo planar imaging. 31:450–453

32. Petropoulos LS, Lampman DA, Morich MA, Liu H (1994) Wide aperture gradient set (WAGS) for fast and high resolution MRI applications. Proceedings of the 2nd Annual Meeting of the SMR, San Francisco, p 1075
33. Brey W. W, Dougherty J L, Mareci TH (1993) A transverse gradient coil with concentric return paths. Proceedings of the 12th Annual Meeting of the SMRM, New York. p 1308
34. Mansfield P, Chapman BLW, Bowtell R, Glover P, Coxon R, Harvey P (1995) Active acoustic screening: reduction of noise in gradient coils by Lorentz force balancing. Magn Reson Med 33:271–281
35. Bowtell R, Mansfield P (1995) Analytic approach to the design of quiet transverse gradient coils. Proceedings of the 3rd Annual Meeting of the SMR, Nice, p 310
36. Cho ZH, Yi JH (1991) A novel type of surface gradient coil. J Magn Reson 94:471–485
37. Herlihy AH, Wong EC (1995) Numerically optimised surface gradient coil design matching RF coil sensitivity for uniform SNR Proceedings of the 3rd Annual Meeting of the SMR, Nice, p 951
38. Martens MA, Petropoulos LS, Brown RW, Andrews JH, Morich MA, Patrick JL (1991) Insertable biplanar gradient coil for MR Imaging. Rev Sci Instr 62:2639–2645
39. Yoda K (1990) Analytic design method of self-shielded planar coils. J Appl Phys 67:4349–4353
40. Pissanetzky S, Elekes A (1992) A fast switching biplanar gradient coil with cylindrical shield. Proceedings of the 11th Annual Meeting of the SMRM, Berlin p 582
41. Bowtell R, Clemence M, Gowland P, Mansfield P (1992) Biplanar gradient coils using the target field approach. Proceedings of the 11th Annual Meeting of the SMRM, Berlin, p 584
42. Petropoulos LS, Martens MA, Brown RW, Thompson MR, Morich MA, Patrick JL (1993) An MRI elliptical coil with minimum inductance. Meas. Sci Technol 4:349–356
43. Chapman BLW, Mansfield P (1995) Quiet gradient coils: active acoustically and magnetically screened distributed transverse gradient designs. Meas. Sci Technol 6:349–354
44. Wong EC (1995) A reduced dB/dt local head gradient coil. Proceedings of the 3rd Annual Meeting of the SMR, Nice, p 950
45. Mansfield P, Harvey PR, Coxon RJ (1991) Multi-mode resonant gradient coil circuit for ultra high speed NMR imaging. Meas Sci Technol 2:1051–1058
46. Nowak S, Schmitt F, Fischer H (1989) Method of operating a nuclear spin tomograph apparatus with a resonant circuit for producing gradient fields. European patent EP 0429 715 B1, 1 December
47. Frie W, Siebold H (1989) Anordnung zum Herstellen von Schnittbildern mit einem Kernspintomographen und Verfahren zum Betrieb der Anordnung. European patent EPA 0389666 B1, 28 March
48. Ideler KH, Nowak S, Borth G, Hagen U, Hausmann R, Schmitt F (1992) A resonant multi purpose gradient power switch for high performance imaging. Proceedings of the 11th Annual Scientific Meeting of the SMRM, Berlin, p 4044
49. Nowak S, Schmitt F (1991) Verfahren zum Betrieb eines Kernspintomographiegerätes mit einem Resonanzkreis zur Erzeugung von Gradientenfeldern. Federal Republic of Germany patent DE 41 27 529 C2, 20 August
50. Fischer H, Nowak S, Schmitt F (1995) Gradientenstromversorgung für ein Kernspintomographiegerät. Federal Republic of Germany patent DE 195 11 833 A1, 30 March
51. Zinke O, Brunswig H (1973) Lehrbuch der Hochfrequenztechnik, vol 1. Springer, Berlin Heidelberg New York, p 5
52. Hong X, Kelley D, Salem H, Hu F, Lindsay K, Lacroix D, Ma Y, Abrue J, Evens R, Roemer P (1996) Dual oblique resonant EPI for cardiac imaging. Proceedings of the 4th Annual Scientific Meeting of the SMR, New York, p 126
53. Fischer H, Nowak S, Schmitt F (1995) Verfahren und Vorrichtung zur Gradientenstromversorgung für ein Kernspintomographiegerät. Federal Republic of Germany patent DE 195 11 832 A1, 30 March
54. Mueller OM, Roemer P, Park JN, Souza SP (1991) A general purpose non-resonant gradient power system. Proceedings of the 10th Annual Scientific Meeting of the SMRM, San Francisco, p 130
55. Mueller OM, Roemer P, Park JN, Souza SP, Watkins RD (1992) A 4 switch GTO speed-up inverter for fast-scan MRI. Proceedings of the 11th Annual ScientificMeeting of the SMRM, Berlin, p 589
56. Souza SP, Roemer P, Peters S, Mueller OM, Rohling KW, Dumoulin CL, Hardy CJ (1991) Echo-planar imaging with a non-resonant gradient power system. Proceedings of the 10th Annual Scientific Meeting of the SMRM, San Francisco, p 217

57. Mueller OM, McFarland TG, Park JN, Wirth WH, Vavrek RM, Roemer P (1993) A new 'quasi-linear', high-efficiency, non-resonant, high-power MRI gradient system. Proceedings of the 12th Annual Scientific Meeting of the SMRM, New York, p 312
58. Mansfield P, Coxon RJ (1985) Inductive circuit arrangements. UK Patent No GB 2184625B
59. Coxon RJ, Mansfield P (1986) A method for the rapid switching of large gradients. Proceedings of the 3rd Conference of the ESMRMB, Aberdeen, pp 45–46

CHAPTER 4

Echo-Planar Imaging Pulse Sequences

P. A. Wielopolski, F. Schmitt, and M. K. Stehling

Introduction

The advent of faster and stronger gradient systems has enormously boosted the acquisition speed and the scope of applications by magnetic resonance imaging (MRI). The higher gradient strengths and faster switching times available with new gradient amplifiers and coil design has made it possible to:

- Image with shorter echo times (TEs) to counteract signal loss of gradient-recalled echo techniques (GRE) in regions with high magnetic susceptibility and extremely short T2* (0.5–2.0 ms). This makes it favorable for the evaluation of lung parenchyma [1].
- Enhance the reliability and utility of magnetic resonance angiography (MRA) with or without contrast agents using very short TEs (1.0–2.0 ms) and high resolution (512 matrix acquisition) and yet maintain reduced sensitivity to signal loss from turbulent flow in poststenotic regions [2, 3]
- Speed up image encoding times and improve time resolution and spatial coverage. This permits adequate characterization of dynamic events such as the first pass of a bolus of contrast through a tissue or the motion tracking in organs and joints using techniques such as ultrashort repeat times (TR) GRE imaging [4, 5]
- In general, reduce drastically the dead time periods during which no MR signal collection occurs. This makes it possible to achieve ultrashort TRs (1.7–3.0 ms) with GRE scans [5] or to reduce the interecho spacing in fast spin-echo (SE) sequences [6–8]

More recently echo-planar imaging (EPI) has made its debut, with particular impact in the clinical arena. Although initially pioneered by Mansfield in 1977 [9], its slowness in gaining acceptance as a useful clinical MRI technique was caused by the stringent hardware necessary to perform the scan. Today EPI is a clinically significant MRI technique. Still considered the fastest and most efficient encoding technique, EPI permits image acquisition times in the order of 30–100 ms [10], and a complete study can be accomplished in a few seconds, with tissue contrast similar to that obtained by conventional SE or GRE imaging techniques. Furthermore, EPI has broadened the number of applications possible for functional MRI and helped to increase the diagnostic quality in uncooperative patients.

This chapter characterizes EPI, describes the main differences with respect to conventional imaging, and illustrates several examples of clinical relevant EPI pulse sequences. The multishot EPI approach, a combination of EPI and conventional imaging, is also discussed in later sections of this chapter. Multishot EPI permits substantial reductions in scan time over conventional imaging protocols yet maintains good image quality without the extreme demands on the gradient hardware needed for good-quality single-shot EPI acquisitions.

Conventional Fourier Encoding

Spatial Encoding

After the application of a single radiofrequency (RF) excitation, the portion of the magnetization rotating in the transverse plane induces a signal in the receiver coil, S(t), that can be expressed by:

$$S(t) = \int\int\int \rho(x,y,z)e^{-t/T_2*(x,y,z)}dxdydz \tag{1}$$

after it has been taken from the resonance frequency ω_o to bandbase by the receiver demodulation circuitry (a multiplication by $e^{i\omega_o t}$). The proton density distribution of the object, represented by $\rho(x, y, z)$, is weighted by an exponential factor including T2*(x, y, z), the transverse relaxation in the presence of field inhomogeneities, a spatially dependent filter that affects the reconstructed images.

Note that S(t) in Eq. 1 has no inherent spatial information, as it is assumed that the main magnetic field B_o is homogeneous. The resonance frequency is proportional to the applied magnetic field through the known relation $\omega_o = \gamma B_o$, where γ is the magnetogyric ratio. The superimposition of a linear magnetic field gradient with a vector component along one direction of interest makes it possible to identify the signal from each spin within the sample based on the resonance frequency at each location. Assuming that the object extends only along one coordinate, for simplicity, the x-axis and the MR signal is read under the presence of a linear magnetic gradient field applied along the same direction, G_x, S(t) then becomes:

$$S(t) = \int \rho(x)e^{-i\gamma G_x xt}e^{-t/T2*(x)}\Delta Vz(x)\Delta Vy(x)dx \tag{2}$$

where $\Delta Vy(x)$ and $\Delta Vz(x)$ represent the contribution to the signal from the projection of all the spins along the y and z coordinates, respectively. The frequency content of S(t), commonly referred to as the bandwidth of S(t), is given by:

$$\text{Bandwith } [S(t)] = \gamma G_x x \tag{3}$$

where γ indicates the magnetogyric ratio divided by 2π (42.57 MHz/T). The maximum frequency found in S(t) is proportional to γ, the gradient G_x, and the size of the object imaged along the x-axis. Note that the bandwidth of S(t) is independent of the strength of the main magnetic field B_o. The magnetic field gradient applied during the signal readout is usually known as the frequency-encoding gradient.

k-Space

It is common to refer to the domain of the signal S(t) as k-space after S(t) has been digitized. k-space is a useful formalism that permits the interpretation of the MR signal from a perspective of the acquisition of spatial frequency data [11–13]. When G_x is a square gradient pulse during the time the S(t) is received, it is convenient to make the substitution:

$$k_x = \gamma G_x t \tag{4}$$

such that Eq. 2 becomes:

$$\overline{S}(k_x) = \int \rho(x)e^{-ik_x x}e^{-t/T2^*(x)}\Delta Vz(x)\Delta Vy(x)dx \tag{5}$$

where $\overline{S}(k_x)$ represents the quantized version of S(t). This expression corresponds to what is known as the imaging equation for a one-dimensional MR experiment. $\overline{S}(k_x)$ is then processed using the inverse fast Fourier transform (IFFT) algorithm to obtain the spin distribution of $\rho(x) \Delta Vz(x) \Delta Vy(x)$ for all the values of x.

The concept illustrated in Eq. 5 can be expanded to encode the spin density $\rho(x, y, z)$ for all three axes by introducing the integral description of the k-space variables:

$$\begin{cases} k_x = \gamma \int G_x(t)dt \\ k_y = \gamma \int G_y(t)dt \\ k_z = \gamma \int G_z(t)dt \end{cases} \tag{6}$$

Assuming that the MR pulse sequence encodes S(t) along the three orthogonal axis, the multidimensional imaging equation can then be written as:

$$\overline{S}(k) = \int \rho(r)e^{-ikr}W(r,T_1,T_2)H(r,k)dr \tag{7}$$

where $k = (k_x, k_y, k_z)$, $r = (x, y, z)$, and W(r, T1, T2) corresponds to the weighting that the particular imaging experiment has on the proton density at each location in the object through T1 and T2. H(r, k) gathers the effects from external factors that modify the resulting intensities on the image, such as filtering effects from signal decay during the readout of S(t) (T2*), geometric distortions from magnetic susceptibility changes, RF homogeneity (B_1) during the excitation and reception process, and variations in the signal intensity during the acquisition itself that pertain to the nature of the MR pulse sequence utilized, and, for example, the influence of physiological motion.

Multidimensional Imaging Encoding

The k-space matrix can be expanded to any dimension depending on the number of axes encoded. Thus for a two-dimensional (2D) representation of the spin distribution a 2D matrix of points must be filled to yield an image of a slice. For a three-dimensional (3D) representation, the collection of a 3D matrix of points will be necessary to produce an entire volume. For both 2D and 3D encoding, an IFFT is applied to recover the proton density distribution. Temporal and chemical shift information can also be included.

In-Plane Phase Encoding

In order to reconstruct a discretized 2D or a 3D representation of the proton density distribution, $\bar{\rho}(x, y, z)$, S(t) must be phase encoded along one or both orthogonal directions to the frequency-encoding gradient. For a 2D imaging experiment two gradients orthogonal to each other are applied to encode the "in-plane" information after a section is selected. In conventional Fourier encoded imaging N_x points equally spaced in time are collected along the frequency-encoding direction under a constant gradient amplitude, for simplicity denoted here as G_x (nonlinear sampling under a time-dependent gradient is also possible, see "The Echo-Planar Readout Module"). The second dimension is encoded by incrementing the phase contribution of the orthogonal gradient to the frequency-encoding gradient, namely G_y, for each acquisition of S(t). This is known as the "in-plane" phase-encoding process, and the number of points required to resolve a sample along this direction, N_y, determine the number of times that the signal S(t) is read. A generic 2D GRE pulse sequences is depicted in Fig. 1a.

k-Space Trajectory

The motion or "trajectory" described along k-space depends solely on the timing of the imaging gradients between the end of the RF excitation and the end of data collection. A single line of data (e.g., all frequency samples along k_x for a single value of k_y, N_x) is obtained per RF excitation during the application of a constant imaging gradient (G_x). The excitation is then repeated at a rate corresponding to the repetition time of the experiment (TR) as many times as necessary to complete the raw data matrix along the second dimension (N_y). To proceed in the k_y direction a phase-encoding gradient is applied prior to the signal readout (G_y) for a fixed time, t_y, and changing amplitude in steps of ΔG_y. The k-space trajectory described thus consists of a series of horizontal lines (Fig. 1b).

To reconstruct an isotropic 2D image the number of points sampled along the frequency and the phase-encoding directions must be the same. Denoting FOV_x and FOV_y as the field-of-view along x and y directions in the image domain, respectively, the relationship between the spatial frequency and the image domains in terms of k-space is given by:

Fig. 1. A Simplified representation of a 2D GRE sequence. B k-space trajectory for data collection. For each RF excitation, N_x points are collected along the frequency-encoding direction. A single line per excitation is read every TR, filling k-space from left to right. N_y phase-encoding steps are required along G_y to complete the data collection, Acquisition time is determined by TR·N_y. TR, repetition time; TE, echo time; α, RF excitation; G_x, frequency-encoding direction; G_y, in-plane phase encoding; G_z, frequency-encoding direction; t_y, in-plane phase encoding time k_x, k_y, spatial-frequency coordinates

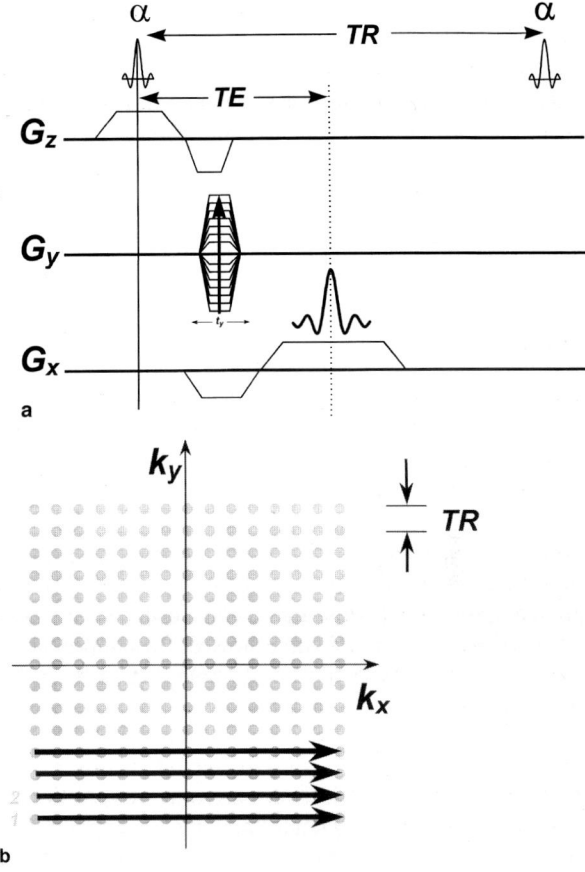

$$\begin{cases} \Delta k_x = \gamma G_x \Delta t = \dfrac{1}{FOV_x} \\[2mm] \Delta k_y = \gamma \Delta G_y t_y = \dfrac{1}{FOV_y} \end{cases} \qquad (8)$$

where Δt is the time between frequency-encoding samples, $\Delta G_y = G_y/N_y$ refers to the increment in the gradient table stepping along the in-plane phase-encoding direction and t_y the time the varying gradient table is applied before the acquisition of S(t) (see G_y in Fig. 1A). In general, both Δt and t_y are fixed parameters, and FOV_x and FOV_y are scaled by changes in the amplitude of the readout gradient, G_x, and the size of the table stepping, ΔG_y.

For a 3D experiment a third dimension is added to the k-space matrix. A phase encoding is incorporated, similar to that used along the in-plane phase-encoding direction, so that slices (also referred to as partitions) can be resolved within the larger volume excited. Denoting the thickness of the volume encoded as FOV_z, then:

$$\Delta k_z = \gamma \Delta G_z t_z = \frac{1}{FOV_z} \tag{9}$$

where ΔG_z and t_z denote the smallest gradient amplitude change of the slice-select phase-encoding table and the application time prior to the signal readout, respectively.

Image Resolution and Tissue Contrast

Equations 8 and 9 can be rewritten in terms of resolution in the image domain such that:

$$\begin{cases} \Delta x = \dfrac{FOV_x}{N_x} = \dfrac{1}{k_x} \\[2ex] \Delta y = \dfrac{FOV_y}{N_y} = \dfrac{1}{k_y} \\[2ex] \Delta z = \dfrac{FOV_z}{N_z} = \dfrac{1}{k_z} \end{cases} \tag{10}$$

Interestingly, Eq. 10 indicates that in order to resolve the smallest feature in an image (a pixel) or in a volume (a voxel) it is necessary to sample all k-space uniformly in each direction. This is analogous to the infinite frequency content of a single spike occurring in time. This fact has considerable implications in the resulting image contrast and overall signal behavior for each tissue that depends on the imaging sequence chosen to collect the data (filtering effects, local geometrical distortion, signal loss, among others; see "Considerations in the Design of Sequences using Echo-Planar Imaging Readouts"). Objects on the order of one pixel (or voxel) show a broad response, meaning that their information is spread equally across the entire k-space matrix. Similarly, the information from objects spanning the entire FOV is concentrated around a small cluster of points. This cluster contains the low spatial frequency components of the object, and it is indicative of the little information necessary to depict larger objects. This cluster of points coincides with the neighborhood around the maximum signal received during the acquisition (time during which the gradient applied during either phase encoding is the lowest, and the signal is refocused as a gradient echo or spin echo along the frequency-encoding direction), and it is referred to as the central portion of k-space. Nonetheless, in many instances the maximum signal does not coincide with the center of the k-space matrix. This is typical for GRE sequences using asymmetric echoes (echo center at far left of the k-space matrix) whenever flow dephasing must be minimized by keeping the TE short.

It is common practice to assign the contrast encoded by the imaging sequence to the central portion of k-space. Image detail, such as edge information, is encoded away from this center. This fact is of extreme importance when small lesions are evaluated with different ultrafast MRI schemes. All these techniques share the idea that contrast is encoded during the collection of the central portion of k-space, and that image resolution is affected by the way in which the magnetization signal varies during data collection at the outer portions of k-space. One objective in MR pulse sequence design is to correctly map the changing magnetization of the MR signal during data collection so that specific spatial frequency components are acquired that can match a contrast that is useful in a clinical setting while producing the least number of artifacts and loss of edge information.

Echo-Planar Imaging

Unlike the single line collection strategy used in conventional imaging, EPI encodes all the information necessary to reconstruct an image in one single shot after the application of the RF excitation. Using the improved gradient and signal reception hardware of newer MR scanners, clinically useful images may be generated rather quickly, within 30–100 ms.

A generic readout module for a GRE-EPI sequence is illustrated in Fig. 2a. At first glance GRE-EPI may be considered an extension of the conventional GRE sequence of Fig. 1a. In essence, an oscillatory gradient is applied along the frequency-encoding direction so that a train of echoes is generated. Each echo is then phase encoded independently and the entire k-space matrix is acquired. The echo spacing is generally denoted as ES.

Although some similarities do exist between conventional encoding and EPI, it is necessary to understand this process more in detail to judge correctly the appearance of EPI images. The relationships between k-space and image domain

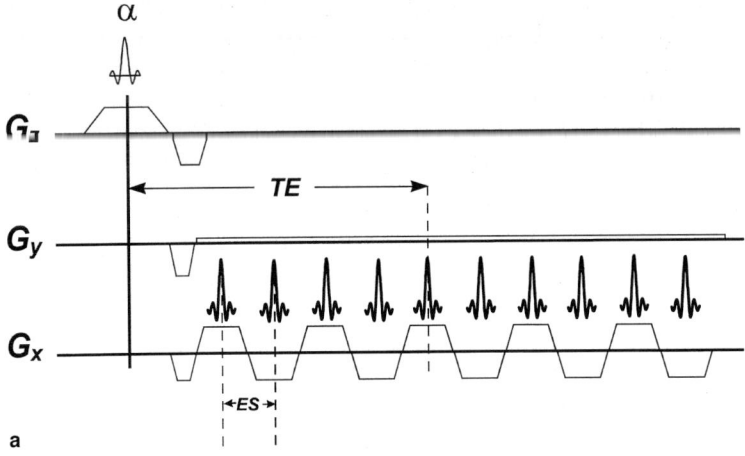

Fig. 2 (a–d). Single-shot GRE-EPI concept. After a single RF excitation an oscillatory gradient is applied along the frequency-encoding direction to generate multiple echoes. These echoes are phase-encoded independently and scan the entire k-space to form an image. Two different phase-encoding schemes are possible. In scheme 1, a constant phase-encoding gradient is applied during the entire readout module (**a**).

Fig. 2 (a–d). (continued) The
k-space trajectory (**b**) describes
a zigzag pattern along k-space,
scanning even and odd lines
from left to right and viceversa.
In scheme 2, a blipped phase-
encoding gradient is used (**c**),
resulting in a similar k-space
coverage (**d**) but with the main
difference that the trajectory is
colinear with the cartesian
grid. k_x, k_y, spatial-frequency
coordinates; *ES*, echo spacing;
TE, echo time. Signal differences between tissues at TE
determine the effective contrast
in the image

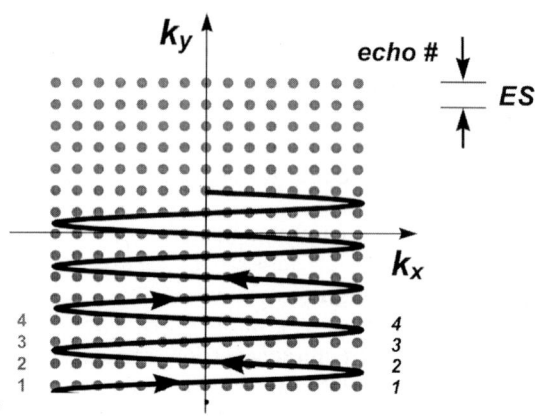

b

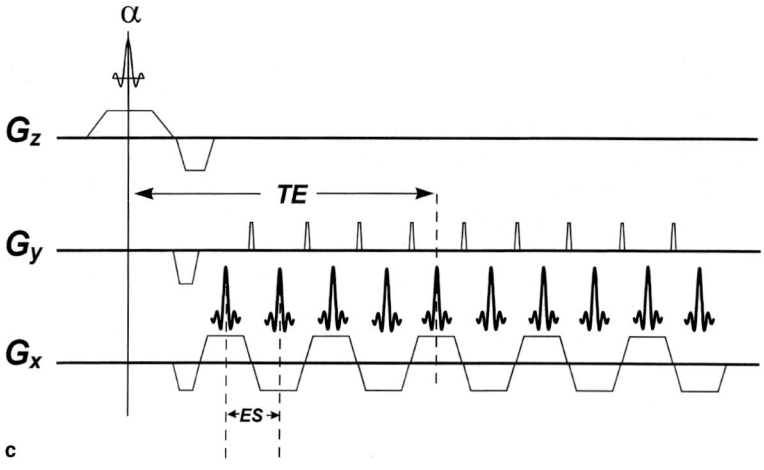

c

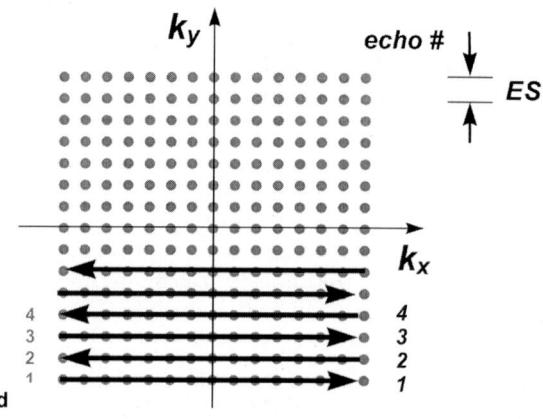

d

are the same as introduced for conventional imaging in the previous section. Below we describe each encoding axis of the basic EPI sequence (Fig. 2a) and draw comparisons to the more conventional GRE sequence.

Frequency Encoding

In conventional GRE techniques a single echo is used to scan one line in k-space (Fig. 1a). In EPI the addition of the bipolar oscillating gradient along the frequency-encoding direction permits the generation of an echo train, and each of the echoes may then be encoded independently along any other orthogonal axis. The oscillating gradient is usually referred to as the EP readout, and several gradient waveforms can be used (trapezoids, sinusoids, or a combination between trapezoidal and sinusoidal ramps with a gradient flattop) as long as a train of echoes is generated. Frequency-encoding artifacts per say are not present; neither T2* decay nor chemical shift artifacts may be appreciated, given that the acquisition time per echo is usually very short, and larger readout bandwidths are used than in conventional GRE scans.

However, there is no analogy between the frequency encoding in EPI and conventional Fourier techniques. The only similarity is that each echo is generated as a GRE using the same bipolar structure as in a conventional GRE sequence (gradient dephasing-rephasing). It must also be taken into account that despite the numerous echoes generated during the oscillatory frequency encoding, the effective echo time that determines the image contrast is related only to the time that the field echo is set to occur for the particular echo to which the center of k-space is assigned. Likewise in the case of SE-EPI the echo that coincides with the RF echo (twice the distance between the 90° and 180° pulses) shows the same signal behavior as that collected with conventional SE imaging; the other echoes generated suffer from T2*decay similarly as in GRE-EPI, but the decay within each echo is very small.

In-Plane Phase Encoding

To achieve the in-plane phase-encoding in EPI one of two approaches may be used to step from one line of k-space to the next. A constant phase-encoding gradient applied over the entire duration of the EP readout, or a phase-encoding "blip" of short duration applied at the end of each frequency-encoding gradient pulse.

Figure 2a,c presents the corresponding GRE-EPI sequences to the phase-encoding strategies above, respectively. The trajectory is slightly different for each, as illustrated in Fig. 2b, d. Note that in the case of a constant phase-encoding gradient the trajectory described along k-space does not match the cartesian grid (Fig. 2b), as compared to the blipped phase-encoding case (Fig. 2d). Thus depending on the trajectory chosen the data are treated differently during image reconstruction, and the error about the high spatial frequency data points may be taken into account to reduce ghosting artifacts [14] (see Chap. 5, 6).

Furthermore, the change in polarity and the time evolution reversal of every second echo of the EP train requires a data reflection about the center of every second line prior to reconstruction.

The echo at which the center of k-space is acquired (image contrast) is controlled by the phase encoding gradient. The center of k-space is reached whenever the area of the dephasing gradient is compensated by the positive, low-amplitude constant gradient (as illustrated in Fig. 2b). In the case of a blipped trajectory the effective echo time occurs when the area accumulated under the blips cancels that of the dephasing gradient pulse.

Observing more closely the GRE-EPI sequence of Fig. 2a, one notes that there is a similarity between the EPI phase-encoding and frequency-encoding processes in conventional GRE imaging. They are completely analogous, and therefore the image behavior along the in-plane phase-encoding direction in EPI is the same as that of a conventional GRE scan along the frequency-encoding direction. This explains the large chemical shift artifacts that are reflected along the phase-encoding direction in EPI (see "Chemical Shift Artifacts"). Chemical shift artifacts are caused by signals which are off-resonance (such as those coming from fat or silicone) and degrade the image quality. This happens because all points of k-space are collected under a single excitation and the phase accumulation from these off-resonance components accrues during the entire EP readout. This chemical shift is proportional to the time between the center of the readout between adjacent phase-encoding steps, or ES. Thus larger chemical shifts are observed as ES increases. This behavior is identical for the blipped phase-encoded GRE-EPI scan of Fig. 2c. Additionally, the low gradient amplitude that is effectively applied during the entire EP readout may be comparable to background field inhomogeneities and create severe geometrical distortions.

Slice Selection

The slice selection in EPI and conventional imaging modalities is the same. The RF excitation is applied under a constant gradient and refocused using a gradient reversal or a 180° refocusing pulse (in the case of a SE sequence). Motion-compensated gradient waveforms can therefore be used to reduce signal dephasing for moving spins (such as in MRA sequences, see Chap. 8). For a 3D sequence, an additional phase-encoding table may be used such as in conventional imaging (placed prior to the EP readout) to generate the necessary sections from the volume excited. Note, however, that if the EP train is used to encode the sections (partitions), images reconstructed along the slice-select direction exhibit the same chemical shift and geometric distortions as described in the previous section for the in-plane phase-encoding direction.

The Echo-Planar Readout Module

This section examines the gradient-time relationships for both the frequency-encoding and the in-plane phase-encoding axis.

Frequency Encoding

Gradient Strength Calculation with Arbitrary Gradient Readout Waveforms

In conventional MRI the MR signal is generally read under a constant gradient. The relationship between the sampling interval Δt, a constant readout gradient amplitude and FOV must comply with the Nyquist criterion, as described in Eq. 8, to avoid aliasing along the frequency-encoding direction. Nonetheless, a constant readout gradient is an arbitrary setting that facilitates data acquisition and reconstruction. In EPI the readout gradient waveform can take any arbitrary form. In general the Nyquist criterion is met when:

$$\int_0^{Tro} G_x(t')dt' = \frac{1}{\gamma FOV_x \Delta t} \tag{11}$$

where, once again, the subindex x is used to indicate the frequency-encoding direction and Tro the acquisition window per echo. For the case of a constant G_x, Eq. 11 reduces to Eq. 8 (e.g., reading the signal of the EP train only during the flattop portion of a trapezoidal readout). Equation 11 states that the gradient-time area under each echo readout must be kept constant independently of the readout gradient waveform to obtain the same FOV for a fixed Δt.

Because gradient amplifiers are not ideal, the finite rise time to maximum gradient strength may cost precious time whenever sampling is performed only on the flattop portion of a trapezoidal EP readout. The need for a short ES is crucial to obtain clinically useful EPI images with the least number of artifacts (see "Considerations in the Design of Sequences using Echo-Planar Imaging Readouts"). A reasonable solution is to sample the signal during the gradient ramps [15, 16]. This can dramatically decrease the readout time per echo, especially when large gradient readouts are used, and the area integral under the gradient ramp is significant in comparison to the readout time per echo.

In the more general case, when the readout occurs during the entire trapezoidal waveform, the amplitude of the readout gradient should be scaled for each case by:

$$factor = \frac{Ac}{A_{TS}} \ (sine\ ramps)$$
$$factor = \frac{Ac}{A_{TL}} \ (linear\ ramps) \tag{12}$$

with respect to the constant readout case. This is illustrated in Fig. 3. The term Ac refers to the unit area under a constant gradient readout of duration Tro:

$$Ac = \begin{cases} (2t_{rs} + Tc) \Rightarrow sine\ ramp \\ (2t_{rl} + Tc) \Rightarrow linear\ ramp \end{cases} \tag{13}$$

The "flattop" portion of the trapezoidal pulses is indicated by Tc, and t_{rs} and t_{rl} denote the time of a sine and a linear ramp, respectively. The unit area under

Fig. 3. Gradient area and amplitude relationships between an ideal EP gradient waveform and more realistic trapezoidal waveforms composed of either sinusoidal or trapezoidal ramps and a "flattop." The relationships consider sampling of the signal during the entire time TRO for all cases (sampling under the varying gradient waveform, e.g., on the ramps). A_c, Area under constant gradient readout; ATS, area under a sine ramp and flattop trapezoid; ATL, area under a linear ramp and flattop trapezoid; G_c, GTS, GTL, gradient amplitudes for a constant, sine ramp trapezoid, and linear ramp trapezoid, respectively; trs, trl, time for sine and linear ramps; Tc, time of flattop

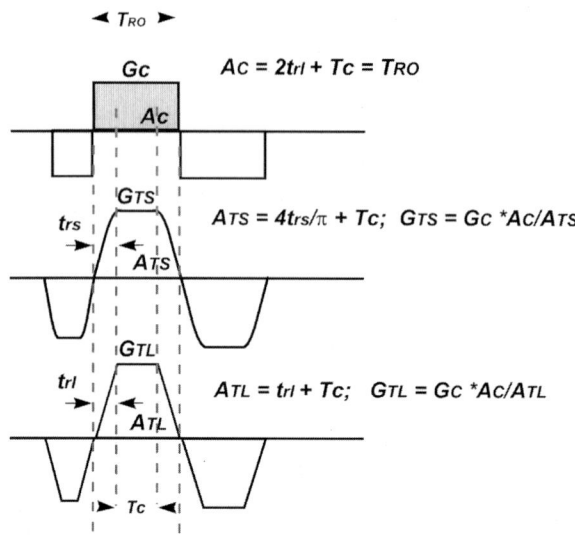

trapezoidal pulses with either sine ramps (A_{TS}) or linear ramps (A_{TL}) is given, respectively, by:

$$A_{TS} = \left(\frac{4 \cdot t_{rs}}{\pi} + Tc \right) \Rightarrow sine\ ramp$$

$$A_{TL} = (t_{rl} + Tc) \Rightarrow linear\ ramp \tag{14}$$

For a pure sinusoidal readout the peak amplitude of G_x must increase to obtain the same FOV as for the constant readout case (maintaining the same readout time). Therefore the amplitude of the sinusoidal gradient must scale by the ratio between the unit area under the sinusoidal gradient during the readout window and that of a constant gradient readout of the same duration. That is:

$$G_{x\_sine} = \frac{Ac}{A_{TS}} G_{x\_constant} = \left(\frac{\pi \cdot 2t_{rs}}{4 \cdot t_{rs}} \right) G_{x\_constant} = \left(\frac{\pi}{2} \right) G_{x\_constant} \tag{15}$$

where the subscripts x_sine and x_constant denote the sine and constant readout cases, respectively. Therefore the maximum gradient amplitude of a sine readout waveform is a factor of $\pi/2$ higher.

Sampling of S(t)

The Nyquist criterion assumes that a constant readout waveform is used, in which case Eq. 8 indicates the appropriate sampling interval Δt to be used to avoid aliasing along the frequency-encoding direction. For any arbitrary gradient waveform, however, two choices must be made with respect to how k-space will be scanned. In either way the end result must produce samples in the k-space matrix that are correctly placed on a cartesian grid prior to performing the 2D IFFT that produces the final image (see Chap. 5).

The two approaches that can be taken to sample S(t) under a varying readout gradient (Fig. 4) are: linear sampling, using a constant sampling interval Δt during the readout period (leading to a variable Δk_x), and nonlinear sampling, using a varying sampling interval during the readout (leading to a constant Δk_x).

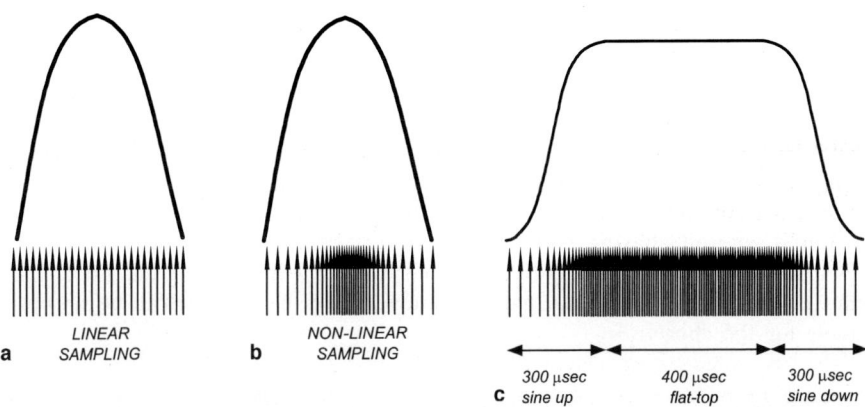

Fig. 4a–c. Sampling schemes. **a** Linear sampling can be used to collect the k-space matrix under any arbitrary waveform, here performed under a sine gradient. This results in a nonlinear scanning of k-space. **b** Nonlinear sampling. Samples are acquired nonuniformily in time leading to linear scanning of k-space. **c** Nonlinear sampling for a trapezoidal pulse with 300 μs sine ramps and a flattop of 400 μs. Note that during the flattop sampling becomes equidistant in time and k-space

Linear Sampling

With equidistant sampling under a varying gradient, a constant increment in time Δt translates into nonlinear increments in Δk_x. This means that to fill the k-space matrix evenly a regridding (interpolation) algorithm must be performed prior to image reconstruction (see Chap. 5). Figure 4a illustrates this case for a sinusoidal readout gradient. Furthermore, to comply with the Nyquist criterion the minimum number of time samples required, N_x, must increase accordingly by ratio between the unit area defined by a constant readout and the unit area of the varying gradient waveform. For the case of the sinusoidal readout the number of samples increases to:

$$N_{x\_sine} = \frac{Ac}{A_{TS}}N_{x\_constant} = \left(\frac{\pi \cdot 2t_{rs}}{4 \cdot t_{rs}}\right)N_{x\_constant} = \left(\frac{\pi}{2}\right)N_{x\_constant} \tag{16}$$

which is, as noted previously the same factor that is necessary to scale the readout gradient amplitude. The subindexes x_sine and x_constant indicate the sinusoidal and the constant gradient readouts, respectively. Thus for a pure sinusoidal readout and a 128 reconstruction matrix the number of samples required to avoid aliasing must be greater than 201 ($128 \cdot \pi/2$ samples). The oversampled signal is then sinc-interpolated to an equidistant k-space grid of 128 points before further processing continues.

There are some disadvantages to linear sampling. Interpolation is computationally intensive and considerably slows the reconstruction process. The size of the on-line memory must increase at least by the multiplicative factor above, becoming especially cumbersome with large data sets and signal reception using phased array coils. Finally, some hardware platforms can support only sampling based on an integer multiple of the base clock period that drives the analog-to-digital converter. To circumvent this sampling restriction the acquisition window is reduced and matched to fit the number of samples necessary to comply with the Nyquist criterion. This reduces somewhat the minimum FOV possible. Taking, for example, a 1000-µs trapezoidal waveform with sinusoidal ramps as shown in Fig. 4c (300-µs ramps and a 400-µs flattop), the number of samples needed to reconstruct a 256 matrix is approximately 330. Assuming a base clock period of 250 ns, the minimum number of samples that can be acquired without aliasing is 400. That is, it is necessary to collect 56 % more data than for the constant gradient readout case. Linear sampling has the advantage over nonlinear sampling that the bandwidth of the receiver can be set optimally for the chosen Δt.

Nonlinear Sampling

The other approach for acquiring S(t) uses a nonlinear sampling scheme [17]. The signal is sampled at equal increments in area under the gradient waveform instead of using constant increments in time. To advance the k_x trajectory in equal increments the following equation must be satisfied at all times:

$$\Delta k_x = \gamma \int_{ta}^{tb} G_x(t)dt = \text{constant} \tag{17}$$

where t_a and t_b indicate the time instance of two adjacent samples. The advantage of this approach is that no data postprocessing is necessary; the nonequidistant sampling in time results in an equidistant coverage of k-space (direct mapping onto the cartesian grid). The number of samples is the same as for the constant gradient readout; the amplitude of the readout gradient must also scale accordingly to accommodate the correct FOV (as reflected by Eqs. 12–15). That is, for the trapezoidal waveform illustrated in Fig. 4c the number of samples required to reconstruct a 256 matrix along the frequency-encoding direction is 256, and the gradient amplitude must scale by a factor of 1.279 to maintain the same FOV as for the constant readout case.

From the latter it is easy to recognize that the nonlinear sampling approach has the inherent advantage over linear sampling of greater flexibility in adjusting the readout window to a desired readout time while keeping the usual number of readout samples. Nonetheless, because of the variable sampling interval it would be optimal to have the bandwidth of the analog filter to match that of each sampling interval to maximize the signal-to-noise ratio (SNR). Most analog filters maintain a fixed filter bandwidth during the entire EP readout.

A General Remark. The addition of nonlinear sampling circuitry has been circumvented by using shorter gradient rise times to a slightly lower gradient amplitude to keep the area under the ramps small and to read the signal using a constant gradient amplitude. By using a constant gradient readout off-center FOV acquisitions along the readout direction can still be performed. It must be kept in mind that dB/dt for the shorter gradient rise time should remain under the threshold of peripheral nerve stimulation (see Chap. 7).

Phase Encoding

Gradient Strength Calculation

As mentioned previously, two approaches may be taken to phase encoding the echo train: using a constant phase-encoding gradient during the entire EP readout or a blipped gradient between echoes. In the case of a constant phase-encoding gradient, such as illustrated in the GRE-EPI sequence of Fig. 2a, its strength can be computed by setting:

$$G_y = \frac{1}{\gamma FOV_y ES} \tag{18}$$

where FOV_y represents the field-of-view along the phase-encoding direction and ES the echo spacing between adjacent echoes. For a triangular blipped phase encoding the amplitude of the blip, G_{bp}, is related to that of a constant phase-encoding gradient by direct comparison between ES and the effective application time of the blip (unit area), $t_{bp}/2$. Thus:

$$G_{bp} = \frac{2G_y ES}{t_{bp}} = \frac{2}{\gamma FOV_y t_{bp}} \tag{19}$$

For a resonant gradient system tuned at 1 kHz the readout time per line during a pure sinusoidal gradient is 500 μs, half the period of the resonance frequency. To obtain an image with isotropic resolution using a 128×128 matrix and a FOV of 250 mm the corresponding gradient strengths for the readout and phase-encoding gradients are 37.80 mT/m and 0.019 mT/m, respectively. To preserve the correct Δk_y increment using a triangular blipped phase-encoding gradient with a blip duration of 100 μs, the amplitude of G_{bp} would have to increase by 20 times, that is, to 0.376 mT/m. For a sinusoidal blip G_{bp} must decrease by the area ratio between a triangular and a sinusoidal blip, leading to:

$$G_{bp} = \frac{\pi}{2} \frac{G_y ES}{t_{bp}} = \frac{\pi}{2\gamma FOV_y t_{bp}} \tag{20}$$

For the example above but using a 100 μs sinusoidal blip, $G_{bp} = 0.295$ mT/m.

Other k-Space Trajectories

EPI may be hampered enormously by such factors as magnetic homogeneity and physiological motion (blood pulsation, see Chapter 8). One way to deal with some of these shortcomings is to reduce the duration of the EP readout. Shortening the EP readout is not an easy task, especially when image resolution must be adequate for scanning specific regions. Therefore various investigators have proposed different ways for scanning k-space. The simplest and most intuitive approach trims the EP readout almost by a factor of 2 using partial Fourier reconstruction techniques. Other approaches that provide some time saving include circular and spiral EPI which only use a circle or a sphere of data for 2D or 3D scans, respectively, to maintain isotropic resolution in each direction.

Partial Fourier Single-Shot EPI

Partial Fourier scanning has been used in the past to halve the imaging time necessary for SE scans [18]. The technique collects half of the k-space data necessary to generate an image and exploits the conjugate symmetry of k-space to recreate the missing part of that raw data [18] (Fig. 5a). An iterative approach referred to as partial Fourier projection onto convex sets (POCS) has also been implemented that does not make implicit use of the conjugate symmetry property but appears to be the most robust method of partial Fourier reconstruction for EPI [19].

Despite the effects of magnetic susceptibility and geometrical distortions in EPI, partial Fourier has been attempted with both SE-EPI and GRE-EPI scans to achieve short TE without a major loss in resolution along the in-plane phase-encoding direction [20, 21]. A shorter TE also helps to reduce flow artifacts for MRA applications based on EPI angiographic sequences (see Chap. 8). With half the scan time per shot, filtering effects from T2* decay are diminished as well. The reduction in scan time per shot can also be used to increase the ES to accommodate a lower readout bandwidth. In this case a smaller FOV is possible along the frequency-encoding direction without a major sacrifice in SNR and imaging time in comparison to full k-space acquisitions (nonetheless, geometric distortions and chemical shift from fat will increase as the phase-encoding gradient must be lowered accordingly from the longer interecho spacing). Partial Fourier encoding has also been used to decrease the image collection time with multishot EPI sequences [22, 23].

Margosian Partial Fourier. This method has been applied quite frequently, it is robust and simple to use when minimal phase errors are present. The method exploits the conjugate symmetry of the Fourier transform and assumes a step function centered at the origin of k-space multiplying the raw data. Under realistic conditions, undesired phase errors that can harm the final reconstructed image may be corrected by collecting several additional lines before the center of k-space is reached. The additional lines are then used to compute a low resolution phase map. The map is then applied to the original data prior to recon-

Fig. 5a–e. Faster k-space acquisition schemes.
a Partial Fourier scanning. Half of the k-space matrix is acquired to speed the readout time nearly by a factor of 2. Although half of k-space is necessary to recreate an image, under realistic conditions some additional lines after the k-space center need to be acquired to account for phase disturbances that need correction before the reconstruction. *Shaded region*, the acquired portion of k-space. Images can be reconstructed with several partial Fourier algorithms.

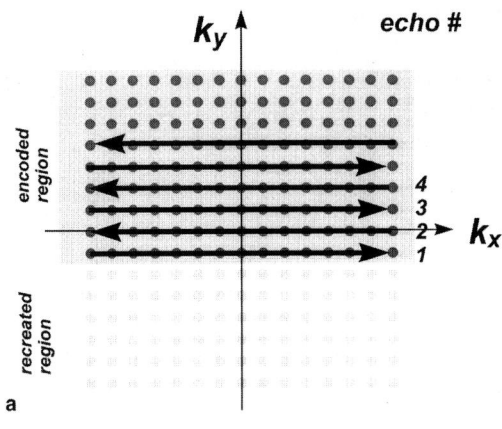

b Circular EPI trajectory can save approximately 27 % of scanning time. Partial Fourier reconstruction can be used to shorten the acquisition even more.

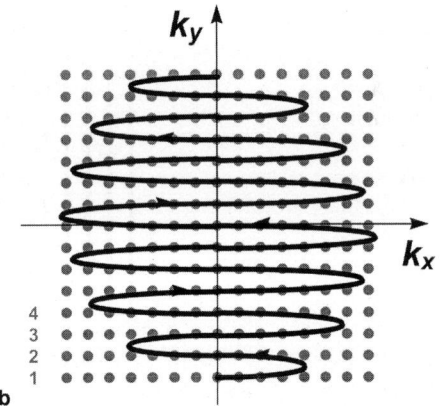

c Spiral k-space trajectory involves the oscillation of two gradient in tandem as shown in (**d**).

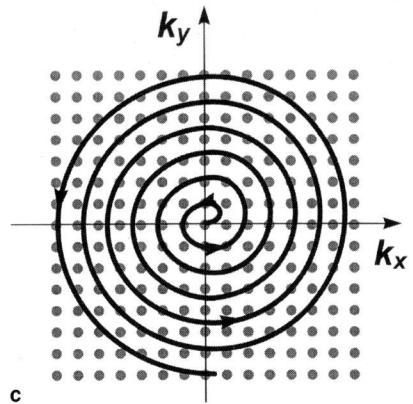

Fig. 5a–e. (continued) **d** The trajectory can save 27% of scanning time. It is inherently flow compensated and can achieve short TE, both necessary for MRA studies. Partial Fourier has not been yet demonstrated.

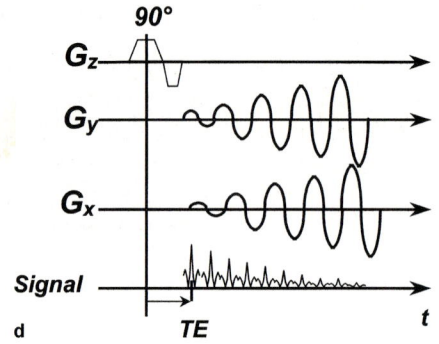

e A square spiral trajectory does not have an inherent time saving but can save on reconstruction time. Partial Fourier could be envisioned.

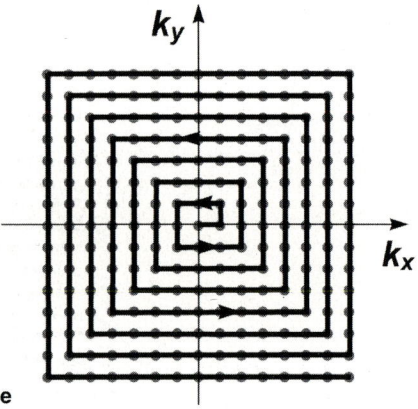

struction to reduce the effect of slowly varying phase errors over the image and to avoid intensity variations and extraneous signal cancellations in the final reconstruction. The resulting image is computed by taking the real part of the 2D IFFT after a phase correction has been applied. Margosian partial Fourier works less well with GRE-EPI than with SE-EPI sequences because of the greater sensitivity to magnetic field inhomogeneities of the former. However, if TE is sufficiently short, phase errors are reduced, improving the results. With longer TE more lines must be collected to obtain a more accurate phase map. The scanning of additional lines imposes a constraint on how short TE can be.

POCS Partial Fourier. More robust partial Fourier methods have been developed that use an iterative approach to recreate the missing k-space data. These methods are less sensitive to rapid local phase changes and work better with GRE-EPI scans than the conjugate synthesis scheme [19]. The algorithm also considers the collection of additional few lines before the center of k-space to generate a low frequency map. In GRE-EPI 1/4 k-space data collection prior to the echo usually shows good immunity to errors in the reconstruction. The computed phase map is applied to the magnitude reconstruction of a hanning filtered version of the truncated data set (one sided filter to eliminate Gibbs ringing). The resulting image is transformed back to obtain a "synthetic" raw data and a composite raw data is then generated by combining the synthetic data with the originally measured data. This is transformed back again to obtain an improved magnitude reconstruction that is multiplied once again by the low frequency phase estimate originally calculated and used as the new synthetic data. This loop is repeated until convergence is achieved. Generally three iterations in the loop are sufficient to obtain the desired image. The SNR is generally better with the iterative approach because the contribution to the signal from the additional points sampled before the echo is not eliminated as in the conjugate synthesis method.

Improving Resolution along the Readout Direction. Partial Fourier reconstruction has been also applied along the frequency-encoding direction. This permits approximately twice the resolution that is possible by the maximum gradient strength when collecting the full data along the frequency-encoding direction for a specific length of the EPI readout module [24]. Because partial Fourier methods can be applied only along one direction, short TEs are not possible in this case (all the k_y data must be collected). Nonetheless, for neuroimaging and functional MRI, long TE scans are typically used and can be practical.

Circular EPI

Similar to EPI, the path through k-space follows the cartesian grid but it is constrained by a circle (Fig. 5b) [25]. Acquisition is approximately 27 % faster than that of a regular EPI trajectory. The time saved is proportional to the area ratio between a square and a circle. The rate at which k-space is traversed along the phase-encoding direction varies substantially, faster at the edges of k-space and slower at the center, at the rate of a typical EPI scan. Thus artifacts are similar but off-resonance spins, such as those of fat, would appear blurred rather than sharp along the phase encoding direction.

Spiral Imaging Encoding

An alternative to image encoding that also involves oscillating the gradients during the acquisition is spiral scanning [26]. To describe a spiral trajectory through k-space (Fig. 5c) two gradients are oscillated in tandem (Fig. 5d). There are some advantages to this approach. Spiral scanning is intrinsically flow compensated, which is interesting for MRA to reduce much of the blurring and displacement artifacts when visualizing flowing spins. Time savings are similar to those in circular EPI. However, it is quite sensitive to static magnetic field inhomogeneities (blurring and ringing), and its advantages and disadvantages over the more conventional EPI encoding require further study. Spiral EPI is discussed in more detail in Chap. 21. Square spiral scanning, initially proposed was a simpler concept in which the trajectory through k-space followed the cartesian grid. The trajectory described is illustrated in Fig. 5e. A square spiral allows no time saving but does not require regridding prior to the reconstruction process. With this trajectory, some form of partial Fourier acquisition may be envisioned involving a combination between a square spiral (collecting the low spatial frequencies) and a one-sided collection of the higher portion of k-space using a normal EPI sequence. This can be of interest to reduce the scan time and mantain a short TE with good flow properties. Blurring of off-resonance components would be a combination of both trajectories.

Considerations in the Design of Sequences Using Echo-Planar Imaging Readouts

Despite some potential artifacts that may occur with EP readouts, as described below, it is very possible to elucidate more robust designs for an EPI sequence where the choice of parameters and imaging orientation can help to produce consistent image quality for each specific region in the body. This also facilitates the correct use of the imaging hardware to attack a specific clinical problem.

Sensitivity to Field Inhomogeneities

Readout bandwidth selection in EPI must be carefully monitored with respect to distortions from susceptibility and chemical shift artifacts. Geometric distortions and signal loss are coupled to the strength of the phase-encoding gradient (directly through ES) and the amount of intravoxel dephasing present for echoes far away from the RF excitation (for GRE-EPI) or the spin-echo time (for SE-EPI).

Because the total duration of the readout period for EPI is several times longer than that for standard pulse sequences (typically $\sim$30–100 ms vs. 5–15 ms), EPI is more sensitive to the effects of static magnetic field inhomogeneities. A constant local gradient induced by the body from susceptibility differences between different tissues (or by a diamagnetic or ferromagnetic material) leads to substantial spin dephasing. For example, consider a negative gradient offset, G_0, superimposed during the readout of a GRE-EPI sequence along the phase-encoding direction, such as depicted in Fig. 6a. As G_0 becomes more negative, the gradient echo moves progressively to the right of k-space along the phase-encoding direction, towards the end of the readout window. Eventually as the strength of G_0 increases such that its phase contribution becomes larger than that of the dephasing gradient alone prior to the ideal center of k-space, the echo disappears from the EP window, and no signal is detected. Figure 6a also depicts the case for a positive background gradient G_0 during the readout period. Under this condition the echo is compressed in time and shifted towards the start of the EP readout. In both cases the consequence is that the image in the region of the inhomogeneous field is initially distorted: the information appears in the wrong physical location, darker or brighter as the echo is compressed (by a positive G_0 gradient) or stretched (by a negative G_0 gradient) and eventually dis-

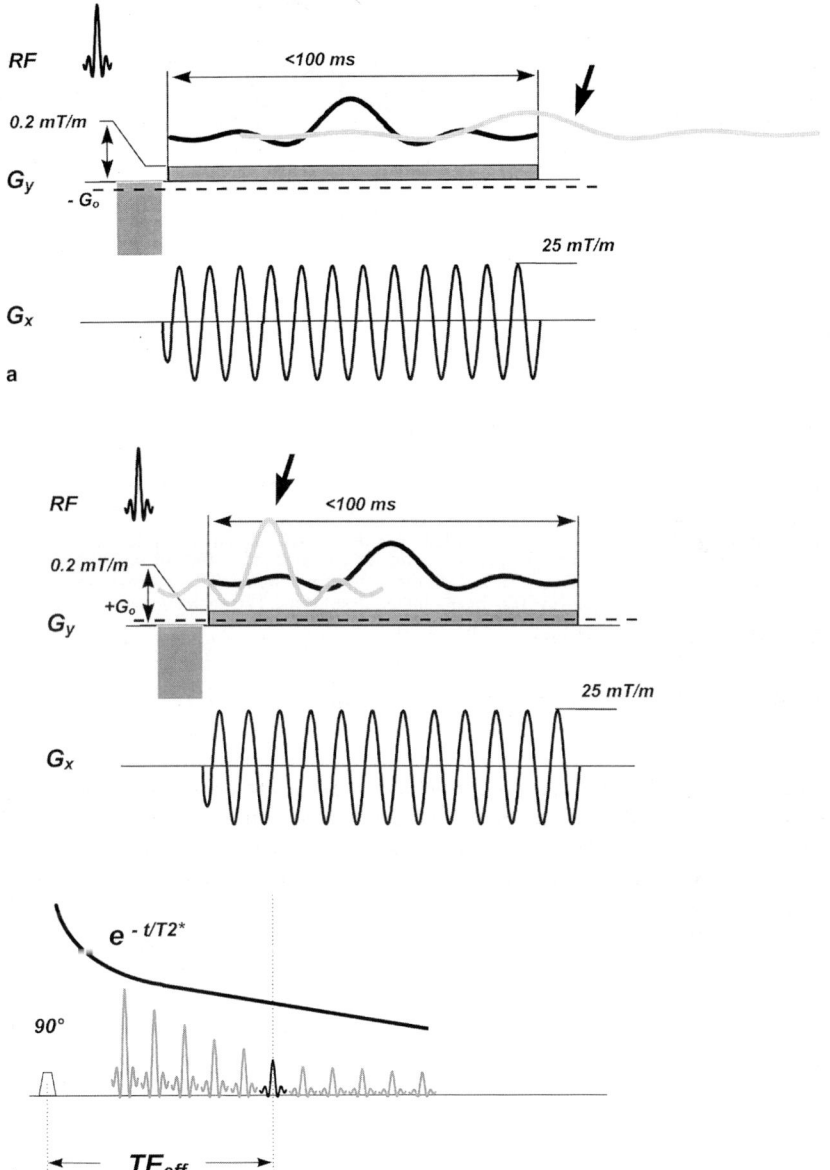

Fig. 6a–c. Potential artifacts that need to be addressed during sequence design. Because the effective phase-encoding gradient applied can have a similar magnitude to the background gradient induced by susceptibility differences or field inhomogeneities, signal loss and geometric distortions can occur. **a** Considering a background gradient with negative amplitude G_o superimposed over the phase-encoding gradient causes a broadened echo to occur (from the lower effective gradient amplitude, local shrinking in the image) towards the end of the EP readout. With positive G_o the echo is compressed and shifted towards the beginning of the EP readout (local expansion in the image). **b** In GRE-EPI the signal decays according to T2* after the RF excitation.

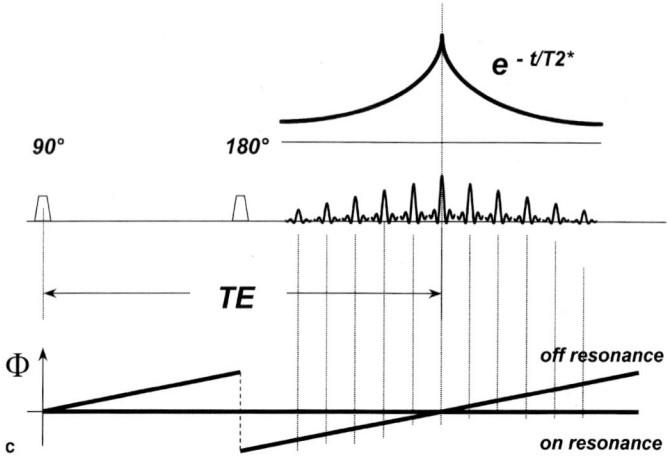

Fig. 6a–c. (continued) **c** In SE-EPI the signal decays according to T2* symmetrically about the spin echo time. All signals are on resonance during the spin echo but slowly dephase away towards the edges of the echo train. TE_{eff}, Effective echo time. Signal differences between tissues at TE_{eff} determine the effective contrast in the image despite the T2* decay. Blurring is higher in GRE-EPI than in SE-EPI, nearly by a factor of $\sqrt{3}$

appears due to signal dephasing (not because of distortion). If the phase-encoding gradient is increased in amplitude, the chance of field inhomogeneities shifting the echo outside the EP window is smaller. Geometrical distortions are reduced accordingly. Correction schemes have been proposed on the basis of a field map to unwarp the distorted images [27, 28].

Because of field inhomogeneities the length of the gradient pulse train is limited by T_2^* decay, which is given by:

$$\left[\frac{1}{T_2^*} = \frac{1}{T_2} + \gamma \Delta B \right] \tag{21}$$

where T2* characterizes the decay of the transverse magnetization in the presence of field inhomogeneities, ΔB a lorentzian distribution that accounts for the susceptibility variations across half a pixel and T2, the intrinsic transverse relaxation decay. Large inhomogeneities result in a shorter T2*, and the signal decays at a faster rate than dictated by T2 in a more homogeneous magnetic field. Because static susceptibility increases quadratically with magnetic field strength (while the magnetization increases linearly) the hardware requirements become more stringent, needing faster and stronger imaging gradients to compensate for the signal loss and filtering caused by a shorter T2* (see "Phase Encoding Blurring").

It must be kept in mind that even as TE is minimally increased in GRE-EPI, the weakest gradient can build up enough phase distortion to cause a dramatic signal loss. Susceptibility artifacts can be problematic in several areas. In the head signal loss can be appreciated at the skull base, near the paranasal sinuses and the anterior orbits. For example, for brain white matter near the sinuses, T2* can be as short as 8 ms. Using T2 = 80 ms for white matter, ΔB_0 would be in the order of 1.5 μT which corresponds to 1 ppm at 1.5 T across the imaging voxel. In the thorax problems are also prominent, as can be noted dramatically at the liver-lung interface. Susceptibility changes between the liver and the thoracic cavity are difficult to overcome, as well as near air-containing bowel loops. Susceptibility effects are reduced by using thin sections or a 3D acquisition [29], and SE-EPI rather than GRE-EPI. A change in slice orientation can also be beneficial. If the geometry of the region to be imaged permits, a rectangular FOV should be used along the phase-encoding direction, to increase the strength of the phase-encoding gradient and hence reduce signal loss and geometric distortions.

Phase-Encoding Blurring

Blurring along the phase-encoding direction arises from the long readout time needed for single-shot EPI to encode the entire raw data matrix relative to the T2* decay of most tissues. Filtering is not significant along the frequency-encoding direction as very little T2* decay occurs during the collection of each single line (0.5–1.2 ms).

For a GRE-EPI sequence the train of echoes decays according to T2* over the entire image acquisition time, as illustrated in Fig. 6b. For this case one can assume an exponential decay over the entire data collection window represented by $e^{-t/T2*}$. This decay produces in the image domain a widening of a voxel with dimension Δy along the phase encoding direction to a voxel with a full width at half maximum (FWHM) given by:

$$\text{FWHM} = \frac{\sqrt{3}}{\pi}(Ta/T2*)\Delta y \qquad (22)$$

where Ta denotes the image acquisition window. Obviously with shorter T2* the FWHM increases. With a SE-EPI acquisition encoding the data during the same EP readout duration as for GRE-EPI, the FWHM results in:

$$\text{FWHM} = \frac{1}{\pi}(Ta/T2*)\Delta y \qquad (23)$$

assuming an exponential decay which is symmetric about the center of the data collection window, a filtering function that can be defined by $e^{|t-Ta/2|/T2*}$. This decay is illustrated in Fig. 6c. The natural T_2 decay is not of importance in this case since it affects only the amplitude of the spin echo, generally collected during the center of the EP readout. From Eq. 23 it can be seen that the filtering effects for a SE-EPI scan are smaller by roughly a factor of $\sqrt{3}$ compared to that of a GRE-EPI scan.

It is interesting to note that in the case of GRE-EPI the filtering effects reduce accordingly with longer TEs (T2* decay starts from the time when the RF excitation is applied) whereas in the case of SE-EPI, filtering is roughly the same for all echo times as T2* affects the data symmetrically from the center of k-space. The filtering function for a fast SE acquisition is similar to that of a GRE-EPI scan with T2* replaced by the natural T2 decay (see Chap. 18, 19, 20). Filtering always affects image quality, increasingly so as the echo train or ES lengthens.

To constrain the resolution loss in pixel size along the phase-encoding direction, the length of the EPI readout should be set so that the FWHM is less than the spatial resolution Δy. If we choose the FWHM to be on the order of 0.1 Δy, the corresponding EP readout lengths for both GRE-EPI and SE-EPI would have to be on the order of 0.18 T2* and 0.31 T2*, respectively. The duration of the readout period can be shortened, for example, by accelerating the gradients (possible only within the physical limits of the gradient system and stimulation threshold) or by reducing the number of phase-encoding lines acquired using a rectangular FOV or a partial Fourier reconstruction to maintain the same resolution. All options reduce T2* effects at the expense of some loss in SNR.

Chemical Shift Artifacts

Chemical shift artifacts using EPI readouts are prominent and appear along any phase-encoding direction. The magnitude of the shift is several times larger than that with standard sequences along the frequency-encoding direction, essentially proportional to the ratio between the read out lengths. Taking fat a chemical shift of approximately 3.3 ppm, the number of pixels along the phase-encoding direction that fat shifts is inversely proportional to the phase-encoding gradient amplitude, G_p, through:

$$\Delta y_{FAT} = \frac{3.3 \cdot 10^{-6} Bo}{Gp} \tag{24}$$

B_o represents the main magnetic field strength and G_p is calculated from Eq. 18 for the case of a constant phase-encoding gradient.

Because of the weak phase-encoding gradient amplitude, the chemical shift from fatty components can be very large (Δy_{FAT} approx. 28 pixels for a 128×128 matrix, Gp ~ 0.019 mT/m, FOV = 250 mm, 64 ms readout time), thus making chemical selective fat saturation pulses or water-only excitation pulses essential for EPI.

Chemical shift artifacts can also be interpreted by looking at the ES of the EP readout in the same way that the sampling interval Δt in conventional GRE imaging determines the readout bandwidth along the frequency-encoding direction.

Because the ES is an indicator of the speed at which k-space is traversed along the phase-encoding direction, another expression for the chemical shift is:

$$\Delta y_{FAT} = \frac{(3.3 \cdot 10^{-6}) B_o \cdot ES}{\Delta k_y} \tag{25}$$

where 1/ES denotes the rate at which k_y is traversed. Chemical shifts become larger as the acquisition bandwidth is lowered (effectively, larger distance between the center of two consecutive echoes), as required to gain SNR.

Ghosting

Odd and even echoes are collected with readout gradients of alternating polarities. Background susceptibility gradients, imperfections in the gradient pulses or any gradient-induced eddy currents can cause slight mismatches between even and odd lines that are manifested in EPI as faint duplicate images of the object, called N/2 or Nyquist ghosts. If severe, these can degrade image quality.

To reduce or suppress the N/2 ghost several points must be taken into account:

- Ensuring gradient stability and minimal eddy currents.
- Matching the analog filter to the rate of data collection to minimize nonlinearities.
- Reducing the effect of the nonlinear behavior of the analog filter. Phase distortions on the signal after filtering are difficult to correct for, and because they exist along the positive time axis, the gradient reversal and subsequent data reflection forms a raw data set with alternating phase errors between even and odd lines.
- Introducing calibration scans using navigator echoes (such as described under "Calibration Scans") to help reduce all the above imperfections. The intensity of the N/2 ghost is reduced by using a nonlinear correction scheme that can take into account the unwanted hardware errors.

There are other conditions that may induce an N/2 ghost that cannot be corrected even with a perfectly tuned system. This is the case when imaging vascular structures. Flow components along the frequency-encoding gradient (see Chap. 8) generate an N/2 ghost with an intensity that depends on the phase difference between even and odd echoes which for constant velocity spins is the same from line to line.

Multishot Echo-Planar Imaging

As discussed above, single-shot EPI is severely limited by susceptibility artifacts and geometrical distortions, especially in the thorax and abdomen where EPI would have the greatest application because of its speed. The length of the EPI readout is constrained because the signal decays rapidly in the presence of short T2* while the spatial resolution is limited by the maximum gradient strength and gradient slew rates for a fixed EP readout length.

Spatial resolution is directly related to the area integral under the readout and the phase-encoding gradient waveforms. To minimize the effects of field inhomogeneities the gradient amplitude and speed would become prohibitively high to decrease the readout time. This is especially difficult with large gradient coils as power requirement and safety issues cannot be ignored. Interestingly, a $\sqrt{2}$ improvement in resolution or in speed is still possible using the same gradient hardware. This is done with an EPI trajectory rotated by 45° in the cartesian coordinate so that both gradients, provide a combined $\sqrt{2}$ increase in the amplitude of the readout gradient for the frequency-encoding axis [30]. After the images are acquired, a 45° counterclockwise rotation is necessary to view the image, resulting from the diagonal scanning of k-space.

Many of the problems related to single-shot EPI acquisitions can be overcome by accumulating the data over multiple excitations using multishot EPI. With multishot EPI the demands on gradient performance are significantly reduced, it is feasible to improve resolution, reduce the effects of T2* and field inhomogeneities and yet mantain the image and diagnostic quality at levels comparable to those of standard pulse sequences yet with much shorter acquisition times.

Multishot SE-EPI has proven to be an alternate approach to faster scanning. Studies have shown that images of high diagnostic quality can be obtained on uncooperative patients. Specifically, T2-weighted multishot SE-EPI has been validated with conventional T_2-weighted SE imaging in the brain on patients with multiple sclerosis [31] and in the abdomen (on an MR system with conventional gradient strengths) [32, 33], demonstrating the potentials of the acquisition technique. The studies yielded comparable sensitivity for small lesion detection with segmented SE-EPI. Other EPI hybrid techniques such as fast SE and GRASE imaging (Chaps. 19 and 20, respectively) are extensions of the segmented EPI approach that have been also conceived to minimize T2* effects, distortions, and chemical shift artifacts. These techniques have been useful for reducing data collection times with a minimum of artifacts using conventional scanners, as illustrated by the common use of T2-weighted imaging in the abdomen in a single breath-hold. However, contrast between lesions and healthy tissue can be hindered by such data collection schemes with the application of many RF pulses causing magnetization transfer (MT) effects, stimulated echo contributions and diminished sensitivity to diffusion and iron deposition as compared to segmented EPI scans that resemble the contrast of standard SE scans.

Two multishot EPI approaches have been reported that encode k-space in two very distinctive ways: the mosaic technique and the interleaved sequential blipped EPI technique. The next two sections discuss the two concepts more closely.

Mosaic EPI

In the mosaic technique the high resolution raw data is composed by tiling several blocks of k-space together (Fig. 7). The tiling can proceed along both the frequency- or phase-encoding directions or both. In either case the choice of tile arrangement determines the degree of freedom possible with respect to the contrast and resolution required. The displacement between the k-space blocks is controlled by the dephasing gradient applied prior to either frequency- or phase-encoding axis depending on the tiling direction selected.

Phase and amplitude discontinuities between overlapping regions must be avoided, particularly when the boundary between blocks is close to the center of k-space. Of particular importance is to perform the tiling in such a way that a smooth variation in amplitude and phase evolution exists across the entire raw data so that blurring and ghosting can be suppressed. To control potential mismatches, additional data lines are added to provide overlap between the blocks. A phase correction is then applied to each block to reduce phase discontinuities at the boundaries. Partial Fourier reconstructions have been demonstrated to reduce the number of shots necessary to form the image.

This method of k-space data collection is not robust. Geometrical distortions and susceptibility artifacts are still problematic (similar to single-shot EPI) and are better accounted for in the interleaved acquisition, as discussed in the following section. The reason for this is related to the effective speed at which k-space is traversed along the phase-encoding direction, which is the same as in the single-shot EPI technique. In this respect good fat suppression is still necessary because the chemical shift artifact is identical. To reduce artifacts the speed at which k-space is traversed along the phase-encoding direction

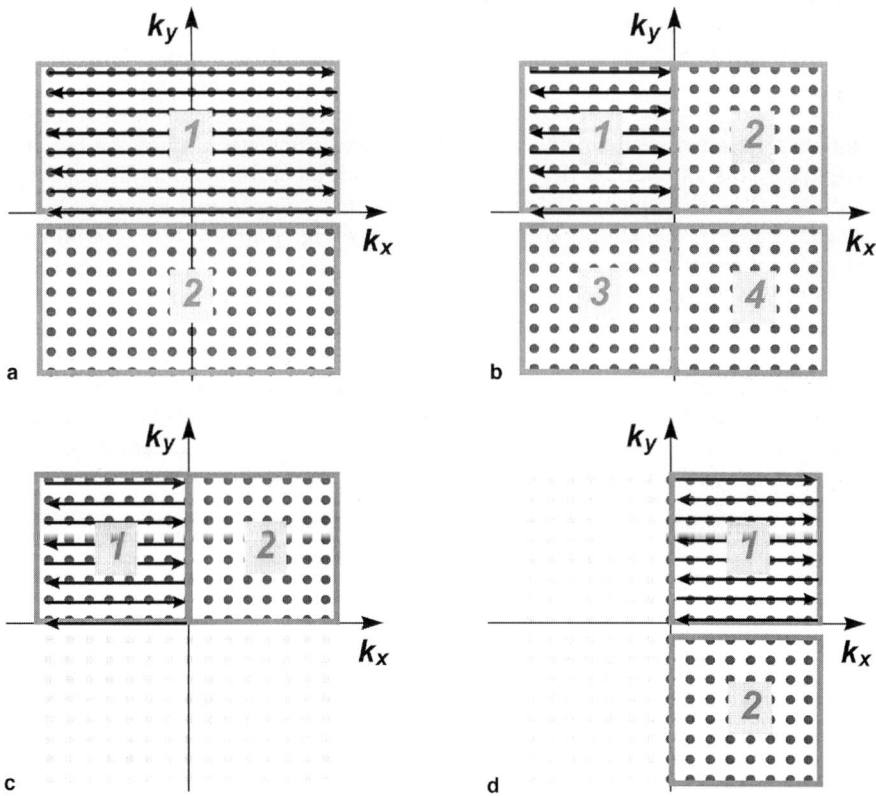

Fig. 7a–d. Mosaic scanning of k-space. The addition of one tile along any particular encoding direction increases the resolution (by a factor of 2 in the cases demonstrated). **a** Two tiles stacked along the phase encoding. **b** Four tiles stacked, two along the frequency-encoding and two along the phase encoding. Partial Fourier mosaic scanning along the phase-encoding (**c**) and frequency-encoding (**d**) directions. The mosaic concept is not robust but may be used under special circumstances, for example, stacking tiles along the frequency-encoding direction to improve resolution (since little T2* decay occurs)

must increase, resulting in a similar technique as described for the hybrid scan (see "Hybrid Imaging").

Interleaved

The first attempts at a multishot interleaved EPI scan were first envisioned by Mansfield and coworkers using the fast low-angle excitation echo-planar technique (FLEET) [34]. FLEET is a segmented GRE-EPI technique involving the acquisition of a double-zigzag trajectory that collects only the right quadrant of k-space using two RF excitations in rapid succession. To ensure that the signal amplitudes of the first and second sweeps are equal (in order to avoid artifacts), the RF excitations are set such that the first excitation is 45° and the second 90°, assuming negligible longitudinal magnetization recovery between the two shots. A different interleaving approach was proposed by Rzedzian with mosaicked echo scan hybrid (MESH) [35]. In this technique two shots are woven together, collecting in one shot every second line of k-space by doubling the amplitude of the phase encoding while in a second shot the remaining lines are encoded similarly but displaced by a single Δk_y value so that the complete k-space matrix was acquired. This approach is depicted in Fig. 8 with its corresponding k-space trajectory. Farzaneh implemented this technique on a conventional scanner [36]. A general segmented GRE-EPI scan is illustrated in Fig. 9 for the case of a blipped phase encoding schema.

The use of an interleaved trajectory effectively reduces the fat chemical shift and the sensitivity to signal loss and geometric distortions from field inhomogeneities. The effect of an interleaved trajectory with respect to the fat chemical shift is to increase the rate at which k_y is traversed by a factor of N_{shot}, where N_{shot} the number of interleaves necessary to fill the raw data. In this case the magnitude of the chemical shift can be reduced in comparison to Eq. 25 by a factor of $1/N_{shot}$, and therefore:

$$\Delta y = \frac{ES(3.3 \cdot 10^{-6} B_o)}{N_{shot} \Delta k_y} \tag{26}$$

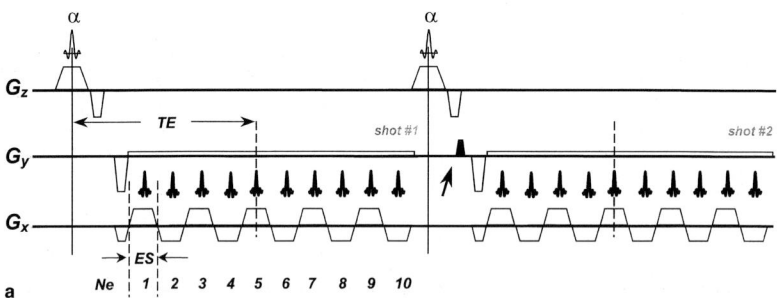

Fig. 8. a Initial implementation of the interleaved GRE-EPI scan using two shots. The phase-encoding gradient is doubled compared to the single-shot case to scan k-space effectively every second line. On the second shot, a small gradient blip of amplitude Δk_y (shaded blip prior to the dephasing gradient) is added to displace k-space by a single line.

Fig. 8. b Resulting k-space trajectory. Geometric distortions, blurring, and chemical shift are cut by a factor of 2. k_x, k_y, Spatial-frequency coordinates; N_e, number of echoes per shot; *ES*, echo spacing

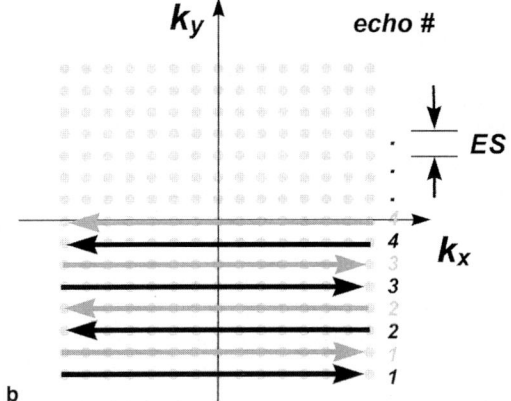

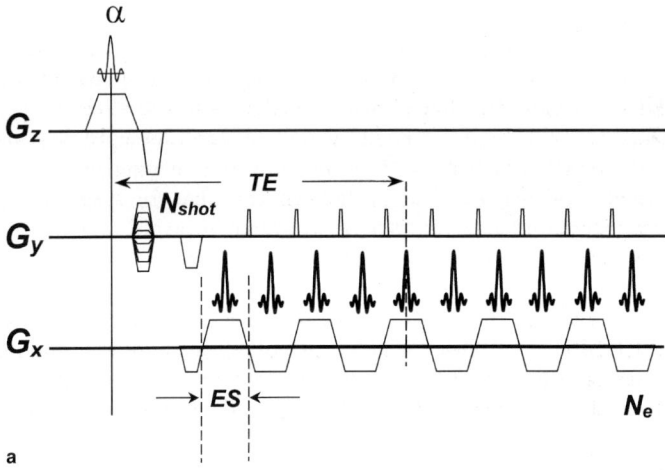

Fig. 9. a A generic multishot interleaved GRE-EPI scan. N_{shot}, the number of shots necessary to acquire all the data, given by (N_y/N_e); N_y, the number of phase-encoding steps; N_e, the number of echoes encoded per shot. The phase-encoding table steps for a single Δk_y per shot.
b Resulting k-space trajectory. The number of k-space segments is equal to N_e and each second segment has the same readout direction for the N_{shot} lines that compose each segment. Geometric distortions, blurring and chemical shift are cut by a factor of N_{shot}

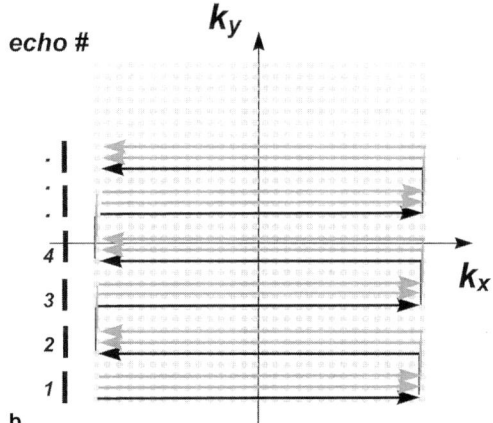

When more than two excitations are used to encode the data, the signal for each RF excitation must remain constant for all interleaves so that ghosting artifacts do not appear along the phase-encoding direction. This is an important consideration for a single slice 2D multishot EPI scan when the interleaves are performed in rapid succession using short TR [33]. In principle, an incremental flip angle series must be used so that the same signal strength is possible for each RF excitation. The FLEET technique, as discussed above, is a particular case where only two RF excitations are used. Assuming that TR is much shorter than the T1 relaxation for the tissue, the flip angle series that must be applied to ensure that the signal for each RF excitation is the same [37] can be approximated by:

$$a_{n-1} = tan^{-1}(sin(a_n)) \tag{27}$$

Because of T1 differences between tissues, a unique incremental flip angle series does not satisfy the condition of equal signal amplitude for all the RF excitations, and a compromise must be found for a particular imaging experiment [38]. In general, a low flip angle excitation would maintain the same signal, rendering essentially a proton density weighted image with the disadvantage of lower SNR. This approach has been used to collect a single slice in the heart in a single heartbeat with higher resolution and reduced susceptibility artifacts [33]. The most robust scenario is to wait until the magnetization recovers between interleaves and use a flip angle that ensures that for a specific TR the longitudinal magnetization has completely recovered to avoid signal variations and hence eliminate ghosting artifacts. Nonetheless, the scan time would be increased.

Another factor that must be taken into account for multishot EPI is that each echo in the EPI readout is different. This implies that not only the amplitude of each echo decays according to T2* but also that a background phase can accumulate in the presence of field inhomogeneities and motion (see Chap. 6, 8), creating some artifacts depending on the phase-encoding strategy used. Because the data collection with multishot EPI is generally interleaved, the amplitude and phase of each echo contributes to generate steplike amplitude and phase discontinuities between k-space segments that may degrade the image quality by introducing some addition ghosting and blurring in the reconstructed images. A smooth phase transition and T2* decay between segments can minimize the discontinuities using echo time shifting [32, 39–42], a method that slides the EP readout according to the current phase-encoding line acquired.

Echo time shifting can smooth the amplitude and phase transitions caused by field inhomogeneities from a steplike function to a linear variation across k-space. This is accomplished by adding a time delay Δt_d before the acquisition of each echo train such that the phase varies linearly as a function of k_y. The time delay Δt_d can be defined as:

$$\Delta t_d = (c_{shot}-1)\left[\frac{ES}{N_{shot}}\right] - \frac{ES}{2} \tag{28}$$

where ES indicates the echo spacing, N_{shot} the number of shots required to fill the entire k-space matrix, and c_{shot} a variable that keeps track of the current shot performed. Figure 10 illustrates the case for an acquisition using ten shots to fill the entire raw data. The echo train is shifted on every shot by a fraction of the readout window ($\frac{ES}{10}$) as stated in Eq. 28. The direct effect of the echo shifting is a slight increase in the blurring and chemical shift but with complete removal of ghosts from phase and amplitude discontinuities.

Hybrid Imaging

A special case of interleaving has been adopted in the hybrid technique [43, 44]. This technique was developed on a conventional scanner to speed the acquisition time by a factor of 2–6. In essence, the hybrid technique uses an oscillatory gradient of small amplitude along the phase-encoding direction (with an amplitude excursion that varies between Δk and several Δk depending on the acceleration factor) to sample several phase-encoding lines during the application of a constant frequency-encoding gradient contrary to the high-amplitude EPI wave form where the oscillatory gradient spans the complete k-space matrix along the frequency-encoding direction.

Fig. 10. Artifact reduction using a sliding EP readout window. On each shot the EP readout is moved from left to right by a time element equal to the ratio between the length of a single echo readout and the number of shots, (N_{shot}) required to collect the entire matrix. In the figure the number of shots is 10. The incremental time shift per shot for the entire EP readout is proportional to $c_{shot} \times ES/10$, where c_{shot} denotes the current shot

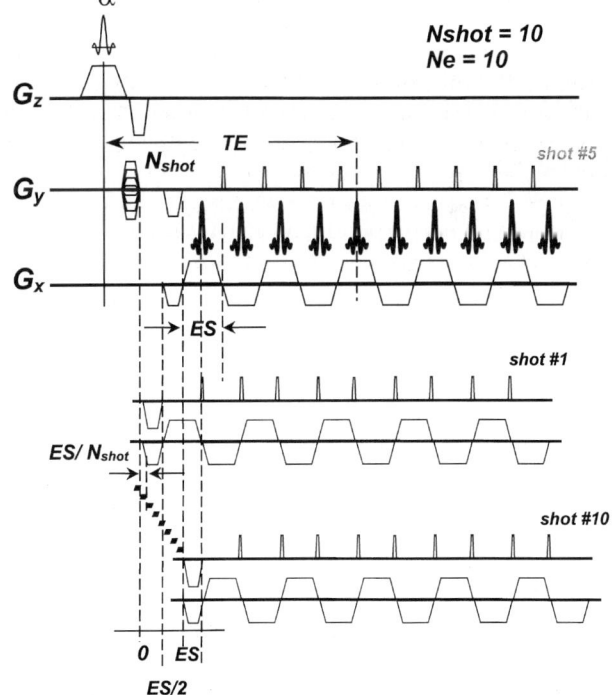

Calibration Scans

Instrumental imperfections and field inhomogeneities introduce phase and time shifts between the even and odd echo signals during the EPI readout that must be corrected prior to image reconstruction to eliminate the N/2 ghost (Nyquist ghost) and artifactual banding. The N/2 ghost is created mainly by sampling the odd and even lines in opposite direction. To minimize these differences the use of navigator echoes has been investigated.

A navigator echo represents a projection of all the spins contained in an imaging plane (for a 2D scan) or an entire imaging volume (for a 3D scan) perpendicular to the direction of the frequency-encoding gradient. The projection data are acquired by collecting the echoes under the EPI readout without the presence of a phase-encoding gradient, generally prior to the EPI readout. By obtaining the reference data, odd and even lines can be corrected separately before image reconstruction to minimize the presence of the N/2 ghost. Several approaches are described below. One approach obtains the reference data from a scan that collects the same number of navigator echoes as number of lines are acquired to form the image (full calibration scan) [45, 46]. Other approaches use only a few echoes to correct the whole raw data matrix [47, 48].

Full reference calibration scan

To produce an artifact-free image using a full reference scan (full calibration scan) the shim over the slice must be better than the inverse of two lengths of the EPI readout for a GRE-EPI scan. For example, for a 64-ms readout a shim of approximately 8 Hz it is necessary to maintain a phase coherence below $\pm 90°$. This is difficult to achieve in many regions in the body. For a SE-EPI acquisition the field homogeneity requirements are halved compared to those needed for GRE-EPI because the data are symmetric about the center of k-space with respect to off-resonant effects. After the reference data are acquired, the projection is normalized, its phase negated and multiplied on a pixel-by-pixel basis with the phase encoded EPI scan. However, because adequate shimming may be difficult over large regions, phase errors present in the projection data translate in the reconstructed images as stripelike artifacts along the phase-encoding direction. This is a problem particularly when the projection data comes from long TE echoes. These long TE echoes accumulate an additional phase from field inhomogeneities, and portions of the projection data may be zero if complete phase dispersion across the voxel occurs, giving rise to a random phase which renders an inconsistent phase behavior between lines. To circumvent this problem it has been proposed to align the echoes by using a constant and a linear phase term to correct all even or odd echo lines, calculated from the data obtained in the full calibration scan [46]. To compute the shift between even and odd echoes (linear phase shift), the echo peak at each projection is detected. The center of symmetry of the data is calculated based on an average of the echo positions between odd and even lines. Even lines in the phase-encoded scan are then folded about this center of symmetry to align all the echoes. This can be performed more precisely in the image domain (see chapter 5, "Linear Phase correction"). To reduce further phase errors an average constant phase term can be computed as well and subsequently applied to all the echoes. Phase correction using a constant and a linear phaseterm is a simplistic approach that does not eliminate the nonlinear phase behavior that the analog filter introduces into the data, leading to some remnant N/2 ghost.

Calibration scan from a limited number of projections

It has been shown that the results of using two navigator echoes to perform the phase correction are more effective in reducing the N/2 ghost than using the data from a full calibration scan in the presence of large field inhomogeneities [47]. To ensure that the phase errors from field inhomogeneities are small in the two-echo reference scan the projections must be acquired during the time of the spin echo in SE-EPI sequences and close to the RF excitation in GRE-EPI scans. Various implementations that collect a two-line reference scan for GRE-EPI and SE-EPI sequences are illustrated in Fig. 11a–d; Fig. 11e depicts the case for a multishot GRE-EPI approach.

For a GRE-EPI scan the reference data can be obtained by using a small RF excitation ($\sim$5°–10°) that samples the projection prior to the application of the 90° excitation to read the imaging data (Fig. 11a). Another approach does not require two RF excitations, as shown in Fig. 11b. The calibration data is collected after the 90° RF excitation, and the rest of the imaging data is acquired subsequently. The effective TE for the image is somewhat longer in this approach, but the longitudinal magnetization can be used completely because a single 90° RF single excitation is applied. The correction proposed by Heid et al. [48] incorporates a reference scan acquiring three lines instead of the usual two that have been used. The generation of a synthetic reference line for the negative by making a linear fit between two positive readouts permits a significant reduction in the N/2 and better behavior in the presence of short eddy current components. Two excitations can be used in SE-EPI scans, but the scan time is doubled because a low flip angle version such as proposed in Fig. 11a is not possible without a large disturbance of the longitudinal magnetization prior to the scan. Instead, the reference data may be acquired following the 90° excitation (Fig. 11c) as a gradient echo. This approach has proven robust.

Another possibility for acquiring the correction data for SE-EPI is to use internal reference lines (Fig. 11d) [49]. When the center of k-space is reached during the EPI readout, the phase-encoding gradient is switched off (only possible for a blipped phase-encoding EPI scan) to permit the collection of an odd and an even line of data that are utilized for the correction. A cross-correlation between the two projections is used to find the phase difference by which all even echoes or odd echoes must be realigned to eliminate the N/2 ghost. However, a discontinuity is created at the center of k-space which can translate into blurring in the image in the presence of off-resonance signals along the phase-encoding direction.

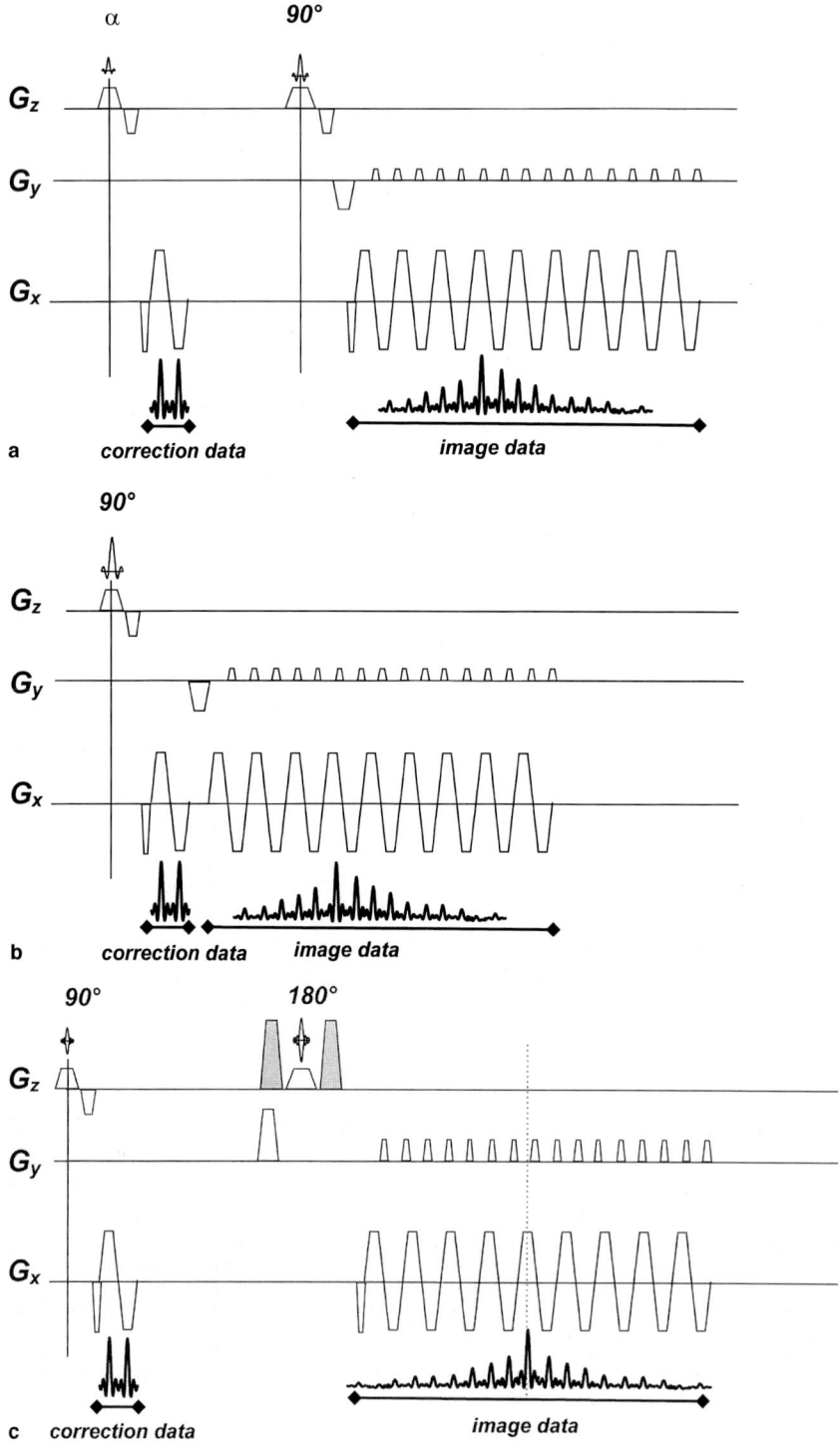

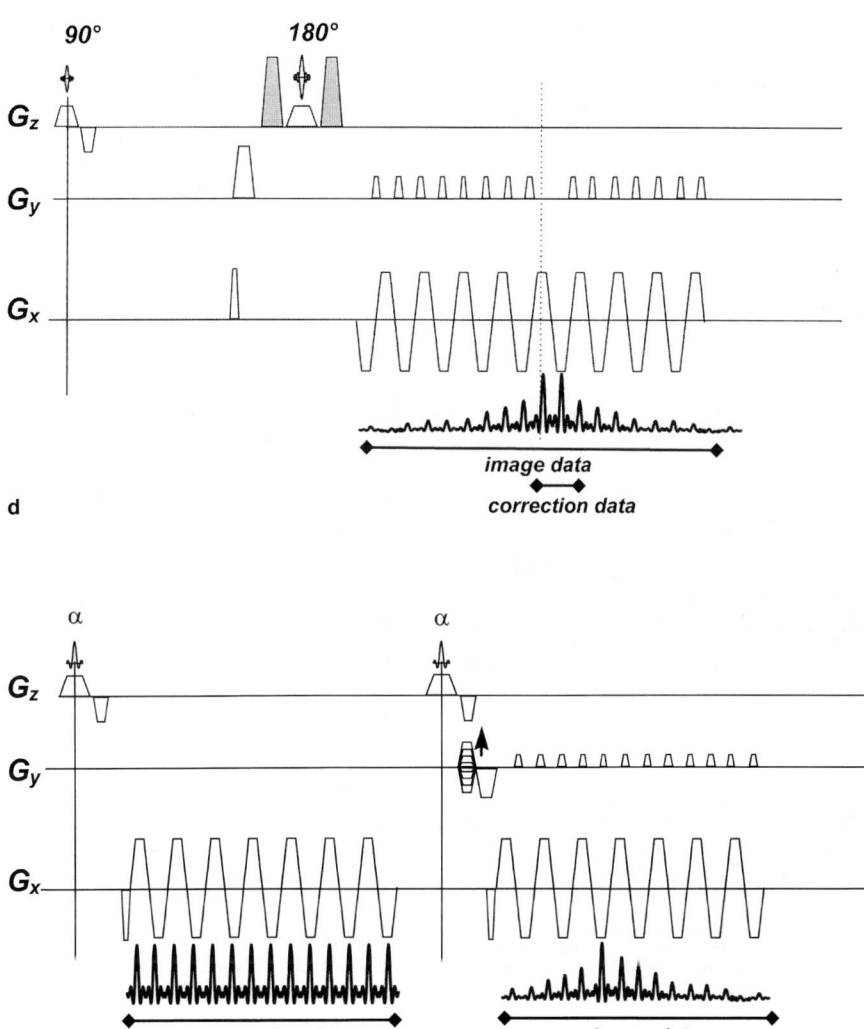

Fig. 11a–e. Strategies for collecting a reference scans for GRE-EPI and SE-EPI to correct for the alignment of even and odd echoes and reduce the N/2 ghost artifact. Navegator echoes are collected without a phase-encoding gradient applied. **a** Two navigator echoes are collected prior to the GRE-EPI image scan using a low flip-angle excitation readout. **b** Navigator echoes collected for a GRE-EPI scan using the entire longitudinal magnetization and collected prior to the image scan (but with a small increase in the minimum TE_{eff}). **c** With SE-EPI the navigator echoes can be formed as gradient echoes after application of the 90° pulse. **d** "Internal" reference lines can be acquired at the same time as the center of k-space is acquired for the image scan. This is done by eliminating a single blip so that two lines are acquired at the center of k-space under a positive and a negative readout. **e** When the number of echoes is small for multishot GRE-EPI scans (or multishot SE-EPI), the projections from all echoes may not suffer significantly from signal cancellation from field inhomogeneities and can all be used to correct all subsequent lines/echoes acquired during the measurement on a one-to-one basis

The calibration data generated from a single slice can be used to correct other slices. Although the center of symmetry varies little between slices, the phase offsets can vary substantially if eddy currents are large, especially with unshielded gradient coils. However, this strategy has been found useful for imaging the thorax by collecting the reference data in a region of greater homogeneity, for example, over the liver, and use it to correct data acquired in the heart.

Calibration scan for multishot EPI

The case of multishot is treated somewhat differently. Figure 11e depicts the case for a generic multishot GRE-EPI scan. Essentially, projections acquired for all echoes/slices set in the scanning protocol at the beginning of data collection, are later used to correct the imaging data. The echo trains for all the shots performed are corrected on a one to one correspondence (similar as in the case full calibration) case with the projections of the echo train acquired at the start of the scan. The phase correction strategy used is the same as in fast SE (turbo SE) scans (see Chap. 19, 20). The above suggestion previously mentioned for imaging the thorax can also be applied. Using the correction data collected in the middle abdomen, for example, effectively avoids phase cancellations in the projection that can lead to stripe artifacts along the phase-encoding direction when long TEs (greater than 12 ms) are encoded.

Echo-Planar Imaging Sequences and Applications

Acquisition Facts and Image Contrast

In general any imaging strategy that has been optimized for lesion detection in conventional protocols can be adapted to EPI, with the advantage of higher immunity to motion artifacts and the possibility to yield clinically useful images on extremely uncooperative or claustrophobic patients. Sequence structures utilized for EPI are in fact direct extensions of the diverse imaging techniques and strategies that have been developed in the past for conventional MRI. The essential concept behind the EPI technique is the replacement of the constant readout gradient used in a conventional sequences by the EPI readout module.

Some contrast differences arise for single-shot EPI, especially for 2D techniques since TR is infinite. In addition, to avoid chemical shift artifacts from fat, chemical shift fat saturation pulses are always applied (a gaussian pulse centered on the fat frequency or a binomial pulse) prior to the excitation and the EPI readout. A water only excitation can be used to eliminate the saturation effects that field inhomogeneities may introduce outside the slice of interest when using non-selective fat saturation schemes (see "Selective Water Excitation").

Because the phase encoding is performed sequentially in a typical EPI readout for GRE-EPI sequences, there is a limit to how short TE can be made to minimize T2* weighting. Centrically ordered phase encoding could be implemented to maintain a short TE to reduce T2* weighting. Nonetheless, the gradient power needed to perform this k-space encoding scheme is tremendous, growing exponentially with increasing phase encoding step. A single-shot centrically ordered scheme cannot utilize the phase accumulation as in normal blipped phase encoding as the phase applied by the previous blip must be rewound by applying the opposite gradient area, plus the area needed for the current phase-encoding step. Unfortunately, the phase encoding gradient contribution cannot be cancelled with RF excitations as in conventional GRE sequences because the echoes assigned for each phase encoding step are formed by gradient reversals. Any phase encoding scheme can be used for conventional imaging because each RF excitation applied resets the transverse magnetization. A SE-EPI scan is inherently centrically reordered in regards to the symmetry of the effect of field inhomogeneities and T2* about the center of k-space. A GRE-EPI scan with centrically ordered phase encoding is possible if k-space is acquired in multiple shots. For a scan using two shots, the acquisition can start at the center of k-space and collect the positive and negative k-space quadrants separately. This approach can be exploited by the mosaic technique (see "Mosaic EPI"). Although the T2* decay is symmetrical, the chemical shift and the evolution of off-resonant components proceed in opposite directions for each shot. In addition, the low-amplitude positive and negative phase-encoding gradients in the presence of magnetic susceptibility and background gradients produce signal loss and geometric distortions which are different for each shot, making this approach somewhat impractical. Nonetheless, with an increasing number of shots encoding k-space, centric k-space acquisitions are more feasible provided that a good fat suppression is possible [50, 51].

Single-shot EPI acquires an image after a single RF excitation. As a result the TR is essentially infinite, and the image exhibits a proton density contrast with moderate T2 (in SE-EPI) or T2* (in GRE-EPI) weighting depending on the choice of TE. Because the contrast generated in conventional imaging depends on the magnitude of the longitudinal and transverse magnetizations during steady-state conditions, such as in the case of fast low-angle shot (FLASH) imaging [52], a more rigorous comparison between single-shot EPI and conventional scans requires a careful choice of parameters so that the signal is comparable in both cases. For example, to obtain T1 weighting a 90° pulse can be applied a time, TR, prior to data acquisition. This can also be achieved by using multiple excitations (such as averaging or using the multishot EPI approach) or a 3D data acquisition. An inversion pulse can also be incorporated to create T1 weighting or to eliminate unwanted tissues from the image. This permits the acquisition of fat-suppressed images using a short inversion time (TI), or suppress tissues with long T1, such as the cerebrospinal fluid (CSF), by choosing a long TI as in the fluid-attenuated inversion recovery (FLAIR) technique. The latter choice helps to enhance lesions with a relatively shorter T1 then CSF but long T2, such as multiple sclerosis plaques. T1/T2 weighting can be obtained by using the EPI equivalent of the fast imaging with steady-state precession (FISP) sequence [53].

In the following sections several EPI sequences are considered, and their potential advantage in the clinical setting are demonstrated with several imaging examples.

Selective Water Excitation

A chemical shift selective fat saturation scheme is always applied to eliminate fat that may superimpose over tissues of interest [54, 55]. This is usually accomplished by applying a frequency selective, spatially nonselective RF excitation. Two spatially non-selective suppression schemes that are used comprise: (a) the application of a gaussian pulse centered on the fat frequency (usually several ms long) or (b) a binomial excitation sequence with short "hard" RF pulses 1-_1_, 1-_2_-1, 1-_3_-3-_1_ excitation pattern the underlined indicating a 180° phase rotation. With a typical binomial excitation the separation between the RF pulses is given by one-half the time that fat spins take to precess 360°, approximately 2.37 ms at 1.5 T. The fat suppression scheme is followed immediately by strong gradient spoiling prior to data collection to eliminate the transverse magnetization of the excited fat spins.

Spectral-spatial excitation schemes [56–58] can improve results dramatically and lead to a more effective fat suppression than the above mentioned strategies. The reason is that fat recovers some of its signal during the time course between the nonselective chemical shift fat suppression pulse and the excitation pulse, time that is completely eliminated using the spectral-spatial excitation. With a spectral-spatial excitation only water spins within the slice excited provide signal, leaving the signal from fat untouched.

Another advantage of the spectral-spatial water excitation can be exploited for MRA (see Chap. 8). When magnetic homogeneity is poor outside the imaging region, the nonselective schemes can suppress water far away from the imaging volume and therefore can render dark signal for blood vessels after time-of-flight effects bring the saturated blood into the slice of interest (similar to those obtained by using a traveling saturation band).

Single-Shot GRE-EPI

A GRE-EPI acquisition is the simplest conception of an EPI experiment. After a chemical selective fat saturation pulse is applied prior to imaging, a selective RF pulse, usually 90° if only a single image is acquired, is used to collect the free induction decay image encoded using the EPI module (Fig. 2a,c). As mentioned in the previous section, a selective water excitation may be used instead to avoid chemical shift artifacts from fat. By keeping TE short, the image contrast is essentially proton density weighted (without any T1 contamination, e.g., for CSF). Examples are shown in Fig. 12 in the brain and Fig. 13 in the abdominal region. Short TEs may be difficult to collect because of hardware limitations, but partial Fourier reconstruction can help to maintain a short TE by acquiring fewer lines before reaching the center of k-space.

With longer TE the image becomes increasingly T2* or susceptibility weighted and can be used for T2*-weighted perfusion studies. Conventional gradient echo imaging has demonstrated that by using long TEs qualitative maps of cerebral blood flow can be acquired during the dynamic bolus injection of a paramagnetic contrast agent. Long TEs with GRE-EPI enhance the signal loss when the contrast agent reaches the blood vessels and the capillary bed using the same susceptibility dephasing mechanism but with the advantage that multiple levels can be obtained with improved temporal resolution. Perfusion studies such as those performed in the brain (Fig. 14) have also been attempted in normally perfused myocardium [59, 60]. The limited immunity to motion artifacts, temporal resolution and multislice capability make GRE-EPI an appealing technique for this purpose. Susceptibility-weighted images have also been found useful in obtaining the blood oxygenation level dependent (BOLD) effect that has been used extensively in the recent years for functional studies of the brain (producing signal enhancement or loss through susceptibility changes during the execution of different functional paradigm) (see Chaps. 15, 16).

With cine GRE-EPI (which uses a reduced RF excitation angle, e.g., 45°, to avoid saturation of the blood pool) it is possible to obtain a series of multiphasic images without the need for cardiac triggering. This permits the observation of beat-to-beat variability, which is not possible with pulse sequences such as con-

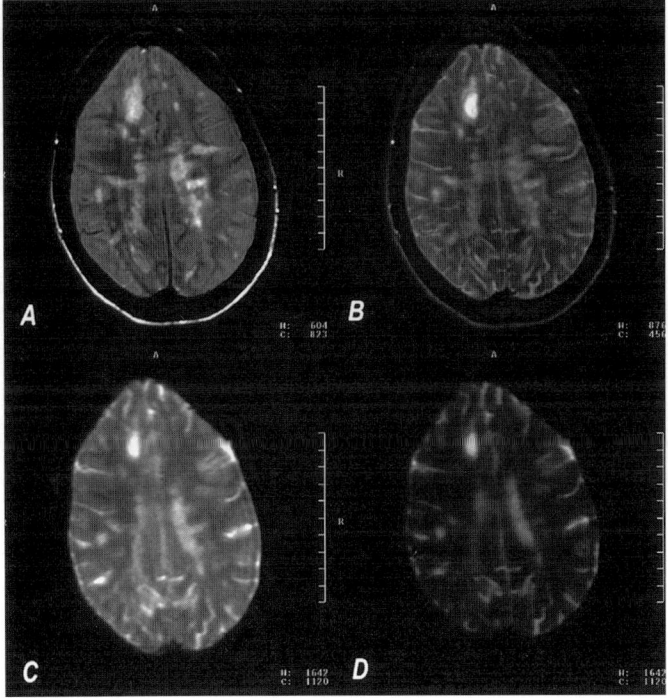

Fig. 12A–D. Comparison between conventional and single-shot GRE-EPI and SE-EPI scans in the brain of a patient with multiple sclerosis. **A** Conventional proton density weighted scan. **B** T2-weighted SE scan. **C** Proton density weighted GRE-EPI scan. **D** T2-weighted SE-EPI scan. Imaging parameters: **A,B** TR = 2400/TE = 15/80 ms, 5 mm thick, scan time of 7 min 44 s, 192×256 matrix, FOV = 250×250 mm; **C,D** 5 mm thick; TE = 22/80 ms, ES = 500 μs, 128×128 matrix, FOV = 250×250 mm (EP readout time = 78 ms, scanner: 38 mT/m, slew rate = 150 mT m^{-1} ms^{-1}). (Courtesy of Steve Warach, Beth Israel Hospital, Boston, USA)

Fig. 13. A Single-shot GRE-EPI in the abdomen. **B** A higher resolution scan was performed at the level of the kidneys using a 128×256 acquisition matrix. Imaging parameters: **A** 6 mm thick, TE = 22 ms, ES = 800 μs, 96×128 matrix, FOV = 200×350 mm, phased array body coil acquisition (EP readout time = 78 ms, scanner: 25 mT/m, slew rate = 80 mT m^{-1} ms^{-1}); **B** 6 mm thick, TE = 22 ms, ES = 800 μs, 96×256 matrix, FOV = 180×280 mm, surface coil acquisition (EP readout time = 78 ms, scanner: 38 mT/m, slew rate = 150 mT m^{-1} ms^{-1})

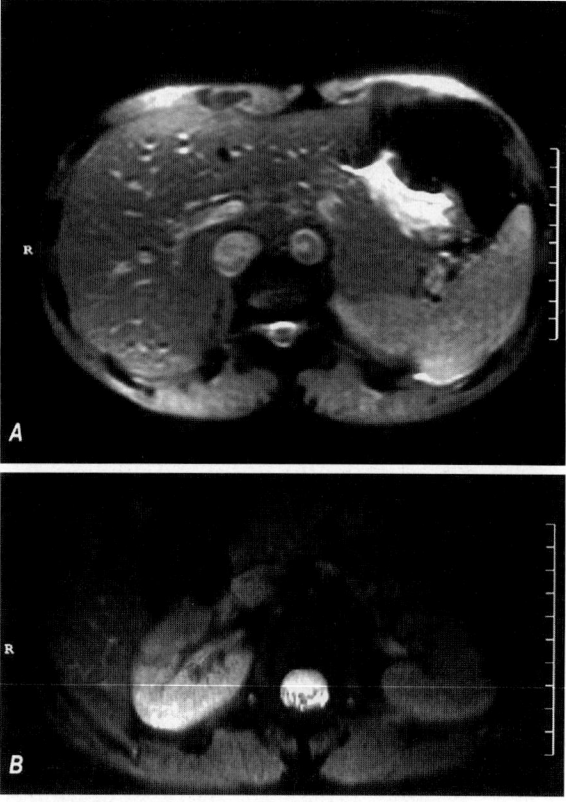

ventional or segmented turboFLASH cine acquisitions, that create a composite image from data acquired over multiple heart cycles. GRE-EPI can be extremely helpful in avoiding motion artifacts in the evaluation of congenital heart disease in children [61, 62].

SE-EPI

In a conventional SE sequence a 90°–180° excitation is used to form the signal. A SE-EPI sequence is formed by the addition of the EPI readout module after the 180° pulse to sample the echo signal. Because the center of the EPI readout coincides with the time of the SE, a SE-EPI sequence is less susceptible to field inhomogeneities and has a symmetric T2* behavior. A basic diagram of SE-EPI is illustrated in Fig. 15.

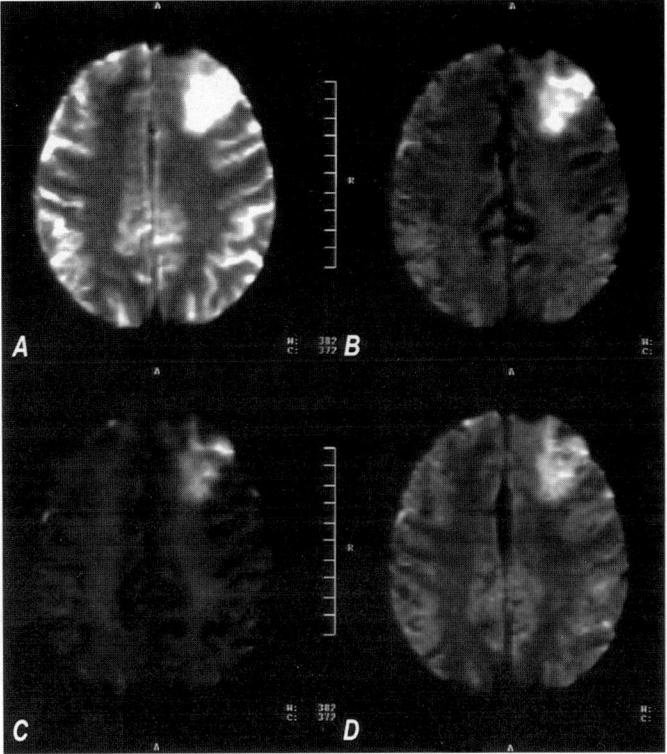

Fig. 14A–D. T2* Perfusion study in the brain of a patient with a frontal tumor. Ten slices were acquired every 2 s after the injection of a 20 ml bolus of Gd-DTPA. Imaging parameters: 6 mm thick, TE = 60 ms, ES = 600 μs, 96×128 matrix, FOV = 280×280 mm (total EPI readout time of 76.8 ms, scanner: 38 mT/m, slew rate = 150 mT m^{-1} ms^{-1}). (Courtesy of Steve Warach, Beth Israel Hospital, Boston, USA)

Proton Density and T2 Weighting

The image contrast is mainly proton density weighted when a short TE is selected. Using partial Fourier techniques (see "Partial Fourier Single-Shot EPI") it is possible to capture the proton density weighting and yet maintain good image resolution. Figure 16 presents an example collected in the brain. Otherwise a short TE GRE-EPI scan could be used, as described earlier. T2-weighted contrast develops as longer TEs are selected. Figures 17 and 18 depict examples in the brain and the liver, respectively.

With conventional SE scans it is possible to generate images in which blood is depicted as black. Dark blood is the result of the well-known time-of-flight effects as the initially excited blood spins by the 90° pulse does not experience the 180° refocusing pulse (specifically when flow is perpendicular to the plane

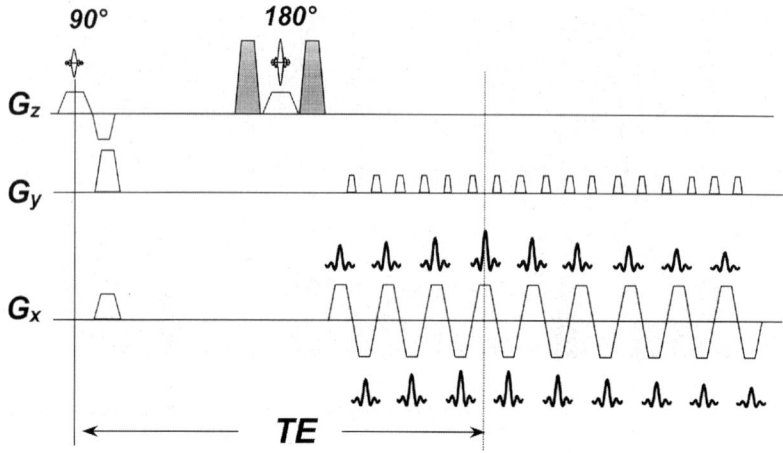

Fig. 15. Single-shot SE-EPI sequence diagram

of section). To obtain a more consistent suppression large balanced dephasing gradients (crushers) are placed around the 180° pulse (Fig. 15). This has been useful in conducting cardiac examinations, helping to eliminate the signal from moving blood and making it possible to acquire in a breath-hold a complete heart volume with good contrast between the blood pool and myocardium. This can aid in the calculation of cardiac output (Fig. 19) by collecting images during systole and diastole in two separate breath-holds. The volume provides the possibility for multiplanar reformation along the heart's short and long axes.

Fig. 16. High-resolution single-shot proton density weighted SE-EPI image in the brain. The data were reconstructed using a partial-Fourier algorithm with eight additional phase-encoding lines collected prior to spin echo and the center of k-space. Imaging parameters: 5 mm thick, TE = 16 ms, ES = 800 µs, 192×256 matrix, FOV = 256×256 mm acquisition (EP readout time = 84 ms, scanner: 38 mT/m, slew rate = 150 mT m^{-1} ms^{-1})

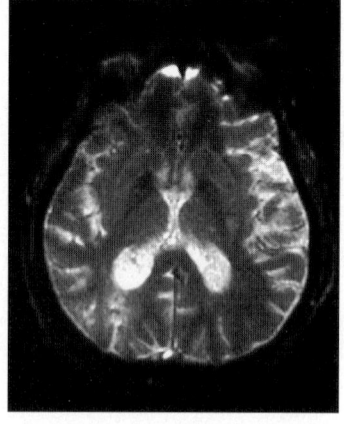

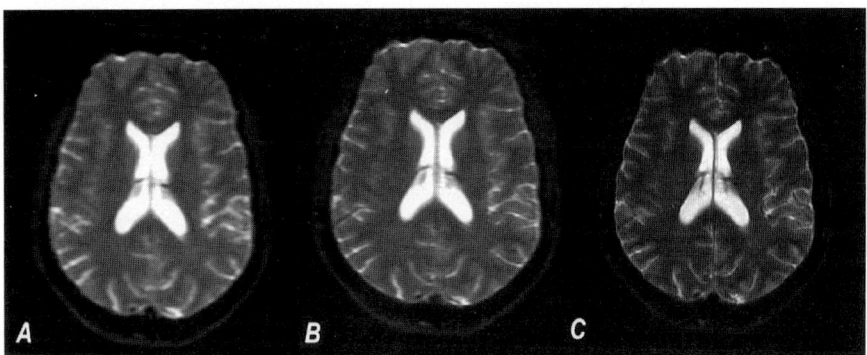

Fig. 17A–C. Single-shot SE-EPI in a healthy brain. Comparison of three different echo times. A TE = 56 ms. **B** TE = 70 ms. **C** TE = 109 ms. Imaging parameters: 5 mm thick, ES = 800 μs, 128×128 matrix, FOV = 256×256 mm (EP readout time = 102 ms, scanner: 25 mT/m, slew rate = 80 mT m^{-1} ms^{-1}). Symmetric data collection was possible in **C**, thus enhancing the spatial resolution compared to **A,B**

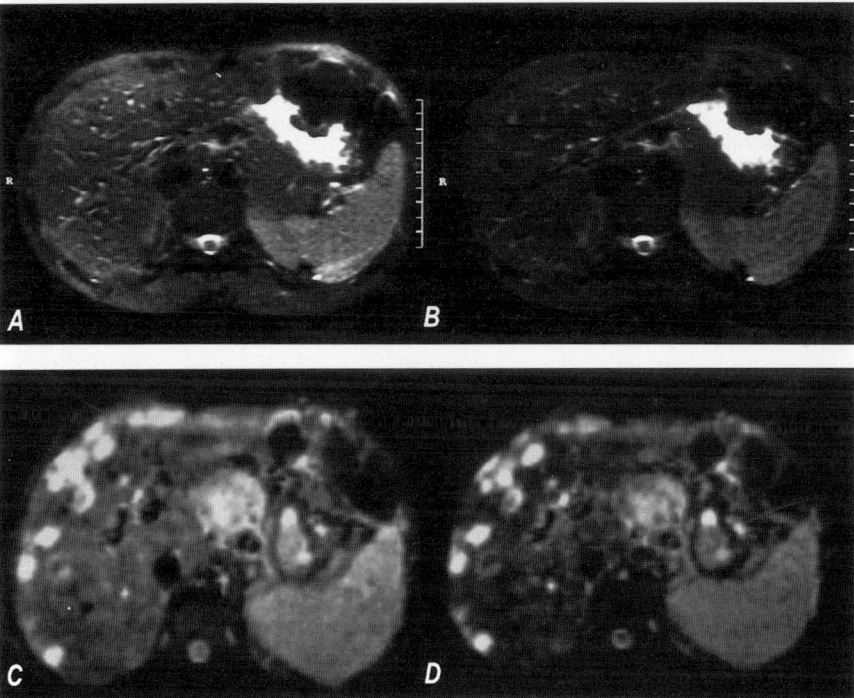

Fig. 18A–D. Single-shot SE-EPI in the abdomen. **A,B** Example in the liver of a healthy subject acquired with TE = 45 ms (**A**) and TE = 75 ms (**B**). **C,D** A patient with multiple cysts and metastases in the liver using TE = 52 ms (**C**) and TE = 100 ms (**D**). Imaging parameters: **A,B** 6 mm thick, ES = 800 μs, 64×128 matrix, FOV = 180×350 mm (EP readout time = 51.2 ms, scanner: 25 mT/m, slew rate = 80 mT m^{-1} ms^{-1}), phased array body coil acquisition; **C,D** 6 mm thick, ES = 500 μs, 128×128 matrix, FOV = 350×350 mm (EP readout time = 64 ms, scanner: 38 mT/m, slew rate = 150 mT m^{-1} ms^{-1}), body coil was used for signal reception

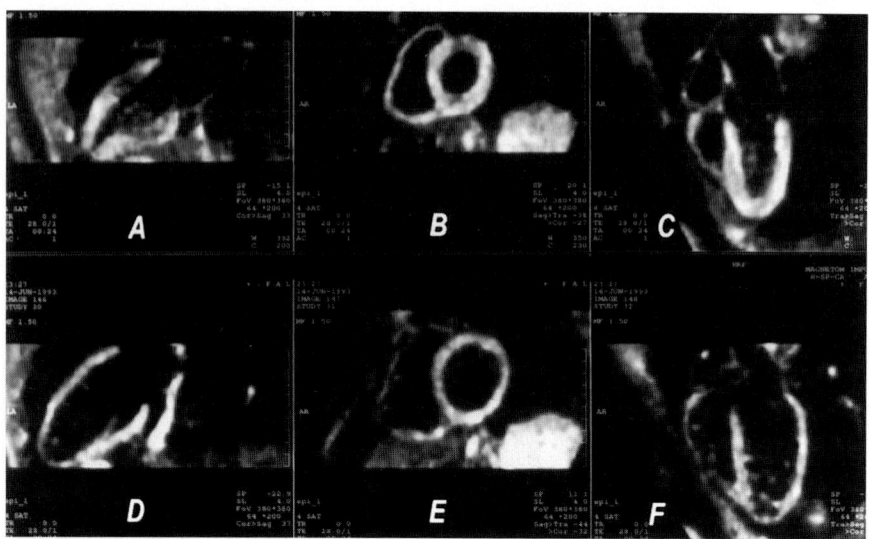

Fig. 19A–F. Multiplanar reformation of two cardiac volumes collected with SE-EPI during systole (A,B,C) and diastole (D,E,F). Twenty transverse slices were collected per breath-hold (20 heartbeats, 24 s) with a SE-EPI sequence with large crusher gradients applied about the 180° (along the slice-select direction) to help dephase the signal from blood and render good contrast between the myocardium and cardiac chambers. Imaging parameters: 4 mm thick, TE = 28 ms, ES = 500 µs, 64×128 matrix, FOV = 190×380 mm (EP readout time = 32 ms, scanner: 38 mT/m, slew rate = 150 mT m^{-1} ms^{-1}), body coil was used for signal reception. A,D,C,F Long axis views. B,E Short axis views

Inner Volume SE-EPI

Susceptibility artifacts can be reduced by augmenting the amplitude of the phase-encoding gradient (see "Phase Encoding"). This is advantageous when imaging the heart, where distortions can be magnified by the already large background susceptibility gradients in the thorax, and in cases in which a bolus of contrast is injected to observe myocardial perfusion (the susceptibility gradients created by the passage of the bolus of contrast can be significant and create local distortions between the blood pool and the myocardium).

To circumvent aliasing along the phase-encoding direction and to use the maximum gradient possible one must apply presaturation pulses to eliminate the signal from unwanted tissues. Another way to overcome aliasing is by using an inner volume excitation in conjunction with a rectangular FOV to increase the strength of the phase-encoding gradient (e.g., by acquiring only 64 phase-encoding steps in 32 ms readout for a gradient oscillation rate of 1 kHz, and a 2:1 rectangular FOV ratio). Blurring decreases as well from the shorter readout time. The inner volume SE-EPI is performed by applying the 90° and the 180° pulses in orthogonal directions [63] (Fig. 20a). The 90° pulse selects the level of interest, and the 180° pulse is applied perpendicularly.

A drawback of this acquisition scheme is that multiple levels cannot be acquired without a recovery time between imaging sections because of saturation effects (other slices experience the inversion pulse). A work around can be performed by using a low-flip angle SE equivalent such as in FATE [64], RASEE [65], and FLASE [66]. In FATE two 180° pulses are applied to drive the magnetization back to the positive z axis while the slice is imaged with a flip angle lower than 90°. Nonetheless, there is a severe drawback for EPI acquisitions related to the separation between the 180° pulses during which the EPI readout is performed, where T1 relaxation effects eliminate the effect of the second 180° pulse (depending on the length of the EPI readout). The RASEE modification is more appealing as a 180° pulse is applied prior to the slice selection, shortening the time between the 180° pulses to approximately TE/2, independently of the EPI readout time (Fig. 20b,c).

Diffusion Weighting

Diffusion is the process of random molecular motion caused by thermal energy. Small molecules such as those of water diffuse rapidly, whereas large molecules such as in proteins diffuse more slowly. Although MR was proposed to measure molecular diffusion in the early 1950s [67], only in the past few years have in vivo measurements become practical [68]. The study of diffusion with EPI has become a clinical reality [69, 70] and has made it possible to observe and diagnose patients in the early stages after stroke (less than 2 h) that are not depicted

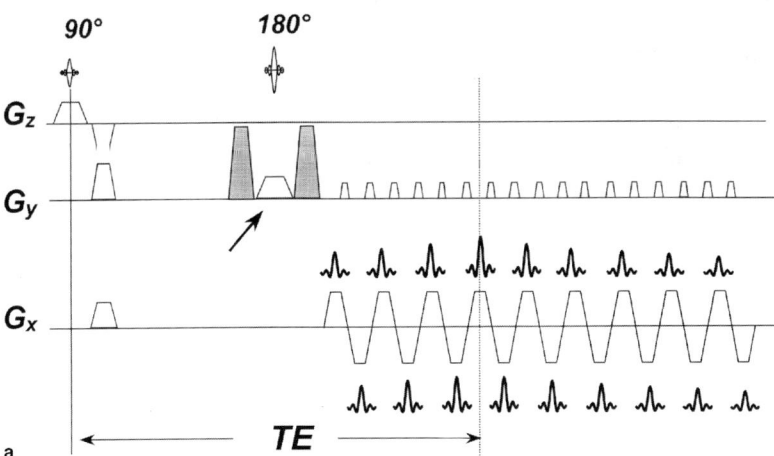

Fig. 20. a Inner volume SE-EPI. The 90° and 180° pulses are applied in two orthogonal orientations to select a smaller imaging volume that can be encoded with a reduced FOV without incurring into aliasing along the phase-encoding direction. *Arrow*, the 180° pulse applied along the phase-encoding direction that confines the FOV to the thickness of the RF excitation profile. The largest phase-encoding gradient possible and rectangular FOV scanning should be used to reduce geometrical distortions. The FATE (**b**) and RASEE (**c**) concepts can be used to optimize the signal for each excitation

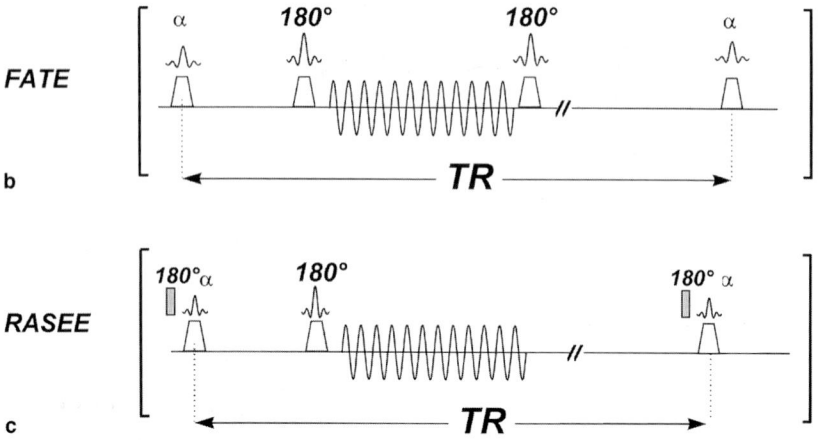

Fig. 20a–c. (continued)

on T1- or T2-weighted images until damage at the cellular level significantly changes the T1 and T2 properties of the tissues involved [71].

A diffusion-weighted image can be obtained using the same SE-EPI sequence structure when a pair of strong diffusion-sensitizing gradients are placed before and after the application of the 180° refocusing pulse (Fig. 21). The strong gradients applied produce an increase in the intravoxel dephasing and loss of signal intensity when diffusion is present. The attenuation factor R which accounts for the signal drop due to diffusion is given by:

$$R = exp\left[-\gamma^2 G_d^2 \delta^2 \left(\Delta - \frac{\delta}{3}\right)D\right] = exp[-bD] \tag{29}$$

where:

$$b = \gamma^2 G_d^2 \delta^2 \left(\Delta - \frac{\delta}{3}\right) \tag{30}$$

where D is given in mm^2/s and b in s/mm^2. A typical diffusion measurement involves repeating the sequence with different gradient strengths and fitting the logarithm of the image intensity [ln(intensity)] vs. b to a straight line whose slope determines D. Figure 22 illustrates the case of a patient with an acute infarction in the brain.

Because diffusion in biological tissues is anisotropic, the collection of a diffusion-weighted image with the diffusion sensitizing direction along any particular axis can yield substantially different results. This is observed in the case shown in Fig. 22. Even within the same subject reproducibility cannot be guaranteed if the orientation of the tissues with respect to the imaging axes changes during scanning. It has been proposed that a diffusion image created by averaging the results from three experiments with the diffusion-sensitizing direction orthogonal to each other can yield more homogeneous and consistent results. Each

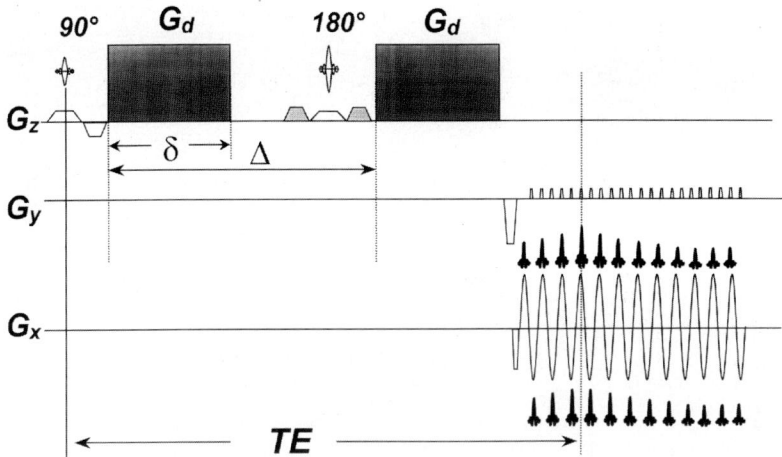

Fig. 21. Simple SE-EPI diffusion-weighted sequence. A pair of diffusion gradients of equal amplitude G_d and timing (equal area) are applied around the 180° RF pulse to dephase and cause signal loss from diffusing protons. Here the diffusion gradients are applied along the slice-select direction

orientation yields one of the diagonal elements of the diffusion tensor matrix (D_{xx}, D_{yy}, D_{zz}), and averaging them eliminates diffusion anisotropy.

In general, an average diffusion-weighted image is formed by collecting three independent scans which are sensitized along the x, y, and z axes, respectively, with the averaged results according to:

$$D_{av} = (\frac{1}{3}[D_{xx} + D_{yy} + D_{zz}]) \tag{31}$$

where D_{av} denotes the averaged or isotropic diffusion coefficient. Nonetheless, EPI has been seen to be sensitive to geometrical distortions and image translation induced by eddy currents generated from the high gradients applied. Thus, averaging the results for a specific b value may not be possible before performing some corrections, especially if a diffusion map is computed from different b values. A more elegant approach has been recently presented that permits the trace of the diffusion tensor to be acquired with a single scan [72]. The principle is readily applicable to EPI and may provide potential advantages. The diffusion-weighted SE-EPI sequence presented in Fig. 23a is one approach that permits a more homogeneous result, but that does not give exactly the average diffusion coefficient D_{av}. Figure 23b illustrates another approach in which the diffusion sensitizing schemes yields the desired result. The diffusion weighting possible with the scheme of Fig. 23b is given by:

$$\ln\left[\frac{S}{S_o}\right] = n_p \gamma^2 G_d^2 \delta^2 \left(\Delta - \frac{\delta}{3}\right) D_{av} \tag{32}$$

where n_p is the number of individual bipolar diffusion gradients used in all axes together prior to the application of the 180° pulse. The respective b value

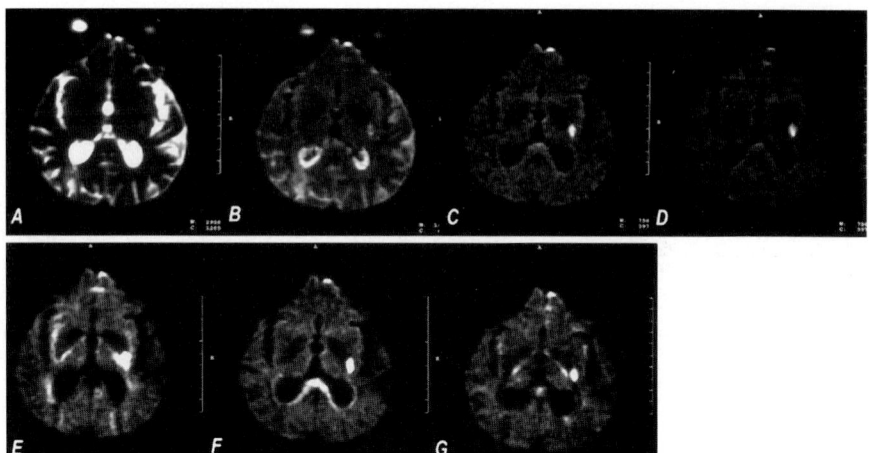

Fig. 22A–G. Acute cerebral infarction. The data are from the same patient as in Fig. 16, showing nonuniform signal intensity in the left globus pallidus, consistent with a stroke that was noted in the low resolution single-shot T2 SE-EPI and better defined on the diffusion-weighted SE-EPI image. **A** T2-weighted single-shot SE-EPI scan with TE = 80 ms. **B,C,D** Diffusion-weighted single-shot SE-EPI image with TE = 100 ms and $b = 310$ s/mm^2 (**B**), $b = 1200$ s/mm^2 (**C**), and $b = 1700$ s/mm^2 (**D**). A region with higher signal intensity than healthy tissue demonstrates decreased diffusion, the region of the infarct. Diffusion anisotropy was also investigated. The diffusion-sensitizing gradients were applied along the x direction (**E**), y direction (**F**), and z direction (**G**) with $b = 1200$ s/mm^2. CSF appears dark because of its high diffusion coefficient while the infarction is bright due to its restricted diffusion. The nerve tracks have directional diffusion and different enhancement depending on the direction of the diffusion gradient. Imaging parameters: 7 mm thick, TE$_{eff}$ = 100 ms, ES = 500 µs, 128×128 matrix, FOV = 300×300 mm (EP readout time = 64 ms, scanner: 38 mT/m, slew rate = 150 mT m^{-1} ms^{-1}). (Courtesy of Steve Warach, Beth Israel Hospital, Boston, USA)

increases linearly with the number of bipolar pulses applied prior to the 180° pulse (off-diagonal elements of the diffusion tensor cancel when all gradient effects are combined). Unfortunately, this technique requires ample gradient power to provide diffusion weighing that is comparable to the diffusion weighting possible by collecting three independent diffusion weighted images for the same TE (the separation Δ between gradients is much smaller than in the traditional case). Average values of b for these schemes that are possible with clinical scanners with a reasonable TE (130–150 ms) vary between 500 and 900 s^2/mm. A short TE is always desirable with the highest diffusion weighting possible to obtain adequate SNR ratio. Values for b that yield good SNR and diffusion weighting for the detection of stroke can be found around $b = 1000$ s/mm^2. Diffusion imaging is treated more in depth in (Chaps. 9, 11, 14).

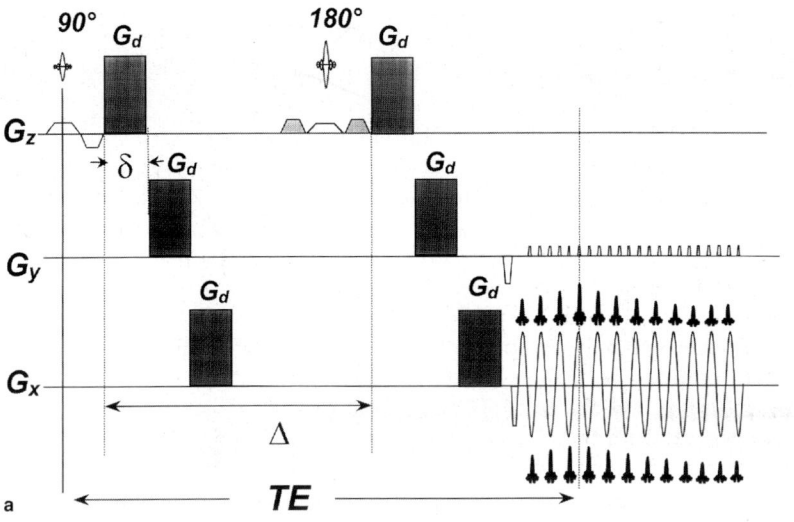

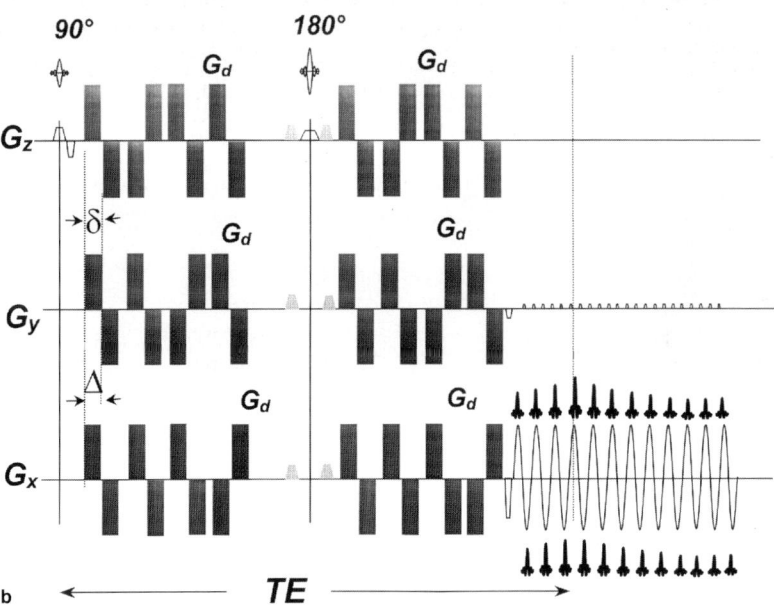

Fig. 23. a Diffusion-weighted SE-EPI scheme that does not show a true average diffusion coefficient, D_{av}, but that helps decrease the anisotropy of the resulting diffusion-weighted images (see Fig. 22e–g). **b** Pulsing diffusion gradient scheme that produces the true average diffusion weighting (eliminates anisotropy and thus directional enhancement). High *b* values using the pulsing diffusion gradient scheme in **b** are extremely difficult to achieve in clinical scanners. G_d, the same gradient amplitude applied along all axes

STEAM Echo-Planar Imaging

T1 weighting

The STEAM sequence applies three RF pulses to form the echo signal through a stimulated echo pathway. The EPI version of STEAM is illustrated in Fig. 24. The first 90° RF pulse tips the longitudinal magnetization (z) to the transverse (xy) plane. The second 90° RF pulse stores half of the magnetization along the z axis while the other half continues to precess in the transverse plane. A SE signal can be acquired immediately after the second 90° pulse and an image generated using a SE-EPI or a GRE-EPI readout. The magnetization stored along z axis during the second RF pulse maintains an imprint of the phase that the spins had and relaxes according to T1 instead of T2. The storage time refers to the interval between the second and third RF pulses and permits to control the T1 weighting that is generated on the MR signal after the third 90° RF pulse. The third 90° RF pulse brings the longitudinal magnetization that was stored back during the second RF pulse to the transverse plane where it is subsequently sampled with the EPI readout module [70, 73].

A STEAM image is T1-weighted although not in the same fashion as in a conventional T1-weighted scans as higher signal is present for tissue with longer T1. Short T1 components, such as fat, can be eliminated from the image effectively

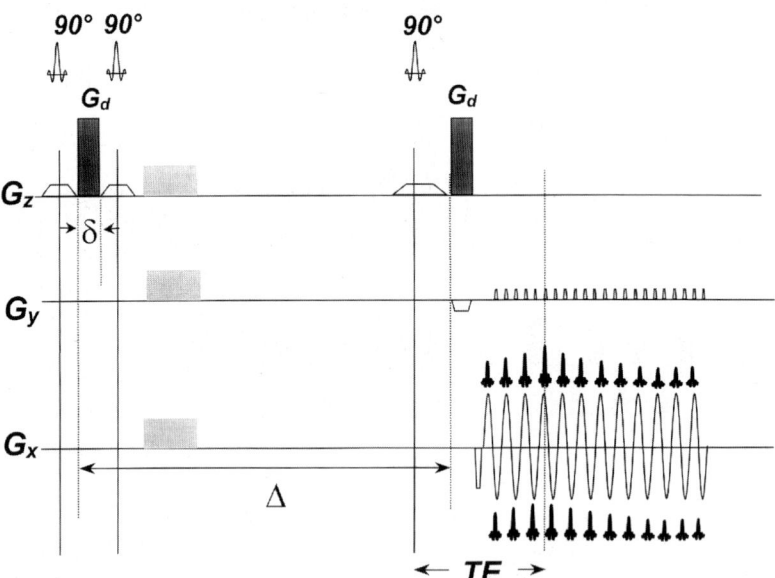

Fig. 24. STEAM-EPI sequence. A pair of diffusion-sensitizing gradients can be applied along either imaging axis to produce the diffusion weighting. STEAM-EPI is advantageous for tissues with long T1 and short T2 as the signal decay is related to T1 and not T2, thus permitting longer diffusion times and larger b values. G_d, the diffusion gradient applied

by choosing a longer storage time. Fat saturation is not necessary when the storage time is about three times the T1 of fat [74], approximately 0.8 s.

Diffusion Weighting

The addition of a diffusion-sensitizing gradient between the first and second RF pulses and another between the third and the EPI readout permits a diffusion-weighted image to be obtained. A limitation of diffusion-weighted SE sequences with long TE is that T2 decay can compromise the SNR in the resulting image. The use of a SE sequence is even more restrictive when short T2 tissues have small diffusion values, which is unfortunately the case with most biological tissues. The use of stimulated echoes for diffusion studies has been proposed [75, 76] to avoid this. These have advantages when working with systems in which T1>T2, a condition that is true for many tissues in the body. This is because the magnetization relaxes with T1 rather than T2 during the storage interval of the STEAM sequence. However, with STEAM only half the original magnetization can be recovered, and hence there is no major advantage in SNR over SE sequences. The STEAM implementation is desirable when time-dependent diffusion is of interest. Because the storage time controls D, a greater diffusion weighting is possible by increasing the storage time. Figure 25 depicts

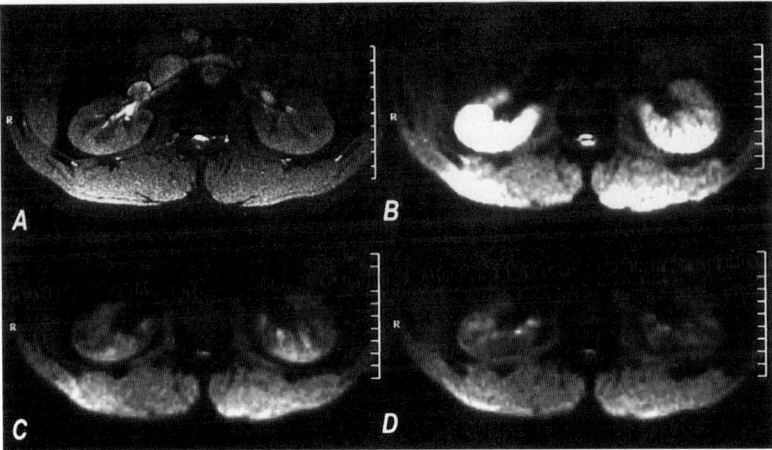

Fig. 25A–D. Anisotropic diffusion in the kidney demonstrated with STEAM-EPI. The diffusion-sensitizing gradient was varied along different axes of the kidney to observe the diffusion anisotropy. **A** Anatomical image using a T1-weighted, fat-suppressed, breath-hold 2D FLASH. **B** Axial slice STEAM-EPI without a diffusion sensitization gradient. **C** Diffusion sensitization in the plane of the renal artery with b of approximately 80 s/mm^2 (heart rate dependent). **D** Diffusion sensitization perpendicular to the plane of section. Four diffusion-weighted images were acquired per breath-hold interval with four different b values and with cardiac triggering (using the RR interval as the storage time). The diffusion images shown are the result of averaging three breath-holds. Imaging parameters: 8 mm thick, TE = 18 ms, ES = 500 µs, 64×128 matrix, FOV = 150×300 mm (EP readout time = 32 ms, scanner: 38 mT/m, slew rate = 150 mT m^{-1} ms^{-1}). (Courtesy of Markus Muller, Inselspital, Bern, Switzerland)

an example demonstrating anisotropic diffusion in the kidneys using STEAM-EPI.

General comments on diffusion weighted EPI

Although the EPI readout permits short image encoding times (32–64 ms), a diffusion-weighted EPI sequence would still be very sensitive to bulk motion from motion occurring between the excitation and the readout time. This contemplates the case of tissue pulsation because of nearby vascular structures and pressure changes (such as the left lobe of the liver being affected by the heart motion). A diffusion-weighted SE-EPI sequence can be very sensitive and complete loss of signal can occur depending on the degree of motion. A STEAM excitation can be in many instances more effective in eliminating bulk motion effects. To reduce the signal attenuation from pulsation a STEAM-EPI sequence can be cardiac triggered. The delay in the cardiac cycle is maintained constant between the R wave and the first RF and the third RF pulses. To store the magnetization quickly along z, the first and second 90° RF pulses can be made nonselective and the third slice selective so that the signal of a particular section is monitored.

Diffusion-weighted STEAM-EPI finds applications such as in breath-hold diffusion-weighted imaging in the heart [77]. Assuming that the heart remains in a similar position between successive heartbeats, the application of the two diffusion-sensitizing gradient pulses can be effective. If small linear translations are present, a linear phase would develop but it would not cancel the signal and interfere with the diffusion weighting. Since the diffusion weighting depends on the separation between the diffusion gradient pulses, the weighting would vary as a function of the subject's momentary heart rate. Preliminary results suggest diffusional anisotropy within the myocardium. It is obviously a major technical challenge to overcome motion artifacts and further studies were suggested to assess the utility of such technique. As in the brain, an infarct in the heart's myocardium may be distinguished from adjacent structures by a decrease in the diffusion coefficient in the infarct (increase in signal intensity).

Using a similar diffusion-gradient scheme as shown in Fig. 23 to make the diffusion-weighted STEAM-EPI image proportional to the average diffusion coefficient is not advantageous here. The reason is that the storage time cannot be used as in the conventional scheme because Δ is defined as the distance between the two gradient of each bipolar pair and not the storage time (compare Figs. 23, 24).

Magnetization Prepared GRE-EPI and SE-EPI

To provide additional T1 weighting to the otherwise proton density, T2*- or T2-weighted images collected with single-shot GRE-EPI or SE-EPI sequences, a magnetization-preparation (MP) period can be included prior to the EPI readout (Fig. 26). As discussed above, to produce a T1 image a 90° pulse can be applied at an interval of TR prior to imaging (saturation recovery). This scheme is not necessary when an imaging section is excited several times, such as in 3D-EPI or averaging multiple excitations.

Complete tissue suppression is possible using an inversion RF pulse for spin preparation prior to image readout [78]. The TI required to null a tissue depends on T1 and is given by T1 ln2. Fatty tissues with their short T1 can be suppressed with a short TI such as performed routinely in short tau inversion recovery (STIR) imaging. An example in the abdomen is demonstrated in Fig. 27 using IR SE-EPI. IR SE-EPI can be used for cardiac perfusion studies (Fig. 28), in which case the signal intensity of perfused myocardium increases after contrast uptake. IR SE-EPI, as opposed to IR GRE-EPI, is advantageous in this particular case because blood signal in the cardiac chambers can be eliminated at any time even during the first pass of the contrast agent, and geometric distortions with SE-EPI readouts are smaller than that for GRE-EPI readouts (especially if an inner volume SE-EPI is used in conjunction with a rectangular FOV).

A particular sequence of interest using an inversion pulse is FLAIR [79, 80]. The concept behind FLAIR is to attenuate the signal of CSF so that when a long TE is selected, lesions characterized by long T2 but shorter T1 than CSF can appear brighter than surrounding white and gray matter in the brain. The FLAIR sequence has been demonstrated to be highly sensitive in detecting lesions in the white matter, such as multiple sclerosis plaques. Small lesions are depicted better because partial volume artifacts from bright CSF are reduced

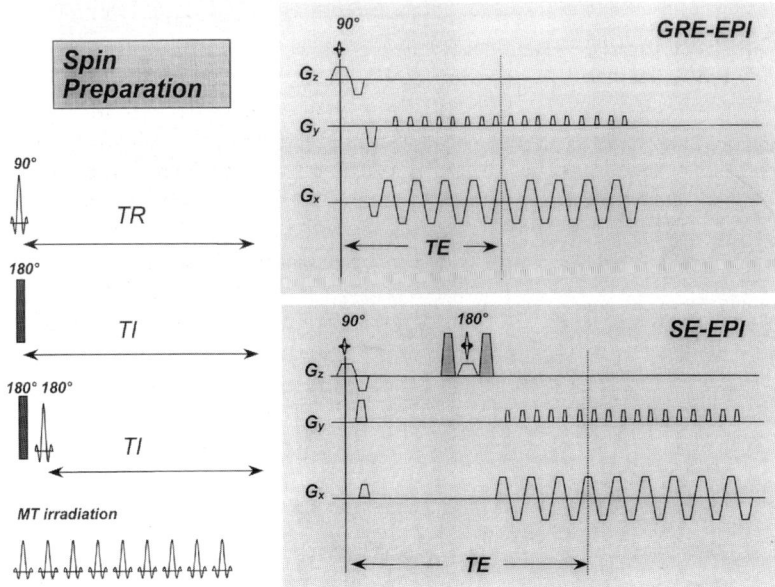

Fig. 26. MP GRE-EPI, SE-EPI sequence. Prior to reading out the MR signal several magnetization preparations can be used, such as a saturation pulse, a selective or a nonselective inversion pulse, a black-blood preparation (inversion-reinversion of the slice and choosing TI to null out the blood signal) or a series of magnetization transfer (MT) pulses. Other magnetization preparations are possible

Fig. 27. IR SE-EPI in the abdomen. Weak diffusion gradients ($b<5$ s/mm^2) are applied to minimize the blood signal of the liver vessels. TI is adjusted to suppress the fat signal. Imaging parameters: 7 mm thick, $TE_{eff} = 59$ ms, $TI = 140$ ms, $ES = 600$ μs, 96×128 matrix, FOV = 262×350 mm, (EP readout time = 57.6 ms, scanner: 25 mT/m, slew rate = 80 mTm^{-1}ms^{-1}), phased-array body coil used for signal reception, (Courtesy of Dr. J. Gaa, University of Mannheim, Germany)

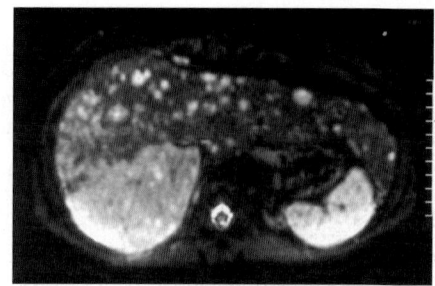

Fig. 28. Breath-hold perfusion study in the heart at a single slice location using the inner volume excitation concept with an IR SE-EPI and a bolus injection of 20 ml Gd-DTPA. Large dephasing gradients were applied along the slice selection about the 180° refocusing pulse reduces the signal from blood. The TI is chosen to reduce the signal from myocardium. Several slices can be acquired if a saturation recovery (a 90° pulse instead) is applied to saturate the imaging slice. Imaging parameters: 6 mm thick, $TE_{eff} = 28$ ms, $ES = 500$ μs, 64×128 matrix, FOV = 190×380 mm (EP readout time = 32 ms, scanner: 38 mT/m, slew rate = 150 mT m^{-1} ms^{-1}), body coil was used for signal reception (Courtesy of Dr. R. Edelman, Beth Israel Hospital, Boston, USA)

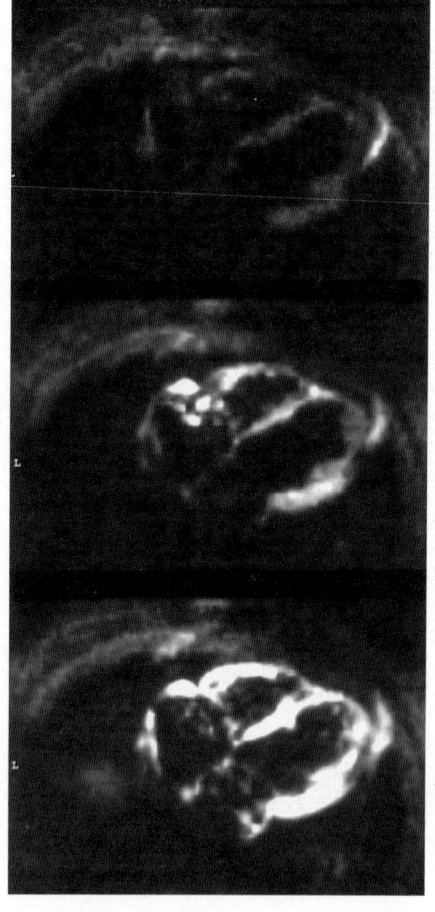

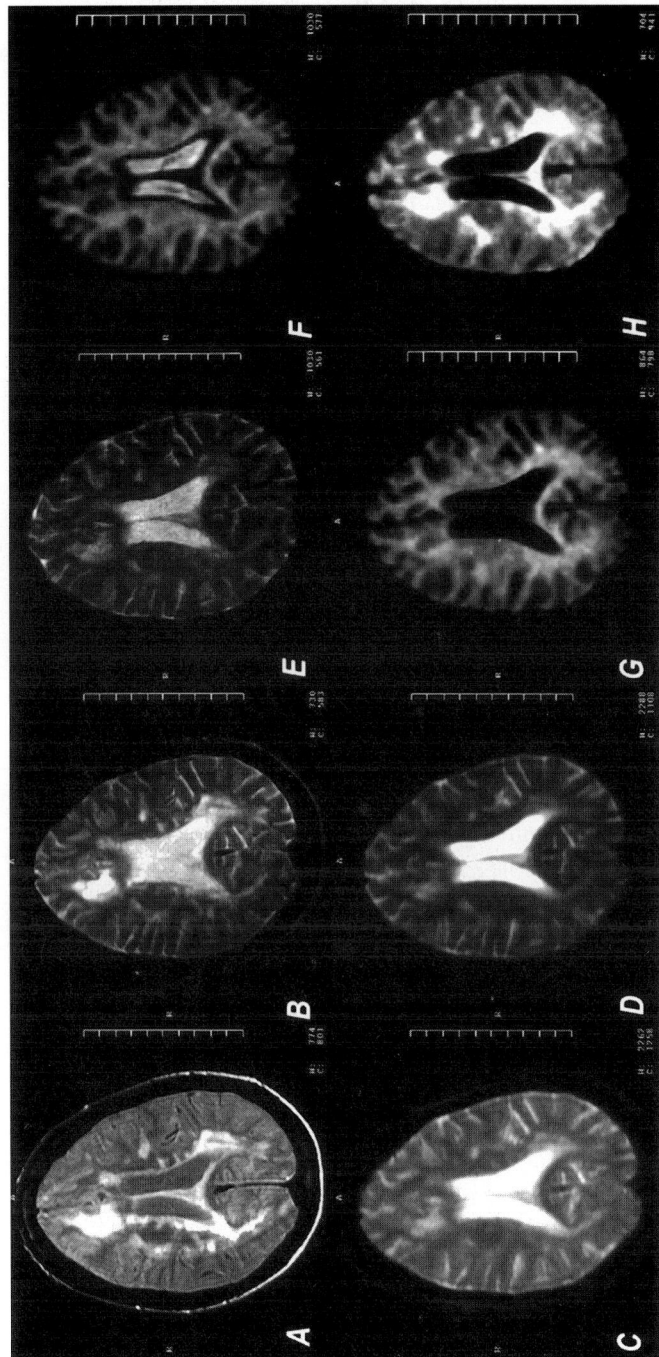

Fig. 29A–H. IR SE-EPI in the brain. Sequence comparison in a patient with multiple sclerosis. Proton density (**A**) and T2-weighted (**B**) SE image with TR = 2400 ms and TE = 15 ms and TE = 80 ms, respectively, 5-mm slices, scan time 7 min 44 s for a 192×256 matrix, FOV = 192×256 mm. **C** Single-shot proton density weighted GRE-EPI image with a 128×128 matrix, FOV = 25 cm, TE = 18 ms, scan time 80 ms per slice. **D** Single-shot T2-weighted SE-EPI with a 128×128 matrix, FOV = 25 cm, TE = 80 ms, scan time 120 ms per slice. **E** High-resolution single-shot T2-weighted EPI with a 192×256 matrix, TE = 80 ms. **F** IR SE-EPI with TI = 800 ms. **G** TI = 1500 ms. **H** TI = 2200 ms. Note that with long TI the signal from CSF is nulled, and multiple sclerosis are enhanced. General EPI readout parameters: TE = 50 ms, ES = 500 μs, 128×128 matrix, FOV = 250×250 mm (EP readout time = 64 ms, scanner: 38 mT/m, slew rate = 150 mT/m m^{-1} ms^{-1}). **E** ES = 800 μs, 192×256 matrix, FOV = 230×270 mm (readout time per slice = 170 ms, scanner: 38 mT/m, slew rate = 150 mT/m m^{-1} ms^{-1})

(Fig. 29). The TI for CSF is in the order of 2.3 s when TR is infinity (shorter TI with finite TR, as in conventional imaging). Because of the long TI the imaging time can be optimized by first applying all the RF pulses needed to invert the signal on each slice and later all the SE-EPI readouts. The spacing between inversion pulses is determined by the length of the SE-EPI readout. The total acquisition time is approximately 2 TI for this scheme. The number of sections possible is dictated by TI and the length of the EPI readout (more slices with shorter EPI readouts). A SE-EPI rather than GRE-EPI is used because of the long TE necessary to reduce the brain signal.

Another possibility for enhancing lesions in the nervous system is to use magnetization transfer (MT) irradiation prior to imaging in conjunction with a T1-weighted scan. A long MT irradiation is applied prior to the acquisition to stabilize the MT effects. After the MT preparation a T1-weighted GRE-EPI or SE-EPI scan can be acquired (using two 90° pulses separated by TR, as discussed above). Because a dead time exists between the two 90° pulses, the MT contrast can be maintained by applying additional MT irradiation between these RF pulses. This strategy also permits the MT contrast to be maintained for all other slices that may be collected for the study.

Multicontrast Single-Shot EPI Sequences

There is an unlimited number of combinations using RF excitations and EPI readouts to produce images with different tissue contrasts. Such combinations make it possible to collect proton density, T1, T2, T2*, diffusion, or MT weighted images rapidly and making it possible to use tissue segmentation programs based on their MR properties for further study. This is more efficient with EPI than for conventional readouts because misregistration artifacts from bulk motion effects are virtually eliminated.

In many cases the matrix size may be limited to maintain the desired contrast and image output. For instance, a multiecho SE scan can be implemented using an EPI readout between 180° RF pulses to obtain images with increased T2 weighting and to generate a rapid T2 map. In this case the matrix size determines the separation between the 180° pulses and influences the effective TE for each of the images collected. A simple way to generate a T2* map is to use a STEAM sequence in which two echoes are encoded after the third RF excitation, one generating an image with the center of k-space collected when the stimulated echo occurs and another at a later time.

The combination of images weighted by proton density, T2, and T1 is possible in a single-shot. This can be performed by using the first 90° pulse to collect a proton density weighted scan using either a short TE gradient echo or a spin echo after the application a 180° pulse. A T2-weighted image can then be acquired using an additional 180° pulse. Because the slice has been already excited, the application of a 90° pulse can then lead to the collection of a T1-weighted image, with an effective TR determined by the distance set between the two 90° pulses. This acquisition strategy is very efficient because the collection of a T1-weighted image by itself requires the application of a 90° pulse a TR prior to image acquisition. Although this set of images can be acquired similarly with a conventional SE technique, EPI is more advantageous in that the proton density and T2-weighted images do not suffer from T1 contamination.

A variant on this scheme that permits the collection of an IR image instead is by using a partial flip angle excitation. For example, with a 45° excitation $\sqrt{\frac{2}{2}}$ of the initial longitudinal magnetization remains unaffected while $\sqrt{\frac{2}{2}}$ is tilted onto the transverse plane, ready to generate a proton density image and a T2-weighted image. The longitudinal magnetization that remains untouched is inverted by the 180° pulse, permitting the acquisition of an IR T1-weighted image. Another variant is a double-echo acquisition combining a spin echo and a stimulated echo using a STEAM-EPI sequence [81]. The first echo may be acquired with proton density or T2 weighting after the second RF excitation while a T1-weighted contrast can be obtained by changing the storage time between the second and third 90° pulses. Diffusion sensitizing gradient can be added after each RF excitation to form two diffusion-weighted images. A low b value can be imprinted on the SE image while a large b value on the stimulated echo by lengthening the storage time. It must be remembered, however, that STEAM provides only half the signal available for each image and the SNR may be limited.

Three-Dimensional Techniques

All the techniques described above can be applied in a 3D mode by incorporating an additional phase-encoding table along the slice-select direction, consequently repeating the experiment with a finite TR [82]. Because SE-EPI is too slow in a 3D modality, the use of 3D is beneficial for acquisition regimes such as in conventional FLASH and FISP techniques to generate either T1- or T1/T2-weighted images quickly. When TR is long, multiple slabs can be acquired to fill in the time gaps between TR and therefore optimize coverage as well as SNR [83]. This makes it possible to collect SE data in a 3D format with large volume coverage with efficient data collection times.

Echo-Volume Imaging

Echo-volume imaging (EVI), initially proposed by Mansfield, has recently been implemented for its potential role in functional imaging studies [84, 85]. The idea of EVI is a direct extension of EPI to 3D imaging using a single RF excitation. The sequence structure incorporates the oscillatory EP readout along the frequency-encoding and phase-encoding axes while for the slice-select phase encoding a constant gradient is applied during the complete readout (or small blips) so that the complete 3D data is encoded. Restrictions in the maximum dB/dt possible have made it possible to encode only low resolution volumes, for example, eight slices with a 64×64 imaging matrix in approximately 120 ms (higher speeds are possible using local gradient coils). Figure 30 illustrates EVI for a constant gradient slice-select phase-encoding. The blipped slice-select

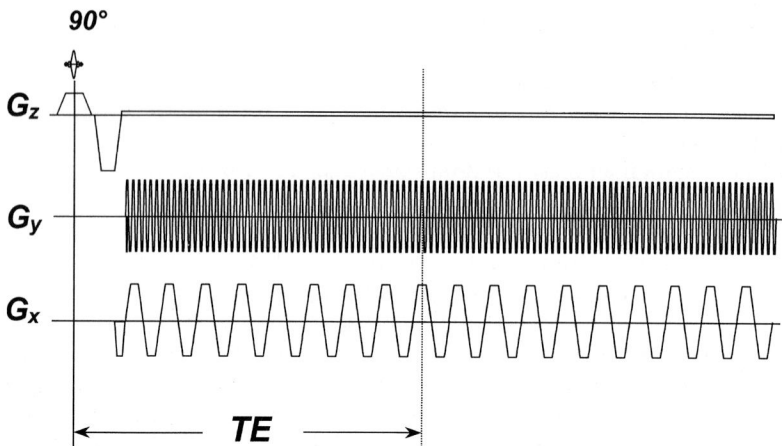

Fig. 30. EVI sequence diagram. A complete 3D data set can be encoded in a single shot with T2* weighting. The sequence can be used mainly for functional MRI studies of brain activation with high temporal resolution and complete volume coverage

phase-encoding direction is possible, but the inaccuracy in applying very short blips of high amplitude can result in ringing and crosstalk between the reconstructed slices.

Because the data are collected under a T2* envelope, a modification has been developed that incorporates multiple 180° refocusing pulses, similar to GRASE and fast SE sequences [86] (see Chaps. 19, 20). This modification permits EVI with scanners with less specialized gradient hardware, as it permits collection of the decaying signal under a T2 rather than a T2*envelope. Between each 180° pulse several in-plane phase-encoding steps are collected for a single phase encoding along the slice-select direction.

The value of EVI in functional imaging studies of the brain focuses on the basic idea that all the slices generated would have the same phase behavior and would eliminate any time delays when evaluating a signal variation occurring throughout the entire volume.

Echo-Planar Spectroscopic Imaging

Spatial and spectral data can be encoded with EPI and produce images of different metabolite components within the proton spectra in short imaging times [87, 88]. Similarly as in 2D spectroscopy, spectral encoding can be carried out with 2D or 3D EPI scans by incorporating an incremental time element between the RF excitation and the EPI readout that is varied incrementally for each shot. Spectral information is then reconstructed by performing a Fourier transformation along the spectral direction to resolve images of the different metabolites. Spectral width and resolution are dictated by the size of the time increments (dwell time) and the number of points sampled. This method has been also employed in the context of a 3D sequence to observe the metabolites in any desired orientation in approximately 30 min with a limited number of sections (4D imaging, three spatial and one spectral dimension) [89]. Diffusion-encoding gradients have also been incorporated to observe the diffusivity of the different metabolites [90].

Applications of Multishot 2D and 3D Echo-Planar Imaging

There are many applications in which single-shot EPI provides a major advantages over multishot EPI techniques. These are related particularly to protocols in which speed (time resolution) is more important than spatial resolution: diffusion, perfusion studies and T2*-weighted images for functional imaging studies, among others. However, higher spatial resolution, reduced geometrical distortions, and reduced signal loss from magnetic susceptibility may be more important clinically in certain applications while keeping scan time short. Additionally, with multishot EPI the demands on gradient performance are significantly reduced, making it more accessible to more conventional MRI scanners.

2D Multishot GRE-EPI and SE-EPI Scans

After a steady-state regime has been established (to ensure that the MR signal is the same for each excitation of the spin system to avoid ghosting artifacts; see "Interleaved"), the constant readout gradient in any conventional GRE or SE technique can be replaced by a blipped interleaved segmented GRE-EPI readout (see Fig. 9). A segmented SE-EPI sequence is presented in Fig. 31. The number of shots necessary to collect the image, N_{shots}, depends on the number of lines selected, N_y, and the number of echoes encoded per shot, N_e:

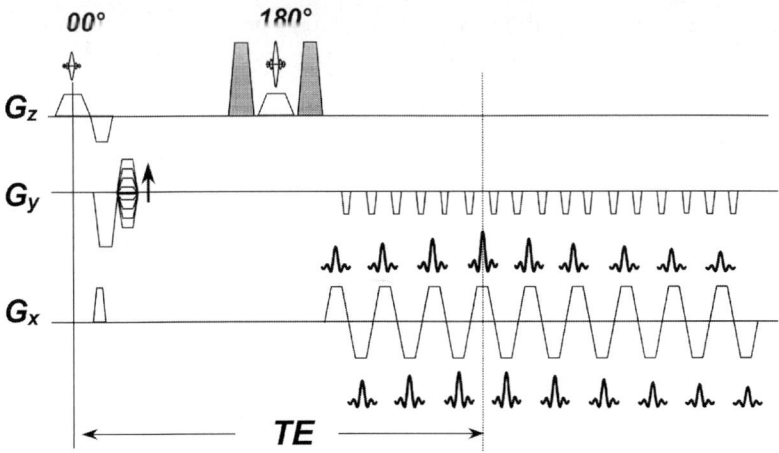

Fig. 31. Multishot segmented interleaved SE-EPI sequence

$$N_{shots} = \frac{N_y}{N_e} \tag{33}$$

The tissue contrast is similar to that of the more conventional GRE and SE techniques, and sequence design can make use of confirmed facts from conventional techniques in routine diagnosis. The major advantages of segmented EPI techniques are robustness and substantially reduced imaging time, permitting breath-hold imaging in the abdomen with T1 or T2 weighting without the MT effects and RF power deposition that fast SE scans induce (see Chap. 19, 20). Figures 32 and 33 present examples in the brain and abdomen, respectively.

Segmented EPI techniques can be made as robust as necessary and perform reliably with respect to image artifacts related to field inhomogeneities or motion. To obtain unartifacted images under any imaging condition the echo

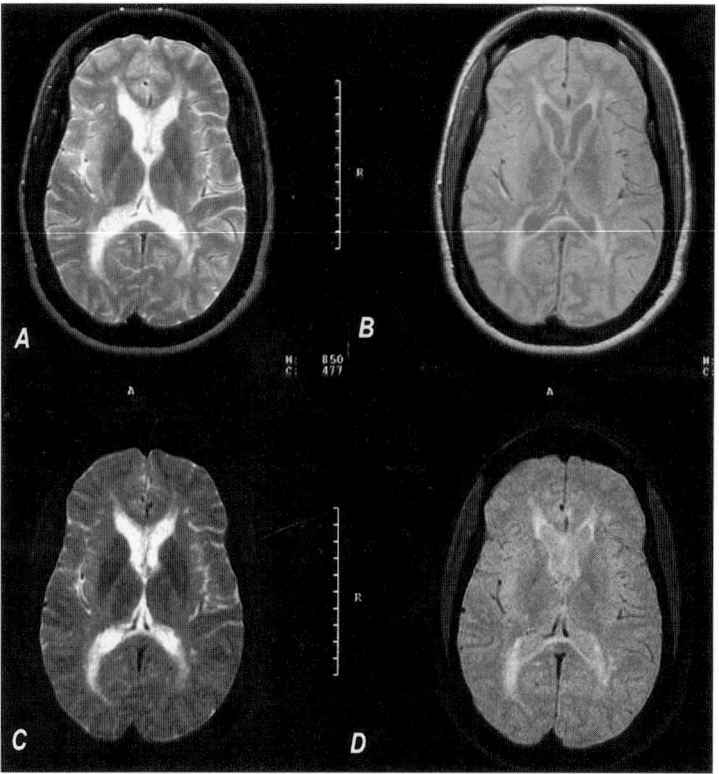

Fig. 32A–D. Comparison between conventional SE and multishot SE-EPI scans on a patient with multiple sclerosis lesions. T2-weighted (**A**) and proton density (**B**) weighted conventional SE image. **C,D** Corresponding multishot T2-weighted and proton density weighted SE-EPI scans. Imaging parameters: **A,B** TR = 2400/TE = 80/15 ms, respectively, 5-mm thick, 192×256 matrix, FOV = 192×256 mm, scan time 7 min 44 s; **C,D** 5 mm thick, TR = 2400/TE = 80/28 ms, ES = 800 μs, 28 echoes per shot, 196×256 matrix, FOV = 256×256 mm, total acquisition time 19 s (EP readout time = 22.4 ms, scanner: 38 mT/m, slew rate = 150 mT m^{-1} ms^{-1})

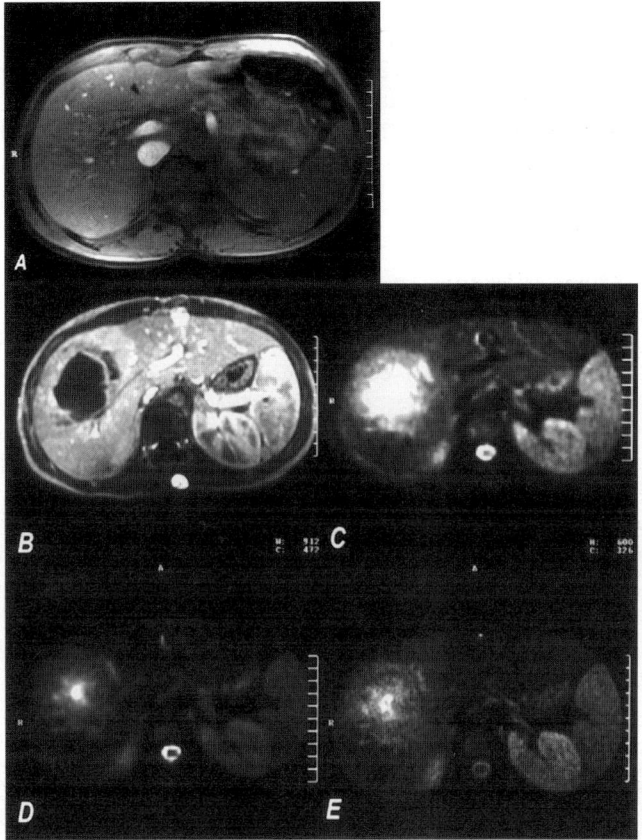

Fig. 33A–E. T1-weighted multishot GRE-EPI in the abdomen. **A** Comparison with the single-shot GRE-EPI scan demonstrated in Fig. 13. One slice from 15 acquired with a fat suppressed T1-weighted multishot GRE-EPI sequence using TR/TE/α = 250/5 ms/90°. A 150×256 matrix was encoded with FOV = 250×240 mm, 6 mm thickness, six echoes per RF excitation ES = 1280 μs (970 Hz/pixel readout bandwidth, EP readout time = 7.68 ms, scanner: 25 mT/m, slew rate = 80 mT m^{-1} ms^{-1}). The images were acquired in a 6-s breath-hold using a body phased array coil. **B** Patient presenting a tumor in the liver scanned with a breath-hold T1-weighted FLASH sequence after administration of Gd-DTPA (TR/TE/α = 110/4.5 ms/80° and a 128×256 matrix). **C** Single-shot SE-EPI image with TE = 50 ms, a 128×128 matrix, one of 20 sections acquired in approximately 3 s. **D** Single-shot SE-EPI with TE = 80 ms. **E** Multishot SE-EPI acquisition with TR/TE = 2000/80 ms, 28 echoes per shot, 252×256 matrix, FOV = 350×350 mm (breath-hold of 20 s). Motion degradation from respiration can be eliminated for all the techniques. **B–E** acquired in the body coil section (EP readout time = 64 ms, multishot EP readout: 22.4 ms, scanner: 38 mT/m, slew rate = 150 mT m^{-1} ms^{-1})

shifting scheme should be implemented (see "Interleaved," Fig. 10). Although some blurring may be present, ghosting from discontinuities in the phase and amplitude of the MR signal between k-space segments can be reduced dramatically. Otherwise, results may be discouraging in many regions of the body, especially in the upper abdomen, close to the diaphragm/lung interface, and at the base of the skull.

Obtaining overall magnetic field homogeneity through shimming becomes more important with longer ES (to provide the necessary resolution and SNR). Shimming is also essential for good fat suppression to eliminate the large chemical shifts that are still present along the phase-encoding direction with lower readout bandwidths. In the presence of flow and pulsatile motion, segmented EPI scans suffer from ghosting. (Motion and flow effects in EPI are discussed in Chap. 8.)

Magnetization-Prepared Multishot 3D GRE-EPI

Short TRs are inevitable for breath-hold 3D scans when a large number of sections and a reduced number of echoes per interleaf are desired to minimize both the sensitivity to flow and susceptibility artifacts. Additionally, the inclusion of fat saturation, presaturation bands, or MT pulses during each TR to improve tissue and flow contrast or suppress unwanted tissues could reduce scanning efficiency by a factor of ½. In these cases magnetization-prepared (MP) acquisitions can provide a greater flexibility for improving contrast by sharing the desired contrast encoded during a magnetization-preparation stage between many lines of k-space. The contrast characteristics and properties of MP techniques have been validated for T1- and T2-weighted imaging in the past with turboFLASH sequences [91, 92]. The extension to segmented EPI provides the potential to encode more data with the same magnetization preparation.

Magnetization preparation could be applied to 2D segmented EPI scans with short TR, but the results would demonstrate ghosting artifacts arising from the dramatic signal changes that can occur during the subsequent RF excitations after the preparation. This can be very pronounced when using an interleaved EPI trajectory (see "Interleaved"). The use of MP acquisitions with short TR multishot EPI 2D scans is therefore not advised; MP scans are more suitable for 3D data collection. More freedom to design a k-space trajectory is possible so that the signal evolution smoothly changes across both phase-encoding directions [93].

A diagram of a multishot 3D MP GRE-EPI acquisition scheme is depicted in Fig. 34. A magnetization-preparation stage precedes the data collection window and any magnetization preparation may be incorporated to encode the necessary contrast. This is necessary because no contrast develops for short TR/TE scans when a k-space segment is collected with a small number of RF excitations closely spaced and a long longitudinal magnetization recovery period is used prior to scanning the next k-space segment. In Fig. 34 TR has been redefined as the time necessary to encode several k-space lines, that is, the time required for magnetization preparation and data acquisition including the longitudinal magnetization recovery. The time between RF excitations has been defined as the excitation spacing (IS).

Many magnetization-preparation schemes can be proposed. For example, T2 weighting can be imprinted by using a nonselectively driven equilibrium scheme [94]. Using the 3D segmented EPI readout, volumetric coverage in the heart is possible in a single breath-hold with improved contrast between blood and mus-

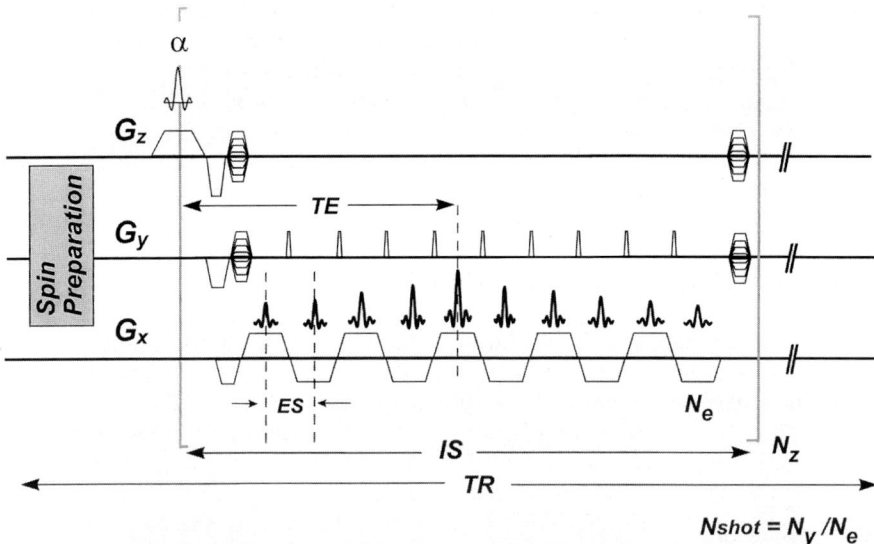

Fig. 34. MP 3D GRE-EPI. Magnetization preparation is applied to encode a specific contrast prior to the EP readout module. A series of RF pulses, separated by an inter-RF spacing (*IS*), is applied to encode all the N_z section-select phase-encoding steps. For each RF excitation an EP readout generates several echoes which are phase encoded independently along the in-plane phase-encoding direction using an interleaved trajectory. TR is defined as the total time necessary per shot. N_y, Number of in-plane phase-encoding lines; N_z, number of sections; N_e, number of echoes; $N_{shot} = N_y/N_e$, number of shots

cle. This is illustrated in Fig. 35, demonstrating a multiplanar reformat along the short and long axes of the heart with good contrast between myocardium and the blood pool. Similarly, MT irradiation can be used to suppress the signal from tissues with water-bound molecules (e.g., to enhance the contrast between blood and muscle). This has been used to suppress the cardiac muscle with the possible advantage that if blood would be carrying an intravascular contrast agent to enhance its T1 relaxation, signal loss from a possible short blood T2 would not affect the MT preparation as compared to the T2 preparation scheme. Figure 36 depicts a reconstruction of the left descending coronary artery using this type of acquisition.

Using a STEAM preparation it is possible to imprint T1 weighting, with the additional advantage that the sensitivity to motion can be adjusted to help eliminate the signal from moving blood, such as illustrated in Fig. 37. Fig. 37 demonstrates several slices from a volume collected in a single breath-hold in the heart during mid-late diastole. Additionally, the MP can consist only of a selective or nonselective inversion pulse to obtain T1 weighting. A proton density weighted scan can be produced by not preparing the magnetization.

Following the magnetization-preparation period all the 3D section-select phase-encoding steps (partitions, N_z) are collected. A section-select encoding is carried out on each RF when the segmentation is performed along the in-plane phase-encoding direction (the contrary when segmentation is performed

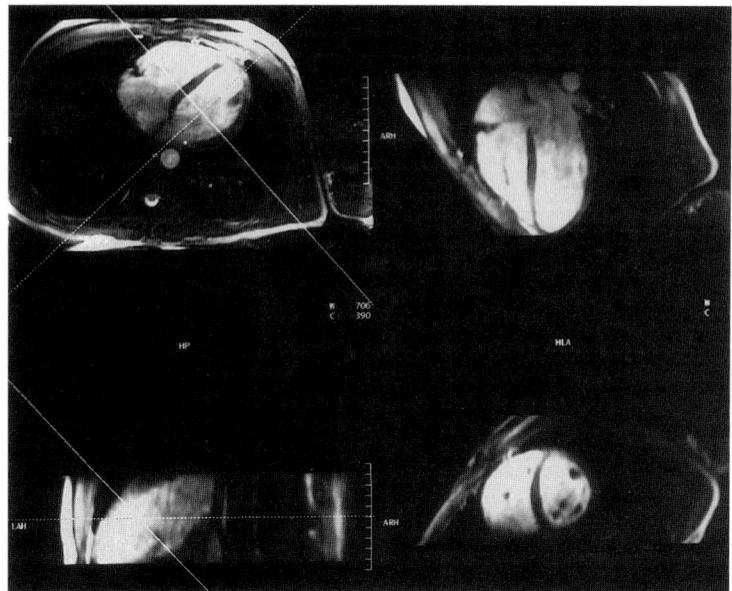

Fig. 35. T2 MP volume collected in a single breath-hold in the heart. Multiplanar reconstructions along both long axes and the short-axis views. The effective TE for the T2-weighted preparation was 80 ms. A trigger delay of 550 ms was selected from the QRS complex, encoding 20 sections with a 126×256 matrix, FOV = 250×340 mm, 6 echoes per RF excitation, IS/TE/α = 8.2/3.4 ms/ 13°, ES = 1100 µs (1090 Hz/pixel readout bandwidth) and a sequential partition encoding. The images were acquired in 26 s with a body phased array coil. (EP readout time = 6.6 ms, readout time per cardiac cycle = 164 ms, scanner: 38 mT/m, slew rate = 150 mT m^{-1} ms^{-1})

along the slice-select phase-encoding direction). In Fig. 34 the echoes are mapped in k-space along the in-plane phase-encoding direction using the interleaved k-space trajectory as illustrated in Fig. 9b [33, 95]. Similarly, the number of shots, N_{shots}, necessary to complete the scan is determined by N_y/N_e, the ratio between the number of lines collected along the in-plane phase-encoding direction and the number of echoes acquired during the interval IS.

3D Multishot SE-EPI

A 3D multishot SE-EPI scan (Fig. 38) can be useful whenever the T2 relaxation of the tissues of interest is long. The sequence can be viewed as an extension of the rapid acquisition with relaxation enhancement (RARE) technique [96] or the more popular fast SE scans [97, 98] using a series of 180° pulses after the initial 90° excitation to encode the data. The constant readout between the 180° pulses used in the RARE and fast SE scans is replaced by the EPI oscillatory gradient waveform to collect several lines.

Similarly as in the MP 3D segmented EPI sequence, each 180° pulse a single section-select phase-encoding step is applied. The echoes are mapped along the in-plane phase-encoding direction using the interleaved k-space trajectory.

The effective TE, defined by the time interval between the 90° RF excitation and the spin echo formed during the center partition, is $IS \cdot N_z/2$, where IS denotes the time between the 180° pulses and N_z the number of sections encoded. Following the same definition for TR as in the previous section and denoting N_y as the number of in-plane phase-encoding lines, the imaging time is determined by the number of shots necessary to encode all the in-plane phase-encoding lines with N_e echoes acquired between the 180° pulses, that is, $TR \cdot N_y/N_e$. This technique has been used to collect 3D MR cholangiograms (Fig. 39), with the possibility of postprocessing using MPR and MIP [99].

Fig. 36. 3D rendering of the right demonstrates (*RCA*), left main (*LM*), and the left descending coronary (*LAD*) arteries. A MT preparation was used in conjunction with an intravascular contrast agent to acquire the complete heart volume in a single breath-hold. A 500-ms MT preparation preceded the data collection on every heartbeat. A 120-mm volume was covered with 56 sections (90 reconstructed) using IS/TE/α = 5.55/1.4 ms/incremental flip angle, 4 echoes per RF excitation with partial Fourier encoding, ES = 1000 µs (1280 Hz/pixel readout bandwidth), a 96×256 matrix, FOV = 180×340 mm, centric partition encoding. The images were acquired in 22 s with a body phased array coil (EP readout time = 4 ms, readout time per cardiac cycle = 155 ms, scanner: 25 mT/m, slew rate = 80 mT m^{-1} ms^{-1})

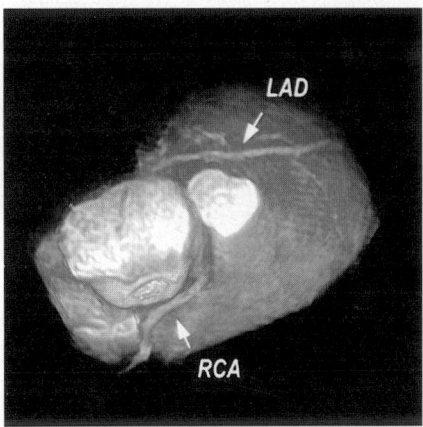

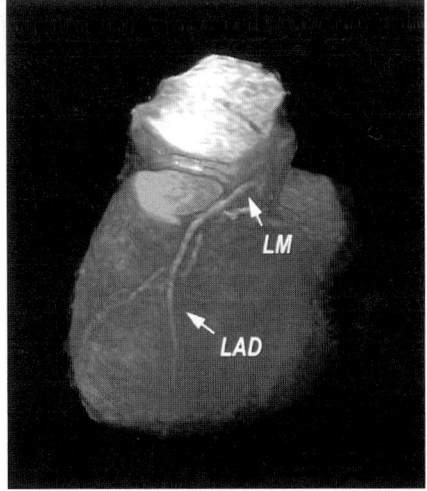

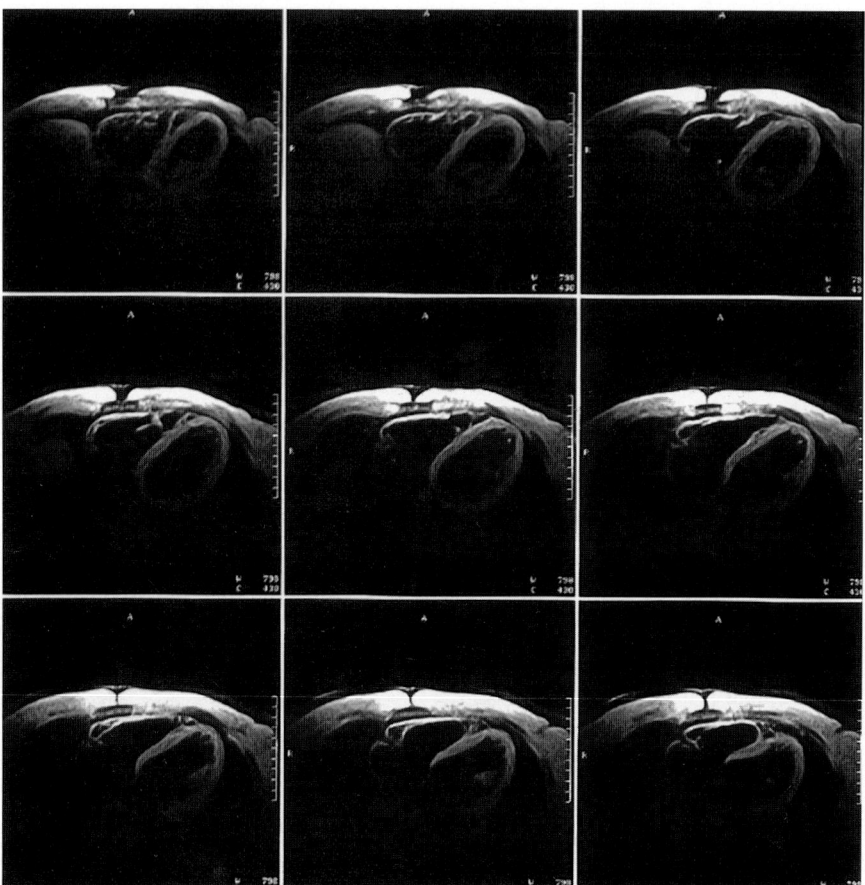

Fig. 37. STEAM 3D multishot EPI in the heart acquired during diastole. Nine adjacent slices from a 16-section 3D data set are displayed. The STEAM preparation consisted of two nonselective 500 µs long 90° RF pulses separated by a 500-µs dephasing gradient and a 15-ms storage time during which a chemical shift fat saturation pulse was applied prior to reading the signal. A trigger delay of 650 ms was selected from the QRS complex, encoding a 126×256 matrix, FOV = 250×340 mm with IS/TE/α = 8.2/3.4 ms/13°, 6 echoes per RF excitation, ES = 1100 µs (1090 Hz/pixel readout bandwidth) and a sequential partition encoding. The images were acquired in 23 s with a body phased array coil (EP readout time = 6.6 ms, readout time per cardiac cycle = 1 ms, scanner: 25 mT/m, slew rate = 80 mT m^{-1} ms^{-1})

Signal-to-Noise Ratio

To collect the data before the signal decays completely by T2* dephasing, the data acquisition rates in single-shot EPI uncomparably higher than in conventional imaging. The SNR is proportional to several imaging parameters (disregarding the contrast generated by each imaging technique), such as indicated in the following expression:

$$SNR \propto \frac{\sqrt{NEX}\sqrt{N_x}\sqrt{N_y}\sqrt{N_z}\Delta x \Delta y \Delta z}{\sqrt{BW}} \qquad (34)$$

where NEX indicates the number of excitations averaged, Δx, Δy, and Δz represent the voxel dimensions, N_x, N_y, and N_z denote the number of points collected along the frequency- and booth phase-encoding axes, respectively, and BW is the acquisition bandwidth, the inverse of the sampling rate Δt. Take into account that, as noted in early sections, the signal bandwidth is proportional to the strength of the gradient applied during the readout. Thus, large readout gradients translate into high readout bandwidths and consequently a reduced SNR and a greater demand for the gradient amplifier.

Maintaining the flip angle, the voxel size, and the number of points identical between a single-shot GRE-EPI and a conventional GRE acquisition, the difference in readout bandwidths is the only factor dictating the difference in SNR. Based solely on the fact that higher acquisition bandwidths are used in single-shot EPI, commonly between 150 and 500 kHz, SNR can be considered several-fold worse. Nonetheless, taking into account that the resolution in single-shot EPI is limited to the gradient power available, SNR can be acceptable because of the larger voxel size.

Although SNR may not be high compared to high flip-angle conventional GRE scans with similar voxel sizes, SNR per unit of time is much higher for single-

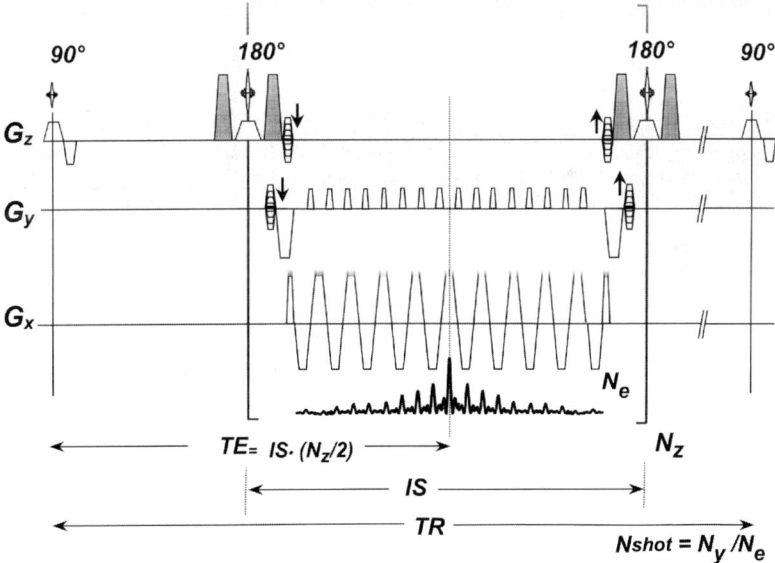

Fig. 38. Fast 3D heavily T2-weighted sequence using a multishot 3D segmented SE-EPI sequence. The series of 180° refocusing RF pulses, separated by an excitation spacing (*IS*) are applied to encode all the N_z section-select phase-encoding steps. During each interval between the 180° RF pulses an EP readout generating several echoes are phase encoded along the in-plane phase-encoding direction using an interleaved trajectory. TR is defined as the total time necessary per shot. N_y, Number of in-plane phase-encoding lines; N_z, number of sections; N_e, number of echoes; $N_{shot} = N_y/N_e$ number of shots,

Fig. 39A,B. Coronal and axial reconstructions of a 3D MR cholangiogram generated in a patient with a tumor and multiple cystic lesions. Breathhold time was 24 s. In total 64 sections were encoded with TR/TE = 3400/634 ms, 11 echoes per RF excitation, ES = 1280 μs (940 Hz/pixel readout bandwidth), IS = 19.8 ms, a 66×256 matrix with FOV = 160×320 mm, sequential partition encoding. Body phased array coil reception (EP readout time = 14.08 ms, readout time per shot = 1.270 s, scanner: 25 mT/m, slew rate = 80 mT m^{-1} ms^{-1})

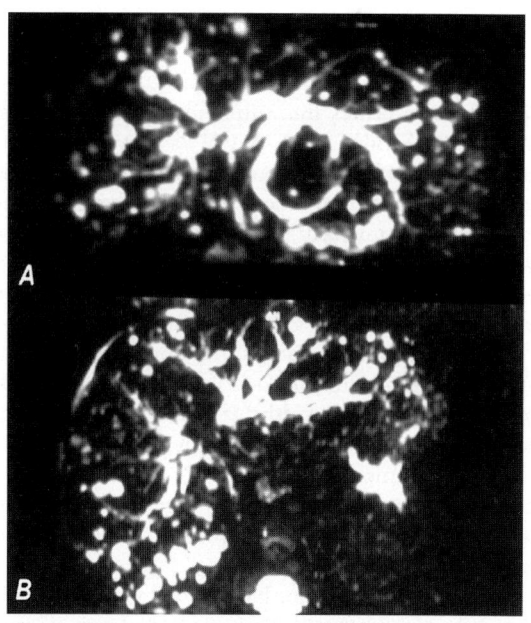

shot EPI. In addition, the fact that all the longitudinal magnetization may be available in the transverse plane after a single RF excitation imploi that some signal could be gained in comparison to conventional techniques when a finite TR may not allow complete recovery of the longitudinal magnetization between excitations (specifically for tissues with long T1, such as the CSF) prior to each RF excitation.

For EPI it is also important to consider that SNR loss may occur in regions with large susceptibility gradients. Thinner slices can circumvent this problem partially and may boost the signal from regions with poor field homogeneity compared to thicker slices. This is typically found when imaging regions such as the base of the brain and near the sinuses, where thinner slices prove to recover some signal that would otherwise be lost from complete phase dispersion across the voxel.

Because SNR can be improved by reducing the acquisition bandwidth, the price that would be paid is an increase in the echo train spacing that augments geometrical distortions from a lower phase-encoding gradient, signal loss and filtering from T2* decay, and ultimately larger chemical shift artifacts. An increase in the main magnetic field does not overcome the SNR problem easily as shorter T2* (which changes quadratically with a change in the main magnetic field) accelerates the signal decay, and correspondingly the acquisition rate and gradient strengths must be increased to a point at which no gain in SNR would be possible. Lower magnetic fields increase T2* and permit lower acquisition bandwidths and some compensation in SNR.

Safety

Neuromuscular stimulations have been reported by several investigators during EPI data collection [100, 101]; this is covered more extensively in Chap. 7. In summary, sensations were classified from very weakly tingling to painful muscle twitching depending on the magnitude of the locally induced electric currents by the rapid oscillation of the magnetic gradient field. These sensations were perceived near the physical extremes of the gradient coil where the gradient field change (and therefore dB/dt) is largest. For instance, the trunk muscles and the peripheral sacrospinal region are typically affected when the head is positioned at the center of the magnet. Similarly, the bridge of the nose may be affected during abdominal imaging. Magnetostimulation experiments with animals [102] and theoretical evaluations [103] show that the threshold for peripheral stimulations is below that of cardiac stimulations, and additional systoles are predicted ten times larger than for peripheral stimulations. Myocardial fibrillation is expected at even higher values. Volunteer experiments using various gradient pulse shapes demonstrate that peripheral stimulations are not dangerous for patients [104].

If higher gradient amplitudes and speed prove interesting for specific applications, the homogeneity of the gradient field (the linearity within the FOV) can be sacrificed so that the maximum dB/dt at the edges of the gradient coil does not exceed the nerve stimulation threshold or the guidelines imposed by the United States Food and Drug Administration. This restricts the use of high gradient amplitudes and short rise times with good linearity over a large FOV with a body gradient coil. Small gradient inserts have recently been built for imaging the head [69] that permit much higher amplitudes, with improved rise times and a power requirement that can be handled by conventional gradient amplifiers, making EPI more accessible for general use. For cardiac applications, for instance, the gradient linearity can be sacrificed along the z direction using a shorter winding so that the linearity extends only to the FOV of interest.

Conclusions

EPI is an extremely versatile image encoding technique that permits a multitude of clinical applications requiring ultrashort imaging times and low sensitivity to motion. With the introduction of commercial MRI systems with EPI capabilities, a comprehensive evaluation of ischemic heart disease can be completed rapidly by combining breath-hold fast imaging of cardiac anatomy and coronary artery MRA with wall motion evaluation using cine and myocardial tagging, first-pass imaging of contrast-enhancement patterns, and possibly diffusion imaging. Other applications include: real time imaging of organ and joint motion, dynamic observation of contrast enhanced studies, temperature monitoring, multisection imaging of the brain or upper abdomen, and functional brain imaging (perfusion, diffusion and cortical activation). In summary, EPI will serve as an adjunct to current imaging protocols to increase diagnostic accuracy.

Although EPI has been known for a number of years, its dissemination as a clinically useful technique has been slow despite its potential capabilities. Advantages that EPI can offer over conventional imaging include:

- Instantaneous image collection that permits real-time observation of dynamic processes such as organ motion, kinematic studies, and follow up of the time course of contrast injections.
- Flexible image contrast
- Reduction in motion artifacts
- Highest signal-to-noise and contrast-to-noise ratios per unit time
- Promises reduced examination times with higher patient throughput and lower cost per examination
- In the near future, the possibility of an interactive imaging system with real-time control that can be used for fluoroscopic imaging in interventional MRI

Although EPI is not likely to replace conventional scanning protocols in the near future, its major potential relies on its high temporal resolution and immunity to physiological motion rather than its limited spatial resolution. By improving coil design or by trading off resolution, speed can be increased and clinical utility preserved, particularly in dynamic studies. The balance between all of these features will be reflected in the suggested imaging parameters of each method as they relate to each specific clinical application. Further studies are still needed to determine the eventual clinical role and cost efficacy of EPI.

References

1. Alsop D, Hatabu H, Bonnet M, Listerud J, Gefter W (1995) Multi-slice, breath-hold imaging of the lung with submillisecond echo times. Magn Reson Med 33:678–682
2. Wielopolski PA, Edelman RR, Finn JP, Schmitt F (1993) High resolution, ultrashort echo time MR angiography with a whole-body EPI imager. J Magn Reson Imaging 3:44
3. Müller MF, Wielopolski PA, Teich-Siewert B, Edelman RR (1996) Magnetoresonanz-angiographie der Aa carotides. Einfluß kurzer und ultrakurzer Echozeiten. Rofo, 164(4)269–356
4. Wielopolski PA, Oudkerk M, de Bruin HG (1996) Three-dimensional MR pulmonary perfusion imaging with gadozentate dimegluinine. Radiology 201(P)230
5. Wielopolski PA, Finn JP, Edelman RR, Schmitt F (1993) Ultrashort TEs for abdominal imaging with a whole body echo planar imaging system. J Magn Reson Imaging 3:73
6. Atlas SW, Hackney DB, Listerud J (1993) Fast spin-echo imaging of the brain and spine. Magn Reson Q 9:61–83
7. Jones KM, Mulkern RV et al (1992) Fast spin-echo MR imaging of the brain and spine: current concepts. AJR 158:1313–1320
8. Kiefer B, Grässner J, Hausmann R (1994) Image acquisition in a second with half-Fourier acquisition single-shot turbo spin echo. J Magn Reson Imaging 4:86
9. Mansfield P (1977) Multi-planar image formation using NMR spin echoes. J Phys C 10:L55–L58
10. Stehling MK, Turner R, Mansfield P (1991) Echo-planar imaging: magnetic resonance imaging in a fraction of a second. Science 254:43–50
11. Twieg DB (1984) Acquisition and accuracy in rapid NMR imaging methods. Man Reson Med 2:437–452
12. Twieg DB (1983) The k-trajectory formulation of the NMR imaging proess with applications in analysis and synthesis of imaging methods. Med Phys 10:610–621
13. Ljungreen SA (1983) A simple graphical representation of Fourier-based imaging methods. J Magn Reson 54:338–343
14. Bruder H, Fischer H, Reinfelder H-E, Schmitt F (1992) Image reconstruction for echo planar imaging with nonequidistant k-space sampling. Magn Reson Med 23:311–323
15. Chen DQ, Marr R, Lauterbur P (1986) Reconstruction from NMR data with imaging gradients having arbitrary time dependence. IEEE Trans Med Imaging 5(3)162–164
16. Zakhor A, Weiskoff R, Rzedzian R (1991) Optimal sampling and reconstruction of MRI signals resulting from sinusoidal gradients. IEEE Trans Signal Processing 19(9):2056–2065
17. Ordidge RJ, Mansfield P (1984) NMR methods. United States patent no 4509015
18. Margosian P, Schmitt F, Purdy D (1986) Faster MR imaging: imaging with half the data. Health Care Instrum 1:195–197
19. Haacke EM Lindskog ED, Lin W (1991) Partial-Fourier imaging. A fast, iterative, POCS technique capable of local phase recovery. J Magn Reson 92:126–145
20. Fischer H, Schmitt FX, Barfuss H, Bruder H (1988) Half Fourier echo planar imaging at 2 teola. In: Book of abstracts: Society of Magnetic Resonance in Medicine 7th Annual Meeting, San Francisco, August 20–26, p 972
21. Schmitt F, Stehling MK, Ladebeck R, Fang M, Quaiyumi A, Barschneider E, Huk WJ (1992) Echo-planar imaging of the central nervous system at 1.0 T. J Magn Reson Imaging 2(4):473–478
22. Davis CP, McKinnon GC, Debatin JF, Duewell S, von Schulthess GK (1995) Single shot versus interleaved echo-planar MR imaging: Application to visualization of cardiac value leaflets. T Magn Reson Imag 5:107–112
23. Wielopolski P, Feyter P de, Jaegere P de, Bruin H de, Oudkerk M (1996) Single breathhold three-dimensional MR coronary angiography. In: Book of abstracts: Society of Magnetic Resonance 4th annual meeting, April 27–May 5, New York, p 451
24. Weiskoff RM, Dalcanton JJ, Cohen MS (1990) High resolution 64 ms instant images of the head. Magn Reson Imaging 8 [Suppl 1]:93
25. Pauly J, Butts K, Luk Pat GT, Macovski A (1995) A circular echo-planar pulse sequence. In: Book of abstracts: Society of Magnetic Resonance. 3rd Annual meeting, Nice, August 19–25, p 106

26. Meyer C, Hu B, Nishimura D, Macovski A (1992) Fast spiral coronary artery imaging. Magn Reson Med 28:202–213
27. Bowtell R, McIntyre DJO, Commandre MJ, Glover PM, Mansfield P (1994) Correction of geometric distortion in echo planar images. In: Book of abstracts: Society of Magnetic Resonance, 2nd Annual meeting, San Francisco, August 6–12, p 411
28. Jezzard P, Balaban RS (1995) Correction for geometric distortion in echo planar images from B0 field variations. Magn Reson Med 34(1):65–73
29. Haacke EM, Tkach JA, Parrish TB (1989) Reduction of T2* dephasing in gradient field-echo imaging. Radiology 170:457–462
30. Kashmar G, Nalcioglu O (1991) Cartesian echo planar hybrid scanning with two to eight echoes. IEEE Trans Med Imaging 10(1):1–10
31. Siewert B, Patel MR, Müller MF, Gaa J, Darby DG, Poser CM, Wielopolski PA, Edelman RR, Warach S (1995) Brain lesions in patients with multiple sclerosis: detection with echo-planar imaging. Radiology 196:764
32. Butts K, Riederer SJ, Ehman RL, Thompson RM, Jack CR (1994) Interleaved echo planar imaging on a standard MRI system. Magn Reson Med 31:67–72
33. McKinnon GC (1993) Ultrafast interleaved gradient-echo-planar imaging on a standard scanner. Magn Reson Med 30:609–616
34. Chapman B, Turner R, Ordidge RJ, Doyle M, Cawley M, Coxon R, Glover P, Mansfield P (1987) Real-time movie imaging from a single cardiac cycle by NMR. Magn Reson Med 5:246–254
35. Rzedzian RR (1987) High speed, high resolution, spin echo imaging by mosaic scan and MESH. In: Proceeding of the Society of Magnetic Resonance in Medicine, 6th Annual meeting, New York, August, p 51
36. Farzaneh F, Riederer SJ, Maier JK, Vavrek R (1989) View-interleaved EPI on a commercial scanner. In: Book of abstracts. Society of Magnetic Resonance in Medicine, p 832
37. Mansfield P (1984) Spatial mapping of the chemical shift in NMR. Magn Reson Med 1(3):370–386
38. Stehling MK (1992) Improved signal in "snapshot" FLASH by variable flip angles. Magn Reson Imaging 10(1):165–167
39. Feinberg DA, Oshio K (1992) Gradient-echo time shifting in fast MRI techniques for correction of field inhomogeneity errors and chemical shift. J Magn Reson 97:177–183
40. Feinberg DA, Oshio K (1994) Phase errors in multishot echo planar imaging. Magn Reson Med 32:535–539
41. Farzaneh F, Riederer SJ, Wright RC (1989) Hybrid imaging with gradient recalled sliding echoes. Magn Reson Imaging 7(1):70
42. Mugler JP III, Brookeman JR (1996) Off-resonance image artifacts in interleaved-EPI and GRASE pulse sequences. Magn Reson Med 36(2):306–313
43. Van Uijen C, Den Boef J, Verschuren F (1985) Fast Fourier imaging. Magn Reson Med 2:203–217
44. Haacke EM, Bearden F, Clayton J, Linga N (1986) Reduction of MR imaging time by the hybrid fast-scan technique. Radiology 166:157–163
45. Schmitt FX, Goertler G (1992) Method for suppressing image artifacts in a magnetic resonance imaging apparatus. United States patent no 5138259
46. Kelley D, Ordidge R (1993) Techniques for phase correction of raw data for EPI with unshielded gradient coils. In: Proceedings of the Society of Magnetic Resonance in Medicine, 12th Annual Meeting, August 14–20, New York, p 384
47. Wong EC (1992) Shim insensitive phase correction for EPI using a two echo reference scan. In: Proceedings of the Society of Magnetic Resonance in Medicine, 11th Annual Meeting, August 14–20, Berlin. p 4514
48. Heid O (1997) Robust EPI phase correction. In: Proceedings of the International Society of Magnetic Resonance in Medicine, 5th Annual Meeting Vancouver, April 12–18, p 2014
49. Jesmanowicz A, Wong EC, Hyde JS (1993) Phase correction for EPI using internal reference lines. In: Proceedings of the Society of Magnetic Resonance in Medicine, 12th Annual Meeting, August 14–20, New York. p 1239

50. Luk Pat GT, Nishimura D (1994) Reducing flow artifacts in echo-planar imaging. In: Proceedings of the Society of Magnetic Resonance, 2nd Annual Meeting San Francisco, August 6–12, p 473
51. Laub G, Deimling M, Petsch R (1994) Segmented volume imaging with multi-echo gradient-echo sequences. In: Proceedings of the Society of Magnetic Resonance, 2nd Annual Meeting San Francisco, August 6–12, p 468
52. Haase A, Frahm J, Matthaei (1986) Flash imaging, rapid NMR imaging using low flip-angle pulses. J Magn Reson 67:258–266
53. Oppelt A, Graumann R, Barfuss H, Fischer H (1986) FISP: a new imaging sequence with rapid pulses for magnetic resonance tomography. Electromedica 54:15–18
54. Joseph PM (1985) A spin echo chemical shift MR imaging technique. J Comput Assist Tomogr 9(4):651–658
55. Dumoulin CL (1985) A method for chemical shift imaging. Magn Reson Med 2:583
56. Meyer CH, Pauly JM, Macovski A, Nishimura DG (1990) Simultaneous spatial and spectral selective excitation. Magn Reson Med 15:287–304
57. Thomasson DM, Purdy DE, Finn JP (1994) Fast spectrally selective excitation in 3D gradient echo imaging. J Magn Reson Imaging 4 :56
58. Thomasson DM, Moore JR, Purdy DE, Finn JP (1994) Minimum-time spatial-spectral pulses using a phase modulated 1-1 binomial pulse design. In: Book of abstracts. Society of Magnetic Resonance, 2nd meeting, San Francisco, August 6–12, p 120
59. Manning WJ, Atkinson DJ, Grossman W, Paulin S, Edelman RR (1991) First-pass nuclear magnetic resonance imaging studies using gadolinium-DTPA in patients with coronary artery disease. J Am Coll Cardiol 18:959–964
60. Wendland MF, Saeed M, Masui T, Derugin N, Moseley ME, Higgins CB (1993) Echo-planar MR imaging of normal and ischemic myocardium. Radiology 186:535–542
61. Chrispin A, Small P, Rutter N et al (1986) Transectional echo planar imaging of the heart in cyanotic congenital heart disease. Pediatr Radiol 16:293–297
62. Chrispin A, Small P, Rutter N et al (1986) Echo planar imaging of normal and abnormal connections of the great vessels. Pediatr Radiol 16:289–292
63. Feinberg D, Turner R, Jakab P, Von Kienlin M (1990) Echo-planar imaging with asymmetric gradient modulation and inner volume excitation. Magn Reson Med 13:162–169
64. Tkach JA, Haacke EM (1988) A comparison of fast spin echo and gradient field echo sequences. Magn Reson Imaging 6(4):373–389
65. Bogdan AR, Joseph PM (1990) RASEE: a rapid spin-echo pulse sequence. Magn Reson Imaging 8(1):13–19
66. Ma J, Wehrli FW, Song HK (1996) Fast 3D large-angle spin-echo imaging (3D FLASE) Magn Reson Med 35(6):903–910
67. Stejskal EO, Tanner JE (1964) Spin diffusion measurements: spin echoes in the presence of a time-dependent field gradient. J Chem Phys 42:288–292
68. Le Bihan D, Breton E, Lallemand D, Grenier P, Cabanis E, Laval-Jeantet M (1986) MR imaging of intravoxel incoherent motions: application to diffusion and perfusion al disorders. Radiology 161:401–407
69. Turner R, Le Bihan D, Maier J, Vavrek R, Hedges LK, Pekar J (1990) Echo-planar imaging of intra-voxel incoherent motion. Radiology 177:407–414
70. Turner R, Le Bihan D, Checnick AS (1991) Echo-planar imaging of diffusion and perfusion. Magn Reson Med 19:247–253
71. Warach S, Gaa J, Siewert B, Wielopolski PA, Edelman RR (1995) Acute human stroke studied by whole brain echo planar diffusion weighted MRI. Ann Neurol 37:231–241
72. Mori S, van Zijl PCM (1995) Diffusion weighting by the trace of the diffusion tensor within a single scan. Magn Reson Med 33:41–52
73. Turner R, von Kienlin M, Moonen CTW, van Zijl PCM (1990) Single-shot localized echo-planar imaging (STEAM-EPI) at 4.7 tesla. Magn Reson Med 14:401–408
74. Muller MF, Prasad P, Siewert B, Nissembaum MA, Raptopoulos V, Edelman RR (1994) Abdominal diffusion mapping with use of a whole-body echo-planar system. Radiology 190:474
75. Tanner JE (1970) Use of stimulated echo in NMR diffusion studies. J Chem Phys 52:2523
76. Merboldt KD, Hanicke W, Frahm J (1985) Self-diffusion NMR imaging using stimulated echoes. J Magn Reson 64:479

77. Edelman RR, Gaa J, Weeden VJ, Loh E, Hare JM, Prasad P, Li W (1994) In vivo measurement of water diffusion in the human heart. Magn Reson Med 32:423–428
78. Stehling MK, Ordidge RJ, Coxon R, Mansfield P (1990) Inversion-recovery echo-planar imaging (IR-EPI) at 0.5 T. Magn Reson Med 13:514–517
79. Maeda M, Itoh S, Yamada H et al (1994) Comparison of the fluid attenuated inversion recovery (FLAIR) with conventional MR imaging in the cortical and subcortical lesions. In: Proceedings of the Society of Magnetic Resonance, 2nd annual meeting, San Francisco, August 6–12, p 538
80. Hajnal JV, Byrant DJ, Kasuboski L et al (1992) Use of fluid attenuated inversion recovery (FLAIR) sequences in MRI of the brain. J Comput Assist Tomogr 16:841–844
81. Börnert P, Jensen D (1994) Single-shot-double-echo EPI. Magn Reson Imaging 12(7)1033–1038
82. Cohen MS, Rohan ML (1989) 3D volume imaging with instant scan. In: Book of abstracts: Society of Magnetic Resonance in Medicine, 8th Annual meeting, Amsterdam, August 12–18, p 831
83. Cohen MS, Hahn P, Saini S (1992) Breath-hold 3D multi-slab volume imaging. In: Society of Magnetic Resonance in Medicine, 11th annual meeting, Berlin, August 8–14, p 102
84. Mansfield P, Howseman AM, Ordidge RJ (1989) Volumar imaging using NMR spin echoes: echo-volumar imaging (EVI) at 0.1T. J Phys (E) 21:274
85. Mansfield P, Coxon R, Hykin J (1995) Echo-volumar imaging (EVI) of the brain at 3.0T: First normal volunteer and functional imaging results. J Comput Assist Tomogr 19(6):847–852
86. Song AW, Wong EC, Hyde JS (1994) Echo-volume imaging. Magn Reson Med 33:668–671
87. Posse S, Tedeschi G, Risinger R, Ogg R, Le Bihan D (1995) High speed 1H spectroscopic imaging in human brain by echo planar spatial-spectral encoding. Magn Reson Med 33:34–40
88. Posse S, DeCarli C, Le Bihan D (1994) 3D echo-planar MR spectroscopic imaging at short echo times in human brain. Radiology 192:733–738
89. Guimaraes AR, Baker JR, Weisskoff RM, Rosen BR, Gonzales RG (1994) 4D echo planar imaging of brain metabolites. In: Book of abstracts: Society of Magnetic Resonance in Medicine, 2th Annual Meeting, San Francisco, August 6–12, p 177
90. Bito Y, Hirata S, Nabeshima T, Yamamoto E (1994) Echo-planar diffusion spectroscopic imaging. Magn Reson Med 33:69–73
91. Haase A (1990) Snapshot FLASH MRI: application to T1, T2, and chemical-shift imaging. Magn Reson Med 13:77–89
92. Li D, Haacke EM, Mugler III JP, Berr S, Brookeman JR, Hutton MC (1994) Three-dimensional time-of-flight MR angiography using selective inversion recovery RAGE with fat saturation and ECG-triggering: Application to renal arteries. Magn Reson Med 31:414–422
93. Wielopolski PA, Manning WJ, Edelman RR (1995) Breath-hold volumetric imaging of the heart using magnetization prepared 3D segmented echo planar imaging. J Magn Reson Imaging 4:403–409
94. Brittain JH, Wright GA, Hu BS, Nishimura DG (1994) Coronary angiography with magnetization-prepared T2 contrast. J Magn Reson Imaging 4:80
95. Butts K, Riederer SJ, Ehman RL, Felmlee JP, Grim RC (1993) Echo-planar imaging of the liver with a standard MR imaging system. Radiology 189(1):259–64
96. Hennig J, Nauerth A, Friedburg H (1986) RARE imaging: a fast imaging method for clinical MR. Magn Reson Med 3:823–833
97. Melki PS, Jolesz FA, Mulkern RV (1992) Partial RF echo planar imaging with the FAISE method. I. Magn Reson Med 26:328–341
98. Melki PS, Jolesz FA, Mulkern RV (1992) Partial RF echo-planar imaging with the FAISE method. II. Magn Reson Med 26:342–354
99. Wielopolski P, Zuo CB, Clouse M, Buff B (1994) Breath-hold 3D cholangiography using RARE and segmented echo planar imaging readouts. In: Book of abstracts: Society of Magnetic Resonance, 2nd annual meeting, San Francisco, August 6–12, p 1448
100. Cohen MS, Weisskoff RM, Rzedzian RR, Kantor HL (1990) Sensory stimulation by time-varying magnetic fields. Magn Reson Med 14:409–414
101. Budinger TF, Fischer H, Hentschel D, Reinfelder H-E, Schmitt F (1991) Physiological effects of fast oscillating magnetic field gradients. J Comput Assist Tomogr 15:909–914

102. Bourland JD, Nyenhuis JA, Mouchawar GA, Geddes LA, Schaefer DJ, Riehl ME (1991). Z-gradient coil eddy-current stimulation of skeletal and cardiac muscle in the dog. In: Proceedings of the Society of Magnetic Resonance in Medicine, 10th annual meeting, San Francisco, August 10–16, p 1276
103. Irnich W (1993) Electrostimulation by time-varying magnetic fields. In: Proceedings of the Society of Magnetic Resonance in Medicine, 12th annual meeting, New York, August 14–20, pg 1371
104. Schmitt F, Wielopolski P, Fischer H, Edelman RR (1994) Peripheral stimulations and their relation to gradient pulse shapes. In: Proceedings of the Society of Magnetic Resonance, 2nd annual meeting, Berlin, August 8–14, p 102

CHAPTER 5

Echo-Planar Image Reconstruction

F. Schmitt and P. A. Wielopolski

Introduction

Echo-planar imaging (EPI), introduced by Mansfield in 1977 [1], permits the measurement of an entire magnetic resonance (MR) image in less than 100 ms. After a single excitation an appropriate gradient sequence encodes the magnetization repeatedly, thus filling the whole k-space. This allows, for example, the freezing of dynamic processes and the observation of these processes in real time. It has been shown that EPI can provide head and body images of biomedically useful quality free of motion and almost unlimited T1- and T2-weighted contrast. The major advantage of EPI is its speed. EPI can acquire a complete set of slices in a time conventional MRI takes to acquire a single slice. This must be kept in mind when comparing EPI with other MRI techniques.

To achieve speed EPI sequences encode the magnetization using a scheme that differs drastically from that used in conventional techniques. First, alternating gradient pulses are applied to obtain gradient echoes. Second, data are typically sampled during varying strength gradient pulses. All this requires different schemes for reconstructing the final image. This chapter describes the common techniques of the EPI reconstruction. A brief introduction of the k-space terminology is followed by a description of the most common EPI k-space trajectories. We then consider the effects of data sampling under varying gradient pulses with respect to time and describe different approaches for obtaining uniform k-space coverage. The reconstruction along the phase-encoding direction can also differ from that of conventional reconstruction, and therefore the interlaced Fourier transform (FT) reconstruction is described. As it is always the case, the real world differs from the ideal, theoretical world; this holds for EPI as well. Several limitations and imperfections existing in the MR scanner hardware must also be considered during the image reconstruction process. Finally, the entire reconstruction scheme is summarized.

We frequently provide information in the form of equations because image reconstruction for MR data acquired under varying gradient pulses is somewhat unusual and more complicated when compared to normal conventional MRI sequence acquiring data at constant gradients only. However, whenever possible we give a graphic interpretation to assist readers who are less familiar with signal processing and FT gymnastics.

k-Space

This section briefly introduces the terminology of k-space, introduced by Ljunggren [2] in 1983. For more detailed information see Chap. 2. Conventional two-
dimensional (2D) magnetic resonance imaging (MRI) is based on a 2D FT [3].
Following the FT algorithm the signal acquired, $S(k_{RO}, k_{PC})$, can be described
mathematically as:

$$S(k_{RO}, k_{PC}) = \int\int S(x,y) \cdot e^{i(k_{RO}x + k_{PC}y)} dx\, dy \tag{1}$$

where:

$$k_{RO}(t) = \gamma \int_0^t G_{RO}(t') dt' \tag{2}$$

$$k_{PC}(t) = \gamma \int_0^t G_{PC}(t') dt' \tag{3}$$

describe the coordinates along the readout (RO) and phase-encoding (PC) k-
space direction, respectively (see Fig. 1). $G_{RO}(t)$ and $G_{PC}(t)$ describe the time
and amplitude dependence of the RO and PC gradient pulses of the imaging
sequence; γ is the gyromagnetic ratio, and i is the complex number defined by
$i = \sqrt{-1}$. The gradient-time integrals of Eqs. 2 and 3 can be interpreted as the
area under the gradient pulse for the time of integration, t. S(x, y) describes
the spatial distribution of the spin density and its relaxation properties such
as the spin-lattice relaxation time, T1, and the spin-spin relaxation time, T2
[4]. In this section we do not explicitly mention the relaxation parameters, but
these should always be kept in mind as they influence image contrast and resolution. An inverse 2D-FT is required to calculate the final MR image, as described
in Eq. 4:

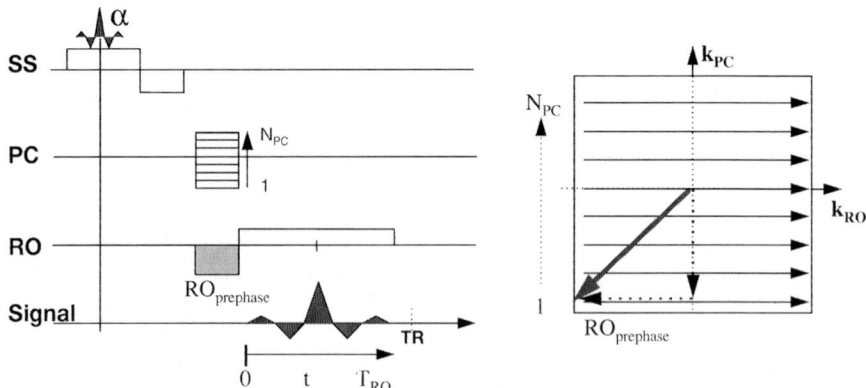

Fig. 1. Conventional 2D-GRE sequence (*left*) and the corresponding k-space trajectory (*right*).
The k-space data lines are acquired from left to right

$$S(x,y) = \int \int S(k_{RO}, k_{PC}) \cdot e^{i(k_{RO}x + k_{PC}y)} dk_{RO} dk_{PC} \qquad (4)$$

The k-space is the coordinate system of the detected MR signal. The path through the k-space and the time succession order of the acquired k-space data is called the k-space trajectory. Many such trajectories are possible for EPI, and each requires its own image reconstruction scheme. Below we present the most common trajectories and describe how the final image is reconstructed.

To demonstrate the special features of EPI we first explain the k-space traversal of a conventional gradient-recalled echo (GRE) sequence (Fig. 1, left). We assume a slice-selective excitation oriented along the slice-selection (SS) gradient perpendicular to the PC and RO gradient directions. The PC gradient starts with a negative amplitude G_1 and is increased gradually to the final positive amplitude G_{NPC}. The gradient amplitude steps are uniform in order to provide an equidistant stepping in k-space (Fig. 1, right). The prephasing lobe of the RO gradient in combination with the first PC gradient amplitude, G_1, define the starting point (lower left edge of k-space) for the first k-space data line. During the time, t (from 0 to T_{RO}), the first line is acquired. The k_{RO} coordinate is proportional to the RO gradient amplitude, G_{RO}, and the time, t, as described in Eq. 5:

$$k_{RO}(t) = \gamma \int_0^t G_{RO}(t')dt' = G_{RO} \cdot t \qquad (5)$$

After the repetition time, TR, the excitation is repeated, and the PC gradient amplitude is increased to amplitude G_2 defining the start position for the second k-space data line. This procedure is repeated until the N_{PC}th PC-gradient amplitude is reached followed by the N_{PC}th data line acquisition. By convention data lines are acquired from left to right when the amplitude of the RO gradient pulse is positive.

For EPI a different scheme is used. The simplest GRE EPI sequence using idealized rectangular RO gradients and infinitesimally short PC-gradient blips is shown in Fig. 2. The major difference between EPI and conventional MRI is that EPI does not require a warp PC gradient as shown for the GRE sequence in Fig. 1. The phase encoding is established by a train of unipolar blips located at the zero crossings of the bipolar RO gradient pulse train. The gradient-time integral over the duration of a blip, T_{blip}, is adjusted to correspond to a step from one k_{PC} data line to the next:

$$\delta k_{PC} = \gamma \int_0^{T_{Blipp}} G_{Blipp}(t)dt = \Delta k_{PC} / N_{PC} \qquad (6)$$

N_{PC} is the total number of k_{PC} data lines to be acquired; Δ indicates a total span (e.g., the total k-space coverage, Δk), and δ indicates the smallest discrete quantity (e.g., δk, which fulfills the Nyquist theorem).The prephasing lobes of the PC and RO gradients of Fig. 2 define the starting point (lower left edge of k-space) of the first k-space data line acquired. During the first positive RO gradient pulse the first k-space data line is acquired, followed by the first blip, which causes a jump of exactly one line in PC direction. The succeeding negative RO gradient pulse causes a backward traversal (from right to left) which corresponds to the

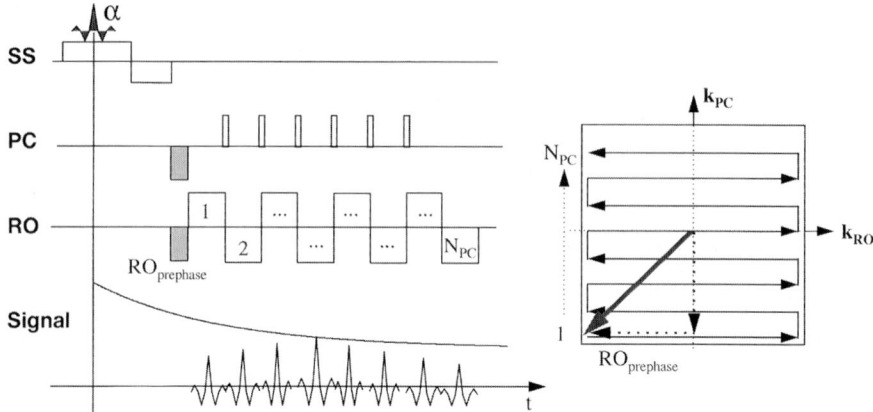

Fig. 2. GRE EPI sequence (*left*) and the corresponding k-space trajectory (*right*). The odd k-space data line traverses forward (from left to right), whereas the even k-space data lines traverse backward (from right to left). This trajectory traversal is characteristic for EPI

second line of k-space. The next blip defines the start of the third k-space data line, which is traversed again from left to right because of the positive polarity of the 3rd RO gradient pulse. This procedure is repeated until the N_{PC}th data line is reached. If we look at the entire k-space traversal and compare it with the traversal of Fig. 1, we see that for EPI every other k-space data line is traversed backwards in k-space. This is one of the major differences between EPI and other conventional MRI techniques and requires special consideration for the image reconstruction.

Common EPI Data Acquisition Modules and Their k-Space Trajectories

Figure 2 shows an idealized EPI sequence using a bipolar rectangular RO gradient pulse train and an infinitesimally short blipped PC gradient. In reality this is not possible. Therefore technically feasible gradient pulse shapes must be

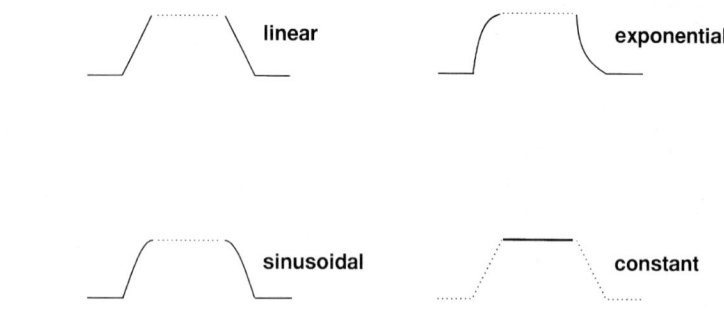

Fig. 3. Common building blocks of gradient pulses

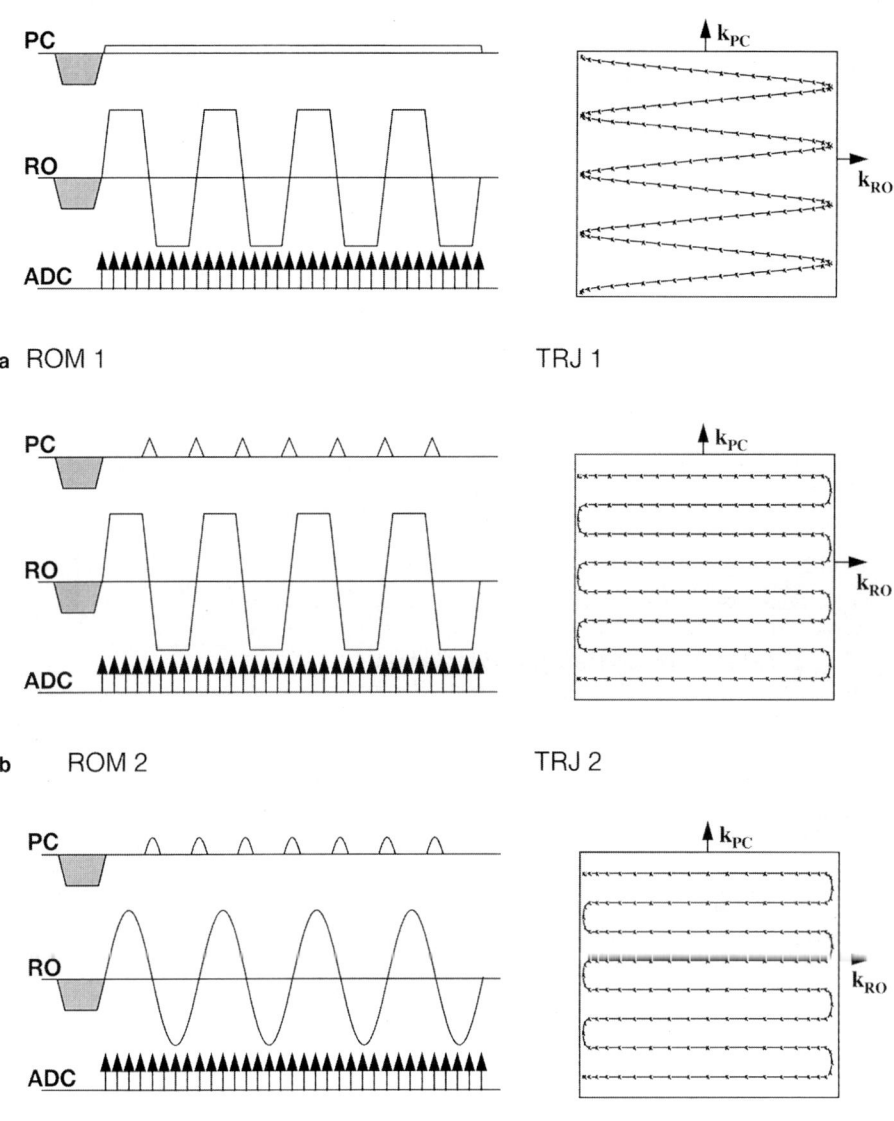

Fig. 4a–f. Possible RO modules (*ROM 1–8*) and its corresponding k-space trajectories (*TRJ 1–8*) combined from the basic gradient shapes of Fig. 3. For the sake of convenience we do not show exponential ramps. The markers on the k-space trajectory indicate the location of the k-space samples when equidistant time-domain sampling is performed. **a** ROM 1. Trapezoidal RO gradient in combination with a constant PC gradient. **b** ROM 2. Trapezoidal RO gradient in combination with a triangular blipped PC gradient. **c** ROM 3. Sinusoidal RO gradient in combination with a sinusoidal blipped PC gradient

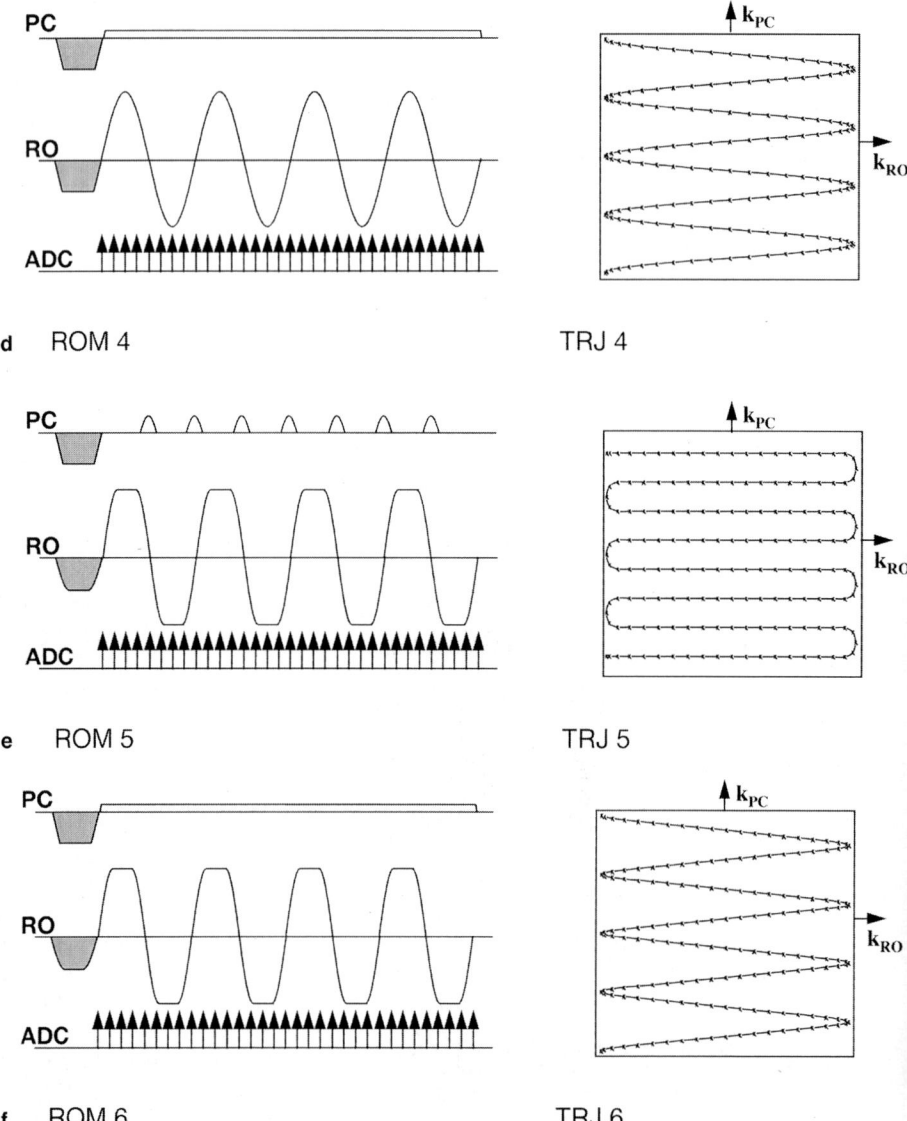

Fig. 4a–f. (continued) **d** ROM 4. Sinusoidal RO gradient in combination with a constant PC gradient. **e** ROM 5. Sinusoidal ramp "trapezoid" RO gradient in combination with a blipped PC gradient. **f** ROM 6. Sinusoidal ramp "trapezoid" RO gradient in combination with a constant PC gradient

applied. Gradient pulse shapes are defined by its slew rate and gradient amplitude possible by the gradient amplifier. The gradient power supply unit available on a particular MRI scanner must provide the required voltage to achieve a certain ramp shape (for further details see Chap. 3). Figure 3 shows some possible gradient shapes, which can have ramps that may be either linear, sinusoidal or exponential. Pure sinusoidal RO gradient pulses are also common for reading out the MR signal. (We describe as "trapezoid" gradient pulses comprising of any type of rise and fall ramp shape in combination with a flat top time, i.e., a constant gradient.)

PC gradients for EPI are typically comprised of triangular or sinusoidal blips or the so-called constant phase encoding. The latter is achieved by a constant PC gradient throughout the entire EPI data acquisition window [5]. The mixture of RO and PC gradient shapes (Fig. 4) define various k-space trajectories which require different k-space regridding schemes; these are described under "Readout Data Sampling and Reconstruction." The differences between blipped and constant phase encoding are evident in Fig. 4. Blipped PC gradients are used to proceed fast from one k-space line to the next while constant PC gradient causes a gradual traversal from one k-space line to the next. Blips are typically performed in a fraction of the RO time per echo, T_{RO}:

$$T_{Blipp} << T_{RO} \tag{7}$$

In Fig. 4 the duration of the blips is assumed to be one-fifth of the total RO period.

Readout Data Sampling and Reconstruction

A major difference between EPI and other MRI techniques is its demand on the speed of several components of the MRI hardware. Data acquisition must be accomplished in a time roughly similar to the tissue T2 relaxation time [6]. To achieve this it is efficient to sample the MR signal during the gradient ramp times. This depends on the flexibility of the data acquisition system, the image reconstruction, and the stability of the gradient power supply unit. Not all vendors of MR systems currently offer this flexibility, which is essential for EPI. If not available on the scanner, the time required to collect the data for a single echo-planar image can be considerably prolonged and make EPI scans clinically useless. For example, let us assume that an echo-planar image of dimension $N_{RO} \times N_{PC}$ is acquired with a fixed gradient rise time, T_{Rise}. The total acquisition time is prolongated by T_{prol}:

$$T_{Prol} = 2 \cdot N_{PC} \cdot T_{Rise} \tag{8}$$

If a typical rise time of 300 μs and $N_{PC} = 128$ Fourier lines are used, the total prolongation is 76.8 ms. This alone is in the order of typical T2 relaxation time of soft tissues of the human body and therefore should be avoided. When the net data acquisition time is added, the result is a total acquisition time per image of far more than 150 ms.

Long data acquisition times for EPI cause image degradation, such as geometric distortions, blurring, and signal loss due to T2* relaxation [6] (see Chap. 6 on EPI artifacts). For the GRE EPI sequence of Fig. 2 this signal loss is described as:

$$S(t) = S_o \cdot e^{-\frac{t}{T2^*}} \tag{9}$$

where S_o is the available signal amplitude right after the slice excitation and T2* is defined as:

$$\frac{1}{T2^*} = \frac{1}{T2} + \gamma \cdot \Delta B_o \tag{10}$$

The term ΔB_o describes the pixel inhomogeneity caused either by limited magnet shimming or by local susceptibility. Shimming can be controlled to improve magnetic field inhomogeneities using electrical shim coils. Typical homogeneities of high field magnets are on the order of ± 5 ppm. Susceptibility boundaries can cause local flux changes on the order of ± 1 ppm, which generally cannot be compensated for by either static [7] or dynamic shimming [8, 9]. Fast data reception is up to now therefore the only efficient way to minimize susceptibility effects.

When data are sampled during time-changing gradient shapes we must consider how sampling affects the trajectory and distribution of samples in k-space. For example, when we assume an equidistant data sampling with respect to time, a nonequidistance in the k-space results. As above, image reconstruction based on the FT requires equidistance between the sampled data. Therefore k-space equidistance must be obtained in some way. This can be achieved in either of two ways: (a) the data are sampled nonequidistantly in k-space and interpolated to equidistant k-space locations, or (b) the data are sampled nonequidistantly in time such that equidistance in k-space results. Both methods are described in the following section.

Uniform Time-Domain Data Sampling

When MR signal data are sampled equidistantly in time during the playout of a time-changing gradient shape, nonequidistance in k-space results. This is illustrated in Fig. 5. Following the definition of k-space, a constant gradient:

$$G(t) = G_o \tag{11}$$

during data reception causes a linearly progressing k(t):

$$k(t) = \gamma \int_0^t G_o(t')dt' = G_o \cdot t \tag{12}$$

and therefore results in equidistant k-space sampling (Fig. 5a) when we assume that the data are sampled at intervals of δt:

$$k_m = k(m \cdot \delta t) = G_o \cdot m \cdot \delta t \tag{13}$$

with:

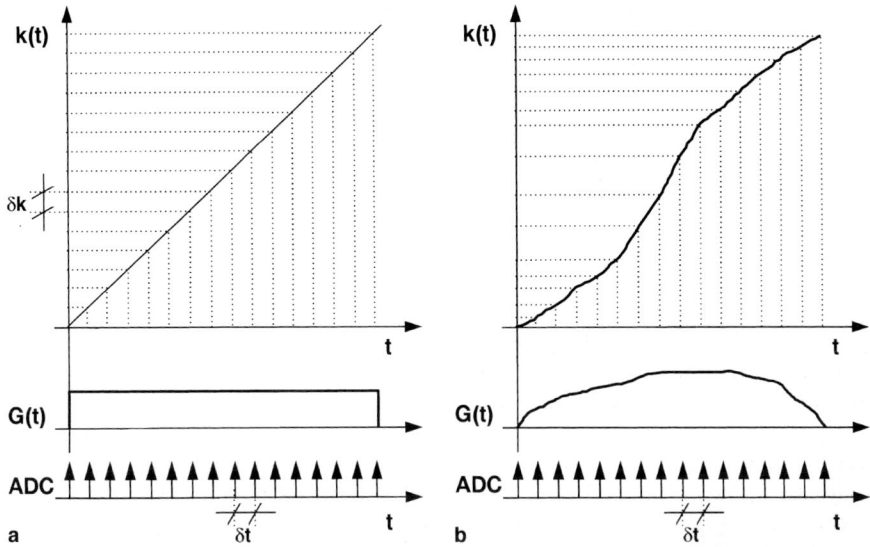

Fig. 5. Equidistant time data sampling of MR signal data for a constant gradient (a) and for a general gradient shape (b) showing gradient amplitude changes over the acquisition time

$$1 \leq m \leq N_{Sample} \tag{14}$$

where N_{sample} describes the total number of data points measured in a single T_{RO} period. For the constant RO gradient. N_{sample} is equal to the number of pixels, N_{RO}, (in RO direction) of the final image matrix ($N_{RO} \times N_{PC}$). However, when a general gradient shape, G(t), is applied:

$$G(t) = G_o \cdot f(t) \tag{15}$$

the resulting k-space is nonequidistantly sampled (Fig. 5b):

$$k(t) = \gamma \int_0^t G_u(t')dt' = G_o \cdot \int_0^t f(t')dt' \tag{16}$$

An important issue of data sampling in general is the Nyquist criteria [3]. This describes how fast (separation of data samples, δt) and how many data must be sampled to avoid aliasing effects. This is of special importance for nonuniform k-space sampling, which is the case in the example of Fig. 5b.

The Nyquist theorem is fulfilled when the following relation holds [5]:

$$N_{Sample} = N_{RO} \cdot \frac{\int_o^{T_{RO}} G_o \cdot dt}{\int_o^{T_{RO}} G_o \cdot f(t) \cdot dt} \tag{17}$$

In a more graphic explanation, the number of samples, N_{sample}, required to avoid aliasing is defined by the gradient-time area ratio of a constant gradient pulse and a nonconstant gradient pulse, both having the same maximum amplitude G_o and duration T_{RO}. From Eq. 17 we can deduce the sampling time, δt, for sampling under an arbitrary gradient waveform which satisfies the sampling theorem:

$$\delta t = \frac{T_{RO}}{N_{Sample}} \tag{18}$$

Let us now consider the specific example of a nonconstant RO gradient to demonstrate how the k-space sampling is evaluated, and how this is the input for the interpolation required to regain equidistance in k-space. Further below we focus on a sinusoidal RO gradient to illustrate the basic ideas behind image reconstruction:

$$G_{RO}(t) = G_{RO} \cdot \sin(\omega \cdot t) \tag{19}$$

with frequency:

$$\omega = 2\pi \cdot f = 2\pi / T \tag{20}$$

and period T. It is assumed that data are acquired during a time $T_{RO} = t_b - t_a$ (Fig. 6). Applying the definition of k-space (Eq. 2) we obtain:

$$k_{RO}(t) = \gamma \cdot \int_{t_a}^{t} G_{RO}(t) \cdot \sin(\omega \cdot t')dt'$$

$$k_{RO}(t) = \frac{\gamma \cdot G_{RO} \cdot T}{2\pi} \cdot \{\cos(2\pi \cdot t_a / T) - \cos(2\pi \cdot t / T)\} \tag{21}$$

Equation 21 shows that k_{RO} varies cosinusoidally with time. If we further assume equidistant time-domain data sampling with intervals δt calculated using Eq. 18 and insert into Eq. 21, we obtain the k-space samples, k_{RO_m}:

Fig. 6. k-Space sampling for a sinusoidal RO gradient. One sine half wave is shown. Data are sampled during the time $T_{RO} = t_b - t_a$. The sampling interval δt is adjusted as shown in Eq. 18. Equidistant time-domain sampling under the sine RO gradient results in nonuniformly distributed k-space samples

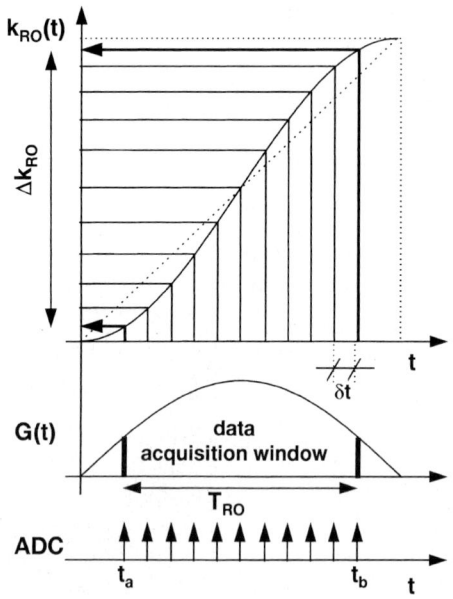

$$k_{RO_m} = k_{RO}(m \cdot \delta t)$$

$$k_{RO_m} = \frac{\gamma \cdot G_{RO} \cdot T}{2\pi} \cdot \{\cos(2\pi \cdot N_a \cdot \delta t / T) - \cos(2\pi \cdot m \cdot \delta t / T)\} \tag{22}$$

Figure 6 illustrates this process of equidistant time domain sampling. Equidistance in the time domains leads to nonequidistance in the k-space domain. The total k-space, Δk_{RO}, covered during the readout period, T_{RO}, is given by:

$$\Delta k_{RO} = \gamma \cdot \int_{t_a}^{t_b} G_{RO} \cdot \sin(\omega \cdot t') dt'$$

$$\Delta k_{RO} = \frac{\gamma \cdot G_{RO} \cdot T}{2\pi} \cdot \{\cos(2\pi \cdot t_a / T) - \cos(2\pi \cdot t_b / T)\} \tag{23}$$

which is equivalent to the area under the gradient pulse for the duration of the data acquisition window, T_{RO}.

As noted above, conventional MR image reconstruction uses a 2D FT that requires equidistantly spaced data so that artifact-free images are obtained. This is illustrated in Fig. 7. A simulated spin-echo (SE) image (not EPI) is shown, with a sinusoidal RO gradient pulse instead of the conventionally applied constant gradient during the RO period is shown. The resulting image (Fig. 7b) shows ringing artifacts and geometric distortion along the (vertical) RO direction. When a proper interpolation is used, the ringing vanishes completely (as shown in Fig. 7a). Clinical images of acceptable quality therefore require further steps in the image reconstruction process, as is shown in the following section.

A major question remains to be answered: how do we achieve the equidistance in the k-space domain when the original data are nonequidistantly distributed over k-space? For this purpose we introduce the concept of rasters, namely the interpolation rasters R_{RO} (for the RO) and R_{PC} (for the PC direction) and the ADC-sampling rasters, R_{ADC}. An RO interpolation raster describes those time points, t_m, for which the k-space is sampled equidistantly:

$$\partial k_{RO} = k_{RO}(t_m) - k_{RO}(t_{m-1})$$

$$k_{RO}(t_m) = m \cdot \delta k_{RO} \tag{24}$$

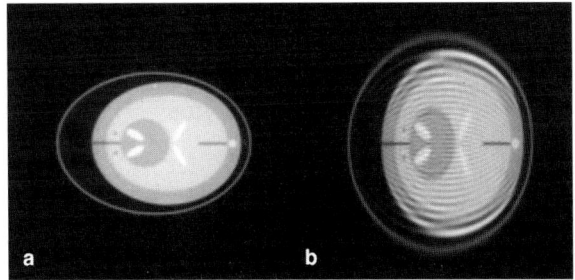

Fig. 7a,b. Image reconstruction of simulated SE MR data acquired under a sinusoidal RO gradient. The RO gradient is sinusoidal. **a** The reconstructed image shows ringing artifacts along the RO direction (*vertical*) when the RO interpolation is not used. **b** After the RO interpolation the ringing is eliminated, and full resolution is restored

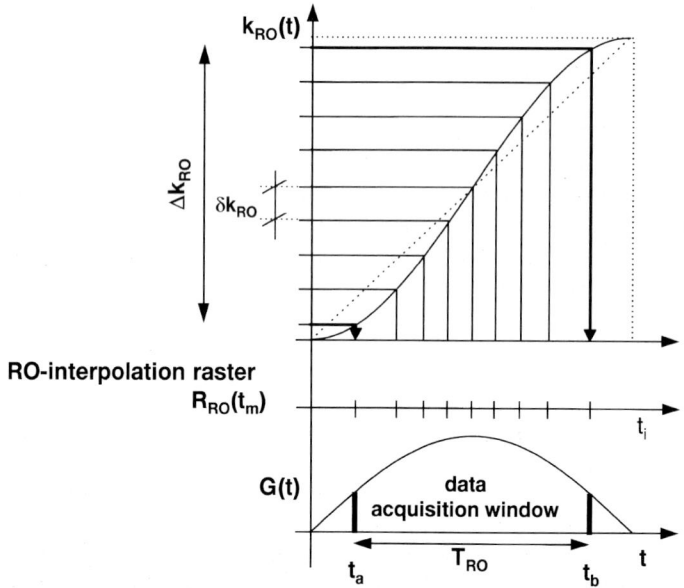

Fig. 8. Geometric construction of the interpolation raster R_{RO}. The covered k-space, Δk_{RO}, is scanned in equidistant steps of δk_{RO} and reflected onto the inverse function (*curved line*) that maps into the correct locations of the time axis

where δk_{RO} is defined as the minimal distance required along the k_{RO} direction so that the Nyquist theorem is fullfilled:

$$\delta k_{RO} = \frac{\Delta k_{RO}}{N_{RO}} \tag{25}$$

with Δk_{RO} given by Eq. 23. What remains now is to calculate the t_m values of Eq. 24. This is done by calculating the inverse function, $k_{RO}^{-1}(t)$, of Eq. 21 by means of Eq. 25:

$$R_{RO}(m) = t_m = \frac{T}{2\pi} \arccos\left\{ \cos\left(2\pi \frac{t_a}{T}\right) - m \cdot \frac{\cos\left(2\pi \frac{t_a}{T}\right) - \cos\left(2\pi \frac{t_b}{T}\right)}{N_{RO}} \right\} \tag{26}$$

A geometrical construction of the interpolation raster is shown in Fig. 8. The covered k-space is scanned in equidistant steps of δk_{RO} and is mirrored by the k-space trajectory, $k_{RO}(t)$ (curved line), onto the time axis. This yields the time points, t_m, which fulfill Eq. 24.

Interpolation

After calculating the RO interpolation raster, $R_{RO}(m)$, we now describe the final step needed to recover uniform k-space coverage: the interpolation. As mentioned above, the interpolation raster describes the time points, t_m, for which the k-space is sampled equidistantly. Therefore the MR signal that we acquire under the sine gradient pulse must be reconstructed exactly at these times, t_m to recreate an image without artifacts. Let $S(t)$ be the continuous MR signal acquired under a single sinusoidal RO gradient. Then the signal sampled at time, $t = m \cdot \delta t$, is described as:

$$\hat{S}(m \cdot \delta t) = S(t) \cdot \sum_m \delta(t - m \cdot \delta t) \tag{27}$$

where $\Sigma\, \delta(t-m\cdot\delta t)$ describes a delta function which is equal to 1 for times $t = m \cdot \delta t$ and 0 elsewhere, and the index m describes the point to be actually sampled. (Note: We define our delta function as an infinitesimally short rectangular pulses of amplitude equal to 1. This is different to the integral definition of the Dirac delta function [3] usually used in the literature.)

The signal to be reconstructed is described as $\hat{S}(t_m)$. Figure 9 shows left (from bottom to top) the interpolation raster $R_{RO}(t_m)$, the equidistant ADC sampling raster, the continuous MR signal, $S(t)$, with the sampled data points (○), $\hat{S}(m \cdot \delta t)$, and the data points to be reconstructed by interpolation (□), $\hat{S}(t_m)$, under the sinusoidal RO gradient pulse $G(t)$. At the right a magnified region of the MR signal is shown centered around the sample that is to be interpolated at $t = t_m$ to be interpolated. In general the process of interpolation can be described as:

$$\hat{S}(t_m) = \sum_{j=0}^{J-1} \hat{S}_{m_o+j} \cdot a_j \tag{28}$$

where J is the total number of neighboring data points to be considered for the interpolation. For each $\hat{S}(t_1)$ to be reconstructed we use the measured data points $\hat{S}_{m_o} \ldots \hat{S}_{m_o+j} \ldots \hat{S}_{m_o+J-1}$ for the interpolation. The interpolation coefficients a_j and the index m_o depend on the time, t_m, for which the signal, $\hat{S}(t_m)$, is to be recovered.

The question is now: What are the optimal interpolation coefficients, a_j? To answer this we must bear in mind that the MR signal is in general a very fast changing signal and therefore requires special attention. Polynomial or cubic spline interpolation [10] does not satisfy the Nyquist theorem adequately. Based on the Nyquist theorem a sinc function interpolation is therefore recommended [11].

The basic idea behind the sinc function interpolation is demonstrated in Fig. 10. Sinc functions with the amplitude $\hat{S}(m \cdot \delta t)$ are centered around times $t = m \cdot \delta t$ having zeros exactly at multiples of the sampling time δt. Only at times of $t \neq m \cdot \delta t$ do the side lobes of the neighboring sinc functions contribute to the signal, $\hat{S}(t_m)$, to be recovered indicated with a box (□). In a mathematical form this is expressed as:

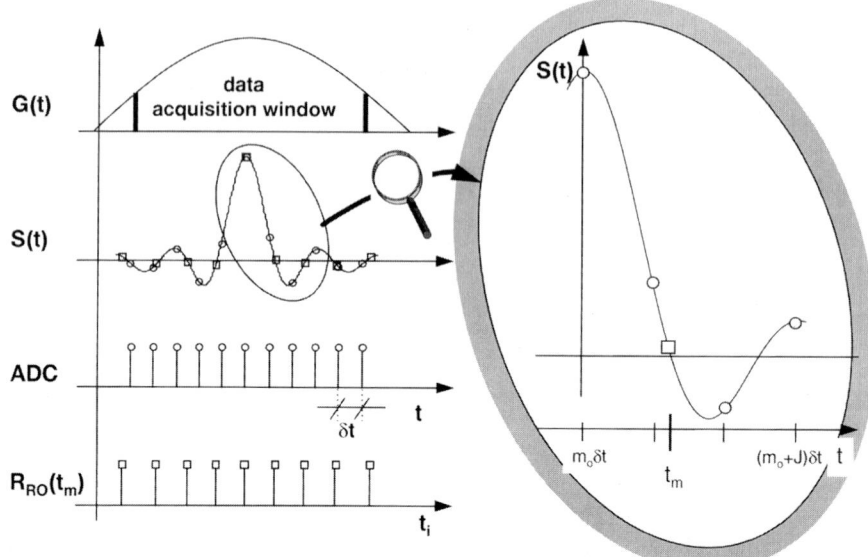

Fig. 9. Interpolation to obtain uniform k-space distribution. *Left, from bottom to top*, interpolation raster, ADC sampling raster, continuous MR signal showing the sampled data points ($\bigcirc$) and data points to be reconstructed by interpolation ($\square$), and the sinusoidal RO gradient pulse. *Right*, a magnified region of the MR signal centered around the sample located at $t = t_m$ to be interpolated. $J = 4$ data points from the acquired dataset, $\hat{S}$, are used to calculate the signal $\hat{S}(t = t_m)$

$$\hat{S}(t_m) = \sum_{j=0}^{J-1} \hat{S}_{m_o+j} \cdot \mathrm{sinc}\left(\frac{t_m - (m_o + j) \cdot \delta t}{\delta t}\right) \tag{29}$$

The interpolation coefficients:

$$a_j(R_{RO}(m)) = \mathrm{sinc}\left(\frac{R_{RO}(m) - (m_o + j) \cdot \delta t}{\delta t}\right) \tag{30}$$

are usually stored as lookup tables because they depend directly on the shape of the RO gradient pulse and the corresponding RO interpolation raster, $R_{RO}(m)$, described by Eq. 26. The lookup tables are stored prior to the start of the sequence execution and help to speed reconstruction. This is important for gaining the fastest reconstruction time possible.

Alternative methods for gaining uniform samples along the RO direction have been proposed in recent past years. One of these, proposed by Zakhor et al. [14], describes an interpolation method based on the maximum likelihood estimator. Other sinc interpolation techniques are described in the literature [11–13, 15].

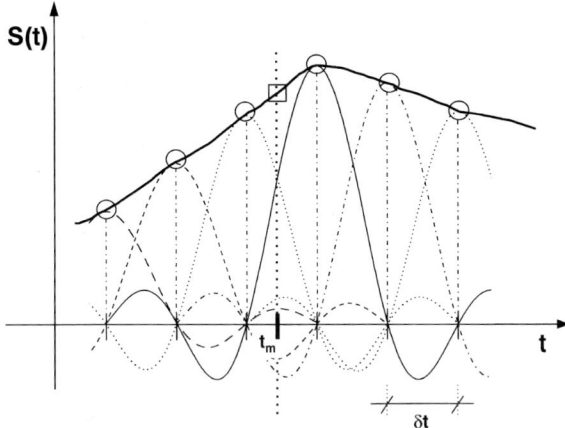

Fig. 10. Graphic description of the sinc function interpolation. Around each regulary spaced data point (○) a sinc function is centered with the amplitude of signal at that time. The signal (□) at the time t_m is calculated by summing all contributions from the sinc functions corresponding to the neighboring samples

Uniform k-Space Data Sampling

The interpolation of the MR signal onto a uniform grid in k-space can be a time-consuming process depending on the length of the interpolation kernel, J. One way to eliminate the lengthy interpolation process is to sample the time-domain data in such a manner that the k-space is scanned uniformly. Ordidge et al. [16] and Howseman et al. [17] described this technique. It poses some demands on the data-acquisition system. Conventional data-acquisition systems address the time points to be sampled equidistantly with sampling times down to 1 μs. For nonequidistant time sampling the ADC must to be triggered with an accuracy of about 100 ns to avoid degradations in the final image.

The condition to achieve uniform k-space sampling is given by the following relation:

$$\gamma \int_{t_m}^{t_{im+1}} G_{RO}(t)dt = \delta k_{RO} \tag{31}$$

where δk_{RO} is defined inith Eq. 25. In a graphic interpretation this means that the area under the RO gradient pulse, $G_{RO}(t)$, measured from a time t_m to a time t_{m+1} must be constant and independent of the time t_m. This is shown in Fig. 11, which selects two different intervals (areas A1 and A2).

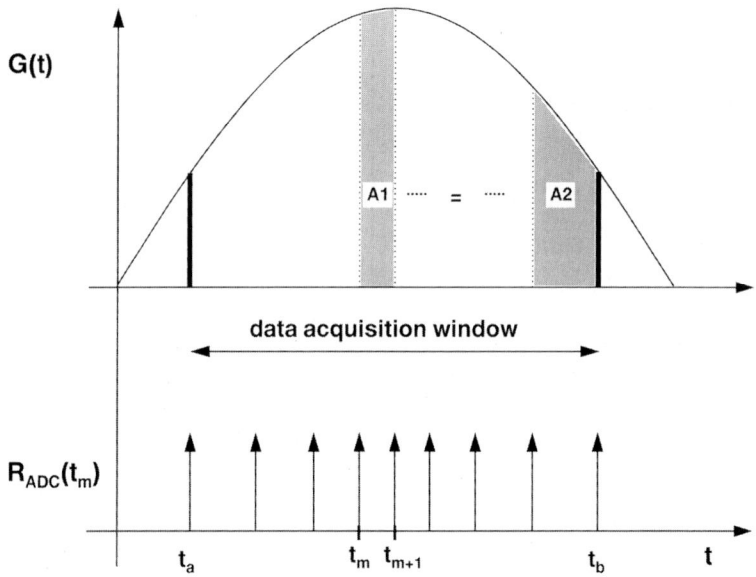

Fig. 11. Nonequidistant ADC triggering. The trigger times are adjusted such that the area under the gradient pulse between times t_m to t_{m+1} is always constant

In the case of a sinusoidal RO gradient pulse, as described in Eq. 19, the ADC raster, R_{ADC}, can be calculated as the interpolation raster, R_{RO}. If we assume the same starting and ending time (t_a and t_b) of the data acquisition window, R_{RO} and R_{ADC} are identical:

$$R_{ADC}(m) = t_m = \frac{T}{2\pi}\arccos\left\{\cos\left(2\pi\frac{t_a}{T}\right) - m \cdot \frac{\cos\left(2\pi\frac{t_a}{T}\right) - \cos\left(2\pi\frac{t_b}{T}\right)}{N_{RO}}\right\} \qquad (32)$$

The number of data samples, N_{sample}, that must be acquired with the nonlinear ADC triggering method differs from the equidistant time domain sampling. Only N_{sample} equal to the matrix size, N_{RO}, are needed. This reduces the reconstruction time as well because fewer data points must be transfered through the data bus of the image processor.

Phase-Encoding Data Reconstruction

With some trajectories the k_{PC} direction shows nonuniformity similar to that along the k_{RO} direction. This is the case with the trajectories TRJ1–TRJ6 in Fig. 4. Nonuniformity occurs when the PC gradient is on during the data acquisition window, T_{RO}. In constant phase encoding (TRJ1, TRJ4, TRJ6) a constant gradient is present over the T_{RO} period whereas for blipped phase encoding (TRJ2, TRJ3, TRJ5), nonequidistance appears only at the outer edges of the k-space (i.e., in k_{RO} direction). Let us consider the trajectory TRJ4, again in order to analyze the principles of the k_{PC} direction (Figs. 12, 13). The sampling pattern in the k_{PC} direction differs from column to column (C1→C2). The ideal k_{PC} lines are shown as dotted horizontal lines. The sign of the deviation, ε, changes when stepped through even and odd data line numbers (i.e., n→n+1). k-Space samples are sampled equidistantly at the center (column C1) and show an alternating pattern (wide↔narrow) for higher k_{RO} values (column C2). In the extreme case the deviation, ε, degenerates to the maximal and minimal values of $\varepsilon = 0$ or $\varepsilon = \delta k_{PC}$, causing singularities which must be considered for the PC data reconstruction.

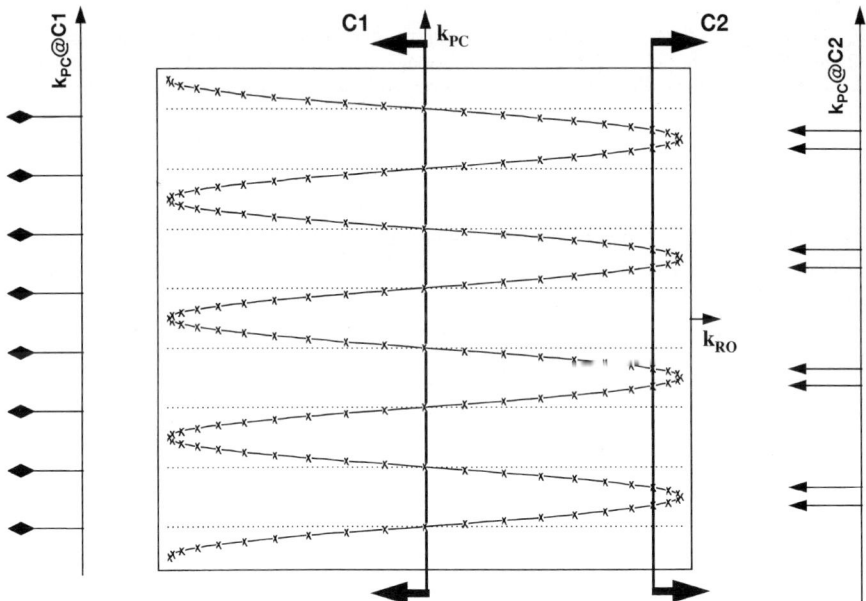

Fig. 12. The k-space trajectory (*TRJ4*) of a sinusoidal RO gradient and a constant PC gradient. The sampling pattern in the k_{PC} direction differs from column to column (C1→C2). K_{PC} samples are placed symetrically around the k_{PC} lines (*dotted horizontal lines*)

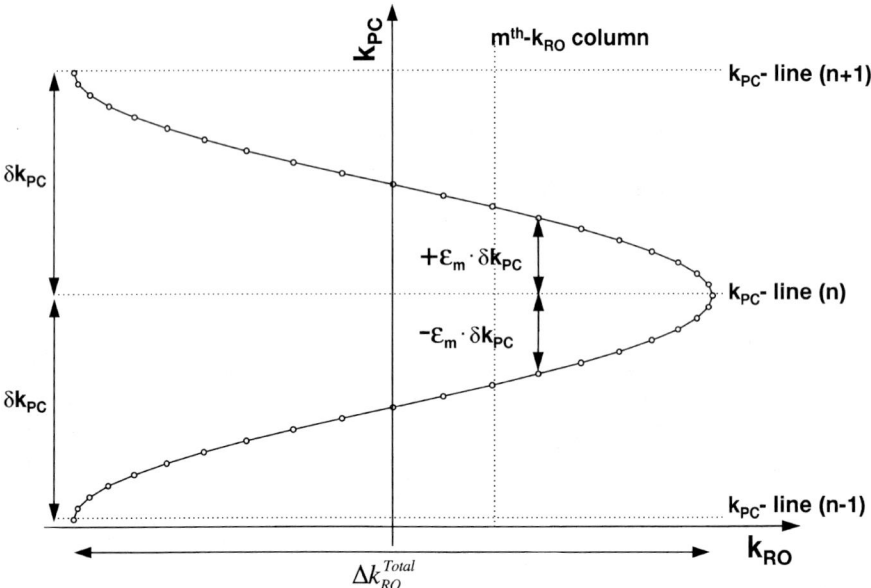

Fig. 13. Two lines of the k-space trajectory (*TRJ4*). Compared to Fig. 12 the ideal k_{PC} data lines (*dotted lines*) are shifted by $\frac{1}{2}$ δk_{PC} to obtain antisymmetric distribution of ε_m. The sign of the deviation, ε_m, changes when stepped through even and odd data line numbers (i.e., $n \rightarrow n+1$)

The Phase-Encoding Raster

There are two basic possibilities for calculating the PC raster. With uniform time-domain signal sampling it can be calculated either before or after the RO data interpolation. However, there are good reasons to apply the PC raster to the RO interpolated data. The reconstruction time is shorter because only N_{RO} data points must be considered, and the above effects of the singularities can be minimized, yielding better signal to noise.

As can be seen from Fig. 13, the PC raster, $R_{PC}(m)$, depends on the RO interpolation raster and can be related through the following expression:

$$R_{PC}(m) = \left(\frac{k_{RO}(R_{RO}(m))}{\Delta k_{RO}^{Total}} - \frac{1}{2} \right) \cdot \delta k_{PC} \tag{33}$$

where δk_{PC} is the minimal required k_{PC} distance to fulfill the Nyquist theorem, i.e., the separation of the k_{PC} data lines as shown in Fig. 13:

$$\delta k_{PC} = \gamma \int_0^{T/2} G_{PC}(t) \cdot dt \tag{34}$$

and Δk_{RO}^{Total} is the total k_{RO} space excursion over the duration, $T/2$, of the entire RO gradient pulse:

$$\Delta k_{RO}^{Total} = \gamma \int_0^{T/2} G_{RO}(t) \cdot dt \tag{35}$$

In summary, the PC raster, $R_{PC}(m)$, contains the deviations from the rectangular k_{PC} grid corresponding to the actual RO raster, $R_{RO}(m)$. The PC raster has a total number of N_{RO} elements.

Interlaced FT

Figure 12 illustrates that the k_{PC} samples are distributed nonuniformly along the k_{PC} axis. The data show an alternating pattern: narrow, wide, narrow, wide, etc. However, uniformity is required to generate an artifact-free image. Bracewell [3] first described in 1978 how these data can be uniquely reconstructed using the "interlaced FT" reconstruction. This idea was reinvented and patented by Sekihara et al. [18, 19] in 1987. The basic idea of the interlaced FT reconstruction is to extract two different data sets, $S_{m1}(k_{PC})$ and $S_{m2}(k_{PC})$, from the original data set $S_m(k_{PC})$ that are sampled equidistantly. The original data set $S_m(k_{PC})$ is the m'th column along the k_{PC} direction corresponding to the m'th-k_{RO} data point (see Fig. 12). Figure 14 shows the process of splitting the data and the complete reconstruction along the PC direction.

For the sake of convenience we have shifted the ideal k_{PC} lines by $\frac{1}{2} \delta k_{PC}$ (see Fig. 13) to obtain an antisymmetric distribution of ε_m. With this simplification, let R_{m1} and R_{m2} be the sampling rasters (along k_{PC}) for the samples shifted by $+\varepsilon_m \delta k_{PC}$ and $-\varepsilon_m \delta k_{PC}$, respectively, expressed as:

$$R_{m1}(k_{PC}) = \sum_{j=1}^{N_{PC}/2} \delta(k_{PC} - \delta k_{PC}(2j + \varepsilon_m))$$

$$R_{m2}(k_{PC}) = \sum_{j=1}^{N_{PC}/2} \delta(k_{PC} - \delta k_{PC}(2j + \varepsilon_m)) \tag{36}$$

Then the splitdata and its corresponding projections (the 1D-Fourier transformed data set $S_m(y)$ is called a projection because it resembles a projection of the object; projections therefore describe signals in the image domain) are described as:

$$S_{m1}(k_{PC}) = S_m(k_{PC}) \cdot R_{m1}(k_{PC}) \qquad\qquad S_{m1}(y) = S_m(y) * R_{m1}(y)$$

$$\xleftarrow{\quad 1D\text{-}FT \quad}$$

$$S_{m2}(k_{PC}) = S_m(k_{PC}) \cdot R_{m2}(k_{PC}) \qquad\qquad S_{m2}(y) = S_m(y) * R_{m2}(y) \tag{37}$$

When we introduce the FT's of the rasters R_{m1} and R_{m2} we finally gain the projections S_{m1}, S_{m2}:

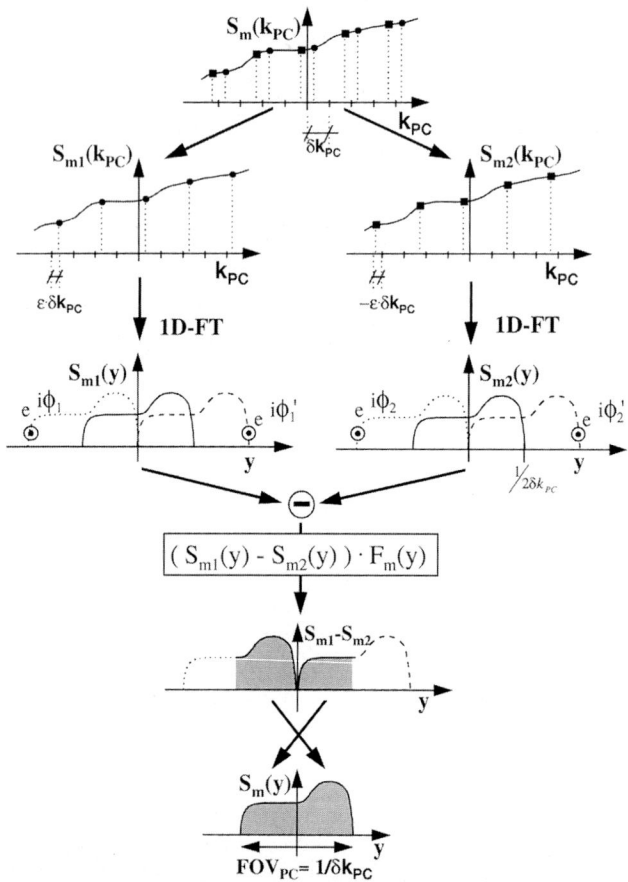

Fig. 14. Interlaced FT reconstruction scheme based on Bracewell. Data are split into two data sets showing uniform samples with twice the sampling width. This causes back folding (aliasing) after the 1D FT indicated by the overlap of the projections. The signal to be retrieved, S_m, can be calculated from the two projections S_{m1} and S_{m2} by subtraction, filtering, and flipping the left versus the right half

$$S_{m1}(y) = S_m(y) * \sum_{j'=-\infty}^{\infty} \delta(y - \frac{j'}{2\delta k_{PC}}) \cdot e^{i\pi j' \varepsilon_m}$$

$$S_{m2}(y) = S_m(y) * \sum_{j'=-\infty}^{\infty} \delta(y - \frac{j'}{2\delta k_{PC}}) \cdot e^{i\pi j' \varepsilon_m}$$

$$(38)$$

where * denotes the convolution operation [3]. From these two data sets we can calculated the true projection $S_m(y)$ by subtracting S_{m2} from S_{m1}, followed by additional filtering as shown in Fig. 14 and described by Eqs. 39 and 40:

Fig. 15. Reconstructed raw data (the signal in the k-space domain) shows increased noise at the left and right side (k_{RO} direction is horizontal) when the k_{PC} raster degenerates (i.e., $\varepsilon_m = 0$ or $\varepsilon_m = \delta k_{PC}$)

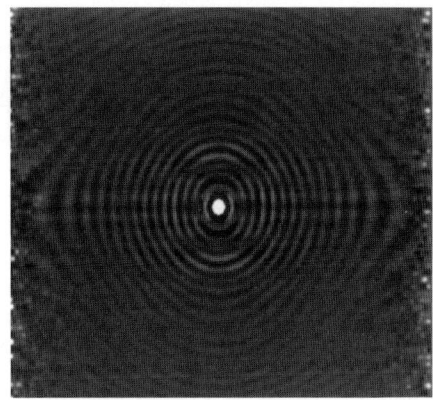

$$S_m^-(y) = (S_{m1}(y) - S_{m2}(y)) \cdot F_{m1}(y) \tag{39}$$

The filter, F_m, depends on the actual deviation from the ideal k_{PC} raster, ε_m:

$$F_m(y) = \frac{1}{-2i \cdot \sin(\pi\varepsilon_m)} \quad \textit{for} \quad y < 0$$

$$F_m(y) = \frac{1}{2i \cdot \sin(\pi\varepsilon_m)} \quad \textit{for} \quad y \geq 0 \tag{40}$$

The true projection, $S_m(y)$, is finally obtained by exchanging the left ($y<0$) with the right ($y \geq 0$) half of the projection $S_m^-(y)$, as shown at the bottom of Fig. 14.

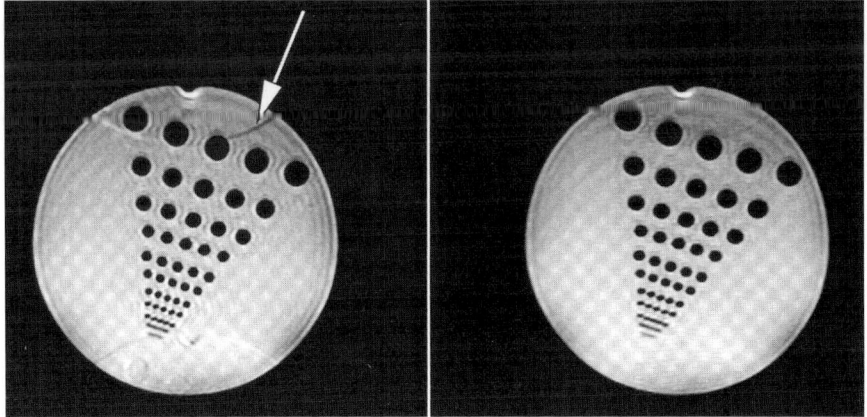

Fig. 16. Reconstructed images demonstrate the effect of the interlaced FT reconstruction. *Left,* without interlaced; sickle-shaped N/2 ghosting artifacts are present. *Right,* reconstructed phantom image shows no ghost when the interlaced FT is perfomed; ringing artifacts along the PC direction are present in these images. This is caused by the asymmetric k-space sampling. The echo appears in the 32nd data line. A 128×128 image matrix is reconstructed. The RO direction is horizontal

In the case of a degenerates k_{PC} raster [i.e., $\varepsilon_m \rightarrow 0$ or $\varepsilon_m \rightarrow \delta k_{PC} \Rightarrow F_m(y) \rightarrow \infty$] the resulting projection $S_m(y)$ is distorted, and typically increased noise is observed at the outer edges of the k-space along the k_{RO} direction when the reconstructed image $S(x,y)$ is back-transformed (via 2D FT) into the k-space as shown in Fig. 15. Therefore it is common to truncate the outermost k_{RO} columns of the k-space when the k_{PC} raster is being degenerated.

The effect of the interlaced FT is demonstrated on simulated raw data (Fig. 16). Without the interlaced FT reconstruction sickle-shaped N/2 ghosting artifacts usually appear (Fig. 16a). The artifacts vanish when the interlaced FT is performed (Fig. 16b). Thus the application of the interlaced FT is always desirable to maintain image quality when the PC gradient is on during the data acquisition window, as it is the case of ROM1–ROM6 in Fig. 4.

Reconstruction Under Real Conditions

EPI is very sensitive to ghosting artifacts. Because the MR signal is sampled under alternating gradients, a data reversal of every other line is necessary. Thus almost any imperfection in the MR system leads to a signal modulation with half the Nyquist frequency, causing a so-called N/2 ghost [5] in the PC direction. For example, one source of the N/2 ghosting is the cutoff characteristic of the analog low pass filter (for other sources of the N/2 ghost see Chap. 6). Due to causality [20] the output signal of the low pass filter is distorted asymmetrically in the positive time direction, causing Gibbs ringing artifacts depending on the steepness of the filter (see Fig. 5 in Chap. 6). In conventional MRI this does not lead to any significant image errors. However, in EPI every second line is reflected with respect to time, so that the distortion occurs alternatingly in positive and negative k_{RO} direction.

Another cause of even and odd echo modulation is the synchronization between the ADC raster and the actual RO gradient pulse. If these are not aligned, severe N/2 ghosting results (see Figs. 2, 3 in Chap. 6). Without correction this leads to severe N/2 artifacts. The suppression of the N/2 ghost has therefore become an important issue in image quality [22].

Reference Scans

The above alternation can be observed on a special raw data set which is collected before, during, or after data acquisition and referred to as navigator scan, correction prescan, calibration, or reference scan. A reference scan [5] is measured by switching off the PC gradient ($G_{PC} = 0$), as shown in Fig. 17, while keeping the timing of the sequence identical. The reference MR data are acquired as regular EPI scans. In the ideal case (i.e., perfect hardware conditions, ideal shim and without T2 effects) we would expect a set of N_{PC}-identical echoes. In reality differences are present, as demonstrated in the raw data set of Fig. 18a acquired with an SE EPI sequence. Echoes are therefore narrow at the center of k-space and broader at the higher k_{PC} data lines. Echo broadening is caused by

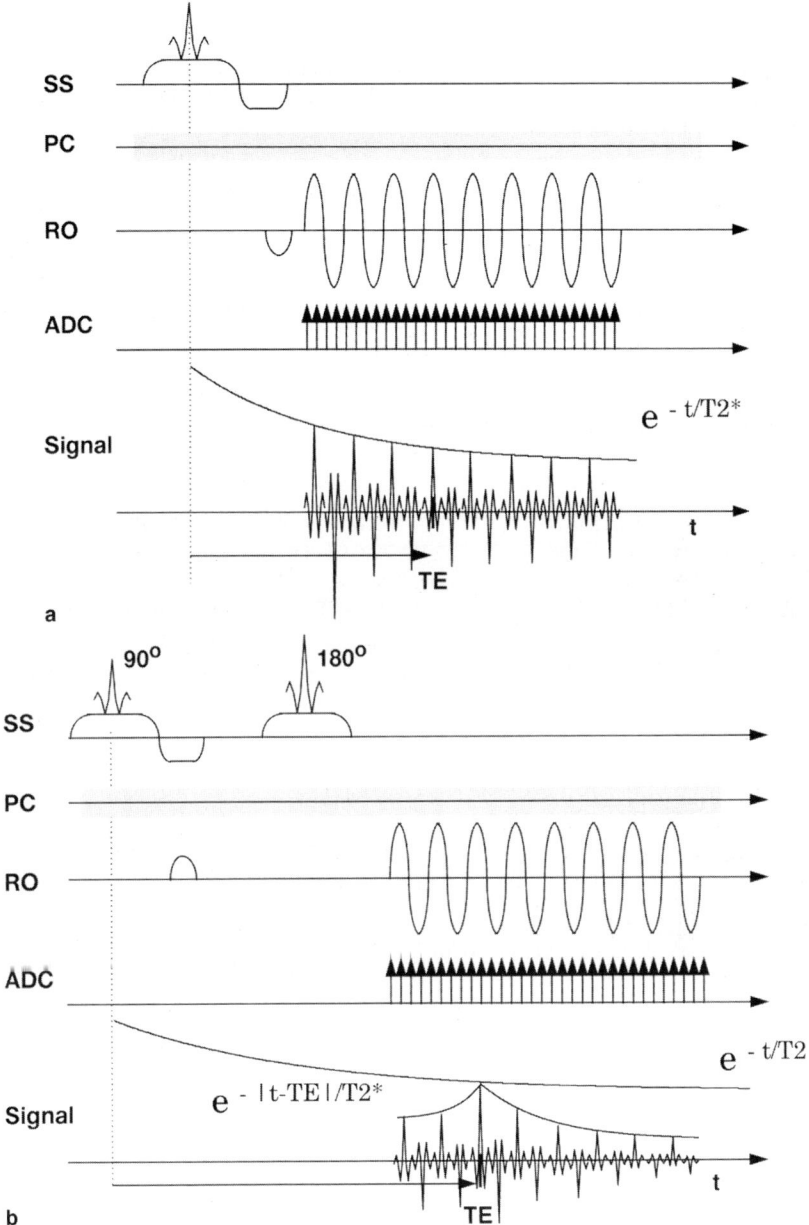

Fig. 17a–b. EPI reference scans based on a GRE and SE EPI sequence. The PC gradient is switched off to avoid the phase encoding of the acquired MR signal. Filters are calculated from the acquired raw data that can minimize the N/2 ghosting artifact effectively. **a** GRE EPI reference scan; the entire matrix size is acquired. **b** SE EPI reference scan; the entire matrix size is acquired.

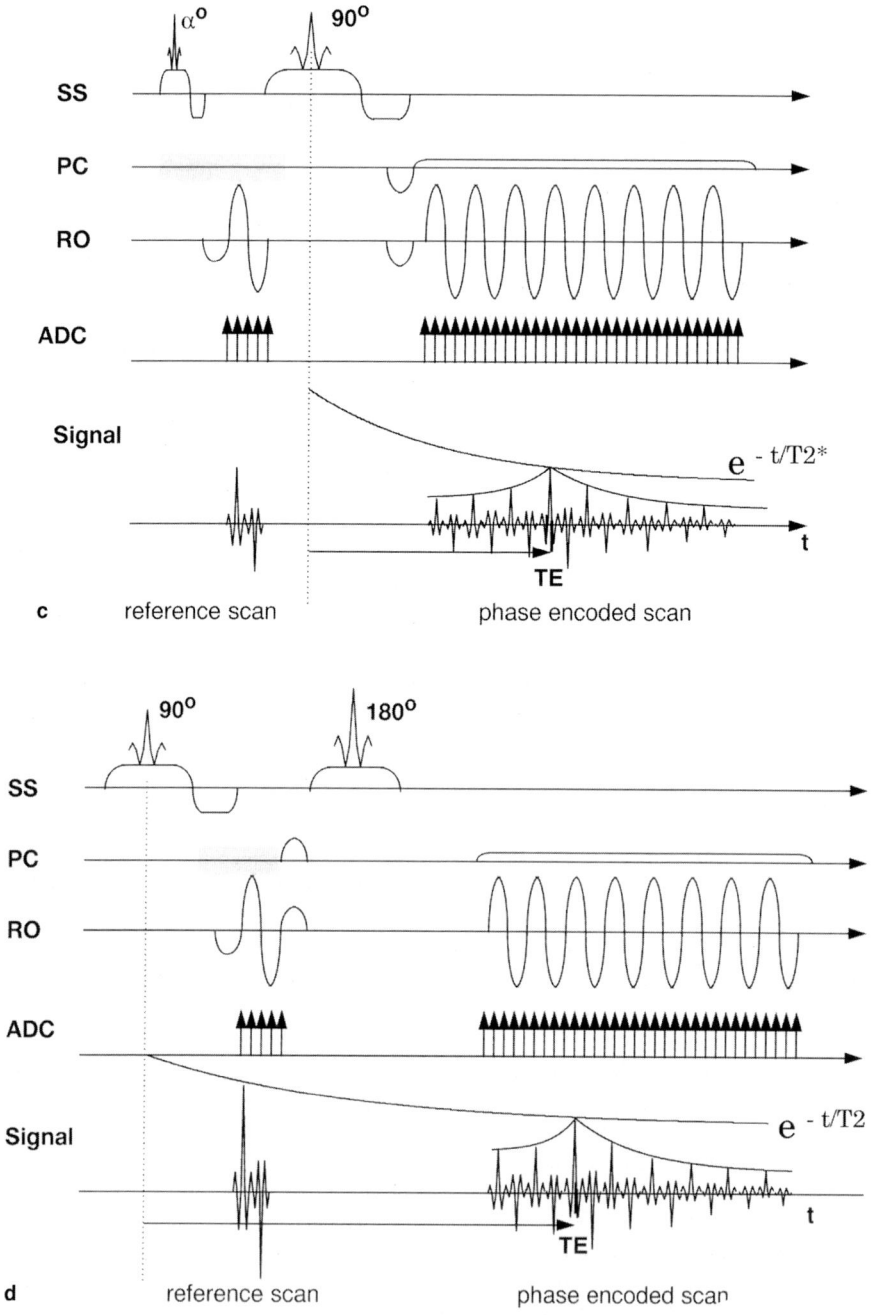

Fig. 17c–d. GRE EPI scan preceeded by a reference scan consisting of only two lines. Low flip-angle RF pulses are applied in order to affect the image scan minimally. **d** SE EPI scan with the acquisition of two reference line between the 90° and 180° RF pulses

B_o inhomogeneity; the spins dephase under this inhomogeneity, become rephased at the echo time, and dephase again. The alternation of the even and odd echoes is generally noticed.

Figure 17a,b shows EPI reference scans for GRE and SE EPI sequences. The switched-off PC gradient is highlighted by the shaded area in Fig. 17. Reference scans of this kind are usually acquired before or after the imaging sequence. For multislice studies it can be measured for all slices or only for the center slice from which the required information to compensate for the even and odd echo alternation is extracted. The total acquisition time for a single reference scan equals the scan time per image for the regular GRE and SE EPI sequences in this case. Therefore reference scans are time consuming and cannot always be performed, for example, for imaging regions of the body which tend to move quickly such as the heart. For this purpose alternatives exist, as shown in Fig. 17c,d. Only two lines of reference scan raw data are acquired reflecting the even and odd alternation (see below). For the GRE EPI sequence the reference data are acquired just prior to the imaging sequence by exciting the spins with a low flip angle RF pulse ($\alpha<10°$) that preserves most of the M_z magnetization for the following imaging scan. The time between the application of the 90° and 180° pulses can be used to place the reference scan for a SE EPI sequence. The echo time is prolongued only by typically 1–2 ms causing no real drawback for clinical applications. A modification of the sequences of Fig. 17c,d has been proposed by Heid [21]. Instead of two reference lines three are acquired, improving the N/2 ghost suppression, when very short eddy currents and large off resonances are present.

Filters Deduced from Reference Scans

As mentioned above, the alternating pattern of even and odd echoes can be reflected in reference scans performed before, during, or after the imaging scan. These scans can provide significant information to yield artifact-free images. Many proposals to achieve artifact-free images have been made in recent years since EPI entered the clinical market. We do not describe these methods and refer the reader to the literature [24, 25]. In this section we describe how the required information can be extracted from the reference scans to compensate for the hardware imperfections.

Constant and Linear Phase Correction

In general echoes of reference scans show variations both in the echo position and in the phase. For example, the shifts can be seen from the reference scan of Fig. 18a. Because the reference scans are merely modified imaging scans, the same echo shifting and phases must be present for the corresponding phase-encoded EPI scan. If the position and the phase at the individual echo peaks are known, for example, by using a parabola fit to the echo peaks (echo shift) or by performing a linear fit [237, 29] to the phase after a 1D-FT, this shift between echoes can be corrected by means of a linear phase correction (Fourier-shift theorem) after a 1D-FT of the time signal. (For uniform time sampling it is important to emphasize that any kind of echo shift correction should be performed prior to the RO interpolation to achieve the best results; see Fig. 21). The phase, Φ_o, of the echo peak can also be calculated by the arc tangent of imaginary (Im) and real (Re) part:

$$\Phi_o = \arctan\left\{\frac{\mathrm{Im}\{S^R(k_e)\}}{\mathrm{Re}\{S^R(k_e)\}}\right\}$$

Even when the shifts, k_e, and phases Φ_o, are very small, i.e., $k_e \ll \delta k_{RO}$ and $\Phi_o \ll \pi$, effects in the final image are visible. Therefore the shift and the phase difference from line to line must be corrected.

Fig. 18. a Reference scan raw data measured with a SE EPI sequence ($G_{PC} = 0$). Broadening of echoes depends on the time difference to the RF spin echo time. The alternation pattern of even and odd echoes is visible, resulting from hardware imperfection during the data acquisition. **b** Nonlinear phase correction applied to the reference scan to show its effect. Echoes are aligned after the self correction. **c** Phantom image reconstructed without any phase correction ($\phi_o = 0$; $\phi_1 = 0$). Strong N/2 ghosting is present. The number of fringes indicate a large shift between even and odd echoes. **d** Phantom image reconstructed with correct constant and linear phase ($\phi_o = 0.1\pi$; $\Phi_1 = -7\delta k_{RO}$) evaluated from a reference scan. Ghosting is almost below the noise level. The remaining ghost can be explained by nonlinear phases due to hardware imperfections. **e** The linear phase is corrected but the constant phase is mismatched ($\phi_o = 0.25\pi$; $\phi_1 = -7\ \delta k_{RO}$). An isointense N/2 ghost is present. **f** The constant phase is corrected but the linear phase is mismatched ($\phi_o = 0.1\pi$; $\phi_1 = -3.4\ \delta k_{RO}$). Fringes appear due to the echo shifting

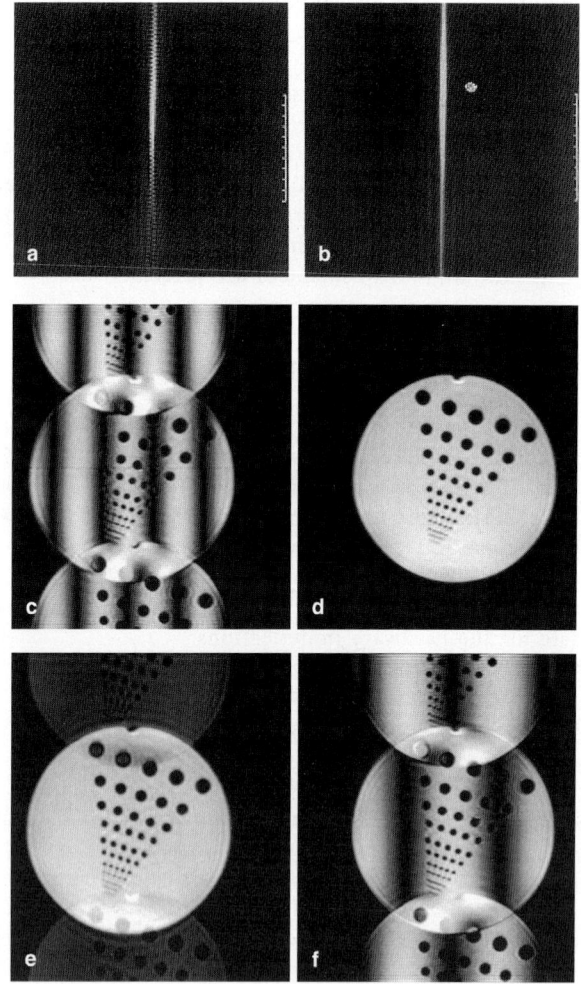

Let $k_o(n)$ be the individual echo shift and $\Phi_o(n)$ be the constant phase of the n'th k_{PC} data line calculated from the reference scan. Let $S_n^{R'}(k_{RO})$ and $S_n^{M'}(k_{RO})$ be the corresponding phase encoded measurement scan affected by the hardware imperfections. The ideal k-space signals (without any distortions due to hardware imperfections) are described as $S_n^R(k_{RO})$ and $S_n^M(k_{RO})$, respectively. The 1D FT signals, depending on the x coordinate of the final image (remember the Fourier correspondence between k-space↔image-space coordinates are: k_{RO}↔x and k_{PC}↔y), are then described as $S_n^R(x)$, $S_n^{R'}(x)$, $S_n^M(x)$, and $S_n^{M'}(x)$, respectively. The following relationship then holds for the shifted echo signal in the k-space and image domain:

$$S_n^{M'}(k_{RO}) = S_n^M(k_{RO}-k_o(n)) \cdot e^{i\Phi_o(n)} \xrightarrow{\text{1D-FT}} S_n^{M'}(x) = S_n^M(x) \cdot e^{i2\pi k_o(n)x} \cdot e^{i\Phi_o(n)}$$

(41)

the shift of the echo can therefore be compensated by means of a filter $F_n^L(x)$ with an inverted phase:

$$F_n^L(x) = e^{-i2\pi k_o(n)x} \cdot e^{-i\Phi_o(n)} \tag{42}$$

$$S_n^M(x) = S_n^{M'}(x) \cdot F_n^L(x) \tag{43}$$

Fig. 18c–f shows reconstructed images with the different constant and linear phase corrections performed. Isointense ghosting appears when the linear phase is corrected exactly, whereas fringes in the ghost appear when the linear phase does not correspond to the echo shift.

Nonlinear Phase Correction

Imaging under realistic conditions may also show nonlinear phase errors. In this section we evaluate correction schemes for these effects. For this purpose let us assume that higher order phase errors exists in the projection data of the reference scans and in the image scans, described as:

$$S_n^{R'}(k_{RO}) \xrightarrow{\text{1D-FT}} S_n^{R'}(x) = S_n^R(x) \cdot e^{i\Phi_n^R(x)}$$

$$S_n^{M'}(k_{RO}) \xrightarrow{\text{1D-FT}} S_n^{M'}(x) = S_n^M(x) \cdot e^{i\Phi_n(x)}$$

(44)

A nonlinear phase filter $F_n^{NL}(x)$ is deduced from the reference scan projection (i.e., merely inverting its phase) compensating these higher order effects:

$$F_n^{NL}(x) = e^{-i\Phi_n^R(x)} \tag{45}$$

Finally the true projections are retrieved by means of this filter:

$$S_n^M(x) = S_n^{M'}(x) \cdot F_n^{NL}(x) \tag{46}$$

Figure 18d shows the resulting image. Compared to the linear phase corrected image (Fig. 18c) the N/2 ghosting is significantly reduced. When we apply the nonlinear phase filter to the reference scan itself and transform these data back to the k-space domain by means of a 1D FT, we can see the effect on the raw data (Fig. 18b). The echoes are now exactly aligned. Only the T2 and T2* effects are present, reflected in the echo magnitude.

Modulation Tranfer Function Deconvolution

MR signals generated by the initial RF excitation are affected by signal deteriorations through several processes defined by hardware imperfections. As long as these processes are linear (i.e., are valid for any k-space sample measured at any time), they can be described by a so-called modulation transfer function (MTF) and corresponding point spread function (PSF). There is a simple relationshp between MTF and PSF [3]. The PSF is defined as the 1D FT of the MTF. In this section we use this formalism to describe the presence of N/2 ghosting, one for the even and one for the odd echo lines.

Let $PSF_e(k_{RO})$ and $PSF_o(k_{RO})$ represent the PSF for the even and odd k_{PC} data lines acquired under positive and negative RO gradients and $MTF_e(x)$ and $MTF_o(x)$ the corresponding MTFs, respectively. Then the following relationships hold for the reference scans:

$$S_{n_e}^{R'}(k_{RO}) = S^R(k_{RO})*PSF_e(k_{RO}) \xrightarrow{\ 1D\text{-}FT\ } S_{n_e}^{R'}(x) = S^R(x) \cdot MTF_e(x)$$
$$S_{n_o}^{R'}(k_{RO}) = S^R(k_{RO})*PSF_o(k_{RO}) \xrightarrow{\ 1D\text{-}FT\ } S_{n_o}^{R'}(x) = S^R(x) \cdot MTF_o(x)$$

(47)

and for the phase-encoded scans split into lines $n_e = 2, 4, 6,...$ N_{RO}, and $n_o = 1,3,5,...N_{RO}$ -1:

$$S_{n_e}^{M'}(k_{RO}) = S_{n_e}^{M}(k_{RO})*PSF_e(k_{RO}) \xrightarrow{\ 1D\text{-}FT\ } S_{n_e}^{M'}(x) = S_{n_e}^{M}(x) \cdot MTF_e(x)$$
$$S_{n_o}^{M'}(k_{RO}) = S_{n_o}^{M}(k_{RO})*PSF_o(k_{RO}) \xrightarrow{\ 1D\text{-}FT\ } S_{n_o}^{M'}(x) = S_{n_o}^{M}(x) \cdot MTF_o(x)$$

(48)

where $S^R(k_{RO})$ is the ideal echo signal of the reference scan and $S^R(x)$ its corresponding 1D-FT. A filter $F_{MTF}(x)$ can be calculated from the reference projections:

$$F_{MTF}(x) = \frac{S_{n_e}^{R'}(x)}{S_{n_o}^{R'}(x)} = \frac{MTF_e(x)}{MTF_o(x)}$$

(49)

We apply this filter to the odd reference-scan projection to show its effect:

$$S_{n_o}^{R'}(x) \cdot F_{MTF}(x) = S_{n_e}^{R'}(x)$$

(50)

By means of this filter we eliminate the "odd" MTF. The resulting projections are affected by only the even MTF. It therefore minimizes the N/2 ghosting but leaves the image in general distorted by only one specific MTF, in our case even MTF. This is always the case for conventional MRI and does not affect the overall image quality.

Deconvoluting the Effects of B_o Inhomogeneity

Due to the long data readout time the echoes in EPI are usually broadened by local B_o inhomogeneity. This effect can be seen in the reference scan shown in Fig. 18a. In the final image B_o inhomogeneity causes geometric image distortions [28] which can be significant especially for EPI due to the extremely small PC-gradient amplitude. In this section we describe an overall distortion correction method based on information that can be extracted from the reference scan.

Assume a constant RO gradient as shown in Fig. 2. If we use the definition of k-space of Eq. 2 and introduce the B_o inhomogeneity, ΔB_o, the reference scan can be described using Eq. 1 as:

$$S_n^{R'}(k_{RO}) = \int \int S(x,y) \cdot e^{iy\left(k_{RO} \cdot x + k_{RO} \cdot \frac{\Delta B_o(x,y)}{G_{RO}}\right)} dx\,dy \tag{51}$$

Performing the integration along the y-axis yields:

$$S_n^{R'}(k_{RO}) = \int S_{P_y}(x) \cdot e^{iy\left(k_{RO} \cdot x + k_{RO} \cdot \frac{\Delta B_o'(x,y)}{G_{RO}}\right)} dx \tag{52}$$

This can be expressed by means of the Fourier convolution theorem as:

$$S_n^{R'}(k_{RO}) = S^R(k_{RO}) * FOU\left[e^{ik_{RO} \cdot \frac{\Delta B_o'(x,y)}{G_{RO}}}\right] \tag{53}$$

$$S_n^{R'}(k_{RO}) = S^R(k_{RO}) * S_n^{B_o}(k_{RO})$$

FOU [...] expresses the 1D FT of the exponential function:

$$e^{ik_{RO} \cdot \frac{\Delta B_o'(x,y)}{G_{RO}}}$$

and $S^R(k_{RO})$ describes the reference scan under ideal condition without any distortions from B_o inhomogeneity and other possible hardware imperfections. Equation 53 then describes the broadening of the echoes of the reference scan as a convolution of $S^R(k_{RO})$ with $S_n^{Bo}(k_{RO})$. The latter can be interpreted as the PSF defined by the B_o inhomogeneity.

The idea is now to use the information of the reference scan taken at a PC data line, $n = n_o$, corresponding to the PC line when the echo of the PC-encoded MR signal occurs and calculate a filter from the projection data which compensates the ΔB_o effects:

$$S_n^{R'}(k_{RO}) \xrightarrow{1D-FT} S_n^{R'}(x) = S^R(x) \cdot S_n^{B_o}(x) \tag{54}$$

$$S_{n_o}^{R'}(k_{RO}) \xrightarrow{1D-FT} S_{n_o}^{R'}(x) = S^R(x) \cdot S_{n_o}^{B_o}(x)$$

$$F_n(x) = \frac{S_{n_o}^{B_o}(x)}{S_n^B(x)} \tag{55}$$

When we apply this filter to the projection of the reference scan itself, as described in Eqs. 54 and 55:

$$S_n^R(x) = S_n^{R'}(x) \cdot F_n(x) = S^R(x) \tag{56}$$

we completely eliminate the effects from the B_o inhomogeneity (Fig. 19). On the left is the measured reference scan, showing the broadening effects caused by the B_o inhomogeneity. After applying the filter all echoes (Fig. 19b) look the same and are perfectly aligned.

Fig. 19a–d. Reference scan of a SE EPI sequence. **a** B_o broadening is visible for echoes away from the RF spin echo. **b** Reference scan after B_o self deconvolution followed by a linear phase correction to eliminate the even and odd echo alternation. Echoes are precisely aligned and look comparable. **c** Reconstructed image without filtering or phase correction. Image appears distorted due to the B_o inhomogeneity responsible for the echo broadening. **d** Reconstructed image after B_o deconvolution, followed by a linear phase correction as described for **b**

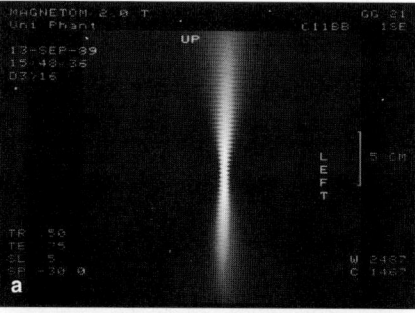

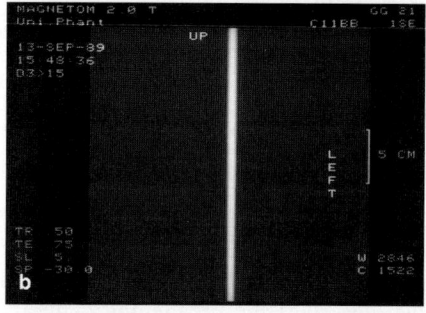

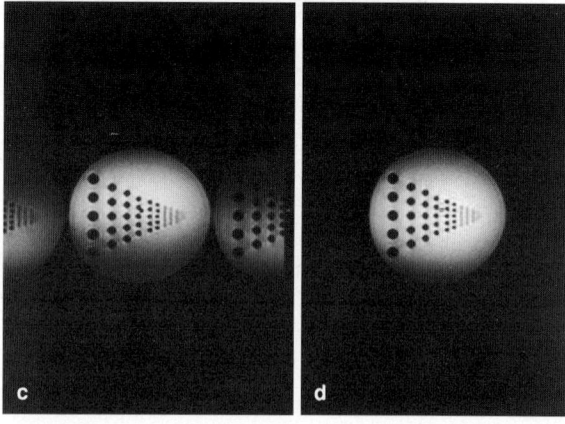

Applying this filter to the phase-encoded raw data set $S_n^{M'}(k_{RO})$:

$$S_n^{M'}(k_{RO}) = S_n^{M}(k_{RO}) * S_n^{B_o}(k_{RO}) \xrightarrow{\ 1D\text{-}FT\ } S_n^{M'}(x) = S_n^{M}(x) \cdot S_n^{B_o}(x) \qquad (57)$$

$$S_n^{M}(x) = S_n^{M'}(x) \cdot F_n(x) = S_n^{M}(x) \cdot S_{n_o}^{B_o}(x) \qquad (58)$$

yields an image affected by the broading of the central echo only, which is virtually nonexistent because the RO time, T_{RO}, per echo is much shorter than the echo time TE. The effect of the filter can be seen in Fig. 19c,d. The original image (Fig. 19c) is geometrically distorted (stretched along the PC direction, which is horizontal) due to B_o inhomogeneity. When the filter is applied, the geometric distortion is compensated (Fig. 19d). Be aware that in Fig. 19c–d PC direction points horizontal.

The filter process based on the reference scan is illustrated in Fig. 20. Reference scan and imaging scan are 1D Fourier transformed independently. From the projection data of the reference scan the appropriate filter or correction phases are calculated and then applied to the projections of the image scan. The final image is reconstructed after the column FT. This type of filtering scheme can also be applied to any kind of fast MRI technique which acquires multiple gradient echoes, such as GRASE [31], turbo-SE, and RARE [32]. These techniques suffer from the scanner hardware imperfection in ways similar to EPI. Instead of N/2 ghosting multiple ghosts along the PC direction may be present.

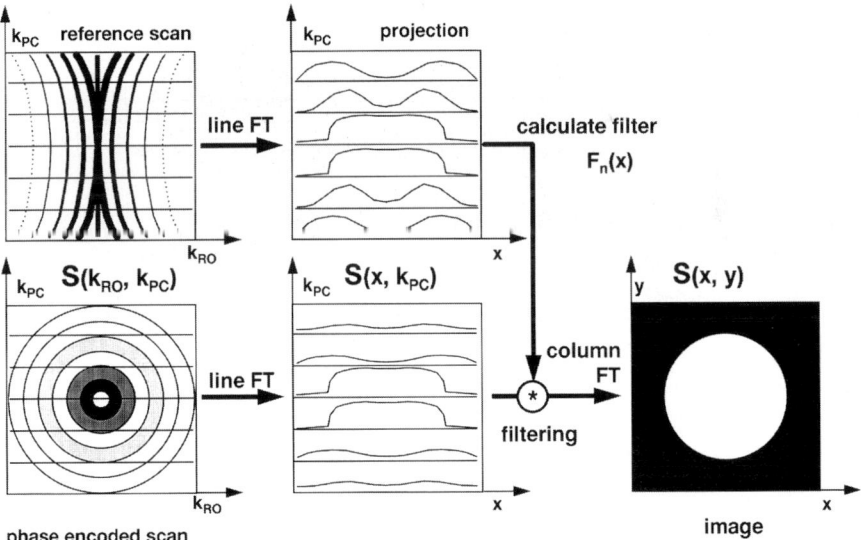

Fig. 20. Reconstruction scheme for EPI when reference scans are used. Usually after the 1D line FT the filters calculated from reference scans are applied. The final image is retrieved after the column FT

The Reconstruction in Total

As discussed above, the complete EPI reconstruction process is divided into several steps. One important step has not yet been described: the reflection of the time signal collected under a negative polarity of the RO gradient. As opposed to conventional MRI, where data are acquired under the same gradient polarity ($G_{RO}>0$ or $G_{RO}<0$), in EPI the echoes are sampled under alternating gradient polarity. This causes a k-space traversal from left to right and reverse when the RO gradient G_{RO} is positive or negative, respectively. The acquired data are usually written in the k-space matrix in the sequence of appearance, thus treated as if they were acquired with a unique G_{RO} polarity. Therefore every

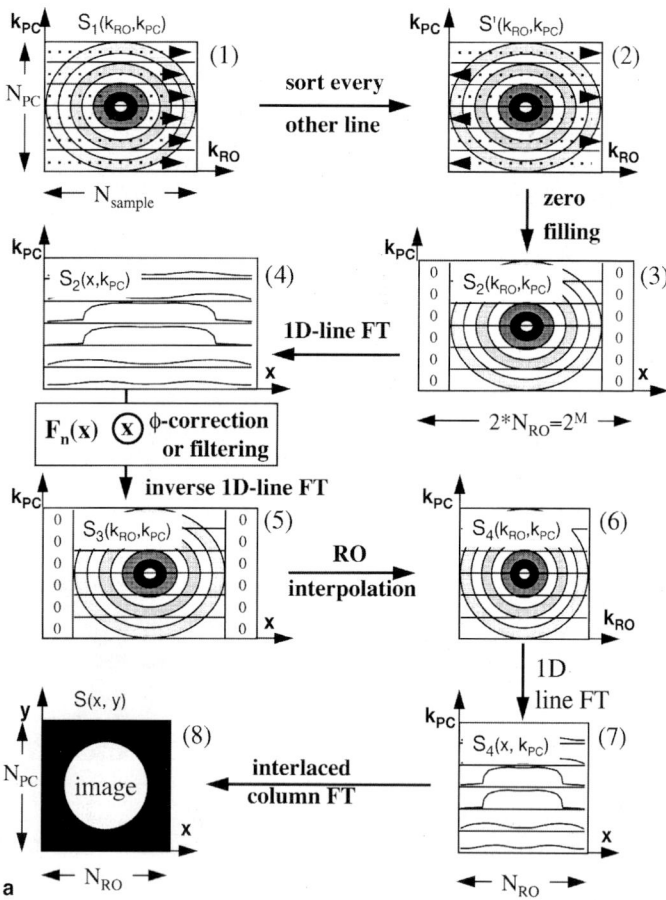

Fig. 21a–c. Overview of the entire EPI reconstruction process. **a** Reconstruction scheme for uniform time-domain data sampling and echo shifting via phase correction

other data line must be time reversed to guarantee the correct order with respect to k-space. This step is shown in Fig. 21 [$S_1(k_{RO}, k_{PC}) \rightarrow S'(k_{RO}, k_{PC})$].

To summarize the EPI reconstruction steps the operations that must be performed after data reflection are: (a) RO interpolation, (b) 1D line FT (forward and backward), (c) phase correction or filtering, and (d) 1D column FT or interlaced FT. The sequence of these steps depends on the k-space sampling technique used (i.e., uniform time-domain sampling or uniform k-space domain sampling). In principle the reconstruction steps for a certain sampling technique can be changed in the order of appearance. However, when the best image quality and the fastest image reconstruction are required, the order described below should be used.

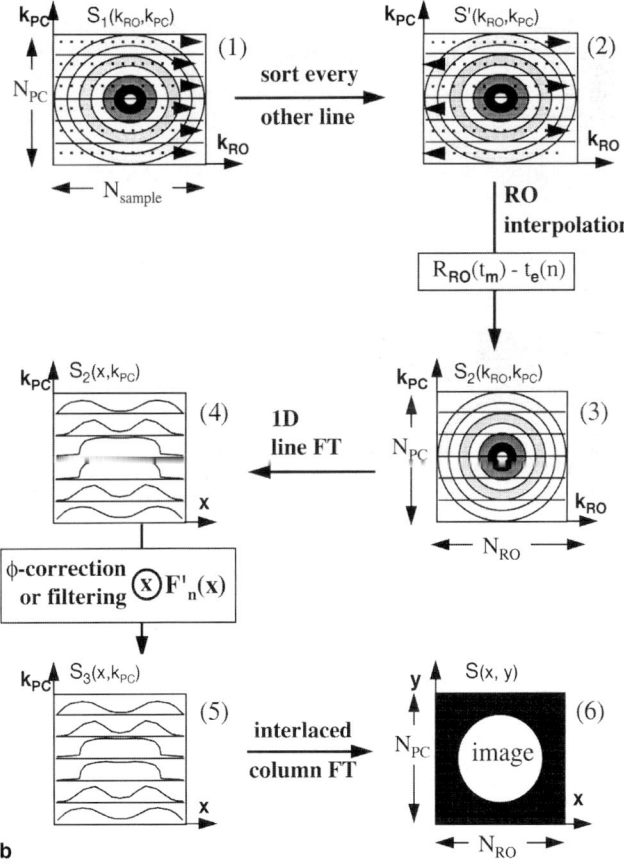

Fig. 21b. Reconstruction scheme for uniform time-domain data sampling and echo shifting via shift of the RO interpolation raster

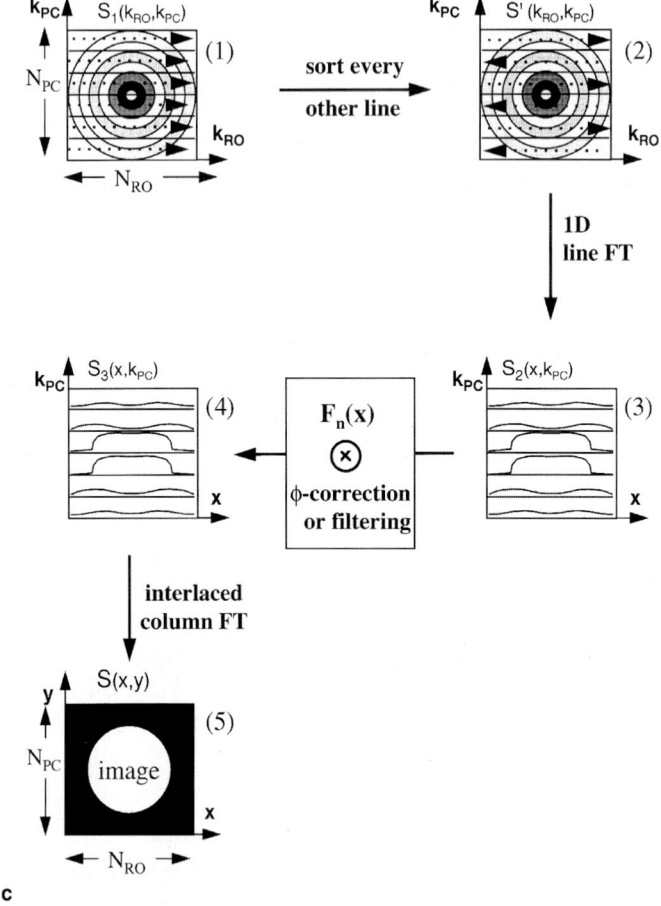

Fig. 21c. Reconstruction scheme for uniform k-space data sampling

Reconstruction Schemes for Uniform Time-Domain Sampling

We follow Fig. 21a for the various reconstruction steps when using uniform time-domain data sampling. The measured plain raw data, $S_1(k_{RO}, k_{PC})$, consists of $N_{PC} \times N_{sample}$ data points. Sorting every other data line in reversed order results in the raw data matrix, $S'(k_{RO}, k_{PC})$, having the k-space samples in the correct order. The data are placed in a zero padded [30] matrix containing $2^M > N_{sample}$ data samples along the k_{RO} direction resulting in the raw data matrix $S_2(k_{RO}, k_{PC})$ which is Fourier transformed along the RO direction to obtain the projection matrix, $S_2(x, k_{PC})$. (To be consistent with the prior section, $S'(k_{RO}, k_{PC})$ always describes the resorted data set.) Zero filling is performed because regular fast FT algorithms are based on 2^M data points. Phase correction or filtering can now be applied based on a reference scan that has been Fourier transformed, for example, as described under "Reconstruction Under Real Conditions." When this operation is followed by an inverse line FT, we obtain the k-space raw data, $S_3(k_{RO}, k_{PC})$, in which data are correctly aligned and filtered to minimize ghosting artifacts. Based on this data set the RO sinc interpolation is applied on the central $N_{PC} \times N_{sample}$ data points, resulting in the uniformly distributed k-space raw data matrix, $S_4(k_{RO}, k_{PC})$. After an additional 1D FT is generated along RO followed by the interlaced FT along the PC direction the final image, $S(x, y)$.

This reconstruction scheme therefore requires three 1D-line FT's to achieve the best image quality. An alternative to this "detour" can be applied when the correction scheme is based only on the echo shifts of a reference scan. When these shifts, $t_e(n)$, are calculated with respect to time, they can be used directly to modify the RO interpolation raster, R_{RO}, as shown in Fig. 21b. The advantage of this scheme is faster reconstruction because there is only one line FT required. To take full advantage of correction phases and filters deduced from reference scans we must calculate new filters and correction phases without the linear phase component as already corrected via the time shift of the RO interpolation raster.

Reconstruction Scheme for Uniform k-Space Sampling

When uniform k-space sampling is used to acquire data (Fig. 21c), the fastest image reconstruction time can be gained. The measured plain raw data set, $S_1(k_{RO}, k_{PC})$, consists of only $N_{PC} \times N_{RO}$ data points. Every other data line is reversed and then 1D Fourier transformed to obtain the projection data set, $S_2(x, k_{PC})$. Performing a phase correction or filtering (based on reference scans), a succeeding interlaced FT results in the final image $S(x, y)$.

To ensure precise equidistance in k-space the ADC sampling interval and actual gradient pulse must be synchronized before collecting reference and image data. Any shifting in the ADC raster in relation to the RO gradient introduces a nonuniformity in k-space that cannot be compensated by phase corrections or filters, and the only possible correction for realigning the ADC raster and RO gradient would be an additional interpolation.

Summary

EPI allows clinically useful MR images to be acquired more rapidly than in any other MRI technique. Although EPI has not yet become fully integrated in clinical practice, it offers new approaches to dynamic processes in which speed is crucial, such as in diffusion and perfusion imaging and in cardiac imaging. For the latter, segmented EPI will be an important imaging technique in the future. In recent years functional MRI has become very popular in brain research. Without the speed of EPI this would have been unthinkable.

Using the full speed that EPI offers is possible only with appropriate reconstruction schemes. We show above that it is essential in EPI to acquire the
data during the gradient ramp periods. This places new demands on the image
reconstruction, such as interpolation to rectilinear k-space grids and alternatively nonuniform time-domain data sampling to achieve uniformly spaced k-
space data. In general for EPI the data can be distributed nonuniformly in the
RO direction, which must be considered in the image reconstruction. A dominant artifact accompanying EPI is the N/2 ghost, which can be minimized
only by special phase corrections and filtering steps. All the correction schemes
developed originally for EPI have now also been adopted for other fast MRI techniques, such as turbo-SE and GRASE imaging, and are essential for the success
of these techniques.

Acknowledgements. The authors appreciate the help of Dr. Hubertus Fischer and Prof. Robert
Turner for carefully reading and correcting the text, as well as for providing images (H.F.) for
this chapter.

Glossary

$S(k_{RO}, k_{PC})$	The measured k-space signal, also called raw data
k_{RO}, k_{PC}	The coordinates in k-space
$S(x, y)$	An MR image
x, y	The coordinates in the image space
i	The complex number equal $\sqrt{-1}$
γ	The gyromagnetic ratio equal to 42.578 Mhz/T
Δk	The span of k-space of the measured raw data: $\Delta k = N \cdot \delta k$ with N = matrix size
δk	Sampling width in k-space
δt	Sampling width of ADC trigger
N_{sample}	Number of measured samples per data line
m	Index describing the actual sample along the RO direction: $1 \leq m \leq N_{sample}$ or $1 \leq m \leq N_{RO}$
N_{RO}	Number of samples in RO direction when either RO interpolation is performed or number of measured samples when equidistant k-space sampling is used. N_{RO} is the number of pixels of the image along RO direction.
N_{PC}	Number of k_{PC} data lines and number of lines of the image
n	Index describing the actual k_{PC} data line: $1 \leq n \leq N_{PC}$
J	Total number of neighboring points to be considered for inter-polation
j	Index for interpolation: $0 \leq j \leq J-1$
$R_{RO}(m)$	RO interpolation raster containing N_{RO} elements
$R_{ADC}(m)$	ADC raster containing N_{RO} elements
$R_{PC}(m)$	PC interpolation raster containing N_{RO} elements
FT	Fourier transformation
1D FT	One-dimensional Fourier transformation
FOU [...]	Fourier transformation of term [...]

$S^{R'}(k_{RO})$ Raw data of measured reference scan (not phase encoded)

$S^{R}(k_{RO})$ Ideal reference scan without any influence from unwanted phases etc.

$S^{M'}(k_{RO})$ Raw data of measured scan (phase encoded)

$S^{M}(k_{RO})$ Ideal measured phase encode raw data without any influence from unwanted phases etc.

$F(x)$ Filter applied in the image domain

References

1. Mansfield P (1977) Multi-planar image formation using NMR spin echoes. J Phys C 10:L55–L58
2. Ljunggren S (1983) A simple graphical representation of Fourier based imaging methods. J Magn Reson 54:338–343
3. Bracewell RN (1978) The Fourier transform and its applications, 2nd edn. McGraw-Hill, New York
4. Bottomly PA, Foster TH, Argesinger RE, Pfeifer LM (1984) A review of normal tissue NMR relaxation times and relaxation mechanism from 1–100 Mhz: dependence on tissue type, NMR frequency, temperature, species, excision, and age. Med Phys 11(4):425–448
5. Bruder H, Fischer H, Reinfelder H-E, Schmitt F (1992) Image reconstruction for echo-planar imaging with nonequidistant k-space sampling. Magn Reson Med 23:311–323
6. Schmitt F, Warach S, Wielopolski P, Edelman RR (1994) Clinical applications and techniques of echo-planar imaging. MAGMA 2:259–266
7. Frese G, Siebold H, Ries H (1985) Aspects of shimming a superconductive whole body MRI magnet. Proceedings of the 9th International Conference on Magnetic Technology, Zurich, pp 249–251
8. Gruetter R (1993) Automatic, localized in vivo adjustment of all fist and second order shim coils. Magn Reson Med 29:804–811
9. Manabe A (1994) Multi-angle projection shim (MAPshim): in vivo shim adjustment up to 2nd order with 0.2 second sequence time. In: Proceedings of the Society of Magnetic Resonance, vol 2, pp 765–765
10. Stöhr J (1976) Einführung in die numerische Mathematik I. Springer, Berlin Heidelberg New York, pp 76–95
11. O'Sullivan JD (1985) A fast sinc function gridding algorithm for Fourier inversion in computer tomography. IEEE Trans Medical Imaging 4(4):200–207
12. Jackson JI, Meyer C, Nishimura D, Macovski A (1991) Selection of a convolution function for Fourier inversion using gridding. IEEE Trans Med Imaging 10(3):473–478
13. Chen DQ, Marr R, Lauterbur P (1986) Reconstruction from NMR data acquired with imaging gradients having arbitrary time dependence. IEEE Trans Med Imaging 5(3):162–164
14. Zakhor A, Weisskoff R, Rzedzian R (1991) Optimal sampling and reconstruction of MRI signals resulting from sinusoidal gradients. IEEE Trans Signal Processing 19(9):2056–2065
15. Trussel HJ, Arnder LL, Moran PR, Williams RC (1991) Correction for nonuniform sampling distortions in magnetic resonance imagery. IEEE Trans Med Imaging 7(1):32–44
16. Ordidge R, Mansfield P (1985) NMR methods. United States patent no 4509015
17. Howseman A, Stehling MK, Chapman B, Coxon R, Turner R, Ordidge R, Cawley M, Glover P, Mansfield P, Coupland R (1988) Improvements in snap-shot nuclear magnetic resonance imaging. Br J Radiol 61:822–828
18. Sekihara K, Kohno H (1987) New reconstruction technique for echo-planar imaging to allow combined use of odd and even numbered echoes. Magn Res Med 5:485–491
19. Sekihara K, Matsui S, Kohno H (1988) Image reconstruction method in NMR imaging. European patent specification, application number: 88110873.2, 7.7
20. Oppenheimer AV, Schafer RW (1975) Digital signal processing. Prentice-Hall, Englewood
21. Heid O (1997) Robust EPI phase correction. In: Proceedings of the Society of Magnetic Resonance in Medicine, p 2014
22. Franconi F, Symms M, Lethimonnier F, Jones R, Schreiber W, Barker GJ (1997) Measurement of ghosting in echo-planar imaging: a multi-center study. In: Proceedings of the Society of Magnetic Resonance in Medicine, p 1807

23. Goldfarb JW, Schmitt F, Fischer H, Haacke EM (1995) A method to remove ghosting result-
    ing from parametric phase distortions in EPI. In: Proceedings of the Society of Magnetic
    Resonance in Medicine, p 759
24. Barnett A (1997) Phase unwrapping algorithm for navigator corrected diffusion weighted
    interleaved echo-planar imaging. In: Proceedings of the Society of Magnetic Resonance in
    Medicine, p 1726
25. Barnett A (1997) Improved reconstruction algoritm for navigator corrected diffusion
    weighted interleaved echo-planar imaging. In: Proceedings of the Society of Magnetic Reso-
    nance in Medicine, p 1727
26. Hong X, Cohen M. Roemer P (1997) Functional EPI with real time imaging processing. In:
    Proceedings of the Society of Magnetic Resonance in Medicine, p 321
27. Hennel F (1997) EPI deghosting by linear phase correction without reference scans. In: Pro-
    ceedings of the Society of Magnetic Resonance in Medicine, p 1808
28. Schmitt F (1985) Correction of geometric distortions in MR images. In: Proceedings of the
    computer assisted radiology (CAR). Springer, Berlin Heidelberg New York, pp 15-25
29. Ahn CB, Cho ZH (1987) A new phase correction method in NMR imaging based on auto-
    correlation and histogram analysis. IEEE Trans Medical Imaging 6(1):32-35
30. Schwartz M, Shaw L (1974) Signal processing, McGraw-Hill, New York
31. Feinberg DA, Oshio K (1991) GRASE (gradient and spin echo) MR imaging: a new fast clin-
    ical imaging technique. Radiology 181:597
32. Hennig J, Nauerth A, Friedburg H (1986) RARE Imaging: a fast imaging method for clinical
    MR. Magn Reson Med 3:823-833

CHAPTER 6

Echo-Planar Imaging Image Artifacts

H. Fischer and R. Ladebeck

Introduction

Echo-planar imaging (EPI) is more sensitive to image artifacts than conventional imaging for two basic reasons; these are (a) reversal of every second echo and (b) the long readout (RO) period.

Every second echo is acquired under a negative gradient. These signals must be reflected with respect to time to make use off all echoes. Any imperfection in the acquired signal leads in this case to an alternate line variation in the raw data. These imperfections can arise, for example, from eddy currents or from the characteristics of the radiofrequency receive path. Alternate line variation in the raw data (or k space) results in a ghost image shifted by half of the field of view (FOV) after Fourier transformation (FT). This artifact is therefore also referred to as N/2 ghosting.

Secondly, the acquisition time is longer than that in conventional imaging. In this time, however, the whole information necessary to reconstruct an image is acquired and not only that for a single line in k space. During this period two gradients are applied: the alternating RO gradient and the phase-encode (PC) gradient. The latter is either a constant or a blipped gradient. Although this gradient is normally referred to as PC gradient, it is in fact a *read* gradient and has the properties of a read gradient (see Fig. 1). The effective acquisition times in RO and PC directions differ in the order of the number of lines, as do the gradient amplitudes. Expressed in bandwidth per pixel in the image, the bandwidth in PC direction is smaller than the pixel bandwidth in the read direction by a factor which is approximately the number of lines of k space scanned.

Several effects are related to the very narrow bandwidth per pixel in the PC direction and the long data acquisition time. These are:

- Large fat–water shift
- Geometric distortions in case of B_o inhomogeneity, induced either by the magnet or by the patient
- Signal loss due to dephasing
- Resolution loss due to filter effect by T2*

The first three of these can be summarized as off-resonance effects. All spins not processing exactly at the reference frequency are affected.

A third effect must be considered. A real gradient coil produces not only the wanted, magnetic resonance (MR) relevant component of the magnetic flux den-

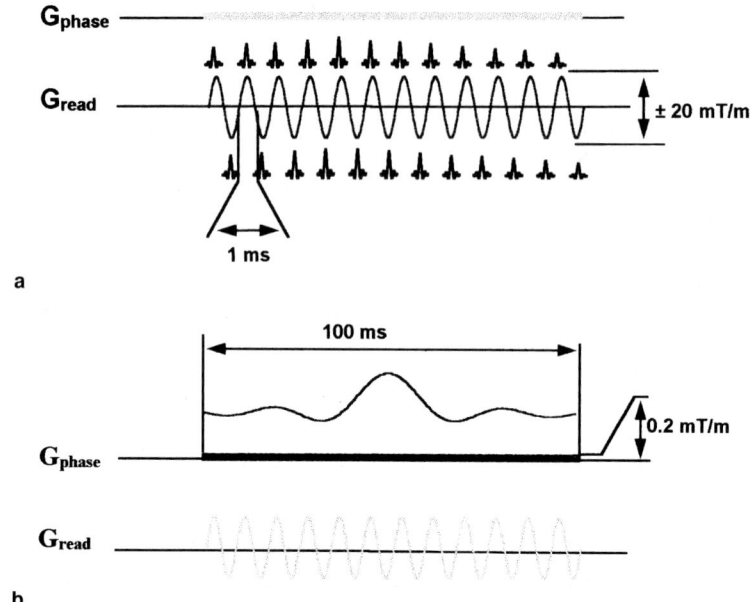

Fig. 1a,b. EPI Readout module. Both imaging directions have the properties of a read gradient

sity but also a concomitant gradient. This might be important for EPI since the two applied gradients differ substantially in amplitude – roughly by the number of lines. The concomitant gradient leads to additional phase accumulation. The resulting artifacts may be a slice shift in the phase direction, in-plane geometric distortion, and additional N/2 ghosting.

By the nature of all artifacts in EPI, they are effective only in PC or low bandwidth direction. No technically induced artifacts arise in the read or high-frequency direction. In general, the shorter the overall acquisition time the fewer artifacts are encountered. It should be noted that the type of PC gradient – continuous or blipped – makes no difference in the artifact behavior in EPI.

N/2 Ghosting

Introduction

A unique problem of EPI is due to the fact that every second line in k space is read under a negative gradient. This negative gradient implies that this line goes backwards in k space, and it must therefore be reversed with respect to time (see Chap. 4). This is the reason that EPI is extremely susceptible to modulations of signal from line to line. Modulations cause a ghost image that is shifted by one-half of the FOV. This chapter discusses all effects that produce differences between odd and even lines in k space.

Eddy Currents

As introduced by Jehenson et al. [9], the effects of eddy currents on the gradient field in the temporal domain can be treated by linear system theory. This means that the eddy currents cause a time delay between the current in the coil and the gradient field, and the amplitude of the gradient field is reduced. Using a sinusoidal read gradient, for example, has both advantages and disadvantages. An advantage is that there is no change in the gradient frequency or in the shape of the gradient; only the overall amplitude of the gradient field may be reduced. This can be easily compensated by an increased current in the gradient coil. A disadvantage is that the gradient field variation is shifted in time. Due to the time reversal of every second line it is obvious that this time shift causes problems.

As shown in Fig. 2, the delayed gradient field causes the magnetization to refocus late. Due to the time reversal of the second line the echo in the second line in k space is shifted by just the same time delay in the opposite direction. Therefore the echoes in k space form a zigzag pattern: this is the first source of N/2 ghosting (Fig. 3).

This problem can be solved by an exact adjustment of the analog-digital converter (ADC) raster to the gradient field. In order to carry out this adjustment an experiment similar to that shown in Fig. 2 should be performed in a well-shimmed magnet. The time determined should be used to delay the ADC triggering in order to be in phase with the gradient field. It is necessary here to discuss the possible sampling strategies. Independently of the gradient shape, it is necessary to have equidistant samples in the k space if a fast FT is be used to reconstruct the image. In standard imaging this is achieved by sampling equidistantly in time and using a constant gradient amplitude. With EPI this would be a severe waste of time since the gradient ramp time is a reasonable amount of the total

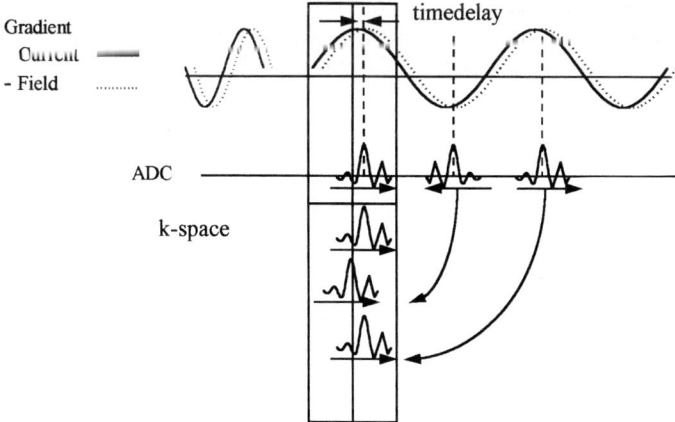

Fig. 2. llustration of a misalignment of gradient and ADC timing. Due to time reversal of every second echo this leads to a zigzag pattern of the echoes in k space

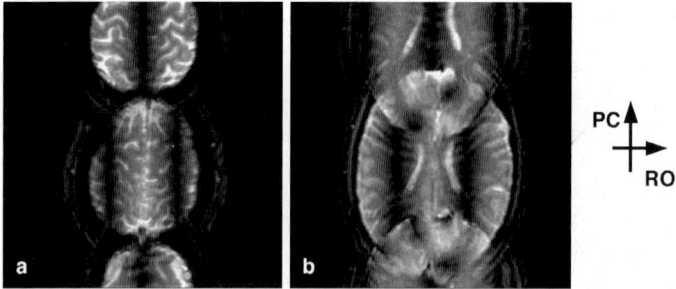

Fig. 3. Effect of misalingned gradient timing. This leads to a time shift of every second echo, thereby introducing a N/2 ghost. The interference pattern in the image and ghost depends on the number of pixels by which the echo is shifted

RO time. Therefore it is necessary to perform sampling during the ramp times of the gradient or merely using a sinusoidal gradient shape. Using a sinusoidal gradient shape, there are two ways of acquiring equidistant samples in k space. Either nonlinear sampling in the time domain can be performed in order to obtain a constant integral of the gradient amplitude, or the data can be sampled at equal time intervals and interpolated afterwards. The latter has the advantage that the interpolation can be combined with low pass filtering, which increases the signal to noise ratio.

Concerning the usable tolerance for the adjustment of the gradient, delay one must distinguish between equidistant sampling in the time and in the k space domain. In the first case all data are sampled with the Nyquist frequency, and transformation to the equidistant k space grid is carried out by interpolation. This is the reason why the shifting of raw data is easy before the interpolation is started, and no undersampling occurs. Thus the gradient delay can be adjusted by postprocessing. In the other case a nonlinear sampling grid in time is used, so that the data already represent the equidistant grid in k space. Here shifting the data by postprocessing would violate the Nyquist theorem. Therefore the adjustment must be exact to a fraction of the sampling clock.

This adjustment poses no major problem if the gradient delay (delay between current and field) is uniform in the FOV. This is usually fulfilled if the eddy currents have the same symmetry as the gradient-producing currents, for example, in the cryostat of a superconducting magnet. If this symmetry is broken, such as by eddy currents in the Faraday screen of a local coil, a spatially dependent raster shift would be necessary, which is impossible. This would lead to N/2 ghosting in special regions of the image.

What else is caused by eddy currents?

If the eddy currents are not exactly symmetrical, the resulting field not only delays and reduces the gradient field but also introduces a B_0 field modulation proportional to the gradient amplitude [9]. If one thinks of the z gradient, for example, misalignment of the gradient coil and the structures where the eddy currents occur (e.g., a shift of the whole gradient coil in z direction) produces asymmetric eddy currents. This means that the field caused by the eddy currents

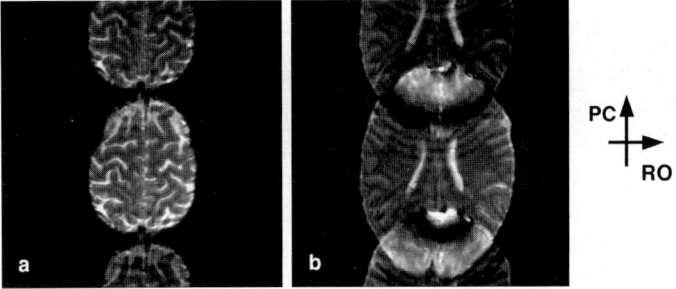

Fig. 4. Image artifact similar to the artifact shown in Fig. 3. A phase variation of 70° was artificially introduced from line to line in the raw data. This leads to N/2 ghosting, but as there is no time shift, the interference pattern is gone. In the overlap region of regular image and ghost image the signal cancels partly due to phase difference

is not only a gradient field but also a B_0 field. Therefore the resonance frequency of the spins is changing from line to line, as the polarity of the B_0 field changes with the polarity of the read gradient:

$$\frac{d\phi}{dt} \propto B(t) \tag{1}$$

According to Eq. 1, the phase (ϕ) of the MR signal differs from even to odd lines, and there is another source of N/2 ghosting. This is shown in Fig. 4.

As the FT is extremely sensitive to phase effects, it is necessary to reduce phase variations to below 1°. This can be carried out very easily with a so-called adjustment scan (same sequence without phase-encoding gradient) that determines the phase difference from line to line depending on the selected gradient amplitude. This phase value is then used to correct every other line.

If the B_0 effects are not uniform in the FOV, there are the same problems as with spatially dependent eddy currents, that is, different phase values between even and odd lines in different regions of the image. In this case a perfect compensation can not be done. Strictly speaking this would no longer be a B_0 effect, as B_0 by definition is homogeneous.

Modulation Transfer Function of the Receive System

An important component of a MR system is the low pass filter. Even with the high bandwidth in EPI it is absolutely essential to cut off the noise associated with frequencies higher than the sampling rate to avoid degradation of the signal to noise ratio due to noise aliasing. Why is a low pass filter a problem in EPI? A low pass filter averages the input values. This averaging can be described as convolution of the input signal with a filter-dependent convolution kernel [20 p. 379]. The effect of this convolution can be visualized by the degradation of a step function. This is illustrated in Fig. 5, which shows the effect of a steep cutoff characteristic in the frequency domain. This filter causes a long signal delay

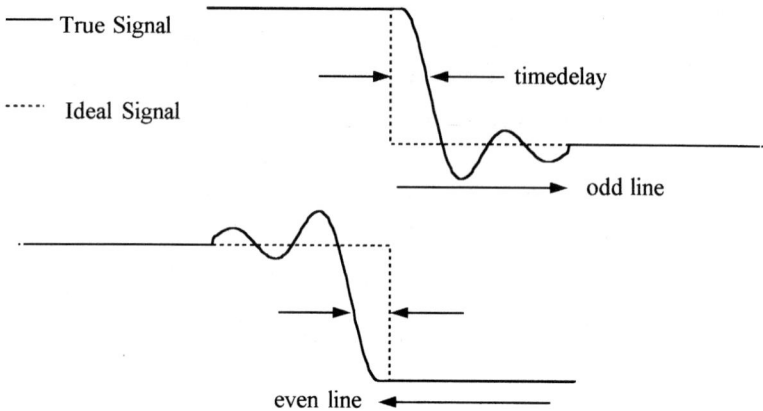

Fig. 5. Signal degradation due to the low pass filter

time and severe oscillations of the signal. Therefore there is again a time shift which causes problems due to time-reversal of every other line. Fortunately, the signal oscillations are only a minor problem. As this time delay is determined by the bandwidth of the low pass filter, its current value scales easily. In order to adjust the ADC timing to the gradient field the filter delay time must be corrected first.

Gradient Offset, No Source of Ghosting

Shim is very important in EPI because the bandwidth in PC direction is low due to the RO time of 50–100 ms. Although the shim is usually adjusted with special sequences, the EPI sequence itself can be used to improve field homogeneity. As discussed by Johnson and Hutchinson [11], if there is an inhomogeneity in read direction, for example, a misadjusted read gradient offset, echoes behave as shown in the Fig. 6. Therefore depending on the size of the misalignment the echoes approach the border of k space. However, there is no N/2 ghost, as there is no periodicity from line to line. This is shown in Fig. 7.

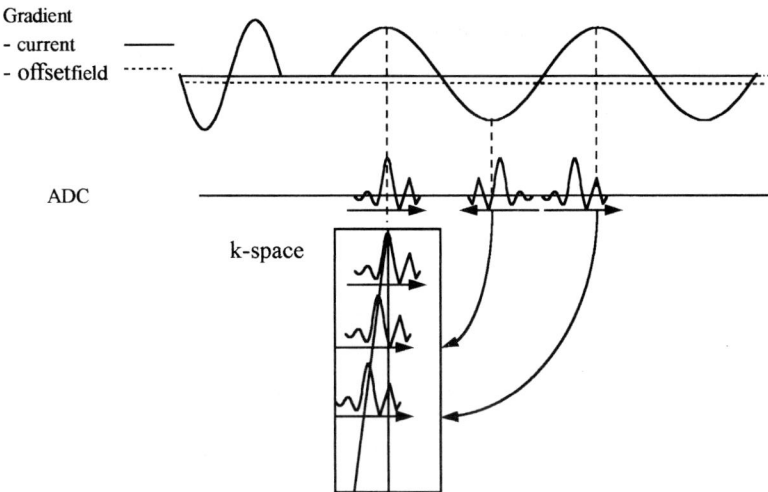

Fig. 6. Effect of a misaligned gradient offset (shim). This leads to a constantly increasing echo shift

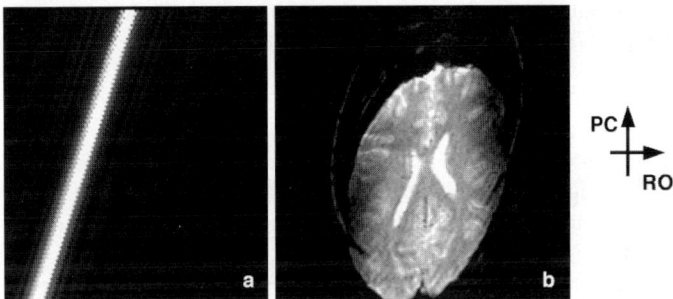

Fig. 7a,b. Image acquired with a misaligned gradient offset of 0.05 mT/m. **a** Magnitude of raw data after reversal of every other line. **b** Corresponding image. Apart from distortion due to low bandwidth there are no further artifacts, especially no N/2 ghosting

Software Correction Methods

As shown above, all ghosting is caused by phase effects, either constant phase shifts, linear phase shifts, or combinations of these. As described for example, by Goldfarb et al. [6], Bruder et al. [2], Sekihara et al. [18], and Zakhor [26], it is possible to remove ghosting by postprocessing. These authors suggest treating the odd and even lines separately. This reconstruction gives two images with N/2 ghosts. If all phases are adjusted properly, the summation of these images cancels the N/2 ghost. These methods work best if there is a region in the image where the ghost does not overlap with the image; then the signal in this region can be minimized.

Artifacts Due to Low Bandwidth

Introduction

The MR signal of spins in fluids or weakly bound molecules after a single excitation pulse decays exponentially with the time constant T2:

$$S(t) \propto e^{-t/T2} \tag{2}$$

T2 is the transverse relaxation time. When an inhomogeneity of the magnetic flux density exists over the volume of the spins, it results in an additional dephasing of the spins in that particular volume [5]:

$$S(t) \propto e^{-t/T2} \, e^{-t/T2'} = e^{-t/T2*} \tag{3}$$

T2' describes the inhomogeneity effect. The effective transverse relaxation time T2* has been introduced as:

$$1/T2* = 1/T2 + 1/T2' \tag{4}$$

If the inhomogeneity is Lorenzian with half-bandwidth ΔB_o, T2' is given by:

$$T2' = \gamma \Delta B_o / 2 \tag{5}$$

with γ denoting the gyromagnetic ratio. In the case of spin-echo, the dephasing due to B_o inhomogeneity is refocused at the time of the spin-echo (which assumed to be zero in the following equation):

$$S(t) \propto e^{-(t+TE)/T2} \, e^{-|t|/T2'} \tag{6}$$

Fig. 8. Signal envelope in EPI FID (a) and EPI SE (b)

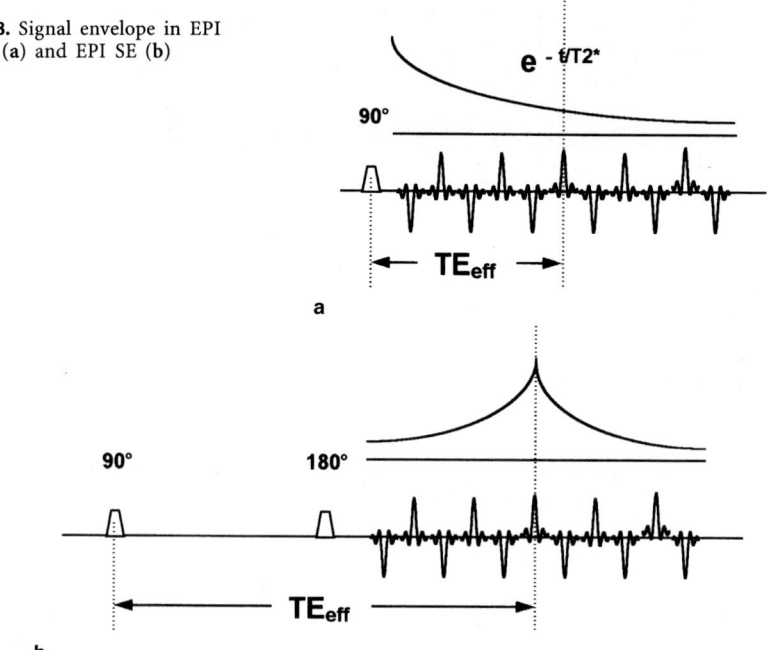

This signal course is sketched in Fig. 8.

In the presence of a field gradient G, and including off-resonance spins, a normalized free induction decay can be described by Ljunggren [12]:

$$S(t) = \int \rho(r) \, e^{i\phi} \, e^{-t/T2^*} \, d^3r \qquad (7)$$

It is integrated over the imaging volume. The term ρ is the spin density, and ϕ is used to describe in general all off-resonance effects:

$$\phi = (\delta\omega + \gamma\Delta B_0)t + \gamma r \int G(t')dt' \qquad (8)$$

In particular, the sources for off-resonance are frequency offset $\delta\omega$, e.g., from spins bound in a different chemical environment, main-field inhomogeneity ΔB_0, and of course the imaging gradients:

$$G = \overline{V}(B_z) = (\partial B_z/dx, \, \partial B_z/dy, \, \partial B_z/dz) \qquad (9)$$

Neglecting for a moment relaxation and off-resonance besides the imaging gradient, i.e., $\delta\omega = 0$, $\Delta B_0 = 0$, and $T2^* = \infty$, and with the definition:

$$k(t) = \gamma \int G(t')dt' \qquad (10)$$

Equation 7 can be written as:

$$S(t) = S'(k(t)) = \int_{\infty}^{\infty} \rho(r) \, e^{ikr} \, d^3r \qquad (11)$$

The integration is thus moved from the imaging volume to infinity. This is valid since the spin density $\rho(r)$ is limited. Equation 11 merely defines the FT: under the assumptions which were made, the spin density is the FT of the signal S'(k(t)).

To describe the actual behavior, the assumptions are dropped. All imaging artifacts can then be derived from Eq. 7. In addition, the finite sampling window is considered. Without loss of generality the discussion is made in the following for the one-dimensional case. In the one-dimensional case, spatial dimension x, corresponding gradient G, the signal is:

$$S'(k(t)) = \text{rect}\,(t/T) \int \rho(x) \, e^{ikx} \, e^{ikd} \, e^{-k/(\gamma GT2^*)} \, x e^{-t/T2^*} \, dx \qquad (12)$$

with k the one-dimensional expression of Eq. 11, and the abbreviation:

$$d = \delta\omega \, /(\gamma G) + \Delta B_0/G \qquad (13)$$

is used. T is the length of the acquisition window. The rect function here is defined by:

$$\text{rect}\,(t/T) = 1 \text{ for } 0 < t < T$$
$$= 0 \text{ otherwise}$$

For the solution of this equation two theorems for FT are needed:

- Convolutions theorem: this says that the FT (F) of the product of two functions g and h is equal to the convolution ($\otimes$) of the single transformed functions:

$$F(gh) = F(g) \otimes F(h)$$

- Shift theorem: if the function g' is the FT of function g, i.e.:

$$F(g(k)) = g'(x)$$

then the following holds:

$$F(g(k)\ e^{ikx}o) = g'(x-xo)$$

Using these theorems, and assuming that T2 is spatially constant (i.e., T2 is not a function of x), the solution of Eq. 11 is:

$$F(S'(k)) = \rho'(x) = \rho(x-d)\otimes PSF(x) \tag{14}$$

with [5]:

$$PSF(x) = \text{sinc}\ (\gamma GTx/2\pi)\otimes(1/((1/\gamma GxT2^\star)^2+x^2)) \tag{15}$$

Equation 14 indicates that the measured spin density ρ' as the FT of S'(k) is the "real" spin density ρ, shifted by a distance d defined by Eq. 13 and convoluted by a function PSF(x). PSF stands for point spread function. The quality of an imaging method in general can be described by the effective PSF. Simply speaking, the PSF is the result of imaging a point (in the mathematical sense), or the way in which a point is depicted by a imaging method. However, it is important to realize that not only the properties of the sequence contribute to the PSF and thus to the image quality but also the imaged object itself, namely by its T2 value. In FT-based imaging methods such as MR imaging the PSF is the FT of the effective modulation transfer function (MTF). To summarize the mathematics, the following contribute to the MTF:

- Finite data acquisition window
- T2 decay
- Local B_o inhomogeneity

The imaging process can be seen this way: the ideal raw data are multiplied by a window function, which describes the finite acquisition window, and by the decaying T2* envelope in the case when a single excitation pulse is used to form the entire image (see Fig. 8).

When the signal is read under the envelope of a spin-echo, the MTF is analogous to Eq. 6. Equation 14 is still valid; the PSF in this case is [5]:

$$\begin{aligned} PSF(x) = \text{sinc}\ (\gamma GT\ x/2\rho)&\otimes Re(1/(1/(\gamma G \times T2+jx))) \\ &\otimes(1/((1/\gamma G \times T2')^2+x^2)) \end{aligned} \tag{16}$$

In practice the k space as defined in Eq. 10 is scanned in the interval $[-\Delta k/2, \Delta k/2]$ at N data points with the span:

$$\Delta k = \gamma \int_T G(t')dt' \tag{17}$$

The offset $-\Delta k/2$ is realized with a prephase gradient lobe. Depending on the properties of the FT, the spatial resolution is:

$$\delta x = 1/\Delta k = 1/(\gamma GT) \tag{18}$$

which is linked to the FOV Δx by:

$$\Delta x = N \ \delta x$$

As described above (see "Introduction"), in EPI we must deal with two gradients. Both are read gradients, and the mathematics reviewed so far applies to both of them. Let T_{RO} be the acquisition time per echo and T_{ES} the echo spacing, where $T_{ES} \geq T_{RO}$. The total acquisition time T_{acq} is the number of acquired lines times the echo spacing, or $T_{acq} = N \times T_{ES}$ [to be exact, $T_{acq} = N \times T_{ES} - (T_{ES} - T_{RO})$]. The pixel bandwidth is the inverse of the corresponding acquisition time:

$$b_{RO} = 1/T_{RO} \tag{19}$$

$$b_{PC} = 1/T_{acq} \tag{20}$$

For example, a continuously sampled EPI train is considered with a RO time per echo and echo spacing of:

$$T_{RO} = T_{ES} = 0.6 \text{ ms}$$

For $n = 128$ lines the total acquisition time is:

$$T_{acq} = 128 \times 0.6 \text{ ms} = 76.8 \text{ ms}$$

The corresponding pixel bandwidths are:

$$b_{RO} = 1667 \text{ Hz}$$
$$b_{PC} = 13 \text{ Hz}$$

Fat-Water Shift

The resonance frequency in MR depends on the flux density at the position of the nucleus. The chemical environment can either enhance or weaken the external flux density. This effect is known as chemical shift. The chemical shift is given as a relative number, i.e., the resonance frequency in one chemical environment relative to the resonance frequency in an other. The absolute frequency difference is proportional to the main flux density:

$$\delta\omega = \gamma\sigma B_o \tag{21}$$

Using a linear field gradient G for frequency encoding, a frequency shift $\delta\omega$ leads to a image shift d of (see Eq. 13):

$$d = \delta\omega/(\gamma G) \tag{22}$$

which in the case of chemical shift is:

$$d_{cs} = \sigma B_o/G$$

Expressed as shift d_{csp} in units of pixels, it is:

$$d_{csp} = \delta\omega/b = \gamma\sigma B_o/b = \gamma\sigma B_o\, T_{acq} \qquad (23)$$

where b is the bandwidth per pixel. The displacement due to the chemical shift – itself sometimes simply called chemical shift – is proportional to the main field B_o and inverse proportional to the pixel bandwidth.

In MR imaging of biological tissue the signal of protons from fat and water is normally visible. The fat protons have a flux density about 3.3 ppm (parts per million) higher than the water protons, or $\sigma = 3.3$ ppm. In conventional imaging G is typically high enough to keep the fat-water shift below 1 or 2 pixels. This is not the case in EPI in the low-bandwidth direction. To continue with the example above, and assuming a magnetic flux density of 1.5 T, the fat-water frequency difference is $\delta\omega = 210$ Hz, and the fat-water displacements due to the chemical shift in units of pixel in frequency and phase direction, respectively, are (see Eq. 23):

$$d_{csp}RO = 210 \;(Hz)/1667 \;(Hz/pixel) = 0.13 \;\text{pixel}$$
$$dcspPC = 210 \;(Hz)/13 \;(Hz/pixel) = 16.1 \;\text{pixel}$$

Thus the shift in read direction is far below 1 pixel and can be disregarded, by comparison with the shift in the phase direction which is more than 16 pixels, or 13 % of the FOV (for 128 lines).

Fat suppression or water-only excitation is absolutely necessary in EPI. The pitfall of incomplete fat suppression in EPI is that the shifted fat image typically appears in the region of interest. For instance, in abdominal imaging the fat rim continues in this case through the liver; Fig. 9 shows an example. Since the chemical shift is so large in EPI, it is also called *chemical shift artifact,* although it is only a shifted image.

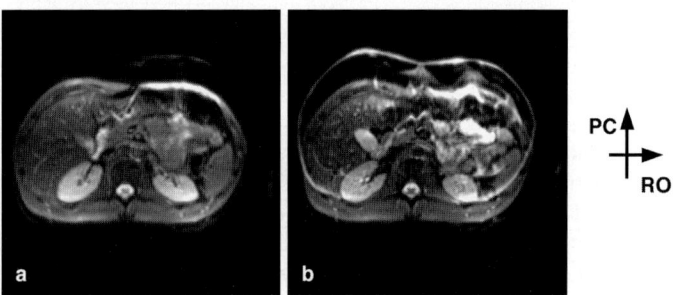

Fig. 9. EPI images of the liver with (a) and without (b) fat suppression

Geometric Distortions and Susceptibility Artifact

A second source of off-resonance in addition to chemical shift is main-field inhomogeneity. The off-resonance arises from a spatially varying main field over the imaging volume. One reason is the flux density inhomogeneity from the magnet: a magnet of finite length has a finite homogeneity. In addition to the inhomogeneity of the main magnetic field based on the magnet imperfection, a second source exists when, in general terms, a sample is brought into a magnet. The magnetic flux density B inside a sample of susceptibility is:

$$B = (1+\chi)\mu_o H \tag{24}$$

where H is the magnetic field strength and o the magnetic field constant (Note: it is common but physically not correct to denote B as field strength). At the intersection of two substances with different susceptibility a local inhomogeneity exists of:

$$\Delta B_o = (\chi_1 - \chi_2)B_o \tag{25}$$

In contrast to the case in chemical shift, the off-resonance effect is not spatially constant, and instead of a shifted image a geometric distortion arises. The amount of the local distortion d is proportional to the field offset B_o and inverse proportional to the gradient strength (see Eq. 13):

$$d = \Delta B_o/G \propto \Delta B_o T_{acq} \tag{26}$$

The geometric distortion is therefore proportional to the data acquisition time and to the absolute value of field inhomogeneity. This might be higher at higher field strength: the common definition of magnet homogeneity is a relative number, namely a value expressed in parts per million. In addition, it is inversely proportional to the gradient amplitude. In EPI of course this means the amplitude in the PC direction since this one is the low-bandwidth direction.

The flux density variation from the magnet varies slowly across the imaging volume. The inhomogeneity from tissues with different susceptibilities is more or less a step function in the field; it cannot be shimmed. It gives typically strong geometric distortions and is probably the largest limitation for EPI in vivo. This type of artifact is called *susceptibility artifact*. This occurs primarily at tissue-air and tissue-bone interfaces. Typical examples inside the human body are the frontal sinus, bowels, and stomach.

Linked with this distortion, which is a stretching or compressing of an image voxel, is a nonuniformity in the image. The brightness of a pixel is proportional to the volume to which it corresponds. In regions where the image is stretched this volume is smaller than in an undistorted region; the signal level is lower. On the other hand, the signal intensity is too bright where pixels are compressed. An example is given in Fig. 10. The images on the left visualize the local B_o inhomogeneity by a technique in which the image is measured by an interference signal of a regular spin echo and a stimulated echo [16]. On the right are the corresponding EPI images.

Only few means are available for reducing the susceptibly artifact. One is the use of thin slices to keep the inhomogeneity across the pixel as small as possible.

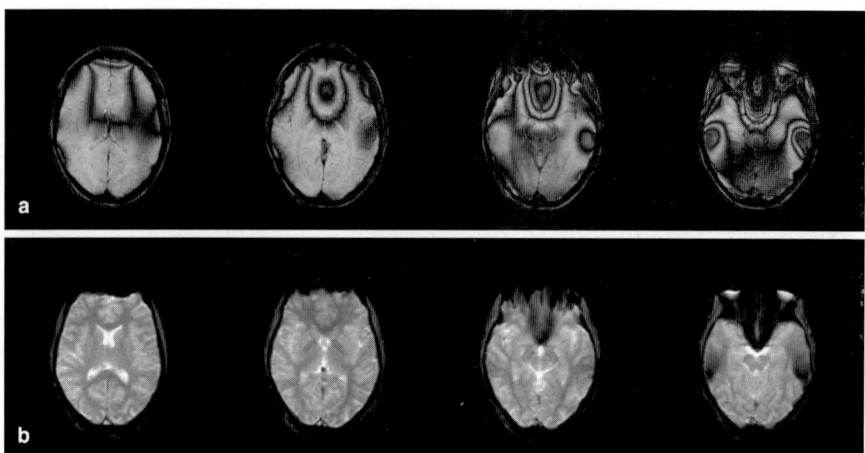

Fig. 10. a Iso-B_o-line image for visualization the local B_o inhomogeneity. **b** Corresponding EPI images

Fig. 11. Slice selection in the head for reduced susceptibility effected images

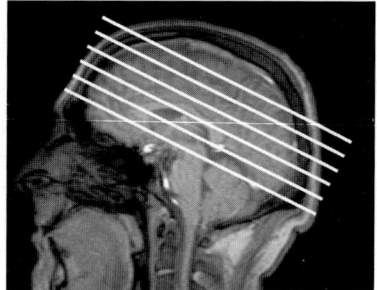

Secondly, in imaging of the head the slices should be selected parallel to the brain basis (see Fig. 11). Another remedy is to fill, for example, the bowels; this has been used successfully in EPI of the abdomen [17].

With knowledge of the B_o distribution it is possible to reduce geometric distortion by postprocessing or suitable corrections during image reconstruction (see for example [1, 10, 19, 23, 24]). However, all these techniques have basic limitations, the first problem is to obtain a reliable field distribution map. Secondly, the signal to noise is in general reduced by these algorithms.

T2*: Signal Loss and Loss of Resolution

As deduced above (see "Artifacts Due to Low Bandwidth: Introduction"), the MR signal course depends on the transversal relaxation time T2 and the local main field inhomogeneity:

$S(t) \propto e^{-t/T2} \, e^{-t/T2'} = e^{-t/T2^*}$ for free induction decay (FID)

$S(t) \propto e^{-(t+TE)/T2} \, e^{-|t|/T2'}$ for spin-echo

$1/T2' \approx \gamma \Delta B_o / 2$

In MR imaging B_o is the field variation across a pixel. For the imaging process this has the consequence that the ideal raw data are multiplied by the signal envelope. This leads to:

- pixel broadening, i.e., image blurring
- decreased pixel intensity

The decreased pixel intensity is a direct consequence of the pixel broadening, the signal is smeared out. This signal loss differs from darker pixel intensity by stretched pixels, as described in the previous section. Here the detected signal intensity is less and cannot be recovered by distortion-correction algorithms. Both effects are of course more pronounced the shorter T2 is and the greater the inhomogeneity is. It should be emphasized again that the PSF reflects not only the properties of the sequence; it also depends on the tissue through the transversal relaxation time T2, on the imaging region by the patient-induced local B_o inhomogeneity, and on the magnet inhomogeneity. Thus the PSF normally varies over the imaging volume. The situation is worst at susceptibility intersections and at the edge of the FOV since here the field inhomogeneity B_o increases in general. The PSF for the example used above is given in Fig. 12. It should be noted that for the same B_o and T2, acquiring the EPI image under the envelope of an spin echo has less effect on the PSF than on acquiring it under a FID. In the former case the dephasing due to B_o inhomogeneity is refocused in the spin echo.

In addition to reducing the local B_o inhomogeneity, as discussed in the previous section, little can be done against these effects. The images of each indivi-

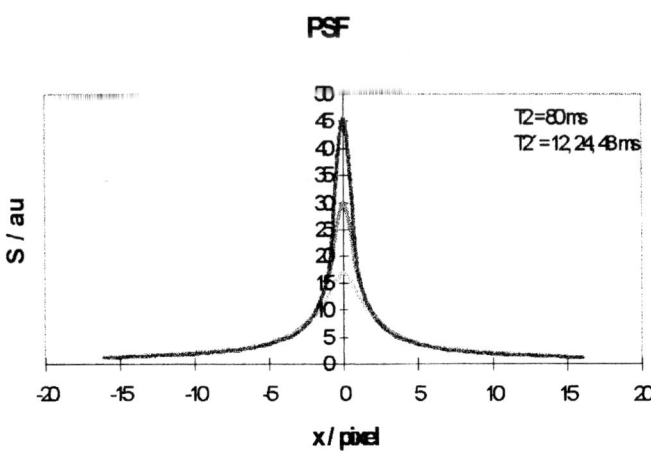

Fig. 12. Examples of PSF. **a** RO time 76.8 ms: T2* roughly 10, 20, and 30 ms. Note the decreased signal intensity and broader lines with the shorter T2*.

PSF: SE vs FID

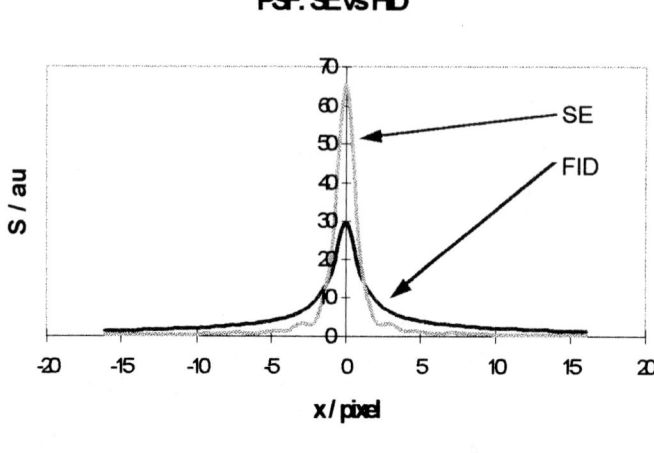

b

Fig. 12. b Difference for FID and SE EPI, with T2 = 80 ms and T2′ = 24 ms. Since the B_o inhomogeneity is refocused during the RO period in the SE case, the PSF is sharper than in the EPI FID

dual tissue are first blurred and then added together; along with noise it is at least a nontrivial task to reduce the effects of the PSF by postprocessing [3]. One iterative approach has been proposed by Haacke [7], and another is discussed by Oshio et al. [15].

Concomitant Field Gradients

Definition

MR imaging makes use of switched magnetic field gradients to obtain spatial information. The field from the gradients is added to the main field, resulting in a spatial dependent resonance frequency. Ideally only a magnetic field component collinear to the main field is generated. Given the main field by definition in z direction, i.e.:

$$B = (0, 0, B_o)$$

the imaging gradient would be (see Eq. 9):

$$G = \overline{V}(B_z) = (G_x, G_y, G_z) = (\partial B_z/dx, \partial B_z/dy, \partial B_z/dz)$$

The resulting field in the presence of all three gradients is:

$$B = (0, 0, B_o+G_xx+G_yy+G_zz) \tag{27}$$

Note: we assume here that the field gradients are strictly linear in space, which is typically fulfilled in the imaging volume.

Norris [13] was the first to point out that the field generated by the gradient coils must satisfy the Maxwell equations for the free space condition. These equations are:

$$\text{div } B = \overline{V} \cdot B = \partial B_x/dx + \partial B_y/dy + B_z/dz = 0$$

and:

$$\text{curl } B = \overline{V} \times B \begin{cases} \partial B_z/dy - \partial B_y/dz \\ B\partial = B_x/dz - \partial B_z/dx = \overline{0} \\ \partial B_y/dx - \partial B_x/dy \end{cases}$$

where $\overline{V}$ indicates the Nabla operator, · the vector product, × the cross product, and $\overline{0}$ the null vector. Applying these equations to the imaging gradients, one obtains the conditions summarized in Table 1 (according Norris [13]).

The concomitant field of the z gradient depends on the gradient design. For example, in case of a Maxwell pair coil (Helmholtz coil but opposite current direction in each coil) we have a = b = –0.5 [14].

In the presence of a concomitant field, the resulting field is no longer purely in z direction as indicated in Eq. 27. Switching, for example, the x gradient, the total field is:

$$B = (G_x z, 0, B_o + G_x x) \tag{28}$$

with a magnitude of:

$$|B| = \sqrt{(B_o + G_x x)^2 + (G_x z)^2} \tag{29}$$

In the case $B_o > (G_x x)$, $(G_x z)$, which is generally fulfilled, this may be expanded to:

$$|B| = B_o + G_x x + (G_x z)^2/(2B_o) \tag{30}$$

The magnitude contains not only the homogeneous main field and the linear field gradient but also the so-called Maxwell term which is proportional to the square of z and to the square of the gradient amplitude and is inversely proportional to B_o. This term leads effectively to a new resonance frequency with an frequency offset ω_{eff} of:

$$\omega_{eff} (G_x) = \gamma G_x^2 z^2/(2B_o) \tag{31}$$

Table 1. Concomitant gradients (note that the Maxwell equation not mentioned in the third column is satisfied trivially)

Axis	Imaging gradient	Condition to be satisfied	Consequence	Concomitant gradient(s)	Concomitant field
x	$Gx = \partial B_z/dx$	curl B = 0	$\partial B_x/dz - \partial B_z/dx = 0$	$\partial B_x/dz$	$Bx = G_x z$
y	$Gy = \partial B_z/dy$	curl B = 0	$\partial B_z/dy - \partial B_y/dz = 0$	$\partial B_y/dz$	$By = G_y z$
z	$Gz = \partial B_z/dz$	div B = 0	$\partial B_x/dx + \partial B_y/dy + \partial B_z/dz = 0$	$\partial B_x/dx, \partial B_y/dy$	$Bx = aG_z x$
					$By = bG_z y$
					$a + b = -1$

The result for the y gradient is similar:

$$\omega_{eff}\,(G_y) = \gamma G_y^2 z^2/(2B_o) \tag{32}$$

For the z gradient one obtains:

$$\omega_{eff}\,(G_z) = \gamma G_z^2\,((ax)^2+(by)^2)/(2B_o) \tag{33}$$

or for the Maxwell pair coil configuration:

$$\omega_{eff}\,(Gz) = \gamma G_z^2 r^2\,(8B_o) \tag{34}$$

with r the distance from z axis, $r^2 = x^2+y^2$.

In summary, for all gradients the Maxwell term:

- Is proportional to the square of the gradient amplitude and therefore independent of the gradient sign
- Is worse at lower field strength since it is proportional to $1/B_o$
- Varies with the square of one spatial dimension

Discussion

The Maxwell term can normally be disregarded in conventional imaging. For example, at 1.5 T the effect of a 10-mT/m x gradient is at a position of z = 15 cm only 0.5 ppm. In EPI, however, this effect must be considered since typically:

- A high read gradient is used.
- The pixel bandwidth in phase direction is extremely low, or the acquisition time is long.

Continuing with the previous example, a gradient amplitude of 25 mT/m gives an effect of 3.1 ppm, which is almost as much as the fat water difference frequency.

In discussing the effect of the concomitant gradient on images in EPI one must consider which gradient is the read gradient. For the following discussion we assume a horizontal bore magnet [25].

Axial Slices

For this orientation either the x or the y gradient is the read gradient with the high amplitude. The dominating effect is an image shift in PC direction. The frequency offset according to Eq. 31 or 32 is proportional to z^2. As in the case of frequency offset due to chemical shift, it results in an image shifted in the PC direction. The shift, however, increases with the off-center position z. With the examples used in this chapter – matrix 128, $T_{RO} = 0.6$ ms, G = 25 mT/m, $B_o = 1.5$ T – the effect at z = 15 cm is as much as 15 pixels. Since this is a uniform shift of the image, it can quite easily be corrected.

The Maxwell term is produced by the read gradient. The phase of the image, i.e., the phase acquired until k = 0, depends also on the z position of the image slice. Apart from the mentioned image shift this phase has no effect on the

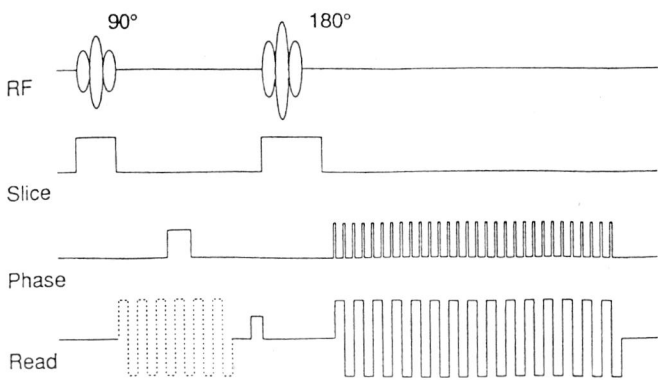

Fig. 13. Schematic pulse sequence with a "prewarping" of the accumulated Maxwell phase. (From Weisskoff et al. [25])

images unless phase information is used, for example, for flow quantification or a three-dimensional implementation of EPI (EPI with a warp gradient in slice direction). When the phase at $k = 0$ is important, a prephasing can be used in the case of spin-echo excitation (see Fig. 13): before the refocusing pulse the read gradient scheme is applied, which is applied after the refocusing pulse until $k = 0$. The phase accumulation due to the read pulses is refocused at the point $k = 0$.

A further effect must be considered when the signal is sampled on the gradient ramps, which is normally performed with a sinusoidal varying gradient. The frequency shift is proportional to G^2, and it therefore changes during the RO period. Slight image blurring and additional N/2 ghosting results in this case.

Finally, the phase accumulation due to the concomitant gradient depends on z^2. The phase variation over a slice must be well below 2π. This limits either the maximum slice thickness or for a given slice thickness the maximum off-center position. The maximum slice shift z_o for a given slice thickness D is:

$$z_o = B_o/(G^2 T \gamma D) \tag{35}$$

In the example of this chapter we have for a slice thickness of 10 mm a maximum allowed slice shift of 73 mm.

Coronal and Sagittal Slices

The effect on coronal and sagittal slices is somewhat more complex. The additional frequency shift is now generally in the image plane, leading to in-plane distortions. For coronal slices using the x gradient as read gradient this produces a frequency shift proportional to z^2 but independent of x. Each line in the images has a slightly different shift. Lines in the middle are unshifted; at the edges they are squeezed or stretched. A schematic drawing is given in Fig. 14. Since the effect varies with the square of z, one remedy against this effect is to limit the

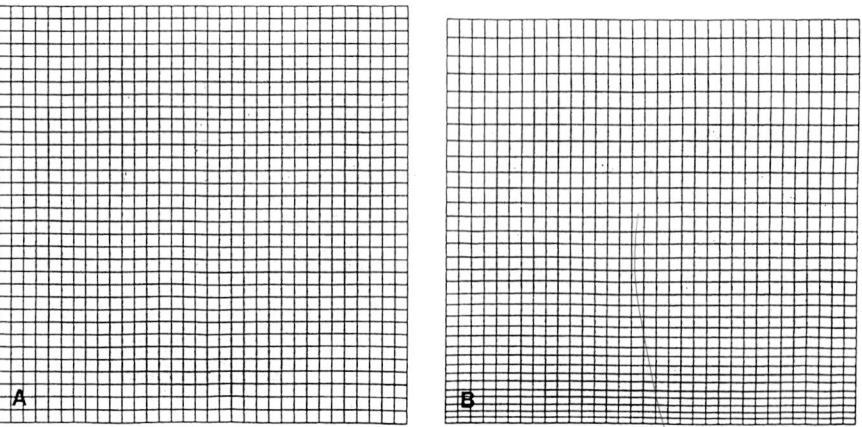

Fig. 14. Schematic representation of image distortion caused in the coronal plane when the image is frequency-encoded with the x gradient. The ancillary Maxwell gradient causes an effective frequency shift that is quadratic with axial position. As a result, pixels at the top and bottom of the FOV are shifted up, thus compressing the image at the bottom, and stretching the image at the top. (From Weisskoff et al. [25])

FOV in this direction. The same holds for sagittal images using the y gradient as read gradient.

When the z gradient is used as read gradient, the Maxwell term is proportional to x^2+y^2, however it is smaller by a factor of 4. One part of this term, namely x^2 in coronal slices and y^2 in sagittal slices, leads to pixel squeezing or stretching, while the other one is responsible for a slice shift in the PC direction, as in the case of axial slices. The phase accumulation for $k = 0$ and the susceptibility to more N/2 ghosting is similar, as discussed in the previous section.

What ways can be used to reduce the effect of the concomitant gradient beyond those that have already been mentioned? First, one can use a high field strength B_0. However, with this the susceptibility artifacts are more dominant. The effect on low field imaging in general is discussed by Norris and Hutchinson [14] and on EPI at 0.2 T by Heid [8]. Second, one can reduce the maximal gradient amplitude. However, for a given resolution the time integral of the read gradient must kept constant see ("Artifacts Due to Low Bandwidth: Introduction"):

$$\int_{T_{RO}} G(t)dt = const.$$

This means that the lower the gradient amplitude, the longer the data acquisition time is, and with this the worse the artifacts of susceptibility and B_0 inhomogeneity are, namely geometric distortions and signal loss due to T2*. The two effects scale oppositely with the RO time. Therefore EPI is always a tradeoff between susceptibility and gradient-induced distortions.

It should be noted that no assumptions are made above for a special gradient coil design (besides the example of the Maxwell coil pair). The discussion is based solely on the Maxwell equations and is independent of the type of magnet, for example horizontal or vertical field.

References

1. Bowtell R, McIntyre DJO, Commandre MJ, Glover P, Mansfield P (1994) Correction of geometric distortion in echo planar images. In: Books of abstracts: Society of Magnetic Resonance, 2nd scientific meeting 411
2. Bruder H, Fischer H, Reinfelder HE, Schmitt F (1992) Image reconstruction for echo planar imaging with nonequidistant k-space sampling. Magn Res Med 23:311
3. Constable RT, Gore JC (1992) The loss of small objects in variable TE imaging: implications for FSE, RARE and EPI. Magn Reson Med 28:9–24
4. Coxon R, Mansfield P (1989) EPI spatial distortion in non-transverse planes. In: Books of abstracts: Society of Magnetic Resonance in Medicine, 8th annual meeting, 361
5. Farzaneh F, Riederer SJ, Pelc NJ (1990) Analysis of T2 limitations and off-resonance effects on spatial resolution and artifacts in echo-planar imaging. Magn Reson Med 14:123–139
6. Goldfarb JW, Schmitt F, Fischer H, Haacke EM, Duerk JL (1995) A method to remove ghosting from parametric phase distortions in EPI. In: Books of abstracts: Society of Magnetic Resonance, 3rd scientific meeting, 759
7. Haacke EM (1987) The effects of finite sampling in spin-echo or field echo magnetic resonance imaging. Magn Reson Med 4:407–421
8. Heid O, Deimling M (1994) Echo-planar Imaging on a low-field system. Radiology Society of North America, 80th scientific assembly and meeting, scientific program, 169
9. Jehenson P, Westphal M, Schuff N (1990) Analytical method for the compensation of eddy-current effects induces by pulsed magnetic field gradients in NMR systems. J Magn Res 90:264–278
10. Jezzard P, Balaban RS (1995) Correcting for geometric distortion in echo planar images from B_0 field variations. Magn Reson Med 34:65–73
11. Johnson G, Hutchinson JMS (1985) The limitations of NMR recalled-echo imaging techniques. J Magn Reson 63:14–30
12. Ljunggren (1993) S. Ljunggren, J. Magn. Reson. 54, 336 (1984)
13. Norris DG (1985) Phase errors in NMR images. In: Books of abstracts: Society of Magnetic Resonance Imaging, proceedings of the 2nd annual meeting, p 1037
14. Norris DG, Huttchinson JMS (1990) Concomitant magnetic field gradients and their effects on imaging at low magnetic field strength. Magn Res Imag 8:33–37
15. Oshio K, Singh M (1989) A computer simulation of T2 decay effects in echo planar imaging. Magn Res Med 11:389–397
16. Schmitt F, Heubes P, Fischer H, Barfuss H, German patent no. 40 04184 (1989)
17. Reimer P, Schmitt F, Ladebeck R, Graessner J, Schaffer B (1993) Evaluation of potential gastrointestinal contrast agents for echoplanar MR imaging. Eur Radiol 3:487–492
18. Sekihara K, Kohno H (1987a) New reconstruction technique for echo-planar imaging to allow combined use of odd and even numbered echoes. Med Phys 5 (6):485
19. Sekihara K, Kohno H (1987b) Image restoration from nonuniform static field influence in modified echo-planar imaging. Med Phys 14 (6):1087–1089
20. Tietze U, Schenk C (1989) Halbleiterschaltungstechnik, 8th edn. Springer, Berlin Heidelberg New York, p 379
21. Twieg DB (1985) Acquisition and accuracy in rapid NMR imaging methods. Magn Reson Med 2:437–452
22. van Hulsteyn DB, Sillerud LO (1987) Transverse relaxation time constrains on resolution in one-dimensional, phase- and frequency-encoded nuclear magnetic resonance imaging. J Magn Reson 71:14–23
23. Wan X, Gullberg GT, Parker DL (1995) Reduction of geometric distortion in echo-planar imaging using a multi-reference scan. In: Books of abstracts: Society of Magnetic Resonance, 3rd scientific meeting, p 103
24. Weisskoff RM, Davis TL (1992) Correcting gross distortion echo planar images. In: Books of abstracts: Society of Magnetic Resonance in Medicine, 11th annual meeting, 4516

25. Weisskoff RM, Cohen MS, Rzedzian RR (1993) Nonaxial whole-body instant imaging. Magn Res Imag 28:769–803
26. Zakhor A (1990) Ghost cancellation algorithms for MRI images. IEEE Trans Med Imaging 9 (3):318–326

CHAPTER 7

Physiological Side Effects of Fast Gradient Switching

F. Schmitt, W. Irnich, and H. Fischer

Introduction

Three types of electromagnetic fields are involved in magnetic resonance imaging (MRI): the static magnetic field, B_o, the radiofrequency (RF) magnetic field, B_1, and the time-varying gradient magnetic field, B_G. Physiological effects resulting from the interaction of these fields with biological tissue are reported in the literature [1]. Effects from strong B_o fields are wide-ranging and often contradictory [2]. At the moment there is no evidence for hazardous or irreversible effects related to exposure to static magnetic fields up to a field strength of 2 T. Studies with whole-body 4-T scanners, however, report unwanted side effects [3] which are not of great concern for further research. All RF power used in MRI is converted into heat within the human tissue [4] due to the conductivity of the tissue.

Visual effects, so-called magnetophosphenes, may occur when the head is exposed to continuous magnetic fields of ≤ 20 mT at frequencies of 50 Hz or below [5, 6]. To date magnetophosphenes have not been reported in humans examined with fast gradients such as those used for fast MRI techniques, including echo-planar imaging (EPI) [7].

Sensory perception of induced effects from time-varying magnetic field gradients were first reported in 1989, although they had been predicted by Budinger as early as 1979 [8]. In view of the technological development over the past decade it is not surprising that it took more than 10 years to observe physiological effects caused by gradient switching. Since its beginning in 1979 MR technology has developed very rapidly. Especially the gradient hardware has undergone dramatic improvement in performance. At the beginning typical gradient amplitudes and rise times were 1 mT/m and 1 ms, respectively. Today the manufacturers of almost every MRI scanner offer whole-body gradients in the range of 20–30 mT/m with rise times as short as 100 µs for EPI. This is a change in the order of a magnitude, and more so in amplitude and rise time.

In 1989 we observed in our laboratory that fast gradient switching can cause neuromuscular sensations. These findings were published by Cohen et al. [9] and Fischer at al. [10] in 1989. The sensations were ranged from weak to painful [11]. These findings led to concern that patients with heart diseases may be harmed in achieving neuromuscular stimulation thresholds. However, subsequent experiments conducted with both animals and human beings and a review of the literature on cardiac pacemakers show that maintaining levels at or slightly above the neuromuscular threshold is safe and entails no cardiac effects. Indeed, gradients least ten times greater than is available today would be required to cause cardiac effects in whole-body imaging. This is far beyond the technical feasibility for whole-body MRI systems. Several investigations in the past decade have considered possible effects due to time-varying magnetic fields [12–21], and the major questions that remain controversial are: (a) Is a hazard associated with the strength of the magnetic flux, B, or its rate of change, dB/dt? (b) What is the threshold value for cardiac excitation in relation to peripheral nerve thresholds?

The IRPA/INIRC Guideline on MRI [22] warns that electric field strengths exceeding 5 V/m may cause ventricular fibrillation, suggesting that the thresholds for nerve and cardiac muscle stimulation are very close to one another.

In addition to stimulatory effects, the gradient can also cause significant acoustic noise. This is important especially with fast MRI techniques such as EPI due to the switching of large gradients. Currently the peak acoustic noise is limited to values below 140 dB (unweighted), a value which can be reached when systems are not optimized to low acoustic noise levels.

This chapter discusses the side effects of fast gradient switching. We first explain why gradient speed and amplitude is so important for MRI and give an overview of gradient coil design and its relationship to magnetostimulation effects. We use the term "magnetostimulation" to describe physiological effects due to gradient switching. In terms of the theory behind magnetostimulation, one can distinguish three different models, none of which fully describes the reality. We then describe the impact of fast gradient switching on humans. We also discuss the various national and international regulatory rules (FDA, BGA, IEC); all of these are based on the field change per unit time (dB/dt).

Experimental results of human peripheral studies are presented to demonstrate the functional relationship of threshold strength, stimulus duration, and. the threshold relationship to stimulus shapes. It has not as yet been possible to produce cardiac stimulation with MRI scanners, and it is very unlikely in the future based on present knowledge. Therefore imaging below the peripheral threshold appears to be safe. Even when operated at or slightly above the threshold, patient safety is guaranteed.

The acoustic aspects of fast gradient switching are presented in the Appendix. Basic principles of the generating forces and the limits of acoustical noise for patients and personnel are described.

Importance of Fast Switching of High Gradient Amplitudes

In MRI the pixel size, δx, is inversely proportional to the gradient-time integral as described in Eq. 1:

$$\delta x = \frac{2\pi}{\gamma \cdot \int_{t1}^{t2} G(t)dt} \tag{1}$$

where γ is called the gyromagnetic ratio, and $T_{RO} = t_2 - t_1$ describes the data-acquisition window (the time when ADC is on) under the gradient $G(t)$ (see Fig. 1). The time integration over the gradient pulse $G(t)$ can be explained as

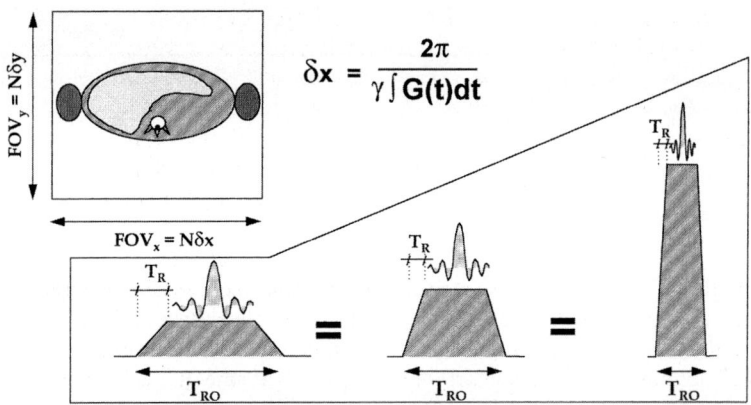

Fig. 1. Resolution in MRI and its consequences on hardware demands. The resolution in MRI is defined by the gradient area under the readout gradient pulse (*shaded area*). When the gradient pulses become shorter, the amplitude must increase, and rise times must become shorter

the area under the gradient pulse. This area must be kept constant for a certain field of view (FOV) or pixel size. Greater speed requires that the gradient amplitude be increased for a trapezoidal pulse shape (Fig. 1).

Below we first present examples of required gradient strength and rise times for standard gradient echo (GRE) MRI and for EPI. These demonstrate the strong demands when moving from conventional MRI to EPI. A typical readout (RO) gradient pulse scheme of a GRE sequence is shown in Fig. 2. For this type of sequence Eq. 1 yields:

$$\delta x = \frac{2\pi}{\gamma \cdot G \cdot N \cdot \delta t} \tag{2}$$

where δt is the ADC sampling time, and N the matrix size. Equation 2 indicates that the gradient strength must be increased in order to reduce the pixel size.

Fig. 2. Readout and RF module of a GRE sequence. Vertical arrows during the time interval $[t_1, t_2]$ indicate the data acquisition period. The achievable echo time (*TE*) depends on the rise time (T_{rise})

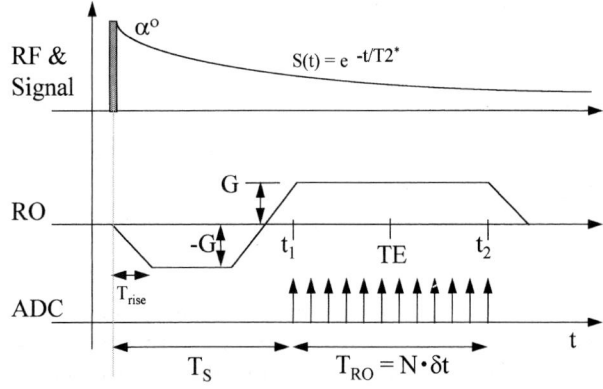

Table 1. Readout-gradient strength (G) and pixel size (δx) calculated for different matrix sizes (N) for the GRE sequence of Fig. 2

N	G (mT/m)	δx (mm)
32	0.6	9.3
64	1.2	4.6
128	2.5	2.3
256	5.0	1.1
512	10.2	0.5
1024	20.0	0.2

Table 1 shows examples of the dependency of the pixel size δx on the gradient strength G and the matrix size N for the RO module shown in Fig. 1. A typical FOV of 300 mm and a RO time T_{RO} of 4 ms was chosen. The prephasing lobe is assumed to have the same gradient strength G as the RO lobe and the echo appears at the center of the RO lobe. Table 1 indicates that submillimeter high resolution MRI, as for example needed for musculoskeletal imaging, in combination with fast MRI techniques may require gradient amplitude in the order of 20 mT/m.

In the RO module of Fig. 2 an echo time TE of 6.5 ms results when a typical rise time of 1 ms is selected. This is still too slow for the fast MRI that is now possible with the latest generation of scanners. Gradient speed is important for achieving shorter echo times (TE) to avoid signal void caused by flowing blood [23, 24] and reduce the susceptibility effects [25]. This is the case in both conventional MRI and in EPI. New applications [26, 27] in MR angiography show that minimum TE times in the order of 1–2 ms are very advantageous for reducing or eliminating turbulent flow artifacts of flowing blood.

EPI places even more demanding requirements in speed and amplitude. The signal to noise ratio and susceptibility are the major obstacles of EPI [28, 29] That implies that the data acquisition time must be compared to the T2* in order to minimize susceptibility effects and gather as much as data during the single free induction decay. Figure 3 shows a typical gradient-echo EPI sequence with a trapezoidal RO gradient pulse train (for further information on sequences see Chap. 4). T2* decay is plotted above the gradient waveform to illustrate the shortening of T2 decay due to local inhomogeneities ΔB_o, as described in Eq. 3:

$$\frac{1}{T2^*} = \frac{1}{T2} + \gamma \langle \Delta B_o \rangle \tag{3}$$

When data are acquired under a T2*-weighted free induction decay, the resulting signal can be described as:

$$S(t) = S_0(t) \cdot e^{-\frac{t}{T2^*}} \tag{4}$$

To reduce signal loss due to susceptibility the echo time must be short compared to the T2* time. A typical T2* time of about 100 ms and a FOV of 300 mm require a RO time per echo (T_{RO}) of 1 ms for a 128×128 image matrix. To achieve this the gradient amplitude must be increased and the rise time shortened. Typical values for the EPI sequence of Fig. 3 are presented in Table 2. Comparing Tables 1 and 2 shows that matrices of 1024^2 are feasible for conventional MRI. However, for EPI the limit in matrix size is reached at about 256^2

Table 2. Readout-gradient amplitude (G) as a function of the matrix size (N) for the trapezoidal GRE-EPI sequence of Fig. 3: echo times (TE) gradient rise times of 100 and 1000 μs

N	G (mT/m)	T_{Rise} = 100 μs (TE, ms)	T_{Rise} = 1000 μs (TE, ms)
32	2.5	21.8	51.5
64	5.0	41.0	99.5
128	10.0	79.4	195.5
256	20.0	156.2	387.5
512	40.0	309.8	771.5
1024	81.1	617.0	1539.5

The start time, T_s, of the data acquisition was set to 2 ms. A readout time, T_{RO}, per echo of 1 ms and a field of view, FOV, of 300 mm was used to calculate the table.

Table 3. Readout-gradient amplitude (G) as a function of the matrix size (N) for the sinusoidal GRE-EPI sequence of Fig. 4: echo times (TE) gradient rise times of 250 and 500 μs

N	T_{Rise} = 250 μs		T_{Rise} = 500 μs	
	G (mT/m)	(TE, ms)	G (mT/m)	(TE, ms)
32	7.8	10.2	3.9	18.5
64	15.7	18.2	7.8	34.5
128	31.4	34.2	15.7	66.5
256	62.9	66.2	31.4	130.5
512	125.9	130.2	62.9	258.5
1024	251.8	258.2	125.9	514.5

The start time, T_s, of the data acquisition was set to 2 ms. The table was calculated for a field of view, FOV, of 300 mm.

because large gradient strengths are required which are far beyond what is technically feasible, and echo times result which have no real medical use.

In addition to trapezoidal gradient pulses, EPI with sinusoidal waveforms is commonly used, with advantages in technical aspects. For more detail see Chap. 3. When sinusoidal gradients are used (Fig. 4, Table 3), Eq. 1 yields:

$$\delta x = \frac{2\pi}{\gamma \cdot G \cdot \frac{\pi}{2} \cdot N \cdot \delta t} \tag{5}$$

This means that when trapezoidal gradient waveforms (Eq. 2) are compared with sinusoidal ones (Eq. 5), the gradient amplitude, G_{sin}, needed for the same resolution δx is:

$$G_{sin} = G \cdot \frac{\pi}{2} \tag{6}$$

This involves even higher gradient strengths for sinusoidal single-shot EPI. A comparison is shown between rise times of 250 and 500 μs, corresponding to sinusoidal frequencies of 1000 and 500 Hz.

Reasonable measurement times for freezing body motion, especially cardiac motion, are on the order of a tenth of a second. Except for long TEs needed to visualize fluid in the human body, typical values range from a few milliseconds to 100 ms. In both approaches, freezing body motion and providing reasonable

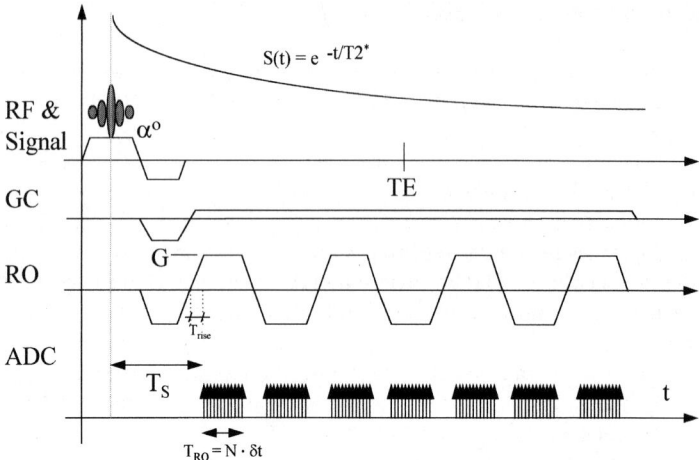

Fig. 3. Trapezoidal GRE EPI sequence. When data are acquired on the flat top only, pause times between the data-acquisition blocks (*vertical arrows*) are present, prolonging the total acquistion time

echo times, whole-body single-shot EPI the appropriate gradient strength is between 20 and 30 mT/m at rise times betweeen 100 and 300 µs. When whole-body MRI scanners are operated inside these limits, magnetostimulation is likely.

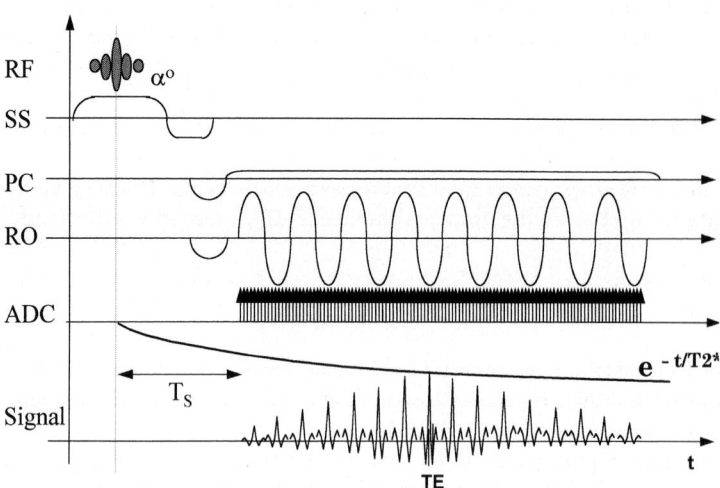

Fig. 4. Sinusoidal GRE EPI sequence. Data are acquired throughout the entire sinusoidal gradient train

Magnetostimulation of Excitable Tissue

In general stimulation can be classified into peripheral and cardiac forms, which are best characterized by their thresholds. Peripheral stimulation is subdivided into sensory, nerve, and muscle or motor stimulation. Sensory stimulation is a very weak sensation and causes no other effects than a weak feeling; it shows the lowest threshold of perception measurable. Muscle or motor stimulation causes muscle twitches and muscular contraction. Thresholds of muscle stimulation are higher than sensory thresholds. Bourland et al. [30] examined peripheral nerve (muscle twitching) and respiratory nerve stimulation on dogs and report peripheral nerves to show lower thresholds than nerves innervating muscles of respiration.

Cardiac stimulation can be subdivided into the threshold for extra systolic excitation and thresholds for fibrillations. From dog experiments it is known that ectopic beats appear earlier than cardiac fibrillations when single stimuli are applied. Ruiz et al. [31] report that the fibrillation threshold is at least 1.4–2 times higher than the threshold for ectopic beats. From these findings it follows that reaching the threshold of additional systoles can induce cardiac fibrillation when the stimulus is applied during the vulnerable phase. Bourland et al. [30] report that the threshold of ectopic beats is about 9.6 times that of peripheral muscle stimulation and about 2.6 times that of respiratory nerve stimulation. They could not produce cardiac fibrillation in dogs, and when scaling their results to humans they concluded that "provoking cardiac arrythmias, and specifically, ventricular fibrillation by pulsed gradients is highly unlikely" [32].

Similar results have been shown by Roos et al. [34] in an open-chest study in dogs. In this study ectopic beats due to magnetostimulation had thresholds about 6.5 times higher than those for peripheral stimulation when the same electrophysiology was assumed for dogs and humans and the thresholds recalculated for human sizes. The rather low cardiac stimulation threshold was explained by the fact that the stimulator coil was in contact with wet cardiac tissue and therefore coupled directly into the tissue. Higher thresholds are expected in "dry" experiments.

Since cardiac magnetostimulation has not yet been reported in humans and is not expected with the current gradient hardware available, we focus on peripheral stimulation, the first sensations that appear. Cohen et al. [34] describe the stimulation as a "small twitch across the bridge of the nose when lying in the prone position with the face pointing directly downward, or in supine position with the face directed upward. Rotating the head slightly to the left or to the right reduces or eliminates the stimulation effects. One subject described small twitch contractions at the base of the spine. Another experienced similar sensations in the lower back occasionally, however, regularly detected twitch contractions on the medial surface of the left thigh." The study was undertaken with a whole-body gradient coil.

In a similar report on a study with ten human subjects Budinger et al. [11] report the stimulation as being noted between the pectoral muscles and the abdomen and in the musculature of the lower back. All subjects described the sensations as electric shock or tap in the buttocks, lower back, or flanks. They were rated as weak, definite, painful (with strong stimuli), or very painful (with extremely high stimulus). The study was carried out with an experimental whole-body EPI gradient coil.

Another whole-body study on 179 persons [25] reports "various types of stimulation. Most of the stimulated regions were about 30–40 cm from the magnet isocenter. Nearly 50 % of these were muscle twitches in the head, chest, abdomen, hips, or arms. Approximately 30 % of the reports were vibrations or pulsations of the nose, forehead, chest, or arm. The remaining 20 % were described as tingling or electric shock in the forearm and/or arms. One subject felt a painful electric shock from both elbows to finger tips when the cervical spine or heart was scanned with hands clasped over the abdomen." For this reason MR vendors offering EPI systems include special instructions in their users' manual for conducting EPI examinations, noting that the hands should not be clasped during EPI scans using the y gradient as the rapidly switched gradient coil.

Schaefer et al. [36] report in a whole-body study on 13 volunteers stimulation sites in the "scapula, bridge of the nose, upper arms, legs, hands, buttocks, head, xyphoid, and on the back." They report that the least pleasant sensation occurs when hands are clasped during a y gradient study. When hands are not clasped the threshold rose by 46 %.

In a volunteer study undertaken with a small stimulator coil placed on palmar surface of the right wrist Mansfield et al. [13] report "the perception of stimulation was sensory at very low levels and at higher levels both sensory and motor, the latter effect producing considerable finger twitch."

Yamagata et al. [37] performed a study with local field coils to evaluate stimulation thresholds of the human forehead and observed that the "somatory sensations were felt around the bridge of the nose."

Gradient Field Design and its Relation to the Location of Magnetostimulation

In MRI the B_z component is the only important component of the gradient field. Therefore gradient coils are optimized to obtain the best B_z field quality. In most MR experiments the transverse field components, $B_\perp$, produced by gradient coils are of no concern, except the effects of the so-called Maxwell terms (see Chap. 6) and magnetostimulation, as described in this chapter. Below we consider actual field geometries generated by gradient coils because these are important for understanding why some coils stimulate more than others.

For superconductive magnets with a cylindrical bore the main magnetic field is along the bore; by definition this orientation is called the z-axis. Gradient coils are therefore typically designed on cylinders. The z gradient comprises cylindrical windings producing a B_z component mainly in the patient access volume. The magnet and the gradients have a finite length, and therefore the B_z component of the gradient coil must drop at a certain distance z_o from the center of the magnet. Typically the maximum flux magnitude B_z is reached outside the FOV (see Fig. 5) to guarantee images without significant geometric distortions. Although z gradients produce transverse field components very close to the coil windings and at the rear and front end of the coil, they do not affect magnetostimulation

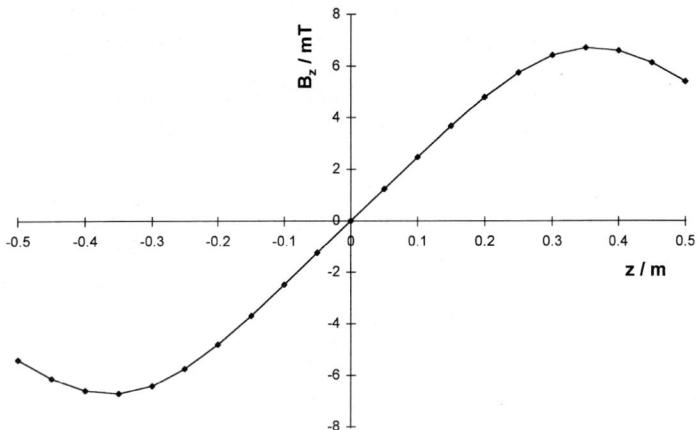

Fig. 5. Magnetic field of a z gradient coil measured along the z axis at x = y = 0

because it lay outside the patient access volume. For more detail on coil design see Chap. 3.

The field distribution is more complex with transverse gradients (x and y). In addition to the z component, transverse coils always produce transverse components B_x and B_y. This is a consequence of Maxwell's equations (magnetic field lines must be closed). Figure 6 shows the z and x components of an x gradient coil as a function of the longitudinal z-axis. Until a certain point $z = z_1$ the B_z component is homogeneous, indicating the edge of the imaging volume. The transverse component B_x reaches its maximum at $z = z_0$. The total field produced by the B_x component is typically larger than those of the B_z component. In general it can be said that an x gradient produces a significant B_x field component, and a y gradient produces a significant B_y field component in addition to the B_z field component, which is MR effective. The other components, B_y of an x gradient and B_x of a y gradient, are only marginal and therefore of no concern for magnetostimulation. A similar description of gradient coil field distribution has been given by Rohan et al. [38].

Understanding the fundamental field distribution of gradient coils, we can now find the location of magnetostimulation when we return to Faraday's law of induction. This describes the relationship between a changing magnetic flux density, B, exposing a conductive matter, for example, human tissue, and the resulting induced electric field, E. In mathematical form this is expressed as:

$$\oint \underline{E} \cdot \underline{ds} = -\frac{d}{dt} \int\int_A \underline{B} \cdot \underline{dA} \tag{7}$$

Each term in the integrals are vectors. The first integral is taken over a closed curve. The element area, dA, and the magnetic flux vector, B, forms a scalar product. Since the magnetic flux B is a vector, $dB/dt = (dB_x/dt, dB_y/dt, dB_z/dt)$ is a vector as well. The plain expression dB/dt is often used in this chapter for

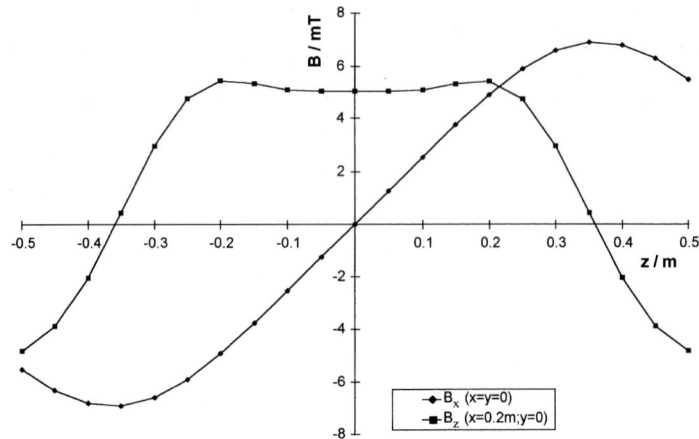

Fig. 6. Longitudinal component B_z and transverse components B_x of an x-axis gradient coil measured along z axis

simplicity where no misunderstanding would arise, but its vector property should always be kept in mind.

Assuming a homogeneous magnetic flux inside a circular loop of radius, r, the magnitude of the induced electric field calculated from Eq. 7 is:

$$E(r) = -\frac{r}{2}\frac{dB}{dt} \tag{8}$$

Equation 8 indicates that the highest electric field is proportional to the flux change per unit time, dB/dt. In the simplified case of a trapezoidal periodic wave of rise time, T_{rise}, we can rewrite Eq. 8 to:

$$E_{max}(r) = -\frac{r\,B_{max}}{2\,T_{Rise}} \tag{9}$$

Equation 9 implies that the location of the strongest induced E field, E_{max}, corresponds to the location of the strongest magnetic flux, B_{max}. This is important for understanding the mechanism of magnetostimulation, as described in more detail below. At this point we use the fact that the location of the highest magnetic flux exposed to the patient defines the most likely location where magnetostimulation may be felt. This has been confirmed by many experiments on humans [38, 39]. Erhardt et al. report in a whole-body study on 179 patients [37] that most of the stimulated regions were about 30–40 cm from the magnet isocenter. This corresponds with B_{max} produced by the gradient coils.

Figures 7 and 8 show the situation for a z gradient and a transverse gradient, respectively. When the head is positioned at the center of the z-coil, magnetostimulation is typically felt at the lower spine, corresponding to the peak field produced by the z gradient coil. Remembering that transverse gradient coils produce transverse field components, $B_\perp$, of the same orientation as the gradient direction, and that $B_\perp$ is typically larger than the amplitude of the MR effective

Fig. 7. Magnetic flux of a z gradient coil and its correlation to the location of magnetostimulation. *Bold line,* location of the magnetostimulation

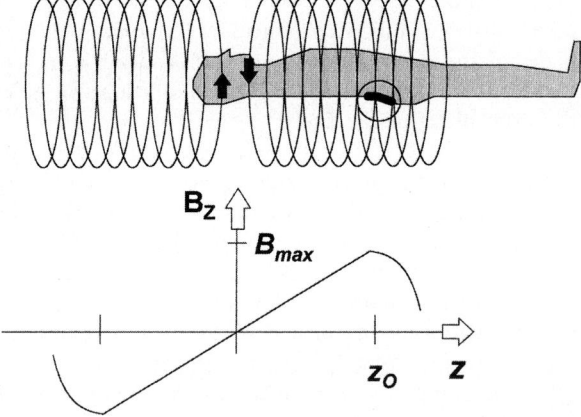

z component and is almost constant over the plane at $z = z_o$, we can now concentrate on these transverse components to understand the location of magnetostimulation with transverse gradient coils. Figure 8 shows simplified saddle-shaped transverse gradient coils. Real transverse gradient coils have a more fingerprint-like appearance. For more detail see Chap. 3. The MR effective z component, B_z, is produced by the inner arcs. The maximum transverse field component, $B_\perp^{max}$, is typically produced at the "eyes" (center of fingerprints) of the saddle coils. The exact location depends on the individual finger print design. Referring to Fig. 8, when the patient is positioned for a cardiac examination, the location of the maximum exposed magnetic flux is at the head and the upper legs, definitely not at the region to be imaged.

When we ask for the most effective flux component with respect to stimulation sensitivity, we can refer to the component producing the maximum magnitude of the flux. For standard fingerprint designs these are given by transverse compo-

Fig. 8. Magnetic flux of transverse gradient coils. The major components responsible for magnetostimulations are the transverse components (B_x for an x gradient and B_y for a y gradient)

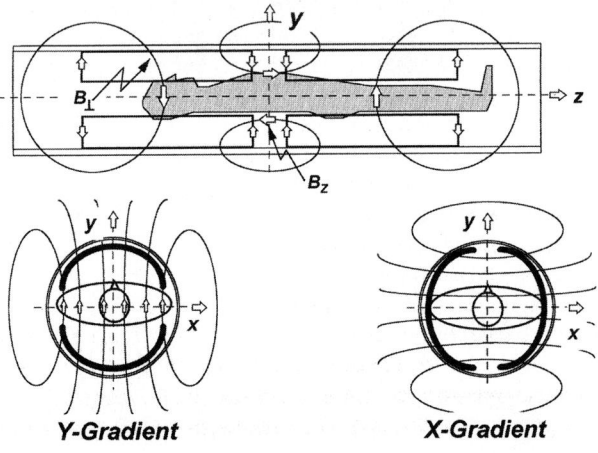

nents of transverse gradients (x, y) and the longitudinal component of the z gradient. The y gradient produces a B_y component passing through the coronal plane of the body. The x gradient produces a B_x component passing throught the sagittal plane and the z gradients produce a B_z component passing through the axial plane of the body.

From Eq. 8 it is seen that the magnitude of the electric field depends on the radius, r, of the idealized body shape. The magnetic flux vector points perpendicularly through the plane of the body. The larger the loop, the higher is the induced E field. This gives a hint to the most effective gradient coil, with respect to magnetostimulation. Figure 9 shows the induced electrical field lines for all three gradient orientations for the whole-body case. Since the body has the largest cross-section in coronal view, the y gradient can produce the largest loop and the highest electric field and therefore has the lowest stimulation threshold. The loop can be enlarged when the hands are clasped.

The x and z gradients have approximately the same stimulation sensitivity, which is significantly lower than that of the y gradient. The relative thresholds depend on the actual coil design, particularly its linearity (see "Prevention of Magnetostimulation").

Magnetostimulation is possible in the head when large enough gradients are switched very fast, and the head is positioned at the maximum magnetic flux, B_{max}, produced by the gradient coils. This was reported by Cohen et al. [35]. We reproduced it with a special whole-body gradient coil generating an amplitude of 37 mT/m (Fig. 22). The x gradient produced the most significant magnetostimulation, with the z gradient a very weak sensation was felt, and the y gradient produced no stimulation. This is opposite to the case in whole-body examinations, where the y gradient is the most sensitive coil. In the head the order of appearance of magnetostimulation differs from that in whole-body

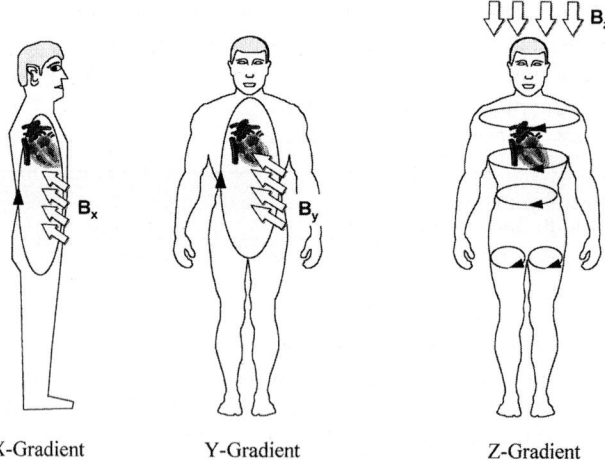

X-Gradient   Y-Gradient   Z-Gradient

Fig. 9. Induced electrical field loops follow the so-called right hand rule. When the thumb points in the B direction, the bended fingers point in the direction of the induced fields

Fig. 10. Magnetostimulations in the head. Magnetostimulations are most likely when the flux points through the sagittal plane

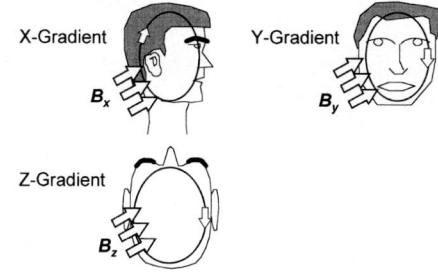

examinations. This is an effect due to the shape of the head, the possible field lines (see Fig. 10), and a number of not yet fully understood physiological aspects. Stimulation can be produced only at the bridge and tip of the nose. A tickling sensation is present during the entire gradient pulse duration. This location seems to have special sensitivity to magnetostimulation. Experiements by Schaefer et al. [38] showed that "typically stimulation sites were in the region where bones were close to the surface. Such anatomy could lead to higher electric fields due to current constrictions." This applies to the bridge of the nose and and to the area around the lower spine bones.

Prevention of Magnetostimulation

As noted above (see "Magnetostimulation of Excitable Tissue"), the location of magnetostimulation corresponds to the point of maximum magnetic flux, B_{max}, produced by the coil inside the patient access region. To minimize or avoid stimulatory effects we must minimize the magnetic flux inside the patient bore. The easiest way to do this is by reducing the linearity volume of the gradient coil. This is explained in Fig. 11. We focus on the z gradient coil only. The results are also transferable to transverse gradient coils. Shortening a z coil, for example, by a certain amount but keeping the gradient strength (slope of the field curve in Fig. 11) reduces both the linearity volume and the maximum magnetic flux. This solution has the disadvantage that the resulting images are geometrically distorted and the selected slice can be curved depending on the linearity and the actual coil design [40]. On the other hand, stimulation thresholds increase with respect to the gradient amplitude when compared to coils having better linearity. The coil can therefore be operated with faster and/or stronger gradient pulses before causing magnetostimulation.

Figure 12 compares two z gradient coils with different linearities. Coil 1 has higher linearity and produces a peak field of 7.4 mT when driven at 30 mT/m. Coil 2 has lower linearity and produces a peak field of 5.0 mT only when driven at 30 mT/m. With the high linearity coil 1 rise times of 120, 160, 200, and 250 μs were measured; with the low linearity coil 2 rise times of 200, 250, and 300 μs were measured. Plotting the rise time of the stimulation pulse train versus the magnetic flux needed to cause magnetostimulation shows a linear relationship.

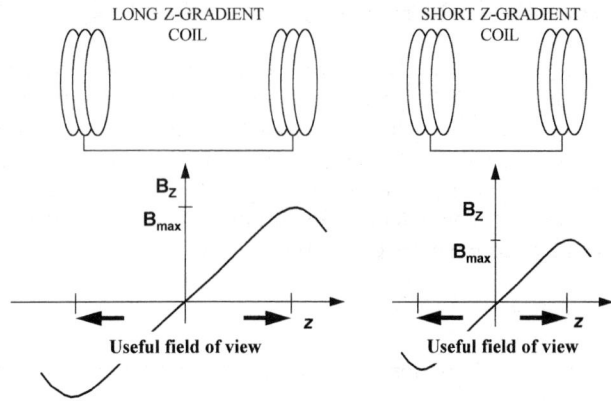

Fig. 11. Magnetic flux produced by a z gradient coil. When the coil length is reduced and its gradient strength (the slope) is maintained, the maximum flux B_z decreases

The threshold values from coil 1 fit into the threshold values of coil 2. This is expected by theory presented below (see "Theoretical Models of Magnetostimulation").

Some clinical applications of EPI are addressed to human brain imaging. Potential applications include perfusion imaging, functional MRI, and diffusion imaging in stroke patients. When concentrating on the head only, head gradient coils are preferred. Head gradient coils [41–43] are generally insertable into whole-body gradient coils. They are smaller versions of the whole-body coils and therefore offer the advantage of decreasing the total field B_{max} produced by the coil, in analogy to Fig. 11. This also reduces stimulatory effects. Stimulation thresholds of head insert coils are much higher than those of whole-body gradient coils. With head gradient coils amplitudes of 50 mT/m at rise times of 100 to 300 μs can be achieved, whereas whole-body coils used in clinical MRI scanners typically produce amplitudes of 25 mT/m at rise times of 200 to 300 μs. Therefore head gradient insert coils offer even faster EPI at higher resolution without encountering physiological side effects because of the head's smaller dimensions than those of the body trunk.

Fig. 12. Threshold comparison for z gradient coils with different linearity. Although different coil designs are used, and the measurements were taken years apart, the data fit very well when referred to the peak flux density produced by the coils and exposed to the subjects

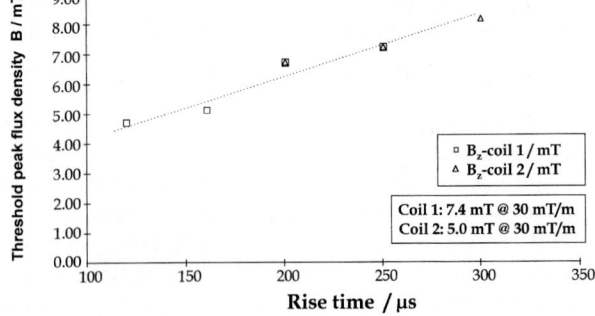

Theoretical Models of Magnetostimulation

According to Faraday's law of induction and Maxwell's laws, a time-varying magnetic flux, dB/dt, produces an electric field, E, which can be calculated by the integral Eq. 7 yielding a special solution for a conductive loop of radius, r, shown in Eq. 8. Silny [20] found that the induced electric field in elliptic bodies depends on the orientation of the applied uniform magnetic field. This effect, which is independent of longitudinal or transverse orientation, yields a coefficient of orientation c, as expressed in Eq. 10:

$$E(r) = -c \cdot \frac{r}{2} \cdot \frac{dB}{dt} \tag{10}$$

with $c = 0.5$ for longitudinal (z gradients) and $c = 1$ for transverse orientation (x,y gradients):

$$0.5 \leq c \leq 1 \tag{11}$$

In a tissue of conductivity, σ, the induced electric field, E, produces a current density, j, defined by Ohm's law as:

$$j(r) = -c \cdot \frac{r}{2} \cdot \sigma \cdot \frac{dB}{dt} \tag{12}$$

For example, a curent density j of 10 mA/m^2 ($c = 1$) is induced into a loop of typical tissue with a conductivity σ of 0.2 S/m and a radius $r = 10$ cm by a flux change dB/dt of 1 T/s.

Reilly [44] introduced another simple model, based on calculations by Durney et al. [45] and Spiegel et al. [46] that considers the human trunk as a conductive spheroid. Using this spheroid model (Fig. 13) the following relationship between dB/dt and induced electric field can be calculated:

$$E = -\frac{dB}{dt} \left(\frac{a^2 u \underline{a}_v - b^2 v \underline{a}_u}{a^2 + b^2} \right) \tag{13}$$

where $\underline{a}_v$ and $\underline{a}_u$ are unity vectors pointing along the major and the minor axis of the spheroid, respectively. The magnetic flux vector, B, points perpenticular

Fig. 13. The electric field E (*bold arrows*) induced by a changing flux B in a spheroid of homogeneous conductivity. Transverse flux B_x produces major electric field components *a* and *b*. Longitudinal flux B_z induces a component *c*

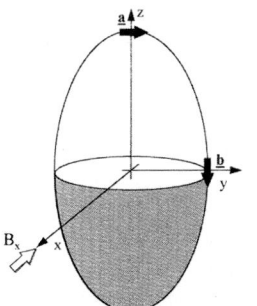
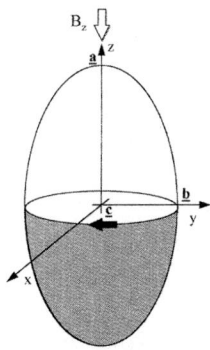

to the elliptical cross-section. A location within the ellipse is described as (u, v).

Under MRI conditions the magnetic field produced by gradient coils is not uniform. The gradient coil produces planes of constant magnetic fields only, with zero levels at the symmetry line and increasing (absolute) values as the distance increases (see Figs. 5, 6). Although it is possible to calculate the electric field with such inhomogeneous magnetic fields using finite element techniques, the problem can be simplified by the following assumption:

$$E_{non-uniform} \leq E_{uniform} \tag{14}$$

An electric field induced by a nonuniform magnetic field is equal to or smaller than the corresponding electric field produced by a uniform magnetic field with a magnitude of the maximum amplitude of the nonuniform field B_{max}. In other words, the assumption of a uniform magnetic field with maximum amplitude yields a worst-case estimation of the induced electric field.

Irnich's Model, Based on Weiss

Reading the articles discussing magnetostimulation, it is surprising to note how little information on cardiac pacing has entered the discussion so far. Therefore the enormous knowledge of cardiac pacing compiled during the past three decades is here applied for the special problem of magnetic stimulation of the heart. This is described first.

The Fundamental Law of Electrostimulation

In 1901 the physicist and physician George Weiss from Paris published a paper [47] in which he tried "to make comparable the different methods of electrostimulation." He found empirically that there is a linear relationship between the charge (current-time integral) needed to reach the stimulation threshold and the duration of current flow; he called this the *formule fondamentale*. The ingenuity of the research in those days is marvelous when considering the delicate and precise experiments required. The results are still valid today and match very well with magnetostimulation results. Their experiments were based on ballistics, precise knowledge of which was essential for military reasons. Figure 14 shows a typical electrostimulation experimental setup of those days. Weiss's experimental finding has been confirmed by numerous other scientists not only for neural but also for cardiac excitation and defibrillation [48]. From these experiments Weiss followed his fundamental law, expressed in a more modern equivalent form as:

$$\frac{Q(\tau)}{Q_o} = \left(1 + \frac{\tau}{\tau_{chron}}\right) \tag{15}$$

and:

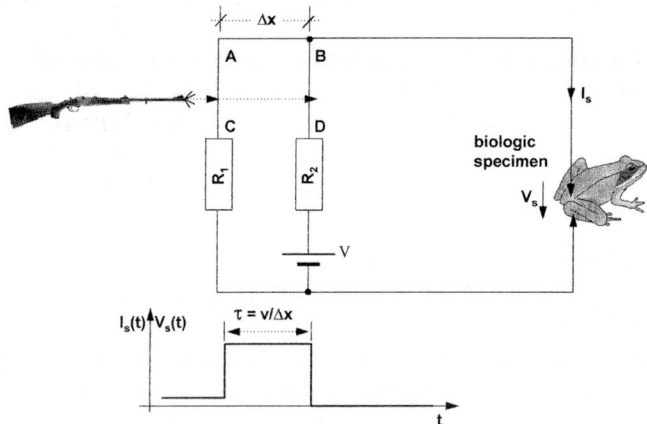

Fig. 14. Principle experimental setup of Weiss based on ballistics to evaluate nerve stimulations. The biological specimen was connected via resistor R_2 and electrodes to the supply voltage V. At the beginning the current was bypassed through resistor R_1. When now the conductor $\overline{AC}$ is interrupted (through a shutgun bullet) the current flows through R_2 and the biological specimen as long as the bullet needs to travel from the conductor $\overline{AC}$ to the conductor $\overline{BD}$. The duration of the pulse is given by the speed, v, and the distance $\overline{AC}–\overline{BD}$. The amplitude of the stimulus is adjusted by the resistors R_1, R_2

$$\frac{I(\tau)}{I_o} = \left(1 + \frac{\tau_{chron}}{\tau}\right) \tag{16}$$

where $I(\tau)$ and $Q(\tau)$ describe the threshold current and charge as a function of the stimulus duration, τ, respectively. Q_o is the minimum threshold for short duration $\tau \rightarrow 0$, and I_o is the minimum threshold charge for long durations $\tau \rightarrow \infty$. The term τ_{chron} is sort of time constant called chronaxie (see below) characterizing the time response of the tissue.

Recently [55] this empirical law from which so-called strength-duration relationships can be derived has found a theoretical justification based on the assumption that opening of sodium pores within the membrane of excitable tissue requires a mechanical impulse, which is produced by an external electric field, E_{ex}. Moving a charged particle, the barrier, from its resting position requires that two conditions have to be fulfilled: (a) The external force, F_{ex}, applied to the particle must be larger than the force, F_{stat}, which binds the particle to its resting state. (b) The time integral over the difference of external and static force over the duration, τ, of the external force must be equal or larger than a minimum mechanical impulse, p_{min}, necessary to open the pore:

$$\int_{\tau} (F_{ex} - F_{stat}) dt \geq p_{min} \tag{17}$$

The forces are supposed to be caused by the electric field. Therefore F_{ex} can be expressed as:

$$F_{ex} = q \cdot E_{ex} \tag{18}$$

were q is the charge of the permeability barrier. Combining Eqs. 17 and 18 yields:

$$\int_\tau E_{ex}dt \geq \frac{p_{min}}{q} + E_{stat} \cdot \tau \tag{19}$$

Using the terms rheobase (E_{rheo} is identical with the static electric field, E_{stat}, fixing the obstacle: $E_{rheo} = E_{stat}$) and chronaxie:

$$\tau_{chron} = \frac{p_{min}}{q \cdot E_{stat}}$$

as introduced by Lapicque [49] in 1909, the fundamental law of Weiss can be transformed into a more general formula given by:

$$\int_\tau E_{ex}dt \geq E_{rheo} \cdot \tau_{chron}\left(1 + \frac{\tau}{\tau_{chron}}\right) \tag{20}$$

If we divide Eq. 20 by τ we can express the thresholds in terms of the average E field, $\bar{E}$:

$$\bar{E} = \frac{1}{\tau}\int_0^\tau E_{ex}dt \geq E_{rheo}\left(1 + \frac{\tau_{chron}}{\tau}\right) \tag{21}$$

were τ is the duration of the exogene electric field E_{ex}. This equation describes a *hyperbolic* strength-duration function.

Equation 21 has the following advantages:

- The primary parameter responsible for stimulation, the electric field, is addressed [17, 50–52, 55]. The electric field is less influenced by changes in conductivity than the current density [53–55].
- The time integral over the electric field guarantees that the average value and not any other specific value (peak, rms value) is considered as being exclusively effective, as observed by Weiss [54] in 1901 and others over the course of the past 80 years [21, 55, 56].
- The linear approach of Eq. 20:

$$\int_0^\tau E dt \; vs. \; \tau$$

is not only the simplest and best fit for experimental results [57] but can be justified theoretically by the assumption of a mechanical impulse necessary for opening the sodium channels within the membrane during electrostimulation [55].

Chronaxie and Rheobase

Figure 15 explains the terms chronaxie and rheobase as introduced by Lapicque. The term "rheobase," which has found general acceptance, is defined as the threshold below which no further excitation is possible, independent of the duration of the stimulus. Its mathematical description is:

$$E_{rheo} = \overline{E}(\tau \to \infty)$$

"Chronaxie" is a type of "time constant" in the decaying hyperbola that determines how fast the rheobase is asymptotically reached. It is defined as the stimulus duration required to stimulate the nerve with a stimulus strength equal to twice the rheobase. It is used exclusively as one of the determining parameters of the *hyperbolic* strength-duration function and not as a time constant of an exponential expression, often called membrane time constant. The chronaxie is a measure of the duration at which the strength-duration curve changes from its long duration to short duration behavior. It is of eminent practical importance for cardiac pacemakers and determines where stimulation takes place with lowest energy. For example, with rectangular pulses energy minimum is exactly at chronaxie; with exponentially decaying pulses it is 1.19 times chronaxie [55].

Chronaxie not only characterizes the specimen but is also a function of electrode size in electrophysiology. It has been reported that chronaxie increases with electrode size [58]. Experimental results on magnetostimulation show prolonged chronaxie values, confirming the electrophyiological findings. A mathematical description of this is given by Panizza et al. [59]. It is obvious that a major difference between electrostimulation and magnetostimulation is the area of interaction. In electrostimulation experiments stimuli are normally applied through small electrodes such as needles. Magnetostimulation is defined by the coil dimensions and is therefore typically exposed to large areas. This implies also that a single type of tissue, i.e., nerve or muscle, cannot be excited by magneto-

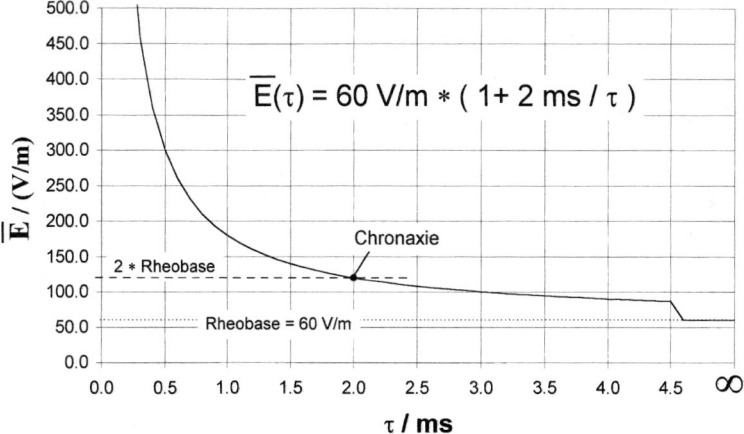

Fig. 15. Hyperbolic strength-duration curve explaining rheobase and chronaxie

stimulation in the same way as transthoracic cardiac stimulation does. All tissue types in the volume of exposure can be excited. They are differentiated by their rheobases, chronaxies, and sensations such as sensory (weak sensation) or motor (muscle twitches) [60].

Stimulation by Time-Varying Magnetic Fields

Combining Eqs. 10 and 20 gives the solution for uniform magnetic fields:

$$\int_\tau E_{ex} dt \leq \int_\tau c \cdot r \cdot \frac{dB}{dt} \cdot dt = c \cdot r \cdot B(\tau) \tag{22}$$

$$B(\tau) \geq \frac{E_{rheo} \cdot \tau_{chron}}{c \cdot r} \left(1 + \frac{\tau}{\tau_{chron}}\right) \tag{23}$$

Equation 23 is in accordance with the calculation of Mansfield and Harvey [13] that it is the maximum variation in magnetic flux density, $B(\tau)$, which is responsible for magnetostimulation. If the stimulation pulse duration, τ, approaches zero (Dirac δ function), the threshold B value reaches a minimum value:

$$B_{min} = \frac{E_{rheo} \cdot \tau_{chron}}{c \cdot r}$$

This means that any stimulation pulse with a flux variation of $\Delta B < B_{min}$ can never cause stimulation, independently of pulse duration. This has been confirmed for pulse durations from 110 μs to 2 ms [61], corresponding to rise times of 55–1000 μs achievable with EPI gradients.

Combining Eqs. 10 and 21 expresses the magnetostimulation in terms of the average value of dB/dt, denoted as $\bar{B}$:

$$\bar{B}(\tau) = \frac{1}{\tau} \int_0^\tau \frac{dB}{dt} dt$$

$$\bar{B}(\tau) = \frac{B(\tau)}{\tau} = \frac{E_{rheo}}{c \cdot r} \left(1 + \frac{\tau_{chron}}{\tau}\right) \tag{24}$$

Equation 24 suggests that regardless of the shape of the magnetically induced pulse the average flux change, $\bar{B}$, or the maximum field excursion, $B(\tau)$, is important. For pulses with long duration the $\bar{B}$ threshold is minimum and can be expressed as:

$$\bar{B}_{\tau \to \infty} = \dot{B}_{rheo} = \frac{E_{rheo}}{c \cdot r}$$

Equation 24 describes the stimulation thresholds in a *hyperbolic* strength-duration curve when expressed in mean threshold, $\bar{B}$. The two equations are identical and do not express different physical or physiological facts. It is only a question of practicability which one is used for defining limiting values.

Equation 23 describes that the magnetic flux required to stimulate is a linear function of the stimulus duration, τ. This linearity has been verified in many experiments. Examples are shown in the experimental part of this chapter.

Reilly's Model, Based on Frankenhaeuser and Huxley

Based on Hodgkin and Huxley's membrane model [62] Reilly used a modified Frankenhaeuser and Huxley model [63] of a myelinated nerve fiber to evaluate nerve stimulation caused by switched magnetic fields. McNeal's method [64] was extended by Reilly et al. [65] to the so-called spatially extended nonlinear node (SENN) model. Myelinated nerve fibers are modeled because they show the fastest conduction rates, shorter action potential durations, and lower electrical thresholds [66], therefore describing the worst case.

An equivalent circuit model for a myelinated nerve fiber is shown in Fig. 16. The individual nodes are described as circuit elements consisting of resistance, R_m, capacitance, C_m, and potential source, E_r, maintaining the transmembrane resting potential. Referring to Fig. 16, Reilly states an equation describing the electrical response of the nerve model as:

$$\frac{dV_n}{dt} = \frac{1}{C_m}\{G_a(V_{n-1}-2V_n+V_{n+1}+V_{e,n-1}-2V_{e,n}+V_{e,n+1})-I_{i,n}\} \tag{25}$$

where $V_n = V_{i,n}-V_{e,n}$ is the voltage across the membrane, $V_{i,n}$ is the potential at the interior of node n, $V_{e,n}$ describes the potential at the exterior of node n, and $G_a = 1/R_a$. The ionic current, $I_{i,n}$, can be described for either a linear or a nonlinear membrane model:

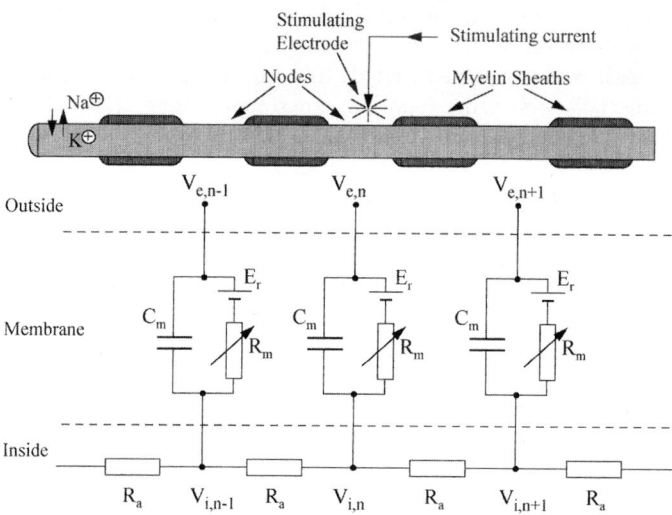

Fig. 16. Equivalent electrical circuit representing a myelinated nerve fiber according to Reilly

$$I_{i,n} = G_m V_m \qquad\qquad linear\ (a)$$
$$I_{i,n} = \pi dW\ (J_{Na}+J_K+J_L+J_P) \quad non\text{-}linear\ (b) \tag{26}$$

W is described as the internodal gap width, d is the axon diameter, and the J terms are ionic current densities. Equation 26a resembles Ohm's law for a linear conductor. Equation 26b is applied for nonlinear ionic current equivalent to the Frankenhaeuser-Huxley membrane [80].

Equation 25 resembles the so-called electrical-cable equation describing the propagation of signals in cables. This model defines an electrical threshold as the stimulus threshold that is adequate to produce a propagating action potential.

Plotting the threshold of stimulation calculated by the SENN model versus the duration of a square wave stimulus yields a strength-duration curve. Based on the electrical equivalent model of the myelinated nerve, Reilly used an exponential relationship described by Blair [67, 68] in 1932 and Lapicque [69] in 1907 to fit his data:

$$\frac{I(\tau)}{I_0} = \frac{1}{1-e^{-\tau/\tau_e}} \tag{27}$$

and:

$$\frac{Q(\tau)}{Q_0} = \frac{\tau/\tau_e}{1-e^{-\tau/\tau_e}} \tag{28}$$

where I, I_0, Q, I_0 describe the same quantities as expressed by with Eqs. 15 and 16. However, τ_e is theoretically described by the time constant, τ_m, defined by the cricuit resistance, R_m, and capacitance, C_m, given as $\tau_e = \tau_m = R_m C_m$. Chronaxie, τ_{chron}, as used in Lapicque's expression, can be calculated from Eq. 27 as:

$$\tau_{chron} = \tau_e \cdot \ln 2 = 0.693 \cdot \tau_e \tag{29}$$

Using R_m and C_m from the assumption of McNeal [81] a threrotical time constant, $\tau_m = 66\ \mu s$ for myelinated nerve fiber results. Fitting the SENN-modeled data with a least means square fit yields time constants $\tau_e = 92\ \mu s$. Reilly reports that this value falls within the reported experimental range [70], although most of the experimentally determined time constants exceed that of the SENN model by a factor of 2. Experimentally evaluated average time constants, τ_e, for neural excitation on peripheral nerves are around 270 μs [18]. From transthoracic cardiac stimulation experiments mean time constants, τ_e, of about 3 ms are reported – values approximately ten times higher than time constants observed for neural [18] and endocardial stimulation. A cardiac excitation or stimulation in this context refers to the production of an ectopic beat.

By means of Eq. 10 and assuming a rectangular stimulus pulse, Eqs. 27 and 28 can be written in terms of $\dot{B}$ and B as:

$$\frac{\dot{B}(\tau)}{\dot{B}_0} = \frac{1}{1-e^{-\tau/\tau_e}} \tag{30}$$

and:

$$\frac{B(\tau)}{B_0} = \frac{\tau/\tau_e}{1-e^{-\tau/\tau_e}} \qquad (31)$$

Instead of fitting the strength-duration curve, either hyperbolically or exponentially, Reilly determined the experimental time constant τ_e in good approximation as:

$$\tau_e \approx \frac{Q_0}{I_0} = \frac{B_0}{\dot{B}_0} \qquad (32)$$

Mansfield's Model, Based on Electrically Equivalent Circuit Model of the Membrane

Around 1932 Blair [85, 86] realized that membranes of excitable tissue can be represented by a parallel resistor, R, and capacitor, C, and derived an exponential expression for the current required for the stimulation. Plonsey et al. [71], Pearce et al. [72], and Mansfield et al. [13, 73] presented similar expressions which relate current, I, duration, t, and membrane time constants $\tau = R \cdot C$. Mansfield et al. modeled breaks in the sheath of the myelin, forming nodes, comprising a selectively permeable mebrane. Through this membrane external currents flow in the case of neural excitation. In the resting state the membrane has a negative potential E of approximately –70 mV due to the potassium concentration in the axoplasm. During excitation the axon potential rises to about +50 mV due to the flow of sodium ions through the membrane. The difference voltage of about 120 mV is called the activation potential V_m. When the transmembrane potential is depolarized by an amount $\Delta V = fV_m$ the neurones are triggered, where f is the threshold fraction in the range of 0<f< 1. During the conduction phase the membrane can be described as a linear electrical circuit shown in Fig. 17. The resistance-area product, r_m, and the capacitance/area ratio, c_m, describe the properties of the circuit. In Mansfield's analysis a magnetostimulation is equivalent to applying an external current generator to the node. The source generator produces a current density $j = j_1 + j_2$.

Assuming a homogeneous tissue cylinder of radius r, the magnetically induced current density is given by:

$$j(t) = c\sigma \frac{r}{2} \left[\frac{dB}{dt} \right] \qquad (33)$$

Fig. 17. Equivalent electrical circuit of a neural node driven by a current generator according to Mansfield et al.

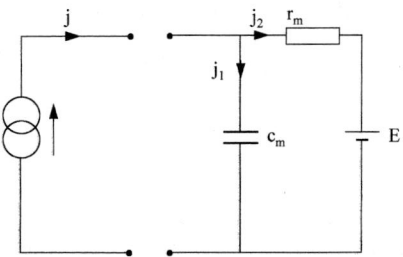

where σ is the tissue conductivity, typically in the range of 0.2–0.5 S/m, and c is a constant to account for the anisotropy as expressed in Eq. 10. Using the Laplace transfom method the following solution for the stimulation current densities, j_s was found:

$$j_s(t) = \frac{K}{\tau_m} \cdot e^{-\frac{t}{\tau_m}} \int_0^t e^{\frac{t'}{\tau_m}} \cdot \left[\frac{dB}{dt'}\right] dt' \tag{34}$$

in which $t_m = c_m \, r_m$ is the membrane time constant and:

$$K = c\sigma \frac{r}{2}$$

Applying a constant magnetic stimulus (i.e., dB/dt = const) the stimulation threshold can be expressed in terms of transient magnetic field at stimulation, B, as a function of its duration, τ, as:

$$\frac{B(\tau)}{B_0} = \frac{\frac{\tau}{\tau_m}}{1 - e^{-\frac{\tau}{\tau_m}}} \tag{35}$$

where B_0 is the minimum threshold for $\tau \to 0$. Equation 34 can be used to compare the effects of different durations and stimulus shapes in neural magneto-stimulation. For example, the stimulus pulse $B(\tau)$ can either be trapezoidal or sinusoidal. In the sinusoidal case Mansfield introduced an effective stimulus duration $\tau_{eff} = T/\pi$ [74], where T is the period of the sine wave. Both trapezoidal and sinusoidal data gained in wrist experiments [78] fit Eq. 35 within experimental errors, although a linear fit proposed by Irnich seems to fit as well. Based on this results, Mansfield et al. conclude that "the magnetic field excursion B rather than dB/dt is the important factor."

Regulatory Limits

Officially recommended limits for time-varying magnetic fields scatter considerably when compared from one country or organization to the other. The major reason for that is that there is no generally accepted theory describing this phenomena. Recommended thresholds are based on experimental findings and worst-case assumptions. Experimental results scatter remarkably due to different experimental setups. Results must often be transfered from a small scale in vitro or in vivo animal study to large-scale human morphology.

Most of the legal limits are based on the change of magnetic flux, dB/dt. There is no clear specification whether the magnitude of the magnetic flux, or its MR effective B_z component must be considered. In the United States the Food and Drug Administration (FDA) [75] and in Japan the Ministry of Health and Welfare [76] distinguish between transverse (G_z) and longitudinal (G_x, G_y) gradient fields.

The major question to be answered in establishing legal limits is whether it is possible to cause stimulation (ectopic heart beats or extrasystoles) or ventricular fibrillation of the heart. Reilly [51] calculates for a large man exposed to a peak dB/dt of 100 T/s in sagittal, coronal, and axial orientation a maximum induced electric field, E = 14.4, 16.0, and 9.9 V/m, respectively. When scaled to the heart an electric field of 12.2, 8.6, and 8.7 V/m is determined. Assuming a conductivity, σ, of 0.2 S/m in the worst case, an induced current density of 2.4 A/m² can be calculated. These values in combination with the assumed electric field rheobase of 6.2 V/m for the myocardial muscle, as proposed by Reilly, and cardiac excitation threshold current densities of 2 A/m², as described by Bernhardt [77], have led to the opinion that magnetic flux changes of this magnitude can cause harm to the patient.

Thresholds are typically classified into two modes: (a) level of no concern or uncontrolled level: using the MR system below this threshold is allowed without any limits; (b) level of concern or controlled level: using the system in this mode requires the presence of a physician, and, for example, cardiovascular function must be supervised.

An earlier German recommendation referred threshold limits to the induced current density, j. The major disadvantage of this is that current densities induced by changing magnetic fields cannot be measured in vivo. Its dependence on physiology, morphology, and electric conductivity is too strong to allow reasonable estimations. The most recent German recommendation [78] specifies thresholds for the electric field and deduced dB/dt thresholds.

The FDA allows dB/dt values above the level of concern when valid scientific evidence demonstrates that "the rate of change of magnetic field for the system is not sufficient to cause peripheral nerve stimulation by an adequate margin of safety (at least a factor of three)."

Limits have been prescribed by the International Radiation Protection Association (IRPA) [79], an association closely related to the World Health Organization (WHO), but these are not obligatory in individual countries. Its recommendations are very conservative. Imaging below a rate of change of the magnetic flux, dB/dt, of 6 T/s is considered of no concern. Patients with changes in the electrocardiogram (ECG) should be monitored when imaged at a dB/dt larger than 6 T/s. A dB/dt of 20 T/s should not be exceeded.

The recommendation of the International Electrotechnical Committee (IEC) will most likely become the European standard [80]. Italy and the United Kingdom describe their legal limits in a similar fashion [81, 82].

Table 4 and Fig. 18 summarize the legal limits of various countries and organizations. The pulse duration, τ, is the duration of a rectangular pulse of the magnetic flux change, dB/dt, which is equivalent to twice the rise time of a magnetic flux pulse B(τ). For sinusoidal pulses τ is the duration of a half period. Unless otherwise stated dB/dt must be calculated as peak or maximum magnetic flux change.

Table 4. Legal limits for time-varying magnetic fields

Country / organization	Recommended thresholds		
	Duration, τ, of dB/dt pulse	Level of no concern (τ in μs)	Level of concern (τ in μs)
USA / FDA (1989) [75]			
For axial gradients (G_z)	τ ≥ 120 μs	dB/dt ≤ 6 T/s	dB/dt < 20 T/s
	12 μs < τ < 120 μs	dB/dt ≤ 6 T/s	dB/dt < 2400/τ T/s
	τ ≤ 12 μs	dB/dt ≤ 6 T/s	dB/dt < 200 T/s
For transverse gradients (G_x, G_y)			If dB/dt is less than 3 times the limits for axial gradients
	Alternative: Demonstrate with valid scientific evidence that the rate of change of magnetic field for the system is not sufficient to cause peripheral nerve stimulation by an adequate margin of safety (at least a factor of three)		
Germany / BfS (1995) [78]			
Recommendations for the rate of change of the magnetic flux, dB/dt	τ ≥ 3000 μs	dB/dt ≤ 6 T/s	dB/dt ≤ 20 T/s
	400 μs ≤ τ < 3000 μs	dB/dt ≤ 6 T/s	dB/dt < 60 000/τ T/s
	100 μs ≤ τ < 400 μs	dB/dt ≤ 2400/τ T/s	dB/dt < 60 000/τ T/s
	8 μs ≤ τ < 100 μs	dB/dt ≤ 2400/τ T/s	dB/dt ≤ 600 T/s
	τ < 8 μs	dB/dt ≤ 300 T/s	dB/dt ≤ 600 T/s
Recommendations for the induced electric field, E	τ ≥ 3000 μs	E < 1 V/m	E < 3 V/m
	400 μs ≤ τ < 3000 μs	E < 1 V/m	E < 9000/τ V/m
	100 μs ≤ τ < 400 μs	E < 400/τ V/m	E < 9000/τ V/m
	8 μs ≤ τ < 100 μs	E < 400/τ V/m	SAR < 0.2 W/100 g
	τ < 8 μs	SAR < 0.1 W/100 g	SAR < 0.2 W/100 g
IEC (1995) [80]	τ ≥ 120 μs	dB/dt < 20 T/s	dB/dt < 20 T/s τ ≥ 3000 μs
	2.5 μs < τ < 120 μs	dB/dt < 2400/τ T/s	dB/dt < 60 000/τ T/s 45 μs < τ < 3000 μs
	τ ≤ 2.5 μs	dB/dt < 960 T/s	dB/dt < 1330 T/s τ ≤ 45 μs

[a] dB/dt must be given as the root means square value τ in μs.

Table 4. Legal limits for time-varying magnetic fields (continued)

Country / organization	Recommended thresholds		
	Duration, τ, of dB/dt pulse	Level of no concern (τ in µs)	Level of concern (τ in µs)
Japan (1991) [76]			
For axial gradients (G_z)	τ ≥ 120 µs	dB/dt ≤ 6 T/s	dB/dt < 20 T/s
	12 µs < τ < 120 µs	dB/dt ≤ 6 T/s	dB/dt < 2400/τ T/s
	τ ≤ 12 µs	dB/dt ≤ 6 T/s	dB/dt < 200 T/s
For transverse gradients (G_x, G_y)		If dB/dt is less than 3 times the limits for axial gradients	If dB/dt is less than 3 times the limits for axial gradients
IRPA (1991) [80]		dB/dt < 6 T/s	6 T/s ≤ dB/dt ≤ 20 T/s 20 T/s should not be exceeded
United Kingdom / NRPB [81]	τ ≥ 3000 µs	dB/dt < 20 T/s	dB/dt < 20 T/s
	120 µs ≤ τ < 3000 µs	dB/dt < 20 T/s	dB/dt < 60 000/τ T/s
	45 µs ≤ τ < 120 µs	dB/dt < 2400/τ T/s	dB/dt < 60 000/τ T/s
	2.5 µs ≤ τ < 45 µs	dB/dt < 2400/τ T/s	dB/dt < 1300 T/s
	τ < 2.5 µs	dB/dt < 950 T/s	dB/dt < 1300 T/s
Italy / Ministero della Sanita (1991) [82]	τ ≥ 10 000 µs	dB/dt^a > 20 T/s	
	τ < 10 000 µs	(dB/dt)^2 * τ < 4	

^{a} dB/dt must be given as the root means square value τ in µs.

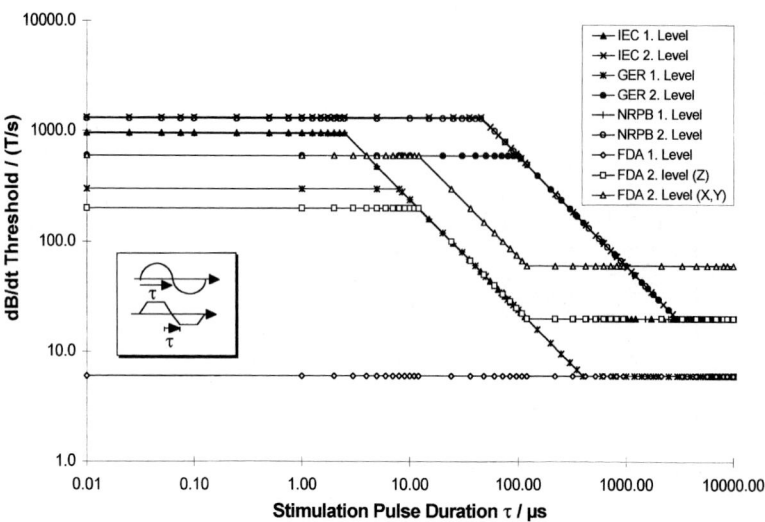

Fig. 18. Recommendations of different countries and organizations for time-varying magnetic fields

Stimulation Experiments and Its Interpretations

This section reports on stimulation experiments demonstrating the functional relation of the stimulation threshold with respect to stimulus duration, stimulus shape, number of stimuli, and other experimental settings. Most of the experiments were performed inside the main magnetic field, B_o. Some were performed outside in free-standing field coils. Nyenhuis et al. [83] have shown that the main magnetic field strength does not affect the stimulation thresholds. Many dog studies and human peripheral stimulation experiments have been performed in the past 5 years. Some of them are referenced in this section. For more details we refer to the literature [51, 75–94, 98, 109]. However, most of the data presented here were collected by the present authors.

Experimental Conditions

Before going into experimental details we must define the meaning of the stimulation duration, τ, and threshold because this is important for the following section. As described above (see "Theoretical Models of Magnetostimulation"), inducing an electric field in the human body is possible only when the magnetic flux, B, changes in time. We therefore consider the duration of a stimulation pulse as the time that a $B(\tau)$ excursion of ΔB takes to change from a value B_1 to another value B_2, where B_1 and B_2 are typically extreme values (maximum and minimum) because this defines the duration of the induced E field pulse.

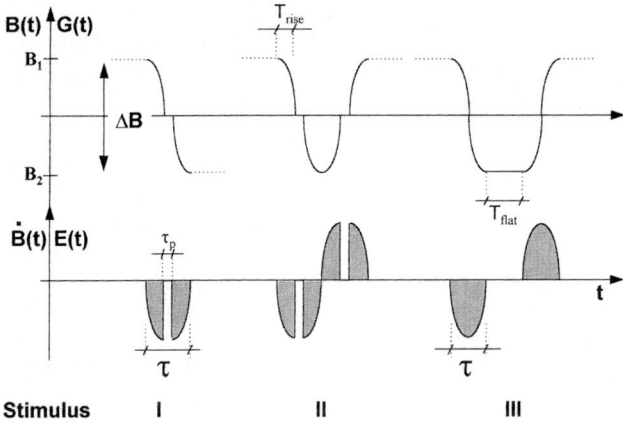

Fig. 19. Definition of stimulus pulses used in this chapter

These stimulation pulses may be repeated with or without changing polarity. Pause times, τ_p, during the field excursion, ΔB, are also included. In the examples of Fig. 19 the stimulus duration, τ, is equal to twice the rise time, T_{rise}, plus the pause time, τ_p, if existing.

The stimulation thresholds are expressed in magnetic flux, B measured in mT, exposed to the patient access volume. Multiple graphs shown in the figure correspond to measurement sessions without moving the subject in and out of the field coil. Under these circumstances the results can be compared directly to an absolute quantitative basis. However, a quantitative comparison is not possible when graphs from different figures are compared because these represent different experimental settings, for example, different field coils or different subject positioning, unless otherwise stated.

When thresholds are expressed in terms of magnetic flux, B, the gradient strength, G, can be used equivalently. The relationship between them is described by:

$$B(r) = S \cdot f(r) \cdot G \tag{36}$$

where S describes the coil sensitivity expressed in mT/(mT/m) and $f(r)$ describes the spatial dependency magnetic flux of the gradient coil ($|f(r)| \leq 1$). Below, when thresholds are expressed in magnetic flux, the maximum flux ($\max\{B(r)\}$) exposed to the volunteer is used.

Volunteers signed written consent forms before beginning the studies. Some experiments were performed with experienced volunteers who had a history of hundreds of studies. Large group studies were performed with unexperienced volunteers. Typically thresholds derived from experienced volunteers are lower than those from unexperienced volunteers. The lowest perception of a magnetostimulation is characterized by a very weak sensation comparable to finger tapping against the wrist, in contrast to a medium magnetostimulation characterized by soft muscle twitching or tingling sensation. For whole-body studies volunteers were positioned feet first and supine, unless otherwise stated. Error bars indicate studies with a group of volunteers, whereas graphs without show experiments of single individuals.

Threshold Amplitude Versus Stimulus Duration

Monophasic Stimuli

Irnich's theory predicts a linear relation between the stimulation-threshold amplitude and its duration. A whole-body experimental study was performed to confirm this relationship. Figure 20 shows the resulting thresholds and the gradient pulse shape, B(t), and the stimulus shape, $\dot{B}(\tau)$. For this study monophasic stimulus were applied with an embedded pause time, as explained in Fig. 19. To achieve a monophasic stimulus the gradient pulse, B(t), is ramped linearly to its maximum value within 2 ms followed by a sinusoidal ramp down in 250 µs. After the pause this pattern is repeated antisymetrically, as indicated with the graph in the upper left of Fig. 20. Linear ramps up and down are applied because the introduced dB/dt is equal or less than 5 T/s and can therefore be neglected when compared to the main sinusoidal stimulus with a dB/dt_{max} of 60 T/s or more.

The stimulus was repeated every 2 s. This enabled the subject to separate the stimulus in time. The experiment was started with a pause time of zero, and the threshold was then determined by increasing the gradient amplitude until the subject reported a sensation. This procedure was repeated with increasing

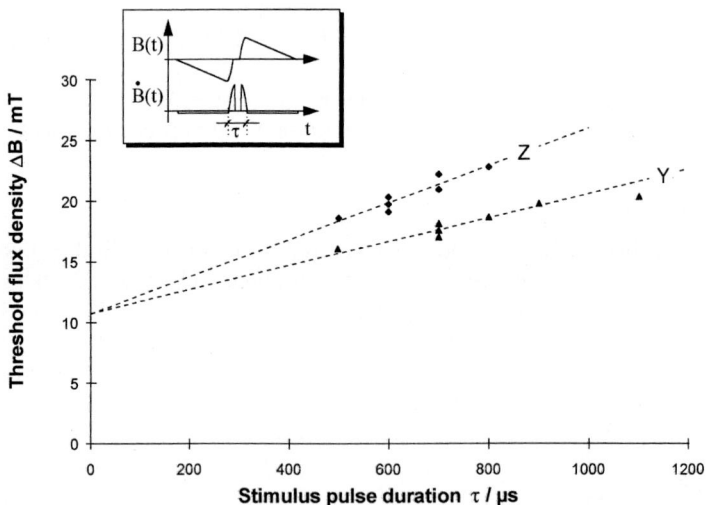

Fig. 20. Peripheral stimulation thresholds acquired in the human body trunk using a whole-body gradient coil. Monophasic stimulus (in dB/dt) are used to demonstrate linear relationship between threshold amplitude, ΔB, and stimulus duration, τ

pause time increments of 100 μs from 0 to 600 μs, corresponding to stimulus durations ranging from 500 to 1100 μs. Figure 20 shows the results of this study for two different gradient axes (y and z). The y gradient showed lower thresholds than the z gradient as explained above ("Magnetostimulation of Excitable Tissue"). Equation 23 indicates that the slope of the stimulation-threshold curves are inversely proportional to the radius of the induced electrical field loop defined by the cross-section of the human body in transversal and coronal flux exposure. Both threshold curves are well correlated with Irnich's linear approach. The correlation coefficient, r^2, was calculated as 0.929 and 0.88 for the y and z gradients, respectively.

Repetitive Multiphasic Sinusoidal Stimuli

Typical MRI sequences consist of repetitive gradient pulses causing multiple stimuli of changing polarity. In the extreme case, as for EPI, the pulse sequence consists of a long sinusoidal gradient pulse train corresponding to a long co-sinusoidal stimulus train. Experimental findings show that independently of the duration of the entire gradient train the threshold amplitude has a linear relationship with the stimulus duration, τ. Figure 21 shows an example of a head study performed with a local head-sized field coil. Instead of gradient field coils a solenoid coil resembling a z gradient and a saddle-shaped coil substituting for an x or y gradient, is applied. The solenoid coil produces B_z components similar to a z gradient. The saddle coil generates transverse components, $B_\perp$, similar to x and y gradients as described above ("Magnetostimulation of Excitable Tissue"). The flux pulse train, B(t), shown in the upper left of Fig. 21, consisted of sinusoidal oscillations with a linearly ramped up and down envelope.

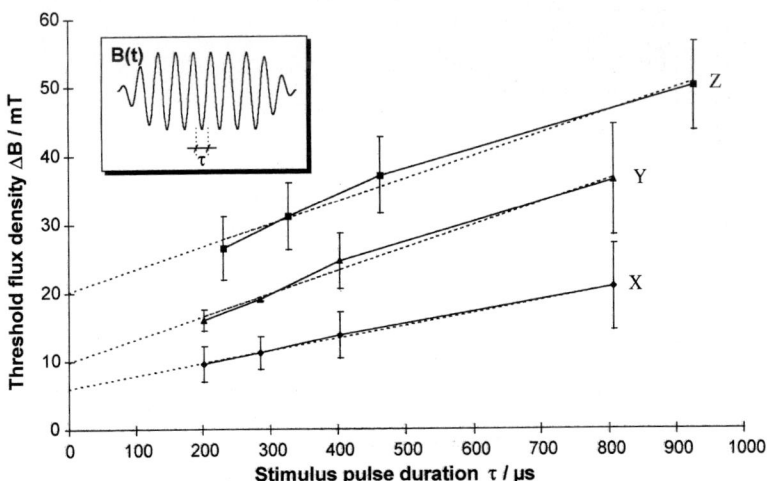

Fig. 21. Peripheral stimulation thresholds acquired in the human head using a local head-sized solenoid (z) and saddle-shaped field coil (x, y)

A frequency range of 540–2480 Hz was covered, corresponding to stimulus durations from about 900 to 200 μs. The total pulse train duration was kept constant at 64 ms. The mean threshold curves as well as its standard deviations are plotted versus the duration $\tau = 2*T_{rise}$. Lowest perception threshold is achieved with the field oriented in the x direction followed by the y direction. Transverse field experiments were achieved by rotating the saddle coil by 90°. The solenoid coil shows the highest thresholds. These findings are consistent with the explanation above ("Magnetostimulation of Excitable Tissue") and with Fig. 10 regarding the induced electric field loops.

A similar study was performed in a whole-body gradient coil to demonstrate the situation for whole-body MRI. This coil consisted of z and x gradients only. Exploring y gradient thresholds was possible when the volunteer turned his body from supine position to lateral. Lying on the side seems to have higher thresholds than supine positioning, as described above ("Magnetostimulation of Excitable Tissue"). Figure 22 shows the resulting threshold curve and its standard deviation to illustrate the variances. In contrast to the experiments of Fig. 20, the y gradient showed higher thresholds than the x gradient during this experiment. This may be due to the fact that the volunteer was examined in lateral position (Fig. 22) rather than in supine position (Fig. 20).

Both studies of head and of body were performed with four volunteers. The stimulation pulses applied for the reported studies are shown in Figs. 21 and 22. The ramp up and down periods lasted 10 ms, and the stationary part always lasted 64 ms. A typical study protocol consisted of a repeated stimulus with increasing amplitudes at intervals of 2 s until the subject reported sensation. The sequence was then repeated for a total of five trials at each frequency and orientation to acquire statistically stable results.

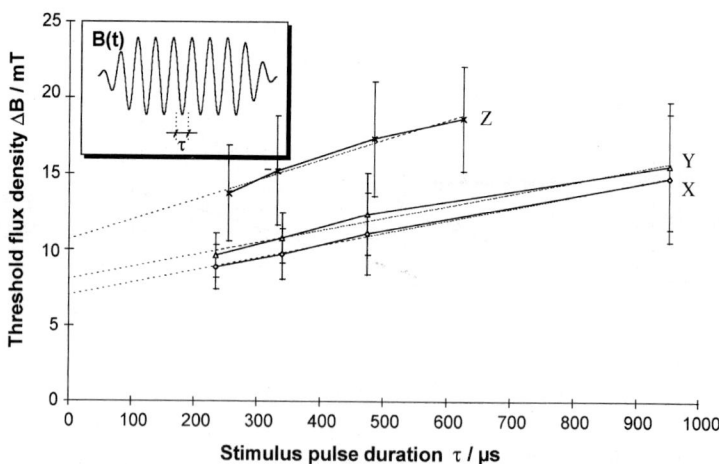

Fig. 22. Peripheral stimulation thresholds acquired in the human body trunk using a whole-body gradient coil consisting of an x and z coil winding. Volunteers were positioned feet first supine when measured for x and z and were laid on the side for y

In both experimental studies the threshold-duration relation followed a linear relationship in good approximation. Fitting the head study experimental data to the linear relation predicted by Irnich yielded a correlation coefficients of $r^2 = 0.997$, 0.990, 0.984 for x, y, and z orientations, respectively. The correlation coefficients for the whole-body experiment were calculated as 0.997, 0.982, and 0.983 for x, y, and z orientations, respectively. Data presented in Figs. 21 and 22 are from Budinger et al. [95].

Threshold Amplitude Versus Number of Stimuli and Phase

Monophasic and Biphasic Repetitive Sinusoidal Stimuli

As shown in the previous section, the threshold value is in good approximation linearly dependent on the stimulus duration. This relationship holds for either a single monophasic or a repetitive sinusoidal stimulus. In this section we show how much the threshold of stimulation changes with respect to the number of stimuli. Figure 23 shows the results of a whole-body study performed to demonstrate this dependency. A sinusoidal y gradient pulse train of 1000 Hz was applied. The number of half waves varied from 1 to 64 with alternating phase. As seen in Fig. 23a, the threshold expressed in magnetic flux density, ΔB, dropped by about 30 % from a single half wave to a train of half waves. The curve saturates at about 32 half waves. Similar findings have been reported by Budinger et al. [11] and by Yamagata et al. [40]. Yamagata et al. stated that the thresholds decrease exponentially up to 10 oscillations and do not change after 30 cycles.

During the same experimental session a study was performed to compare bipolar sinusoidal with unipolar sinusoidal half waves. The results are also

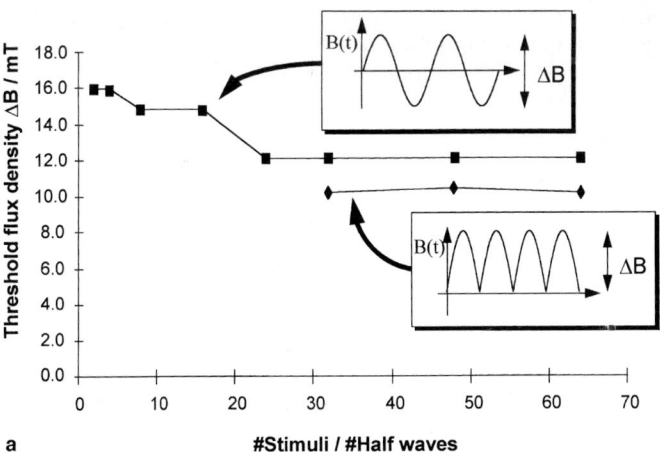

a   #Stimuli / #Half waves

Fig. 23. a Magnetostimulation threshold as a function of the number of stimuli for monophasic and biphasic sinusoidal gradient field pulses obtained with a whole-body y gradient coil. A gradient frequency of 1 kHz was applied. Thresholds are expressed as flux density, B, in mT

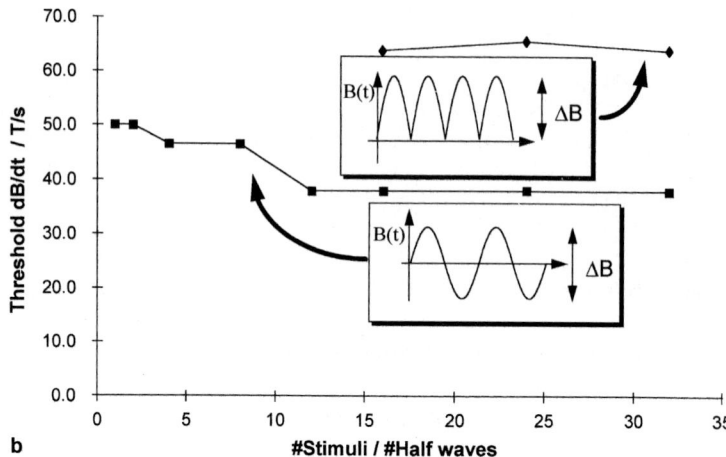

Fig. 23. (continued) **b** Magnetostimulation threshold as a function of the number of stimuli for monophasic and biphasic sinusoidal gradient field pulses obtained with a whole-body y gradient coil. A gradient frequency of 1 kHz was applied. Thresholds are expressed as flux change, dB/dt, in T/s

shown in Fig. 23a. Monophasic stimulus have about the same stimulation sensitivity when referred to total magnetic flux change, ΔB (Fig. 23a). When the results are expressed in peak dB/dt (Fig. 23b), we see that monophasic half waves require about twice the dB/dt of the biphasic pulses. This is consistent with Irnich's and Mansfield's theory predicting that the total field excursion, ΔB and not dB/dt defines the magnetostimulation thresholds.

Monophasic Stimuli with Different Sinusoidal Rise Times. Mansfield's and Irnich's theory predict that the magnetic flux excursion, ΔB and not the peak dB/dt characterizes the stimulation thresholds. This implies that the magnetostimulation threshold is independent of the stimulus pulse shape. To confirm this a stimulation experiment was performed with a whole-body z gradient coil. The applied stimuli were the same as discribed above in Fig. 20. Two different rise times of 250 µs and 190 µs, corresponding to a sinusoidal ramp pulses of frequency of 1000 and 1315 Hz, were applied, respectively. Figure 24a shows the results of the study. Threshold flux, ΔB, is plotted versus the stimulus duration, τ, which is equal to twice the rise time plus the pause time. Dashed lines indicate that the results linearly fit with the stimulus duration. However, the two rise times have different threshold levels. This is in contradiction to Mansfield's and Irnich's theory. Interesting to note is the fact that stimuli with higher intrinsic peak dB/dt (1315 Hz) show higher thresholds than stimuli with lower peak dB/dt (1000 Hz). This is also in contradiction to Reilly's theory, which concludes that the higher the dB/dt, the lower is the threshold.

Biphasic Stimulus with Different Sinusoidal Rise Times. When biphasic stimulus are applied, the thresholds are independent from the rise times of the sinusoidal

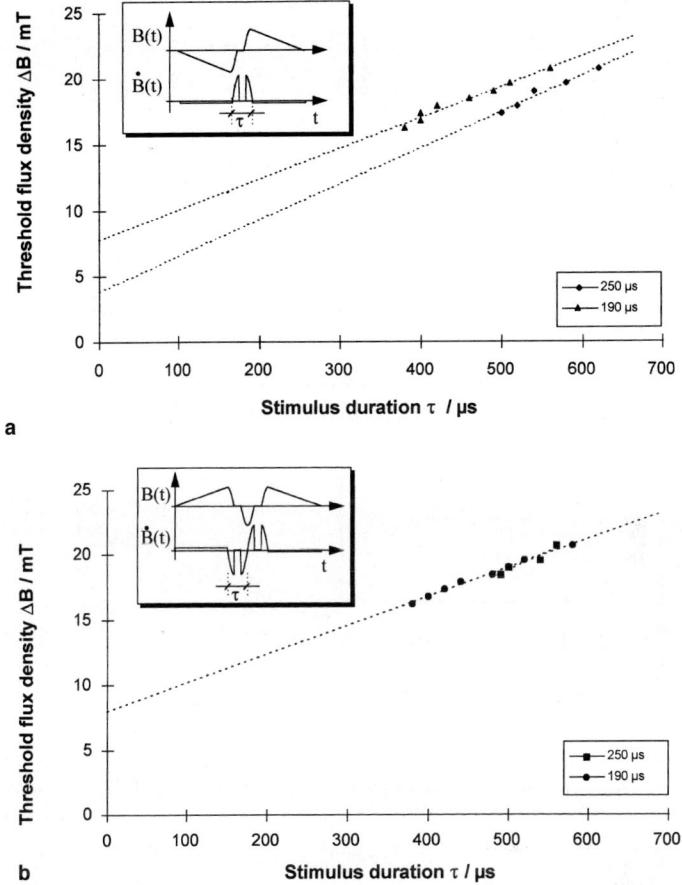

Fig. 24. a Magnetostimulation threshold comparison of monophasic stimuli with different sinusoidal gradient rise times of 190 and 250 μs. For further explanation see text. **b** Magnetostimulation threshold comparison of biphasic stimulus with different sinusoidal gradient rise times of 190 and 250 μs. For further explanation see text

ramps (Fig. 24b). This experiment was repeated several times to verify the findings. Based on the stimulus applied for this study it can be concluded that biphasic stimuli show thresholds independent of the stimulus shape.

Multiphasic Stimulus with Different Sinusoidal Rise Times. When the number of alternating stimuli is increased, the faster rise time stimuli (1315 Hz) show higher thresholds than the slower stimuli. Figure 24c,d shows results with 3 and 41 dB/dt stimuli. The qualitative finding of Fig. 24a is confirmed. Similarly to our finding, Irnich [96] found a higher cardiac threshold in dogs for the higher frequency stimulus when sinusoidal stimuli of 200 Hz, 133 Hz and 100 Hz are compared.

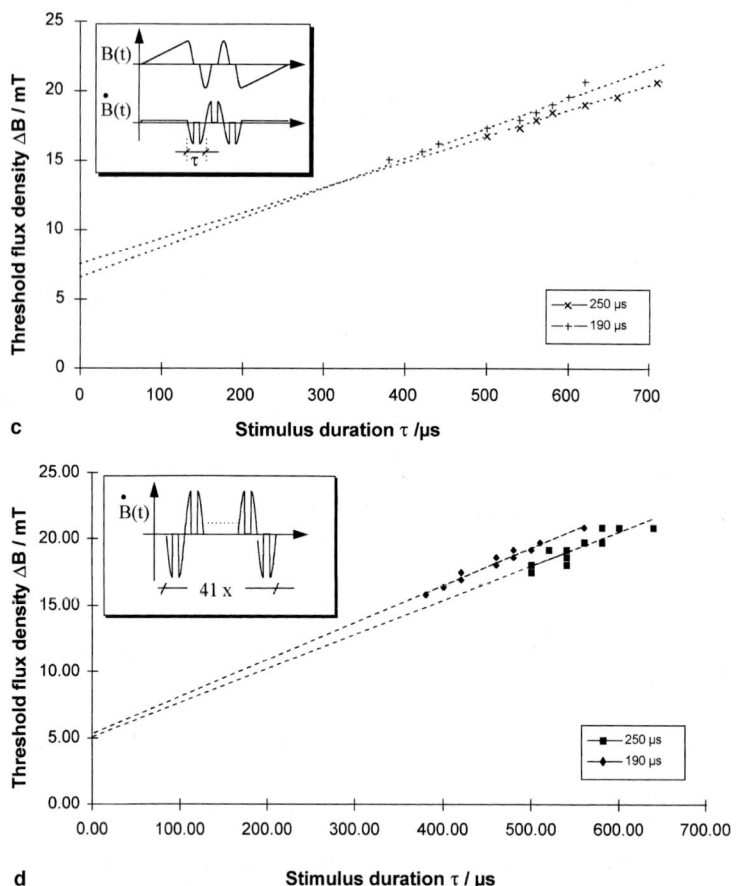

Fig. 24. (continued) **c** Magnetostimulation threshold comparison of three alternating stimuli with different sinusoidal gradient rise times of 190 and 250 µs. For further explanation see text. **d** Magnetostimulation threshold comparison of 41 multiphasic stimuli with different sinusoidal gradient rise times of 190 and 250 µs. For further explanation see text

Threshold Amplitude and Stimulus Pulse Shape

A controversy among the various manufacturers characterized the introduction of EPI in recent years concerning the threshold dependency of sinusoidal and trapezoidal EPI gradient pulse trains. It was stated that trapezoidal pulses of a certain rise time have higher thresholds than sinusoidal pulses with the same rise time and are therefore beneficial for whole-body EPI [13]. Here we describe a comparative study in 19 volunteers for a y gradient. Volunteers were positioned feet first and supine, and they did not change position after the start of the study. Both trapezoidal and sinusoidal gradient pulses were measured under this

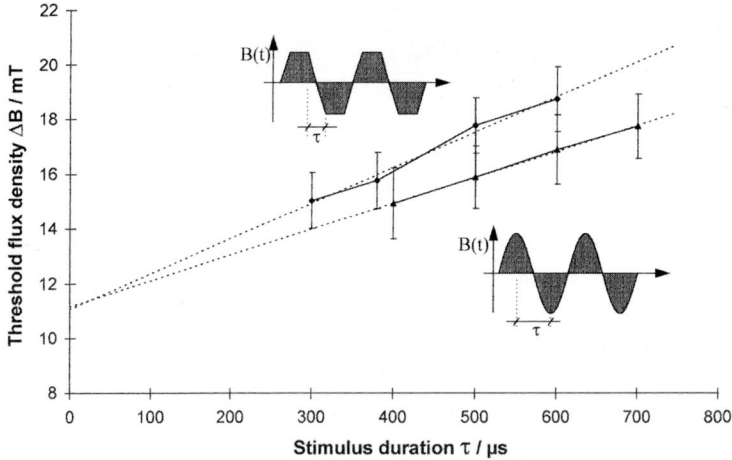

Fig. 25. Y gradient threshold comparison between sinusoidal and trapezoidal gradient pulse trains. Mean value data are shown taken from 19 subjects

experimental setting. Gradient rise times ranged from 150 to 350 µs, corresponding to stimulus durations from 300 to 700 µs.

Figure 25 shows that the threshold for sinusoidal pulse trains are indeed lower than those of trapezoidal pulse trains, when referred to the same stimulus duration, τ, equal to twice the rise time. Each threshold curve is well correlated with the linear relationship predicted by Irnich (dashed line of Fig. 25). Correlation coefficients are calculated as 0.998 and 0.986 for sinusoidal and trapezoidal pulse shapes, respectively. Both fitted lines intersect with the vertical axis at about the same B_0 value of 11.1 mT. This is in coincidence with the theory based on Weiss because for infinitesimally short stimulus durations the ramp shapes are considered equal. Therefore the two shapes, sinusoidal and trapezoidal, must intersect at the same ordinate.

From the pure magnetostimulation threshold point of view, sinusoidal pulses are therefore less advantageous for EPI than trapezoidal pulses. However, for both EPI and conventional MRI the achievable gradient strength is less important than the area under a gradient pulse because it describes the minimum FOV and resolution as described above ("Importance of Fast Switching of High Gradient Amplitudes"). Therefore the acquired magnetostimulation thresholds are recalculated in terms of the FOV ratio, FOV_{sine}/FOV_{trap}. This is shown in Fig. 26. The FOV ratio is plotted versus the pulse duration of a gradient pulse (trapezoidal pulse with linear ramps or trapezoidal pulse with sinusoidal ramps). Pulse durations ranging from 600 to 1000 µs are used for the calculations. Ratios are calculated based on the stimulation thresholds. It is assumed that a flat top inserted into a periodic pulse does not affect the thresholds. This is demonstrated with Fig. 26. Values below a FOV ratio of 1.0 indicate an advantage for sinusoidal ramps; values above indicate an advantage for linear ramps. For short pulse

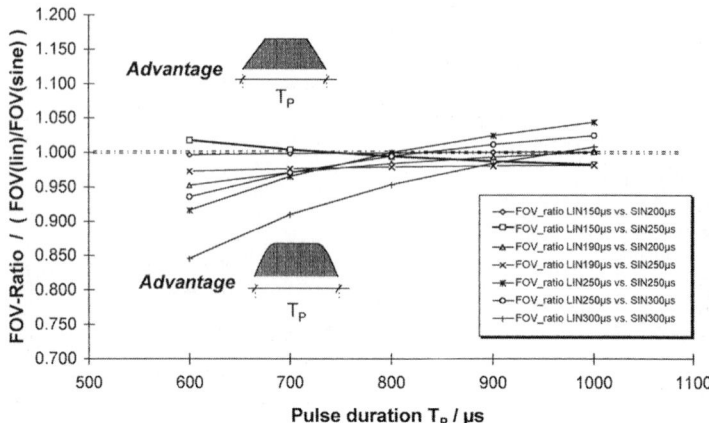

Fig. 26. FOV ratios calculated from magnetostimulation threshold of Fig. 25. Data points below the ratio value of 1 indicate an advantage for sinusoidal gradients

duration, T_P, sinusoidal ramps are more advantageous. This is a general advantage for EPI because speed is the most relevant issue when EPI is applied.

Yamagata et al. [40] performed a similar study in 1991 using a head coil. They compared sinusoidal and trapezoidal pulse trains of period durations of 800 and 1425 μs, corresponding to 1.25 and 700 Hz. The trapezoidal pulses had a rise time of 100 μs always. The fast pulse experiment (800 μs) did not show significant differences (dB/dt = 71 and 86 T/s for sinusoidal and trapezoidal pulses, respectively), whereas the slow experiment (1425 μs) showed 30 % lower thresholds for the sinusoidal pulse train.

Threshold Amplitude and Its Dependency on Pause Times

As was shown in Fig. 24, pause times inserted into the changing phase of a gradient pulse (i.e., at the zero crossings) has an effect on the magnetostimulation thresholds. This is explained by the fact that the total duration of the stimulus is prolonged, and therefore the average dB/dt is reduced (see Eq. 24). The question remains: what happens with thresholds when the stimulus is separated such as stimulus III of Fig. 19?

To evaluate this we first compared stimuli II and III of Fig. 19. A z gradient coil was used for this study. Rise times of 200 μs were applied. Figure 27 shows the thresholds plotted versus the pause times. Pulse and stimulus shapes are shown in the graph as well. A pause time between the changing phase of the gradient pulse (stimulus II) caused a rapid increase in thresholds. At a pause time of 220 μs the limit of the gradient system was already reached. On the other hand, a prolongation of the flat top (stimulus III) did not affect the thresholds.

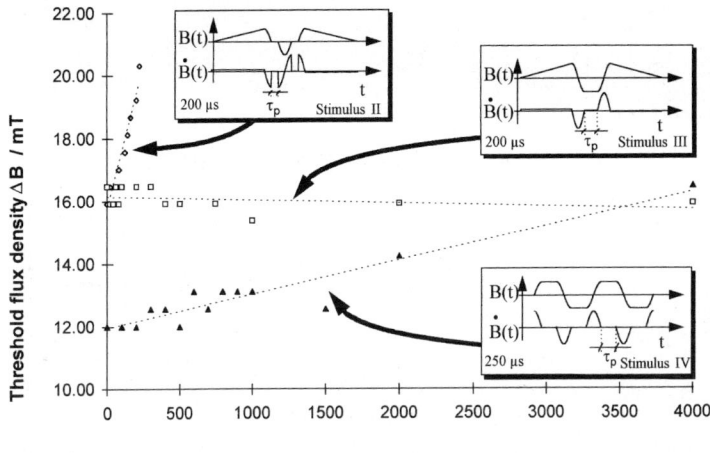

Fig. 27. Dependency of magnetostimulation thresholds on pause times. A z gradient was used for this study. The sinusoidal gradient rise time was 200 μs (stimuli II and III) and 250 μs (stimulus IV). Experiments with stimulus II and III were performed in one session whereas the stimulus IV was performed in a separate session. Therefore experiments cannot be directly compared on a quantitative basis. In order to visualize the results we have overall lowered the curve, corresponding to stimulus IV by 2 mT. This corresponds to the fact that periodic stimuli show lower thresholds than single stimuli (see Fig. 23), and that shorter rise times show lower thresholds than longer rise times

However, when a train of stimuli of 64 oscillations with sinusoidal rise times of 250 μs was applied (stimulus IV) thresholds increased with the flat top pause time but less rapidly than the stimulus with pause times at the zero crossings. This threshold curve becomes saturated after a certain flat top pause time. We could not reach this saturation value because of the duty cycle limits of the gradient system. From an electrophysiological point of view the saturation threshold is reached when a single stimulus (i.e., a single rise or fall time of the gradient train) causes a magnetostimulation.

Experiments with stimuli II and III were performed in one session, whereas stimulus IV was performed in a separate session. Therefore experiments cannot be directly compared on a quantitative basis. To visualize the results we lowered the overall curve corresponding to stimulus IV by 2 mT. This corresponds to the fact that periodic stimuli show lower thresholds than single stimuli (see Fig. 23).

Both pause times described above can be used to reduce stimulatory effects with EPI sequences. This is demonstrated in Fig. 28 which shows a GRE EPI sequence. A pause time can be inserted during the zero crossing phase of the slice-selection gradient. During the readout period a flat top time can be inserted. This allows lower bandwidth EPI acquisition and results in better the signal to noise ratio, at the price, however, of a longer total data acquisition time.

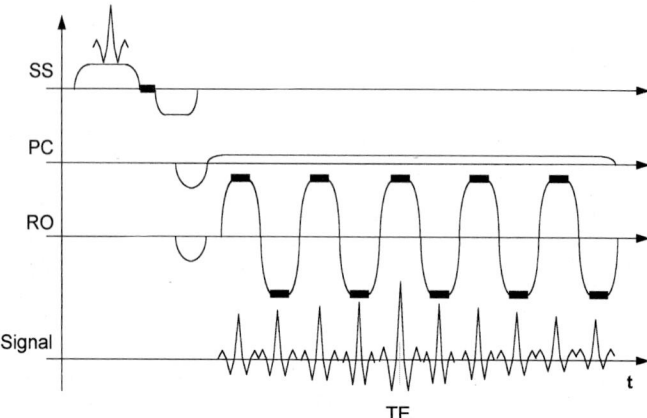

Fig. 28. GRE EPI sequence used for low bandwidth acqusition. Pause times (*bold lines*) in SS direction and in RO direction can reduce magnetostimulation sensitivity. For further information see text

Mixed Gradient Orientations and Its Effect on Stimulation Thresholds

For clinical MRI the orientation of the acquired images depends on anatomy. For imaging of the head more or less orthogonal transverse, sagittal, or coronal orientations are used. For imaging of the spine the sagittal orientation is generally used in combination with slices parallel to the vertebrae and the vertebral discs. The latter orientation is typically single-oblique, tilted axial to coronal. Cardiac imaging, however, requires double-oblique orientation when imaging along the long and short axis of the myocardium or visualizing the four-chamber view.

For oblique and double-oblique imaging the logical gradients (phase-encode G_{PC}, readout G_{RO}, slice-select G_{SS}) are spread over several physical gradients (G_x, G_y, G_z) and result in a linear combination of the logical gradients. This relationship can be described by a matrix operation as shown below. It is assumed that the initial orientation is transversal:

$$(G_x, G_y, G_z) = \begin{pmatrix} \cos\theta & \sin\theta \cdot \sin\phi & -\sin\theta \cdot \cos\phi \\ 0 & \cos\phi & \sin\phi \\ \sin\theta & -\cos\theta \cdot \sin\phi & \cos\theta \cdot \cos\phi \end{pmatrix} \cdot \begin{pmatrix} G_{PC} \\ G_{RO} \\ G_{SS} \end{pmatrix} \tag{37}$$

where ϕ describes the angle from sagittal to coronal orientation and θ describes the final angle to coronal. This is usually written as:

$$\begin{aligned} \angle\phi &= SAG > COR \\ \angle\theta &= \quad\quad > TRA \end{aligned} \tag{38}$$

Using double-oblique orientations in combination with EPI raises the question of how the thresholds depends on the tilt. From Figs. 9 and 13 it follows that a gradient axis perpendicular to the coronal plane (the y gradient) produces the

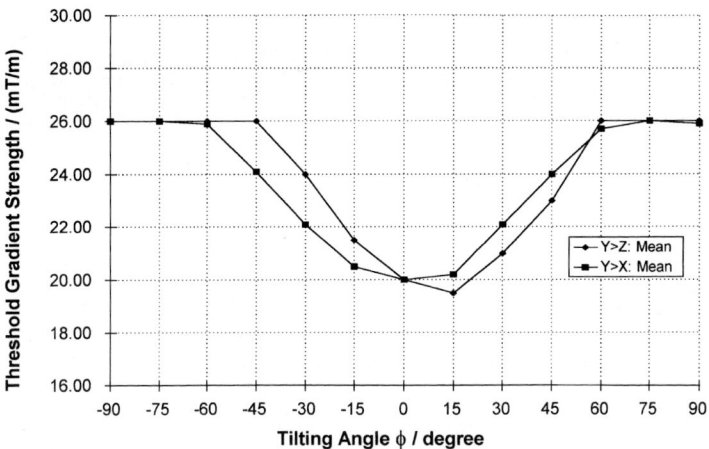

Fig. 29. Mixed gradients and its affect on thresholds. Two studies are shown (Y>Z and Y>X). The minimum threshold at angle 0° correspomds to the y gradient only

highest electrical field and therefore shows the lowest stimulation thresholds. This was confirmed with experiments carried out by Abarth et al. [97]. Their first study of ten volunteers (Fig. 29), explored the single-oblique case. A typical GRE EPI sequence with a sinusoidal readout gradient pulse train of 64 cycles of 833 Hz was applied. The maximum gradient strength achievable was 25 mT/m. For volunteers who did not perceive stimulation, a conservative stimulation threshold of 25.1 mT/m was assigned. Two experiments are plotted in Fig. 29: case I, tilting from Y to X; case II, tilting from Y to Z. Under these circumstances two gradients were on simultaneously described as:

$$\text{Case I:}\quad \begin{aligned} G_y &= G_{RO} \cdot \cos\phi \\ G_x &= G_{RO} \cdot \sin\phi \end{aligned} \qquad\qquad (39)$$

$$\text{Case II:}\quad \begin{aligned} G_y &= G_{RO} \cdot \cos\phi \\ G_x &= G_{RO} \cdot \sin\phi \end{aligned} \qquad\qquad (40)$$

In the second experiment (Fig. 30) seven volunteers were studied under double-oblique orientations. Under these circumstances three gradients were simultaneously switched on. The gradient strength can be calculated from Eq. 37. It is important to note that as the absolute angles approach 0° for oblique and double-oblique measurements the y gradient component increases. Therefore we can conclude that magnetostimulation thresholds decrease as the contribution of the y gradient to the overall gradient strength increases. Simultaneous switching of any gradient does not affect the lowest value of the threshold observed with the y gradient alone. Peripheral stimulation in a whole-body gradient coil is defined by the y gradient alone. Only minor deviations from 0° orientation (y gradient) were observed.

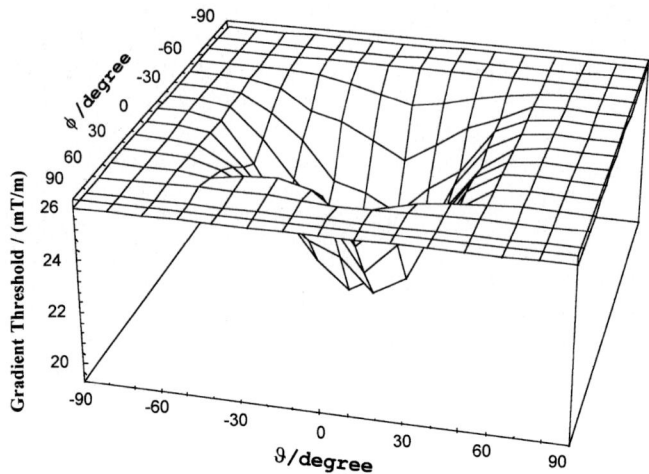

Fig. 30. Magnetostimulation thresholds for mixed gradients. The study represents double-oblique EPI. The minimum threshold is reached when the y gradient amplitude is at its maximum

Discussion

Irnich's theory is based on empirical findings from Weiss explored in 1901 and by Lapicque in 1909. A hyperbolic strength-duration function can be derived based on the assumption that opening of sodium pores requires a mechanical impulse caused by an external electric field. In Irnich's theory stimulation occurs when the external force is larger than the static force needed to hold the barrier in its resting state. Magnetostimulation thresholds are best described in terms of magnetic flux excursion, $B(\tau)$, which holds a linear relationship to the stimulus duration, τ. Equivalently, thresholds are expressed in average flux change, $\bar{B}$, as an inverse function of τ. Rheobase and chronaxie are the characteristic parameters describing nerve excitation. Chronaxie, τ_{chron}, is defined as 0.69 times τ_e, the "membrane time constant" based on exponential strength-duration models. Both rheobase and chronaxie are applicable to peripheral and cardiac excitation. In the latter they are used to adjust intensities in cardiac pacemakers. The linear relationship between stimulus duration and amplitude-time product was proposed and confirmed in many peripheral nerve stimulation experiments ("Stimulation Experiments and Its Interpretations"). Different stimulus pulse shapes show different thresholds when referred to the same rise time.

Mansfield's model is based on a simple electrical circuit of the membrane of a myelinated nerve originally described by Blair et al. in 1932. His theory allows prediction of thresholds for arbitrary pulse shapes. A magnetostimulation is equivalent to applying an external current generator to a nerve node, causing a breakdown in negative resting potential. An exponential strength-duration curve can be deduced from this model. When the stimulus duration, τ, is short compared to the tissue time constant, τ_e, the threshold is a linear function of the maximum excursion in B. Therefore Mansfield et al. state that $B(\tau)$ rather than dB/dt is the important factor describing neural activation. Comparing trapezoidal and sinusoidal stimulation thresholds by means of the equivalent rise time shows good agreement with their theory.

Reilly's SENN model of a myelinated nerve is based on an electrical circuit describing the propagation of signals similar to the signal propagation in electrical cables. A magnetostimulation threshold is defined as the stimulus adequate to produce a propagating action potential. The SENN model allows the simulation of arbitrary stimulus pulse shapes. A strength-duration relationship can be fitted to this simulation data. When time constants, τ_e, are compared, SENN-modeled τ_e values are shorter than those observed experimentally, typically by a factor of 2, and about 50 % longer than the membrane time constant based on resistance and capacitance of the equivalent circuit. Reilly concludes from experiments and his simulation that peripheral nerves have tissue time constants, τ_e, of about 200 µs and an electric field rheobase of 6.2 V/m for a myelineated nerve of 20 µm diameter. Cardiac tissue shows a much longer τ_e of about 3000 µs. However, following his explanation on safety aspects cardiac tissue does not show higher electric field rheobase values.

Common to all three models is the fact that the relevant stimulation force is the induced electric field in the biological tissue. Reilly and Mansfield fit their results to exponential strength-duration curves. Irnich fits the data to a hyperbolic strength-duration relationship. Table 5 summarizes the formulae for the strength-duration expressions of electrostimulation, expressed in current, I, and charge, Q, and for magnetostimulation expressed in terms of the magnetic flux, B, and its rate of change, dB/dt.

Differences between the hyperbolic and exponential approaches are remarkable. Taking the same rheobase and chronaxie for each model, Q_o or B_o (see Table 5) differs in the two approaches. For rectangular pulses energy is lowest at chronaxie in the hyperbolic approach, whereas it is nearly twice chronaxie in the exponential case. This is important for cardiac pacemakers. The membrane

Table 5. Summary of strength-duration relationships used in the literature to describe electro- and magnetostimulation

Strength-duration expression	Electrostimulation	Magnetostimulation
Hyperbolic (used by Weiss, Lapicque, Irnich)	$\dfrac{Q(\tau)}{Q_o} = 1 + \dfrac{\tau}{\tau_{chron}}$	$\dfrac{B(\tau)}{B_0} = 1 + \dfrac{\tau}{\tau_{chron}}$
	$\dfrac{I(\tau)}{I_o} = 1 + \dfrac{\tau_{chron}}{\tau}$	$\dfrac{\dot{B}(\tau)}{\dot{B}_0} = 1 + \dfrac{\tau_{chron}}{\tau}$
Exponential (used by Blair, Pearce, Mansfield	$\dfrac{Q(\tau)}{Q_0} = \dfrac{\tau/\tau_e}{1 - e^{-\tau/\tau_e}}$	$\dfrac{B(\tau)}{B_0} = \dfrac{\tau/\tau_e}{1 - e^{-\tau/\tau_e}}$
	$\dfrac{I(\tau)}{I_0} = \dfrac{1}{1 - e^{-\tau/\tau_e}}$	$\dfrac{\dot{B}(\tau)}{\dot{B}_0} = \dfrac{1}{1 - e^{-\tau/\tau_e}}$

Charge (Q) flux density (B) current (I) and rate change of the flux (dB/dt) are equivalent counterparts in electro- and magnetostimulation.

time constant cannot be determined by real membrane parameters. It is determined empirically as with chronaxie. Experiments in cardiac stimulation and defibrillation, rather, support the validity of the hyperbolic than the exponential approximation. When the data available from the literature are fitted to the linear relationship, correlation coefficients close to 1 are obtained. Therefore a linear relationship (Eq. 23) seems to be at least as good as an exponential relationship. This was confirmed by Mouchowar et al. [71] as well.

Are there cardiac risks? Reilly calculated the rheobase electric field for myelinated fibers of 20 μm diameter to be 6.2 V/m. The chronaxie times for nerves are reported to range between 20 and 600 μs, with values typically around 100 μs. Mouchawar et al. [15] performed an interesting study with dogs to evaluate closed-chest cardiac stimulation with a pulsed magnetic field. They concluded that the response to magnetic fields is the same as that produced by direct electrical stimulations and found a rheobase electric field of about 30 V/m.

Compared to peripheral nerves, cardiac muscle fibers show a much higher rheobase of approximately 60 V/m [98] and a chronaxie of about 2 ms (membrane time constant 2.9 ms). This is about ten times higher than the 6.2 V/m assumed by Reilly [99]. This fact is important for predicting cardiac thresholds and safety legal limits. The current regulatory recommendation of most countries are based on Reilly's assumption of the rheobase threshold of 6.2 V/m and therefore lead to very conservative thresholds.

It is surprising to note that these important facts have not yet entered the discussion on magnetostimulation because they have a direct effect on legal limits. This is demonstrated with Fig. 31, which shows the hyperbolic strength-duration curves of peripheral nerves and cardiac muscles based an rheobases of 6.2 V/m (Reilly's assumption) and 60 V/m (lowest possible electric field for sinusoidal cardiac stimulation [98]). Assuming a typical gradient rise time of 250 μs corre-

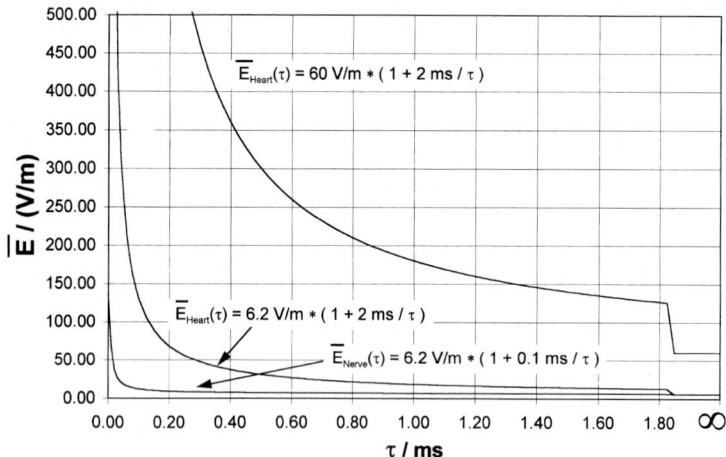

Fig. 31. Hyperbolic strength-duration curves for peripheral nerve and myocardial muscle fibers. The cardiac thresholds are plotted twice to show the differences in myocardial rheobase values of 6.2 and 30 V/m

sponding to a stimulus duration of 500 μs, cardiac stimulations are expected at about 4 times and 40 times the peripheral threshold based on Reilly and Irnich, respectively. Dog and human peripheral experiments performed by Bourland et al. [94] yield a difference by a factor of 20 between sensory and cardiac threshold corresponding with a rheobase of 60 V/m.

An investigation by Irnich [98] demonstrates that the cardiac threshold variability is surprisingly low. Although data were compiled for in vitro and in vivo experiments from different species, the standard deviation as a percentage of the mean was only 23 %, indicating that excitation of cardiac fibers obeys a rather strong and common law. This is confirmed by experimental and clinical experience that pacing thresholds are rather uniform. Drugs can occasionally lower thresholds but not below 80 % of the normal value [100]. Change in electrolyte concentration can reduce it to 85 % of its normal value [64]. Consequently, following these findings, it is therefore not necessary to consider "hypersensitive" patients by means of excessive safety factors.

A safety limit philosophy should contain all relevant factors under "worst-case" conditions. It therefore seems wise to choose the orientation factor c of Eqs. 10 and 11 equal to 1 to eliminate orientation considerations of the gradient field. The nonuniformity of the magnetic field, which we have not quantified, also increases the stimulation thresholds. Taking into consideration the stability of thresholds of excitable cells, a safety factor of 3 as proposed by Reilly [17] is sufficient when formulating limits for MRI applications. It is interesting to note that a FDA draft version of a primer on medical device interaction with MRI systems [101] reports that "current FDA guidance limits the Time Rate of Change of Magnetic Field (dB/dt) to levels which do not result in painful peripheral nerve stimulation."

Although there is still a lack of information about the functional relationship between stimulus shape and thresholds we can conclude from experiments performed up to now that levels close to or slightly above the peripheral stimulation threshold are save. For manufacturers of MR equipment it therefore remains to determine these peripheral thresholds for individual coil designs based on experimental studies or theoretical calculations in order to define the limits for scan operation.

Appendix: Acoustic Noise Generated by Fast MR Gradients

Gradient acoustic noise is of great concern for patient comfort and for patient safety [102–105] when large gradients are switched very rapidly. The acoustic noise is caused by the so-called Lorentz force. When a current passing through a wire is exposed to a magnetic field, a force perpendicular to the current and the magnetic field is generated. Mathematically this is expressed by the vector product (x):

$$\underline{F} \sim \underline{I} \times \underline{B} \tag{41}$$

where F is the force, I is the electric current, and B is the magnetic flux. All quantities are described as vectors.

In MR scanners the main magnetic field, B_o, and the current through the gradient coils generate a deformation of the coil structure. This effect causes vibrations similar to a loudspeaker and therefore produces acoustic noise. The amplitude of the acoustic noise is largest when a maximum current in combination with a minimum rise time is pulsed through the coil. The highest noise level that can be generated occurs when all three gradient axes are pulsed at the same time. The National Electrical Manufacturer Association (NEMA) [106] describes this type of noise as the maximum gradient acoustic noise (MGAN) in contrast to the maximum clinical acoustic noise (MCAN), which is produced under clinical MRI conditions. The latter occurs by applying clinical sequences with high gradient duty cycles and gradient currents in combination with minimum rise times.

Figure 32 illustrates the forces to a wire carrying a current, I, exposed by a magnetic flux, B (upper left and right) The situation for an z gradient is shown in the lower figure. Upon application of a positive current to the z gradient, the right end of the gradient coil is expanded whereas the left end is contracted. Changing the polarity causes an alternation of contraction and expansion. For bipolar gradient-pulse trains the coil oscillates and thus produces oscillatory acoustic noise as well. In general, gradient coils have several modes of oscillations (eigenmodes) [107–109] depending on their geometrical dimensions and material properties such as weight and stiffness.

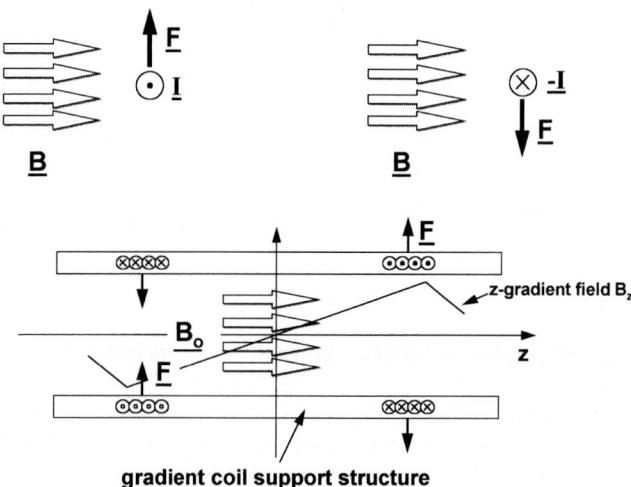

gradient coil support structure

Fig. 32. Lorentz forces on a wire carrying current, I, exposed to a magnetic flux, B. *Above*, a force pointing upward when the current points towards the observer. When the current is directed away from the observer (*–I*), the force points downward (*upper right*). For a z gradient coil both cases are present simultaneously (*below*). For a postive current (generating an elevation of the flux at positive z positions) the coil is expanded on the left side and contracted on the right side. When the current polarity is changed, the contraction and expansion are altered. This causes compression and depression of the air inside the gradient bore and produces acoustic noise

With the introduction of fast MRI techniques, especially EPI, the acoustic noise became more and more relevant because it reaches noise levels that can cause harm to both patients and personnel. Therefore limits for maximum acoustic noise set by several organizations must be applied to MRI. The NEMA [106] describes a standardized procedure for the measurement of the acoustic noise produced by MR gradients. A trapezoidal bipolar gradient pulse train (without eddy current compensation) of maximum amplitude and minimum rise time must be applied simultaneously for all three axes to measure the MGAN at defined spatial positions. To measure the MCAN the worst-case clinical sequence must be used, which is represented by the worst-case acoustic combination (minimum echo time, minimum repetition time, minimum slice thickness, minimum FOV, and oblique scan planes). The NEMA leaves it up to the manufacturer to measure the MGAN or the MCAN.

In the United States and Japan the Occupational Safety and Health Administration (OSHA) [110] sets the limit for the unweighted peak sound pressure level (SPL), L_{Peak}, to 200 Pa (or 140 dB referenced to 20 μPa). An A-weighted rms SPL average value of 90 dB(A) is the limit for occupationally exposed individuals averaged over 8 h per 24-hour day [or 105 dB(A) over 1 h]. This value is considered very conservative when applied to infrequent exposure which are typical for MR examinations.

An European standard [111] requires that the unweighted peak level be below 140 dB and the A-weighted level below 99 dB(A) for patient examination. If necessary, acoustic noise protection equipment must be used. For personnel various local regulations apply concerning acoustic noise exposure which may vary from country to country within the European Union.

References

1. Shellock FG, Kanal E (1994) Magnetic resonance bioeffects, safety, and patient management. Raven, New York
2. Budinger T (1981) Nuclear magnetic resonance (NMR) in vivo studies: known thresholds for health effects. J Comp Assist Tomogr 5:800–811
3. Redington R, Dumoulin C, Schenk J (1988) MR Imaging and bioeffects on a whole body 4.0 tesla imaging system. Proceedings of the Society of Magnetic Resonance in Medicine, p 4
4. Bottomly PA, Edelstein WA (1981) Power deposition in whole body NMR imaging. Med Phys 8:510–512
5. Barlow H, Kohn H, Walsh E (1947) Visual sensation aroused by magnetic fields. Am J Physiol 148:372–375
6. Lovsund P, Nillson S, Reuter T, Oberg P (1980) Magnetophosphenes: a quantitative analysis of thresholds. Med Biol Eng Comput 18:326–324
7. Mansfield P (1977) Multi-planar image formation using NMR spine-echoes. J Phys Chem Solid State Phys 10:L55–L58
8. Budinger T (1979) Thresholds for physiological effects due to to RF and magnetic fields used in NMR imaging. IEEE Trans Nucl Sci NS-26:2821–2825
9. Cohen MS, Weisskoff RM, Kantor ML (1989) Evidence of peripheral stimulation by time-varying magnetic fields. Proceedings of the Radiological Society of Northern America (RSNA), 75th Anual meeting Scientific program: 1188
10. Fischer H (1989) physiological effects by fast oscillating magnetic field gradients. Proceedings of the Radiological Society of Northern America (RSNA), 75th Anual meeting Scientific program: 1189

11. Budinger TF, Fischer H, Hentschel D, Reinfelder H-E, Schmitt F (1991) Physiological effects of fast oscillating magnetic field gradients. J Comp Assist Tomogr 15:909–914
12. Bureau Central de la Commission Electrotechnique International (1991) Draft IEC standard medical electrical equipment. II. Particular requirements for the safety of magnetic resonance systems for medical diagnosis. IEC/SC 62B, Geneva
13. Mansfield P, Harvey (1993) Limits of neural stimulation in echo-planar imaging. Magn Reson Med 29:746–758
14. McRobbie D, Foster MA (1985) Cardiac response to pulsed magnetic fields with regard to safety in NMR imaging. Phys Med Biol 30:695–702
15. Mouchawar GA, Bourland JD, Nyenhuis JA, Geddes LA, Foster KS, Jones JT, Graber GP (1992) Closed-chest cardiac stimulation with a pulsed magnetic field. Med Biol Eng Comput 30:162–168
16. National Radiological Protection Board (NRPB) (1983) Revised guidance on acceptable limits of exposure during nuclear magnetic resonance clinical imaging. Br J Radiol 56:974–977
17. Reilly JP (1989) Periphal nerve stimulation by induced electric currents: exposure to time-varying magnetic fields. Med Biol Eng Comput 27:101–110
18. Reilly JP (1992) Electrical stimulation and electro-pathology. Cambridge University Press, Cambridge
19. Roth JR, Basser P (1990) A model of the stimulation of a nerve fiber by electromagnetic induct. IEEE Trans Biomed Eng 37:588–597
20. Silny J (1987) Zur Gefährdung der vitalen Funktion des Herzens im magnetischen 50 Hz-Feld. Medizinisch-technischer Bericht des Instituts zur Erforschung elektrischer Unfälle. Berufsgenossenschaft Feinmechanik und Elektrotechnik, Cologne
21. Wessale JL, Bourland JD, Tacker WA, Geddes LA (1980) Bipolar catheter defibrillation in dogs using trapezoidal waveforms of various tilts. J Electrocardiol 13:359–366
22. International Non-Ionizing Radiation Committee of the International Radiation Protection Assocation (IRPA/INIRC) (1991) Protection of the patient undergoing a magnetic resonance examination. Health Physics 61:923–928
23. Bradley WG, Waluch V (1985) Blood flow: magnetic resonance imaging. Radiology 154:443–450
24. Laub GA, Kaiser WA (1988) MR angiography with gradient motion refocusing. J Comp Assist Tomogr 12(3):377–382
25. Lüdeke KM, Röschmann P, Tischler R (1985) Susceptibility artefacts in NMR imaging. Magn Reson Imaging 3:329–343
26. Wielopolski PA, Finn JP, Edelman RR, Schmitt F (1993) Ultrashort TEs for abdominal imaging with a whole body echo planar imaging system. Proceedings of the Society of Magnetic Resonance in Medicine, San Francisco, p 73
27. Wielopolski PA, Edelman RR, Finn JP, Schmitt F (1993) High resolution, ultrashort echo time MR angiography with a whole-body EPI imager. Proceedings of the Society of Magnetic Resonance in Medicine, San Francisco, p 45
28. Edelman RR, Wielopolski P, Schmitt F (1994) Echo-planar imaging. Radiology 192:600–612
29. Schmitt F, Warach S, Wielopolski P, Edelman RR (1994) Clinical applications and techniques of echo-planar imaging. MAGMA 2:259–266
30. Bourland JD, Nyenhuis JA, Mouchawar GA, Elabbady TZ, Geddes LA, Schaefer DJ, Riehl ME (1991) Physiological indicators of high MRI gradient-induced fields. Proceedings of the Society of Magnetic Resonance in Medicine, WIP. p 1276
31. Ruiz EV, Russo JA, Savino GV, Valentinuzzi ME (1985) Ventricular fibrillation threshold in the dog determined with defirbrillating paddles. Med Biol Eng Comp 23:281–284
32. Bourland JD, Nyenhuis JA, Mouchawar GA, Elabbady TZ, Geddes LA, Schaefer DJ, Riehl ME (1992) Gated, gradient-induced cardiac stimulation in the dog: absence of ventricular fibrillation. Proceedings of the Society of Magnetic Resonance in Medicine, Berlin, vol 1, p 4804
33. Roos MS, Budinger TF, Brennan KN, Wong STS (1992) Coil electric field effects in neuro muscular stimulation experiments. Proceedings of the Society of Magnetic Resonance in Medicine, p 4036
34. Cohen MS, Weisskoff RM, Rzedzian RR, Kantor ML (1990) Sensory stimulation by time-varying magnetic fields. Magn Reson Med 14:409–414
35. Ehrhardt JC, Lin CS, Magnotta VA, Baker SM, Fisher DJ, Yuh WTC (1993) Neural stimulation on a whole body echo-planar imaging system. Proceedings of the Society of Magnetic Resonance in Medicine, vol 3, p 1372
36. Schaefer DJ, Bourland JD, Nyenhuis JA, Foster KS, Wirth WF, Geddes LA, Riehl ME (1994) Determination of gradient induced, human peripheral nerve stimulation thresholds for trapezoidal pulse trains. Proceedings of the Society of Magnetic Resonance in Medicine, p 101

37. Yamagata H, Kuhara S, Seo Y, Sato K, Hiwaki O, Ueno S (1991) Evaluation of dB/dt thresholds for nerve stimulation elicited by trapezoidal and sinusoidal gradient fields in echo-planar imaging. Proceedings of the Society of Magnetic Resonance in Medicine, works in progress, p 1277
38. Rohan ML (1992) Stimulation by time-varying magnetic fields. Proceedings of the Society of Magnetic Resonance in Medicine, Berlin, p 587
39. Schmitt F, Wielopolski P, Fischer H, Edelman RR (1994) Peripheral stimulation and their relation to gradient pulse shapes. Proceedings of the Society of Magnetic Resonance in Medicine, San Francisco, p 102
40. Schmitt F (1985) Correction of geometrical distortions in MR images. Proceedings of the Computer Assisted Radiology, CAR. Springer Berlin Heidelberg New York, pp 15–23
41. Schmitt F, Fischer H, Ladebeck R (1988) Double acquisition echo-planar imaging. Proceedings of the 2nd European Congress of NMR in Medicine and Biology, Berlin
42. Bandettini PA, Wong EC, Hyde JS (1992) Echo-planar imaging of the human brain using a three axis local gradient coil. Proceedings of the Society of Magnetic Resonance in Medicine, p 105
43. Kilian V, Sellers M, Hentzelt H, Bömmel F, Carlberger T, Schuster H, Schmitt F, Haase A (1996) A Comparison of different head gradient coil designs. Proceedings of the Society of Magnetic Resonance in Medicine, p 1396
44. Reilly P (1992) Principles of nerve and heart excitation by time-varying magnetic fields. Ann NY Acad Sci 649:96–117
45. Durney CH, Johnson CC, Massoudi H (1975) Long wavelength analysis of plane wave irradiation of prolate spheroid model of a man. IEEE Trans Microwave Theory Tech 23(2):246–253
46. Spiegel RJ (1977) Magnetic coupling to a prolate spheroid model of a man. IEEE Trans Power Appar Syst 96(1):208–212
47. Weiss G (1901) Sur la possibilité de rendre comparable entre eux les appareils servant à l'excitation électrique. Arch Ital Biol 35:413–446
48. Irnich W (1990) The fundamental law of electrostimulation and its application to defibrillation. Pacing Clin Electrophysiol 13:1433–1447
49. Lapicque L (1909) Definition expérimental de l'excitabilité. Soc Biol 77:280–283
50. Irnich W (1973) Physikalische Überlegungen zur Elektrostimulation. Biomed Tech 18:97–104
51. Lepeschkin E, Jones JL, Rush S, Jones RE (1978) Local potential gradient as a unifying measure for thresholds of stimulation standstill, tachyarrythmia and fibrillation appearing after strong capacitor discharges. Adv Cardiol 21:268–278
52. Winfree AT (1990) The electrical thresholds of ventricular myocardium. Cardiovasc Electrophysiol 1:393–410
53. Knisley SB, Smith WM, Ideker RE (1992) Effect of intrastimular polarity, reversal on electric field stimulation thresholds in frog and rabbit myocardium. J Cardiovasc Electrophysiol 3:239–254
54. Lepeschkin E, Jones JL, Rush S, Jones RE (1978) Local potential gradient as a unifying measure for thresholds of stimulation standstill, tachyarrythmia and fibrillation appearing after strong capacitor discharges. Adv Cardiol 21:268–278
55. Bourland JD, Tacker WA, Geddes LA, Chafee V (1978) Comparative efficacy of damped sine wave and square wave current for transchest ventricular defibrillation in animals. Med Instrum 12:43–45
56. Tacker WA, Geddes LA (1980) Electrical defibrillation. CRC, Boca Ration, pp 74–85
57. Mouchawar GA, Geddes LA, Bourland JD, Pearee JA (1989) Ability of the Lapicque and Blair strength-duration curves to fit experimentally obtained data from a dog heart. IEEE Trans Biomed Eng 36:971–974
58. Irnich W (1980) The chronaxie time and its practical importance. Pacing Clin Electrophysiol 3:292–301
59. Panizza M, Nilson J, Roth BJ, Basser PJ, Hallet M (1992) Relevance of stimulus duration for activation of motor and sensory fibers: implications for the study of H-reflexes and magnetic stimulation. Electroencephalogr Clin Neurophysiol 85:22–29
60. Bourland JD, Nyenhuis JA, Noe WA, Schaefer DJ, Foster KS, Geddes LA (1994) Motor and sensory strength-duration curves for MRI gradient fields. Proceedings of the Society of Magnetic Resonance, San Francisco, vol 1, p 1724
61. Harvey PR, Mansfield P (1993) Avoiding peripheral nerve stimulation: switched gradient waceform criteria for optimum image resolution in EPI. Proceedings of the of the European Society for Magnetic Resonance in Medicine and Biology, Tenth Annual Scientific Meeting and Exhibition, Rome, p 422

62. Hodgkins AL, Huxley F (1952) A quantitative description of membrane current and its application to conduction and excitation in nerve. J Physiol 117:500–544
63. Frankenhaeuser B, Huxley AF (1964) The action potential in the myelineated nerve fiber of Xenoppus leavis as computed on the basis of voltage clamp data. J Physiol 171:302–315
64. McNeal DR (1985) Analysis of a model for excitation of myelinated nerve. IEEE Trans Biomed Eng 32:329–337
65. Reilly JP, Freeman VT, Larkin WD (1985) Sensory effects of transient electrical stimulation – evaluation with a neuroelectric model. IEEE Trans Biomed Eng 32-1001–1011
66. Ruch TC, Patton HD, Woodbury JW, Toiwe AL (1986) Neurophysiology. Saunders, Philadelphia
67. Blair HA (1932) On the intensity-time relations for stimulation by electric currents. I. J Gen Physiol 15:709–729
68. Blair HA (1932) On the intensity-time relations for stimulation by electric currents. II. J Gen Physiol 15:731–755
69. Lapicque L (1907) Consideration préalables sur la nature du phenomene par lequel l'electricite excite les nerfs. J Physiol Pathol Génér 9:565–578
70. Reilly P (1988) Electrical model of neural excitation studies. APL Technical Digest 9:44–59
71. Plonsey R, Fleming D (1969) Bioelectric phenomena. McGraw-Hill, New York, p 380
72. Pearce JA, Bourland JD, Neilsen W, Geddes LA, Voelz M (1982) Myocardial stimulation with ultrashort duration current pulses. Pacing Clin Electrophysiol 5:52–58
73. Mansfield P, Morris P (1982) NMR imaging in biomedicine, Supplement 2: Advances in magnetic resonance, pp 314–332
74. Harvey PR, Mansfield P (1994) Avoiding peripheral nerve stimulation: gradient waveform criteria for optimum resolution in echo-planar imaging. Magn Reson Med 32:236–241
75. Federal Register of the United States of America (1989) Medical Devices: Draft Guidance for Premarket Notification Submissions for Magnetic Resonance Diagnostic Devices; Availability vol 53, no. 233, 48981
76. Ministry of Health and Welfare, Medical Department, Japan, Group of Medical Equipment Development (1991) About the treadment of clinical test concerning the submission of approval of NMR-CT instruments. March 28. 1991
77. Bernhardt JH (1985) Evaluation of human exposures to low frequency field. The impact of proposed frequency radiation standard on military operations. Lecture series 138, Advisory Group for Aerospace Research and Development (NATO), Surseine, France
78. Bundesamt für Strahlenschutz: Empfehlung zur Vermeidung gesundheitlicher Risiken bei Anwendung magnetischer Resonanzverfahren in der medizinischen Diagnostik (1995) Empfehlung der Strahlenschutzkommission, verabschiedet in der 131. Sitzung am 22. Juni 1995, geändert in der Sitzung am 27. Juni 1996
79. International Radiation Protection Association (IRPA) in Health Physics (1991) Protection of the patient undergoing a magnetic resonance examination 61:923–928
80. International Standard of the International Electrotechnical Comission (IEC) (1995) Medical electrical equipment. II. Particular requirements for safety of magnetic resonance equipment to medical diagnosis. Equivalent ot the proposed European norm EN 60601-2-33
81. National Radiation Protection Board (NRPB) Document of the NRPB (1991) Principles for the Protection of Patients and Volunteers During Clinical Magnetic Resonance Diagnostic Procedures Vol 2 No. 1, pp 17–21
82. Gazzetta Ufficiale (1991) Decreto Ministeriale 1 agosta Autorizzazione alla installazione ed uso di apparechiature diagnostiche a risonanza magnetica. Serie generale no 194, supplemento. Rome 20 August, Ministero della Sanita, Italy
83. Nyenhuis JA, Bourland JD, Schaefer DJ, Foster KS, Schoelein WE, Mouchowar GA, Elabbady TZ, Geddes LA, Riehl ME (1992) Measurement of cardiac stimulation thresholds for pulsed z-gradient fields in a 1.5 T magnet. Proceedings of the Society of Magnetic Resonance in Medicine, p 586
84. Rohan ML (1992) Stimulation by time-varying magnetic fields. Proceedings of the Society of Magnetic Resonance in Medicine, p 587
85. Nyenhuis JA, Bourland JD, Schaefer DJ, Foster KS, Schoelein WE, Mouchawar GA, Elabbady TZ, Geddes LA, Riehl ME (1992) Magnetic measurement of cardiac stimulation thresholds for pulsed z-gradient fields in a 1.5-T. Proceedings of the Society of Magnetic Resonance in Medicine, p 586
86. Bourland JD, Nyenhuis JA, Schaefer DJ, Foster KS, Schoenlein WE, Elabbady TZ, Geddees LA, Riehl ME (1992) Gated, gradient-induced cardiac stimmulation in the dog: absence of ventricular fibrillation. Proceedings of the Society of Magnetic Resonance in Medicine, p 4804

87. Nyenhuis JA, Bourland JD, Mouchawar GA, Elabbady TZ, Geddes LA, Schaefer DJ, Riehl ME (1991) Comparison of stimulation effects of longitudinal and transverse MRI gradinet coils. Proceedings of the Society of Magnetic Resonance in Medicine, WIP. p 1275

88. Bourland JD, Nyenhuis JA, Mouchawar GA, Elabbady TZ, Geddes LA, Schaefer DJ, Riehl ME (1992) Physiologic indicators of high MRI gradient-induced fields. Proceedings of the Society of Magnetic Resonance in Medicine, p 1276

89. Yamagato H, Kuhara S, Seo Y, Ato K, Hiwaki O, Ueno S (1991) Evaluation of dB/dt thresholds for nerve stimulation elicited by trapezoidal and sinusoidal gradient fields in echo-planar imaging. Proceedings of the Society of Magnetic Resonance in Medicine, works in progress, p 1277

90. Schaefer DJ, Bourland DJ, Nyenhuis JA, Foster KS, Licato PE, Geddes LA (1995) Effects of simultaneous gradient combinations on human peripheral nerve stimulation thresholds. Proceedings of the Society of Magnetic Resonance and the European Society for Magnetic Resonance in Medicine and Biology, p 1220

91. Eberhardt KEW, Abart J, Storch TH, Huk WJ, Richter I, Zeitler E (1995) Clinical investigation of stimulation threshold of no healthy adults using sinusoidally oscillating gradients. Proceedings of the Society of Magnetic Resonance and the European Society for Magnetic Resonance in Medicine and Biology, p.1221

92. Schaefer DJ, Bourland JD, Nyenhuis JA, Forster KS, Wirth WF, Geddes LA, Riehl ME (1994) Determination of gradient-induced, human peripheral nerve stimulation thresholds of trapezoldal pulse trains. Proceedings of the Society of Magnetic Resonance, p 101

93. Schmitt F, Wielopolski P, Fischer H, Edelmann RR (1994) Peripheral stimulation and their relation to gradient pulse. Proceedings of the Society of Magnetic Resonance, p 102

94. Bourland JD, Nyenhuis JA, Noe WA, Schaefer DJ, Foster KS, Geddes LA (1994) Motor and sensory, strength-duration curves for MRI gradient Fields. Proceedings of the Society of Magnetic Resonance, San Francisco, vol 1, p 1724

95. Budinger TF, Roos MS, Wong STS, Brennan KM (1993) Neuro-musculare stimulation by oscillating magnetic fields. (unpublished)

96. Irnich W (1976) Elektrotherapie des Herzens – physiologische und biotechnische Aspekte. Schiele & Schön, Berlin, pp 68–73

97. Abart J, Eberhardt K, Fischer H, Huk W, Richter E, Schmitt F, Storch T, Zeitler E (1997) Peripheral nerve stimulation by time varying magnetic fields. J Comput Assist Tomogr 21:532–538

98. Irnich W (1994) Electrostimulation by time-varying magnetic fields. MAGMA 2:43–49

99. Reilly P (1990) Peripheral nerve and cardiac excitation by time-varying magnetic fields: a comparison of the thresholds. Report MT 90–100, Office for Science and Technology. Center for Devices and Radiological Health, Food and Drug Administration, Rockville

100. Lüderitz B (1986) Herzschrittmacher, Therapie und Diagnostik kardialer Rhythmusstörungen. Springer Berlin Heidelberg New York

101. Center of Device and Radiological Health (CDRH) of the Federal Food and Drug Association (FDA) (1997) A primer on medical device interaction with MRI systems. Feb. 7. http://www.fda.gov//cdrh/ode/primer6f.html#mri

102. Quirk ME, Letendre AJ, Ciottone RA, Lingley JF (1989) Anxiety in patients undergoing MR imaging. Radiology 170:463–466

103. Hurwitz R. Lane SR, Bell RA, Brant-Zawadzki MN (1989) Acoustic analysis of gradient-coil noise in MR imaging. Radiology 173:545–466

104. Goldmann AM, Gossmann W, Friedlander PC (1989) Reduction of sound levels with anti-noise in MR imaging. Radiology 173:549–550

105. Sellers MB, Pavlidis JD, Carlberger T (1996) MRI acoustic noise. Int J Neuroradiol 2(26):549–560

106. National Electrical Manufacturers Association (NEMA) (1989) Acoustical noise measurement procedure for diagnostic magnetic resonance imaging devices. Standards publication no MS 4. NEMA, Washington

107. Haiying L, Junxiao L (1996) Gradient coil mechanical vibration and image quality degradation. Proceedings of the Society of Magnetic Resonance, p 1393

108. Hedeen RA, Edelstein W (1996) Characterization and prediction of gradient acoustic noise in MR imagers. Proceedings of the Society of Magnetic Resonance, p 1389

109. Sellers M (1996) A new method of quantifying the acoustic noise of MRI devices. Proceedings of the Society of Magnetic Resonance, p 1390

110. 29CFR Ch. XVII, § 1910.95; pg 204-219. (7-1-1990 Edition): Occupational noise exposure, Occupational Safety and Health Administration, Department of Labor, 200 Constitution Avenue, N.W. Washington, DC 20210

111. European Standard (1997) Medizinische elektrische Geräte, Teil 2: Besondere Festlegungen für die Sicherheit von medizinischen Magetresonanzgeräten; DIN EN 60601-2-33 Juni 1997

CHAPTER 8

Echo-Planar Imaging Angiography

P. A. Wielopolski, O. P. Simonetti, and J. C. Duerk

Introduction

Speed continues to be one of the most powerful features that echo-planar imaging (EPI) can offer relative to other magnetic resonance imaging (MRI) techniques. For most conventional MRI sequences, data acquisition is still slower than many dynamic physiological processes, often yielding images plagued with motion artifacts that can obscure important information. On the other hand, EPI can ensure successful scanning of uncooperative patients and the study of anatomical regions in which normal physiological motion severely compromises image quality. Additionally, a large number of slices can be acquired in few seconds, reducing many studies to a single, short breath-hold acquisition. Keeping these features in mind, coupled with the continuing development of magnetic resonance angiography (MRA), EPI angiographic techniques may be used to obtain dramatic reductions in scan time that could permit rapid screening of large vascular territories and later assessment by higher resolution MRA techniques.

Motion artifacts can be significant even with acquisition speeds on the order of 30–100 ms per shot, specifically when in-plane motion and flow velocities lead to significant displacements during the EPI readout. Theoretical analysis and simulations have shown that EPI is highly sensitive to motion and flow occurring during the signal encoding [1, 2]. On the other hand, experimental validation has been scarce, and its use in clinical routine imaging has also been extremely limited. Other factors unrelated to motion that reduce the image quality of EPI acquisitions, such as magnetic field inhomogeneity, are an enormous problem in abdominal and thoracic examinations where speed is important.

Despite the above difficulties MRA using EPI techniques have recently been evaluated [3, 4]. Several recent techniques have been devised that may render EPI adequate for several indications. This chapter describes and illustrates the effects of flow in single-shot and multishot EPI techniques and reviews some potential MRA applications that have been explored to date.

Effects of Flowing Blood

This section summarizes the effects that have been commonly observed in conventional MRA sequences in the presence of moving spins that are also noted in EPI acquisitions. EPI is merely another image-encoding scheme, and more conventional MRA acquisition strategies can be used with slight modifications.

Flowing blood modulates the MR signal in different ways depending on the imaging sequence selected. The changes are usually reflected in the reconstructed images by observing the following effects:

Signal Loss (Dephasing, Wash-Out). In conventional spin-echo (SE) imaging, washout and signal loss occur when spins initially excited in the slice of interest move out of the slice during the time interval between the 90° and 180° pulses. This property of SE scans can be used to reduce ghosting artifacts related to amplitude and phase modulation of the blood signal during pulsatile conditions. This effect is also evident in single-shot SE EPI. The latter can be useful for generating "black blood" contrast, usually referred to as black-blood MRA [5]. Signal loss may also occur through spin dephasing. Signal cancellation at the time of the echo (TE) arises when a uniform phase distribution across the imaging voxel exists. This can be observed equally in SE and in gradient-recalled echo (GRE) techniques and also in their EPI counterparts. The effect is observed most commonly in GRE scans, the preferable imaging technique for MRA applications.

Signal Enhancement (Wash-In). Inflow enhancement occurs when the repetition time between RF excitations is long enough to allow partially saturated spins to be replaced by fully magnetized spins from outside the imaged slice (imaging volume). In single-shot GRE EPI a single RF excitation is used to read the signal from spins which are virtually fully magnetized, thus yielding poor flow contrast. The use of preparatory RF excitations over the volume of interest can provide the inflow enhancement that has been observed in more conventional MRA techniques. Multiple RF pulses are applied for multishot EPI techniques, and therefore they exhibit inflow enhancement depending on TR and flip angle similar to conventional time-of-flight (TOF) MRA sequences.

Vessel Misregistration. Also known as the oblique flow artifact, this is another TOF effect that is seen whenever signal loss from other mechanisms is not complete. The artifact stems from the difference in time of encoding at the various positions along each of the imaging axes. The position of a moving spin is defined at three distinct times during the imaging sequence: at the RF pulse, at the center of the phase-encoding pulse, and at TE. Depending on the direction and magnitude of the motion components, specific for spins moving obliquely through the slice-selection and phase-encoding axes, the encoded position at TE may lead to severe misregistration and distortion of the vessel lumen. The oblique flow artifact is present similarly in EPI acquisitions, but the effects on the resulting image are not simple shifts, as discussed below, and it is complicated by the unique spatial encoding scheme of EPI.

From the list above, the first two items can be used to obtain flow contrast. The effects of vessel misregistration and signal loss from dephasing are deleterious and have been studied extensively to gain a better understanding of the effect of motion under different k-space trajectories.

In general, flow effects can be understood by looking at the effect that moving spins exert on the phase of the MR signal. Thus in the following sections the flow-induced phase change on each imaging axis is discussed. Several motion compensation techniques that have been proposed theoretically to help reduce signal loss and vessel misregistration are also discussed.

Phase Effects of Flow

Sampling the MR signal from moving spins throughout a time-varying readout gradient and phase encoding by either a constant gradient or a series of short gradient pulses or "blips" result in motion artifacts that may be considered unique to EPI.

Phase Accumulation Under a Magnetic Gradient Field

The phase accumulation for moving spins, $\Phi_r(t)$, under the influence of a time-varying magnetic gradient field $G_r(t)$, can be expressed as:

$$\Phi_r(t) = \gamma \int_0^t G_r(t')r(t')dt' \tag{1}$$

with γ indicating the gyromagnetic ratio ($\gamma=2.6746\times10^8$ rad/s) and $G_r(t)$ the effective gradient experienced. The position of a moving spin, indicated by $r(t)=[x(t)\ y(t)\ z(t)]$, is defined by:

$$r(t) = r_0 + v_r t + a_r t^2/2 + \ldots\ldots\ldots \tag{2}$$

where r_o, the spatial position vector $[x_o\ y_o\ z_o]$ represents the starting position of the moving spin at the time $G_r(t)$ is applied. The terms v_r and a_r represent the velocity and the acceleration vector components (first and second moments) based on the point of expansion t, respectively. The inclusion of flow effects into the imaging equation leads to [6]:

$$s(t) = \int_r \int_v m(r,v)e^{-i2\pi(k_r(t)r + k_v(t)v)}\,drdv \tag{3}$$

The indexes r and v indicate the position and velocity fields, respectively, and $m(r,v)$ denotes the magnetization of the moving spin. The k-space parameters $k_r(t)$ and $k_v(t)$ are defined as:

$$k_r(t) = \frac{\gamma}{2\pi} \int_0^t G_r(t')dt'$$

$$\tag{4}$$

$$k_v(t) = \frac{\gamma}{2\pi} \int_0^t t'G_r(t')dt'$$

Phase Accumulation Under a Constant Magnetic Gradient Field

Evaluating Eq. 1, the phase induced from the application of a rectangular uni-polar magnetic gradient along the x-axis of constant amplitude A and duration T in the presence of motion results in:

$$\Phi_r(t) = \gamma A[x_o T + v_x T^2 / 2 + a_x T^3 / 6 + \dots\dots\dots]$$ (5)

From the above equation it is seen that the sensitivity to velocity is proportional to the gradient amplitude multiplied by the gradient duration squared. Likewise, in spins moving with constant acceleration the contribution is proportional to the gradient amplitude and the gradient duration cubed.

The cause of spin dephasing in conventional GRE and EPI techniques is the same (intravoxel phase cancellation); nonetheless the effects are accentuated for the latter for higher order motion terms that can be magnified several-fold as a result of the longer echo times and effective readout windows used. If signal loss from dephasing does not occur, the large phase variation over k-space may produce a form of Gibbs ringing (enhancement of high spatial frequencies).

Flow compensation techniques reduce the phase sensitivity to motion in conventional MRA to suppress signal dephasing and misregistration artifacts by nulling first (and higher) order gradient moments. Flow compensation has also been attempted for EPI MRA sequences [7]. Nonetheless, flow compensation techniques must take into account that EPI retains "phase-memory," i.e., the spin system remembers its previous history at each value of the in-plane phase-encoding line, contrary to conventional GRE scans in which the phase evolution starts from zero with the application of each RF excitation. The following sections discuss potential artifacts that may be observed for single-shot and multishot GRE EPI sequences for each imaging axis and explore solutions that have been proposed.

Flow Effects Along the Slice-Selection Axis

Spin dephasing along the slice-selection axis in single-shot and multishot EPI is identical to that in conventional MRA sequences. A single-shot GRE EPI sequence with first-order moment nulling along all axes is depicted in Fig. 1a. This can be compared to a conventional GRE sequence, presented in Fig. 1b. The comparison of the two modalities indicates that the moment nulling along the slice-selection axis is identical. Thus conventional motion compensation by gradient moment nulling [8, 9] can be applied to the EPI slice-selection gradient to compensate for any intravoxel phase dispersion from flowing spins for any desired moment. Velocity compensation waveforms already designed for conventional SE can be ported to SE EPI if the latter is used for depicting flow (or to evaluate the T2 properties of arterial and venous blood in the presence of motion).

Nonetheless, some differences exist between single-shot EPI and conventional MRA sequences. Single-shot EPI is less sensitive to artifacts from motion along the slice-selection axis than conventional MRI for two reasons: (a) the high-performance gradient system required for EPI can be used to reduce the slice-selec-

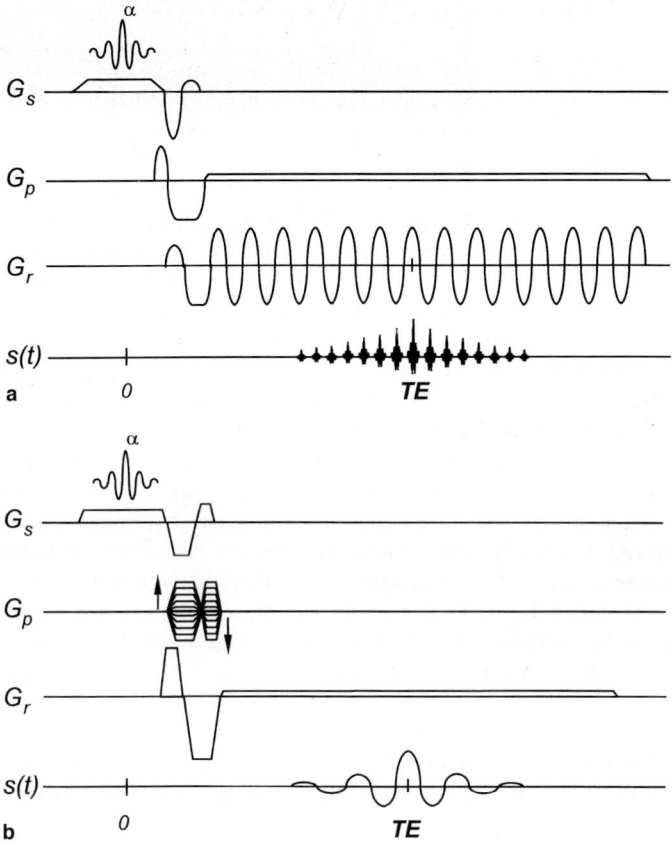

Fig. 1. a Velocity-compensated GRE EPI sequence. **b** Velocity-compensated conventional GRE. Along the section-selection direction the RF and velocity-compensation gradient waveforms are analogous. Similarly, motion compensation along the phase-encoding axis for EPI using a constant phase-encoding gradient is identical to that of the frequency-encoding axis in the conventional GRE sequence. Along the frequency-encoding direction only the odd echoes are velocity compensated while all even echoes maintain a small but constant phase shift during the EPI readout. *a*, RF excitation angle; *Gr*, readout gradient; *Gp*, phase-encoding gradient; *Gs*, section-selection gradient *s(t)*, signal

tion gradient duration and refocusing, thereby reducing gradient moments and motion-induced dephasing, (b) the slice-selection gradient waveform is applied once for the acquisition of the entire image, as opposed to once for every line in a conventional MRA acquisition. Thus the possibilities for line-to-line variations in phase or amplitude due to temporal changes in motion along the slice-selection direction do not exist in single-shot EPI.

A constant, spatially uniform velocity results only in a constant phase shift within each voxel, and therefore signal loss from dephasing is not likely to occur. The case of multishot EPI is similar to that of conventional MRA

Fig. 2. Effect of flowing spins perpendicular to the slice-select direction. Mean flow velocity was set to 95 cm/s. Note the absence of flow artifacts. A 5-mm transverse section was encoded in 64 ms using a fully velocity-compensated GRE EPI sequence, 128×128 matrix, TE=14.9 ms, FOV=250 mm, echo spacing of 500 μs, and a sinusoidal readout waveform

sequences and signal cancellation, and ghosting may be problematic as a result of the multiple RF excitations that are necessary to encode the image.

A flow phantom setup has been investigated to validate the effects of flow perpendicular to the slice selection on single-shot GRE EPI sequences. The flow phantom consisted of two tubes with flowing liquid in opposite directions and a peak flow velocity of 95 cm/s. Figure 2 demonstrates a cross section of both tubes acquired under flowing conditions using a velocity compensated GRE EPI sequence such as depicted in Fig. 1a. No flow artifacts are evident.

Clearly the well-behaved characteristics of flow along the slice-selection axis permit the implementation of EPI MRA techniques when the plane of section is completely perpendicular to the flow direction. In fact, TOF [3, 10–12], phase contrast [13–16], and velocity quantification [17–19] angiographic techniques using single-shot and multishot EPI have readily been described in the literature. Flow with components along the other two imaging axes is more troublesome for EPI, and the effects are discussed in more detail in the following sections.

Flow Effects Along the Phase-Encoding Axis

Analogies

The phase-encoding direction in EPI is analogous in many respects to the frequency-encoding axis in conventional imaging sequences. Thus flowing spins with components along this axis show behavior similar to that observed on conventional MRA sequences. The EPI sequence with constant phase-encoding in Fig. 1 illustrates this point, noting the similarity between the phase-encoding waveform and a conventional GRE frequency-encoding waveform using first-order moment nulling. The same observations can be made in the case of a blipped EPI sequence in which the constant phase-encoding gradient is replaced by small gradient bursts ("blips") between adjacent echoes of the EPI readout.

Since the phase accumulation due to velocity is proportional to the gradient applied and time squared (see Eq. 5), a blipped phase-encoding gradient is somewhat easier to compensate than a constant phase-encoding gradient due to its smaller contribution to the phase of moving spins. Blipped phase encoding is also preferred for phase encoding as it helps to simplify image reconstruction.

Although there are similarities between conventional frequency-encoding and the EPI phase-encoding process, two points must be taken into account: the duration of a conventional frequency-encoding waveform is only about 2–15 ms, while the EPI phase-encoding waveform varies between 30 and 100 ms. The long gradient duration exacerbates the same flow-dephasing effects, displacement artifacts, and quadratic blurring which occur with a conventional frequency-encoding gradient waveforms. For constant-velocity moving spins, the phase accumulated is proportional to the gradient strength but quadratic with time. Thus flow effects can be large and tend to worsen with longer echo times, echo spacing, and echo train lengths.

Point Spread Function

The sensitivity to flow for sequences with similar TE but different interecho spacing is not obvious. There are three phase terms that contribute to produce signal loss and broadening of the point spread function (PSF) [8]. Taking the case of a single-shot EPI sequence using a constant phase-encoding gradient, these phase terms are as follows.

A constant phase term given by $\frac{1}{4}\gamma G[v_p TE^2]$ can be compensated independently of TE and EPI readout length. This phase term is the major cause of intravoxel dephasing and consequent signal loss in regions with turbulence.

A linear phase shift, given by $\gamma G[v_p TE]t$, introduces a displacement of a moving spin by $v_p TE$ in the image, making it appear at position $y_o + v_p TE$, where y_o indicates the position at the center of the RF excitation and v_p the velocity component of a moving spin along the phase-encoding axis. This linear-phase shift term is the same for different EPI readout lengths. This is because the product between the area of the phase-encoding gradient and the echo spacing is constant for a specific field of view (FOV). The displacement can be reduced only if a rectangular FOV is applied, contrary to the frequency-encoding case in conventional MRA.

A phase term changing quadratically in time, $\frac{1}{2}\gamma[G_p v_p]t^2$, acts as a complex filter and leads to a loss in resolution in the reconstructed image [20]. Phase errors induced by this term are larger towards the end of the readout window because of the quadratic dependence in time, and therefore a greater filtering effect is observed for longer EPI readouts.

Figure 3 compares the PSF for stationary and flowing spins along the phase-encoding direction in single-shot EPI using a blipped phase-encoding trajectory. The phase accumulation for blipped single-shot EPI is considerably smaller than that for a constant phase-encoding gradient, essentially a factor inversely proportional to the ratio between the echo spacing and the blip duration. Thus flow along the frequency-encoding direction in conventional GRE sequences has a broader PSF than flow along the phase-encoding direction with a blipped single-shot EPI sequence and identical acquisition window. The PSF continues to broaden to a point that flattening and ringing are introduced from the high degree of phase asymmetry induced by flowing components. Initially a double peak is apparent (Fig. 3e).

Fig. 3a–e. PSF for single-shot for spins flowing with a constant velocity along the phase-encoding axis. **a** Basic GRE EPI sequence utilized for the simulations. PSF for the stationary condition (**b**) and for a 25 cm/s mean flow velocity and an echo spacing of 0.5 ms (**c**), 1.0 ms (**d**), and 1.5 ms (**e**), respectively. The effective TE occurred half-way through the acquisition matrix with the blip amplitude scaled to G/(number of frequency-encoding samples) an a blip duration of one frequency-encoding sample. Simulation performed for a 64×64 matrix with a FOV=240 mm. Additional peaks start to appear in the PSF with larger velocities or echo spacing. This effect is noted in E, and it is similar to Gibbs ringing, resulting from the high degree of phase asymmetry induced by flowing spins. Peak value of each PSF is shown, scaled with respect to the PSF of the stationary condition α; RF excitation angle, Gp, in-plane phase encoding gradient, Gr; readout gradient; $s(t)$, signal

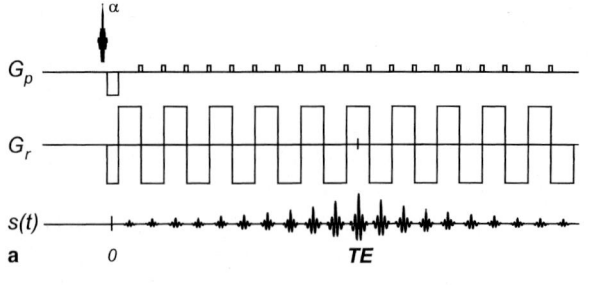

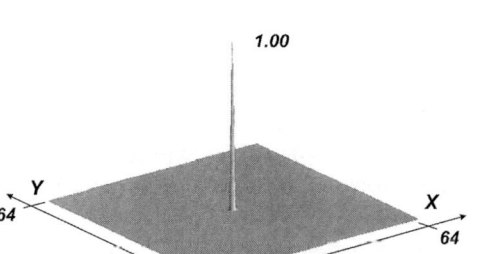

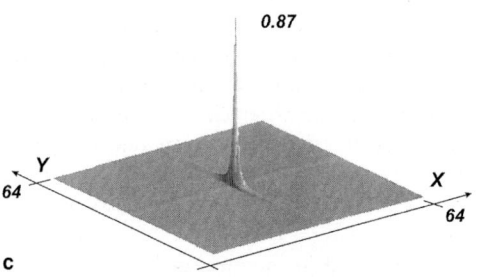

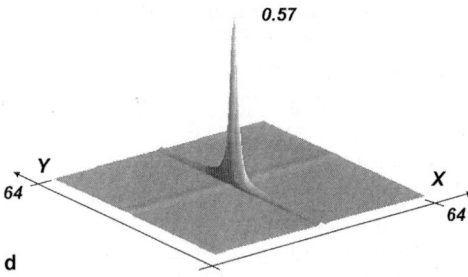

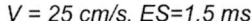

$V = 25$ cm/s, ES=1.5 ms

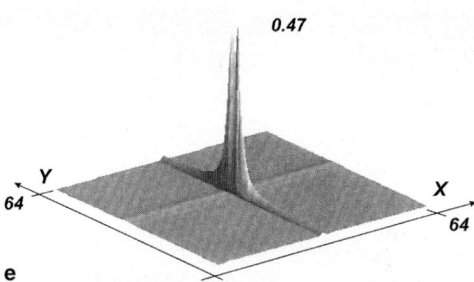

Motion Compensation

Dephasing due to motion along the phase-encoding axis accumulates over the duration of the acquisition (Fig. 4), illustrating the phase trajectory for constant-velocity moving spins using a blipped phase-encoding gradient. The constant phase offset at the center line can be compensated using gradient moment nulling exactly as applied to the frequency-encoding axis in conventional imaging. This effectively shifts the phase trajectory to cross zero at the centerline echo (k-space center). Conventional gradient moment nulling ensures that the phase shift caused by spins moving at constant velocity is zero at the center line echo. However, this technique cannot compensate for the complex blurring and signal loss from the quadratic component of the phase evolution throughout the acquisition. This quadratic dephasing is most severe late in the acquisition, at one far edge of k-space. The quadratic blurring is directly related to the duration of the phase-encoding gradient, i.e., the echo train length. Keeping this time as short as possible is an important consideration to reduce the sensitivity to motion artifacts along this axis. Increasing the speed of the gradient hardware can be an expensive solution, otherwise, k-space segmentation using a multishot GRE EPI must be used.

Fig. 4. Phase trajectories for flow along the phase-encoding axis in single-shot GRE EPI without (**a**) and with (**b**) conventional first-order gradient moment nulling and a blipped phase encoding. The addition of motion compensation permits the acquisition of the center k-space line with reduced flow sensitivity and a more symmetric phase evolution about this point

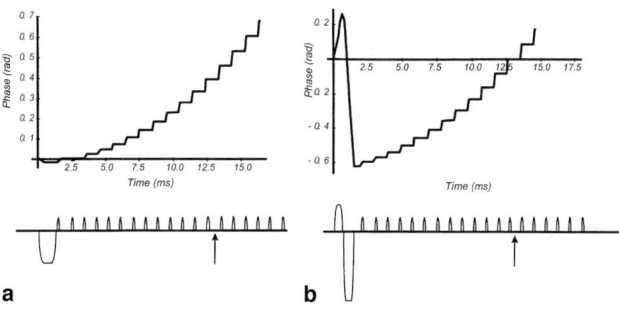

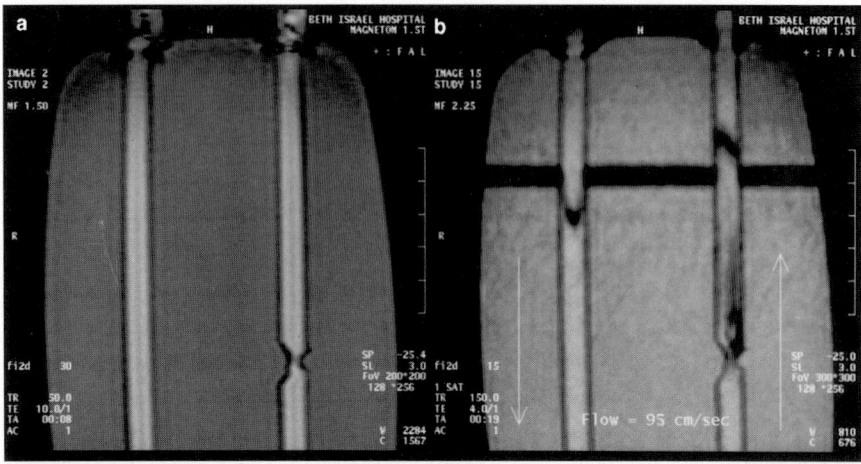

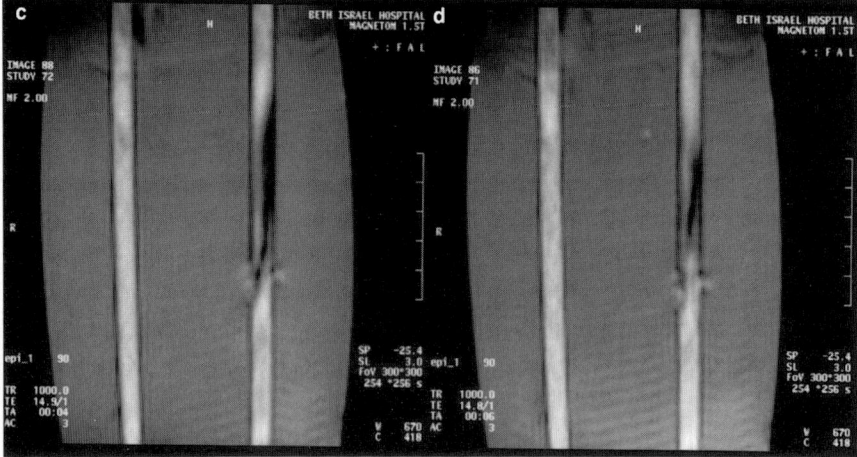

Fig. 5. a Coronal section of the phantom acquired with GRE EPI with stationary fluid. **b** Parabolic flow profile with a mean velocity of 95 cm/s demonstrates using a bolus tracking sequence with TE=4 ms. **c** No flow compensation using GRE EPI with TE=14.9 ms. **d** Using the same TE with compensation along the phase-encoding axis demonstrates the benefits of moment nulling parallel to the flow direction, illustrating a smaller signal loss in the poststenotic region. With flow, blurring of the stenosis is increased in comparison to the stationary case. The blurring present at the stenosis in **c,d** arises from misregistration of flowing spins prior to the stenosis that are mapped over the stenosis due to the longer TE utilized. Filtering also takes place from the same group of flowing spins being at a different positions for each echo readout. The stenosis consisted of a 6-mm-long irregular constriction with a maximum 70 % obstruction by area along 2 mm of the plastic tubing. For the GRE EPI sequence a 3 mm section was selected and encoded in 51.2 ms with a 64×256 matrix, FOV=240×320 mm, echo spacing of 800 µs (250 µs ramps with a 300 µs flattop), centerline echo occurring after 22 % of raw data were acquired

Fig. 6a–c. Displacement of flowing spins with velocity components along the slice-selection and phase-encoding axes. **a** Diagram illustrating the slice encoded with respect to the flowing tubes. Velocity components exist only along the slice-selection and the phase-encoding direction with the phase-encoding direction selected from left to right. **b** The stationary condition. **c** Parabolic profile develops under flowing conditions, here depicted with an average flow velocity of 95 cm/s. Flowing spins are shifted outside the tube lumen, indicative of the displacement occurring between the center of the RF excitation and the effective TE when the center of k-space is encoded, in this case TE=14.9 ms. Acquisition parameters as in Fig. 2, using a fully velocity-compensated flow sequence as in Fig. 1

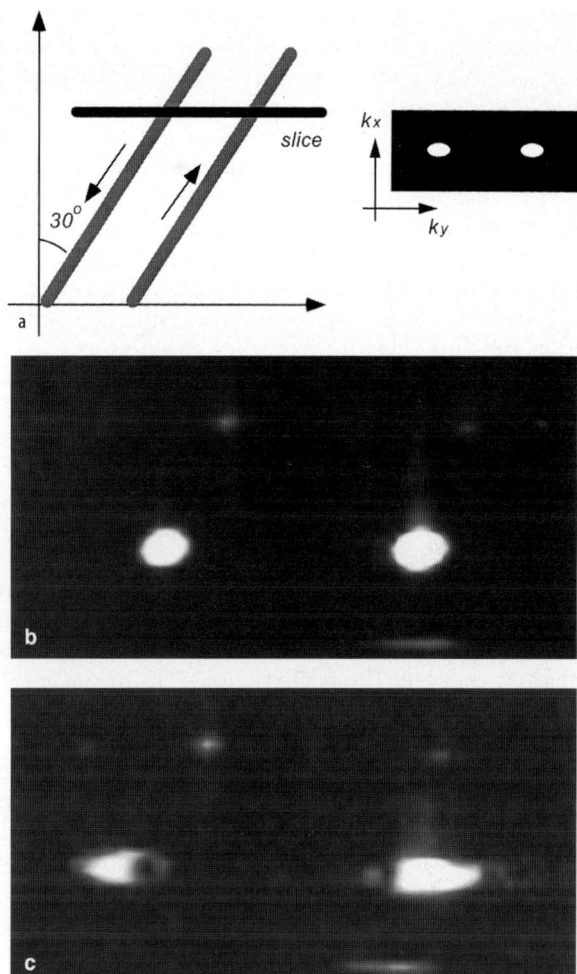

Despite blurring, moment nulling can help reduce the signal loss due to intra-voxel dephasing in poststenotic regions. This is illustrated in Fig. 5, depicting single-shot GRE EPI images acquired on a flow phantom with flow directed along the phase-encoding axis. An irregular stenosis is present with a maximum occlusion of 70 % of the transverse area. Figure 5a demonstrates the phantom under stationary conditions. Figure 5b depicts the phantom under flowing conditions with a mean flow velocity of 95 cm/s, calculated from the displacement of tagged spins. Poststenotic signal loss can be observed along the frequency-encoding (flow) direction even when utilizing a velocity-compensated GRE sequence. Figure 5c illustrates the poststenotic signal loss occurring with single-shot GRE EPI without flow compensation. There is evidence of greater signal loss in the image acquired without gradient moment nulling than in the velocity-compensated sequence (Fig. 5d). Blurring over the stenosis is present from the misregistration of spins at the longer TE and from the change in spin location for each echo readout. A short TE, highly asymmetric, needs to be selected to visualize the poststenotic signal loss reduction at high flow velocities with the velocity-compensated GRE EPI sequence (and to avoid signal loss from susceptibility artifacts at longer TE with a more symmetric data acquisition).

The effective TE is determined by the time at which the accumulated area of the phase-encoding gradient returns to zero. Thus TE is dependent not only on the time required to sample each phase-encoding line but also on the number of lines acquired before the center line. An asymmetric echo in EPI implies the acquisition of fewer lines before the center line occurs, analogous to asymmetric echo sampling along the frequency-encoding axis in conventional MRI. This trick provides the same benefits of shorter TE, reduced gradient moments, and consequently less dephasing from turbulent flow (Fig. 5). Unfortunately, some loss in signal-to-noise (S/N) ratio and resolution is associated with any degree of asymmetry, but most observable when the echo asymmetry is high [21]. Specialized reconstruction algorithms which exploit the natural conjugate symmetry of the MR data, such as in partial Fourier imaging [22–24] can compensate somewhat for these effects.

Flow displacement in EPI is similar to that encountered in conventional MRA pulse sequences [25]. The artifact is always present and is related to the temporal difference between the slice selection and the time during which the center of k-space is encoded. The relatively long TEs of single-shot GRE EPI make it particularly obvious when the flow components are present along the slice-selection and phase-encoding axis only. This is demonstrated in the phantom images of Fig. 6. Flow is now oriented at an angle of 30° from the sagittal towards the transverse slice orientation, as depicted in the diagram. Under flowing conditions, a parabolic displacement may be observed, similar to that encountered in conventional MRA sequences along the frequency-encoding axis.

Displacement artifacts can be significant in single-shot EPI at normal blood flow velocities, as seen in the images of a normal volunteer (Fig. 7). Figure 7a,b

---

Fig. 7a–f. In vivo demonstration of flowing effects in the abdominal aorta with flow components along the slice-select and phase-encoding directions. **a** The flow direction orientation of the aorta with respect to a transverse slice, approximately 12° from the coronal to the transverse axis. **b** The small velocity component that may develop along the frequency-encoding direction from a small tilt of 5° from the sagittal plane. Flow in the inferior vena cava is nearly perpendicular to a transverse section. **c** Single-shot flow compensated GRE EPI scans triggered to acquire data during late diastole (trigger delay=0 ms). **d** Trigger delay of 200 ms, close to peak systolic velocities in the aorta. The signal from the aorta appears completely outside the vessel during systole, less so during diastole when flow velocities are smaller. Note that the signal from the inferior vena cava suffers minor misregistration during systole since flow components are perpendicular to the selected slice. Using multishot GRE EPI, as depicted in diastole (**e**) and systole (**f**) a considerable reduction in misregistration and blurring in the aorta can be noted. Acquisition parameters in **c,d** considered a 60×256 matrix, TE=14.9 ms, FOV=210×280 mm and an EPI readout time of 48 ms using an echo spacing of 800 μs (250 μs ramps with a 300 μs flattop), centerline echo occurring after 23 % of raw data were acquired. For the multishot GRE EPI used velocity compensation was for all axes, and 14 echoes were read per shot, with a 140×256 matrix acquisition, TE=8 ms, FOV=210×280 mm, an echo spacing of 800 μs (250 μs ramps with a 300 μs flattop) with the echo occurring at the center of k-space

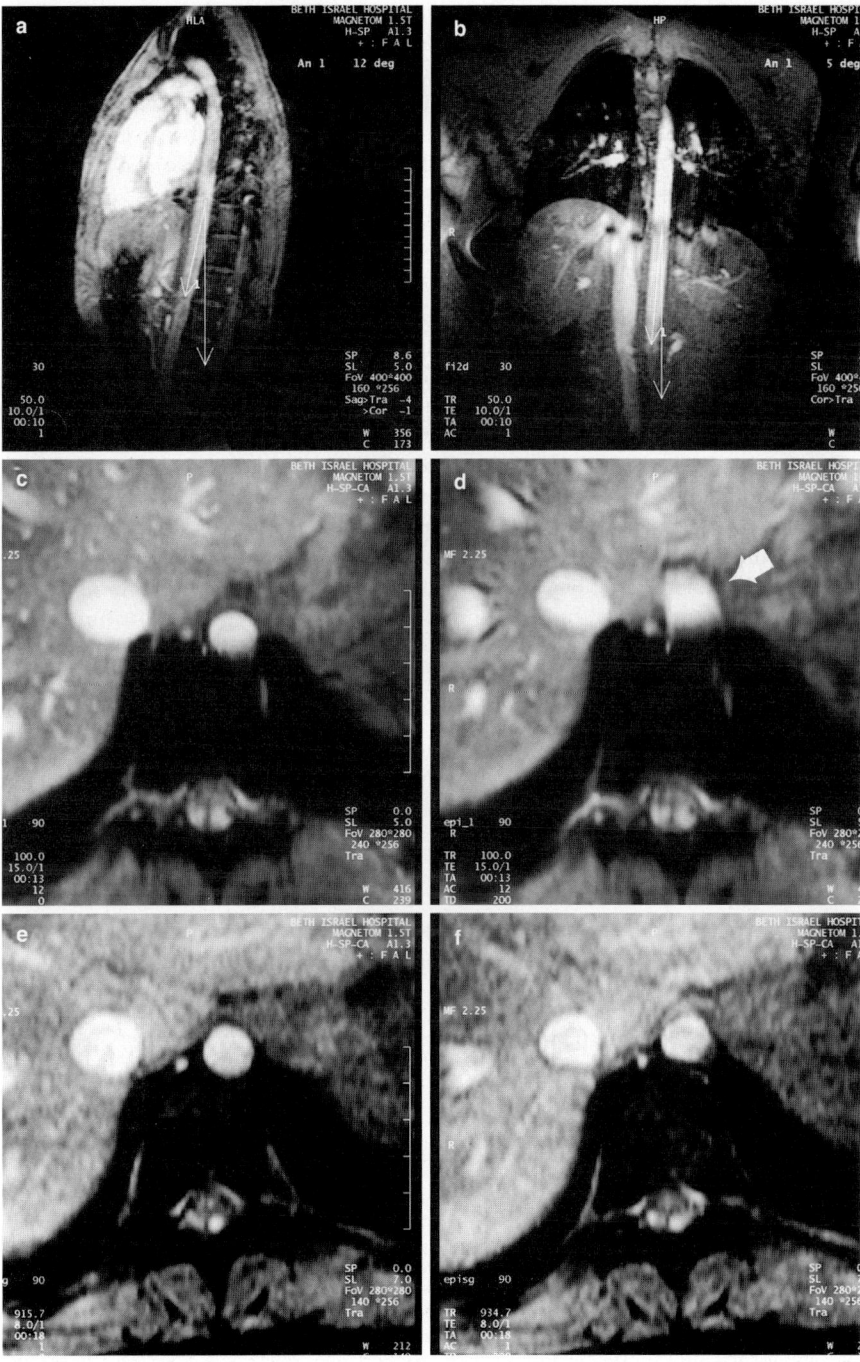

illustrates the relative orientation of the flowing components along the abdominal aorta with respect to the transverse section selected for the evaluation. Figure 7c,d depicts the flow displacement occurring during late diastole and peak systole, respectively, showing a large displacement even for the latter despite the relative small flow components along the phase-encoding direction. Flow in the inferior vena cava is fairly constant during any phase of the cardiac cycle and maintains its lumen (untriggered acquisitions may thus be used to image the venous vasculature). Displacement artifacts are reduced by shortening TE, preferably using a multishot EPI approach (Fig. 7e,f).

A solution has been proposed to eliminate both the displacement and the quadratic blurring due to constant velocity motion along the phase-encoded direction in "blipped" EPI sequences only [2]. The solution considers the replacement of each unipolar gradient blip with an asymmetric bipolar blip (similar to that used along the in-plane phase-encoding table as illustrated in the conventional GRE sequence of Fig. 1b). These bipolar pulses are designed to be first-order moment nulled about the center line echo time. This removes the quadratic phase component due to a linearly changing position (constant velocity). Figure 8 illustrates this technique of velocity compensation at every echo. Although theoretically interesting, to date this solution has remained unattainable even on commercial whole-body EPI imaging systems for single-shot EPI due to excessive gradient speed and amplitude requirements (due to physiological stimulation limits). With current hardware the EPI readout would be extremely long and could introduce more severe flow artifacts. The implementation of this approach is more feasible for multishot GRE EPI with a reduced number of echoes (e.g., 6–12 echoes per shot).

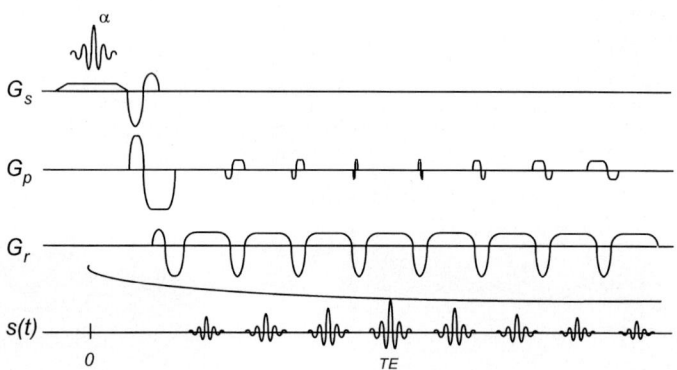

Fig. 8. GRE EPI sequence using bipolar phase-encoding blips to compensate for dephasing and misregistration from constant-velocity moving spins along the phase-encoding axis. Each bipolar blip is calculated with respect to the effective TE, and its function is to impart a negative phase shift that maps constant velocity flowing spins to the same encoded position for each readout. Additionally, the frequency-encoding waveform also intends to eliminate the constant phase induced from constant velocity moving spins along this direction at the center of each echo. All echoes are also encoded in the same direction, contributing to eliminate ghosting artifacts that are usually present from hardware imperfections and when data reflection occurs on every second line in single-shot EPI sequences (N/2 ghost). α, RF excitation angle; Gr, readout gradient; Gp, in-plane phase encoding gradient; Gs, section select gradient. s(t) signal

Multishot EPI

Multishot EPI reduces the severity of dephasing, blurring, and misregistration artifacts as it permits shorter TEs and acquisition windows. However, despite the decreased sensitivity to flow effects each echo of the multishot EPI echo train may have a different phase, and blurring and flow displacement remain. Multiple high-intensity ghosts can be noted along the phase-encoding direction if high flow velocities exist or the echo spacing increases to a point that phase differences are not negligible between encoded echoes.

Ghosting is caused by the phase discontinuities present at the junctions between k-space segments, creating a steplike appearance in the phase behavior along the phase-encoding axis when the data are acquired in a sequential inter-leaved fashion [1, 6]. Similar ghosting is also present from the phase accumulation from field inhomogeneities, the alternating phase from off-resonance spins (such as fat), and decaying magnetization. Although blurring and flow displacement may increase slightly, the amplitude of the ghosts can be reduced substantially by "sliding" the EPI readout with respect to the RF pulse in successive shots of the multishot acquisition [1]. This has the effect of smoothing and blending the motion-induced phase from one view to the next, further reducing any discontinuities in the raw data. The shift is performed in equal time incre-

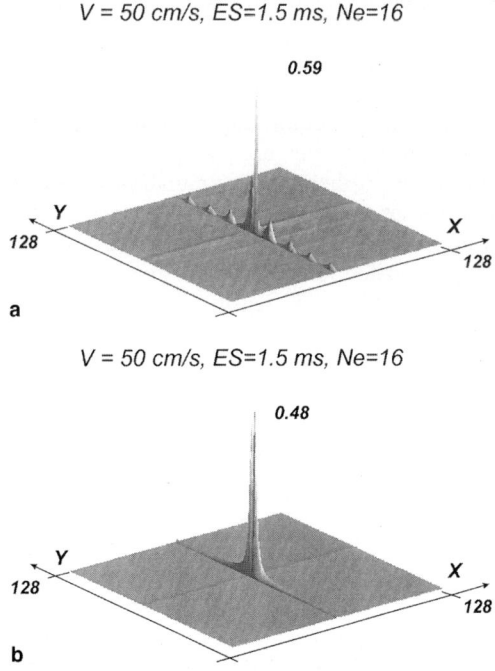

Fig. 9a,b. PSF for multishot EPI for constant velocity flowing spins at 50 cm/s parallel to the phase-encoding axis. **a** Multishot GRE EPI acquisition using 16 echoes per RF excitation, echo spacing of 1.5 ms, 128×128 matrix, and FOV=240 mm. The PSF demonstrates multiple ghosts propagating along the phase-encoding direction arising from phase discontinuities between adjacent k-space segments. The number of ghosts is equal to the number of shots minus one. The spacing is proportional to the inverse of the number of shots utilized to acquire the image $\left(\frac{\text{FoV}}{\text{Nshot}}\right)$. **b** With a sliding window approach ghosts can be eliminated but at a broader PSF approximately at the same location. Peak value of each PSF is shown, scaled with respect to the stationary condition. In **b** the PSF starts splitting with larger velocities. This is demonstrated as well in the case of single-shot GRE EPI in Fig. 3. The phase-encoding table was applied during the duration of the dephasing gradient. *Ne*, number of echoes acquired per shot; Nshot, number of shots

ments that depend on the number of shots necessary to encode the complete raw data matrix. The size of the time increments is calculated by taking the ratio between the echo spacing and the number of shots. Using a sliding readout window is equivalent essentially to a single-shot EPI acquisition in which the same acquisition matrix is acquired, but the echo spacing is chosen so that it is inversely proportional to that of the multishot acquisition by the number of shots used (so that the readout window to complete the scan and echo times are the same). Ghosting is depicted in Fig. 9a and the ghost suppression using the sliding readout window in Fig. 9b.

If the sliding window technique cannot be implemented, multishot GRE EPI sequences should make use of the maximum readout bandwidth possible for the desired FOV (to reduce as much as possible the echo spacing) or use a limited number of echoes per shot. It may be stated that flow effects are similar for EPI readouts of the some lengths (number of echoes vs readout bandwidth). The balance between the two options is weighted by the S/N ratio required versus acquisition speed. It must be kept in mind that ghosting and blurring are unnoticeable if a vessel runs parallel to the phase-encoding direction. In this case blurring and ghosting may end up superimposed on the stenosis if present along a vessel.

Special k-Space Trajectories

Centric phase-encoding order and spiral trajectories can also help to reduce flow dephasing and the displacement artifact [26]. With these techniques a very short TE can be achieved by acquiring the center of k-space at the beginning of the acquisition window. Nevertheless, centrically ordered single-shot EPI is impractical as the phase-encoding blip amplitudes become prohibitively high as the scan progresses towards the high k-space values. A single-shot centrically ordered scheme cannot utilize the accumulation of phase that is characteristic of a constant or a blipped phase-encoding gradient. Thus the phase imparted by the previous blip must be rewound by applying the opposite gradient area, in addition to the area needed for the current phase-encoding step. Centric ordering in multishot GRE EPI is more feasible with current EPI hardware. The acquisition is performed in two shots by starting each shot at the center of k-space and working outward with a blipped phase-encoding trajectory [27, 28].

Centric ordering is sensitive to the off-resonance effects of poorly suppressed fat because of the opposite shifts experienced along the phase-encoding direction. Furthermore, the distortions along the phase-encoding direction are different for each half of k-space scanned, as the background gradient never changes its polarity. Furthermore, spatial misregistration from flowing spins also have opposite directions for each shot and can lead to flow ghosting.

A spiral trajectory is also sensitive to off-resonance effects but has several advantages over the blipped centric approach. The gradient moments of a spiral trajectory are small near the origin of k-space, smoothly varying and circularly symmetric over k-space. Additionally, rewinding is inherent in a spiral trajectory and does not require the extreme hardware requirements to achieve low flow sensitivity.

Flow Effects Along the Frequency-Encoding Axis

Analogies

The frequency-encoding axis in EPI does not have a conventional MRI analog in terms of flow effects. Therefore the analysis of the EPI trajectory on flowing spins along this axis is quite interesting.

In conventional imaging the position encoded for a spin moving along the frequency-encoding direction depends on TE and the magnitude of the flow components. Thus:

$$r(TE) = r_o + v_r TE + a_r TE^2/2 + (\ldots\ldots) \tag{6}$$

where r_o denotes the location of the flowing spins at the time of the center of the RF pulse, and v_r and a_r the velocity and acceleration components along the readout direction, respectively.

With constant flowing conditions the displacement is the same throughout the acquisition, and the overall effect, for example, in the case of a group of spins moving with a parabolic flow profile is that of a parabolic displacement. This can be seen in Fig. 5b where a parabolic flow profile can be observed after the application of a tagging saturation band prior to image encoding in the flow phantom.

With pulsatile flow the changing velocity translates into a change in the displacement and phase at the time of the echo, thus generating blurring along the frequency-encoding direction and ghosting along the phase-encoding direction that are related to the periodicity of the motion itself [29].

Point Spread Function

Although the time separation between echoes (also referred to as the echo spacing) is generally less than 1 ms in single-shot EPI, the time at which each of the echoes is formed increases constantly for each readout window. Thus the position for each echo follows:

$$r(TE_1) = r_o + v_r TE_1 + a_r TE_1^2/2 + (\ldots\ldots)$$
$$r(TE_2) = r_o + v_r TE_2 + a_r TE_2^2/2 + (\ldots\ldots) \tag{7}$$
$$r(TE_n) = r_o + v_r TE_n + a_r TE_n^2/2 + (\ldots\ldots)$$

where the subindex accompanying TE indicates the line number acquired during the EPI readout. Each echo is phase-encoded independently during the same shot, and the changing position from echo to echo gives rise to a change in the slope of the phase evolution of moving spins from one phase-encoded line to the next, resulting in a two-dimensional (2D) blur along both the frequency- and phase-encoding directions.

A different type of ghost also appears along the phase-encoding direction. While the first moment at the center of each echo readout is relatively small, its values alternate between odd and even echoes as the gradient changes polarity. This alternation of velocity sensitivity gives rise to a single ghost that propagates along the phase-encoding direction and appears displaced by half the FOV, thus called an N/2 ghost. The phase difference between odd and even echoes is given by:

$$\Delta\Phi = \gamma v \int_{te}^{to} G(t)dt \tag{8}$$

where te and to indicate the time at the center of an even echo and an odd echo, respectively. When the integral is evaluated for an ideal EPI waveform, a very well-known expression is obtained:

$$\Delta\Phi = \gamma v G \frac{T_{read^2}}{4} \tag{9}$$

which is the phase accumulation for constant velocity flowing spins during the application of a bipolar gradient pulse, in this case of duration T_{read}, the readout time per echo. When gradient rise times are considered, the readout waveform becomes trapezoidal. Denoting Tr as the gradient rise time (linear), the phase difference becomes:

$$\Delta\Phi = \gamma v G \left[\frac{2}{3}Tr + \frac{T_{read^2}}{4} + Tr \cdot T_{read} \right] \tag{10}$$

If the flow velocity is large enough that the phase difference between the echoes of two adjacent phase-encoding lines is π, the signal within a vessel disappears completely and appears only as a ghost. Figure 10 demonstrates the 2D blur and N/2 ghost theoretically for three different readout lengths for single-shot and multishot EPI readouts. It is noted that the PSF widens with increasing echo spacing or flow velocity. Additionally, the N/2 ghost becomes more evident as the constant phase difference between odd and even echoes increases. It can be also noted that the PSF does not appear in the center, indicating that not only 2D blurring but vessel lumen displacement occurs in the same flow direction.

Figure 11 illustrates the 2D blurring, N/2 ghost, and the displacement as seen in the flow phantom with flow oblique to the slice-selection and frequency-encoding axes. Figure 12 illustrates the effects in the abdominal aorta acquired with the same EPI sequence as in Fig. 7 but with the phase- and frequency-encoding directions swapped (interchanged). Blurring and displacement is greatest during peak systole when flow velocity and acceleration effects are the greatest. The 2D blurring is not obvious if the vessel runs parallel to the frequency-encoding direction, but the effects can be noted by the artifactual increase in the vessel lumen with faster flow. An additional ghost may appear if a triphasic flow pattern develops during the EPI readout. This is not likely to occur in vivo.

Fig. 10a–g. EPI flow artifacts for spins flowing along the frequency-encoding direction. PSF for the stationary condition (**a**) and for a 25 cm/s mean flow velocity and an echo spacing of 0.5 ms (**b**), 1.0 ms (**c**), and 1.5 ms (**d**). A 2D blur is observed with increasing intensity of the N/2 ghost with larger echo spacing and flow velocities. Ghost arises from a constant phase difference between odd and even echoes. The effective TE occurred at the center of k-space, and the readout gradients were scaled accordingly to obtain a FOV=240 mm for a 64×64 image

$V = 0$ cm/s

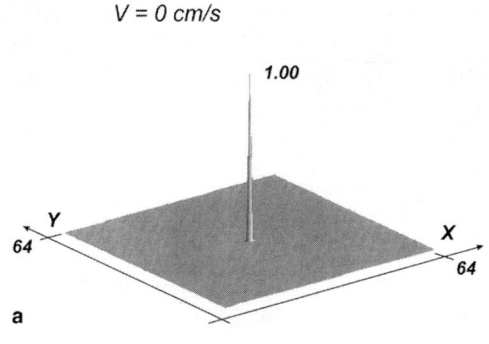

a

$V = 25$ cm/s, ES=0.5 ms

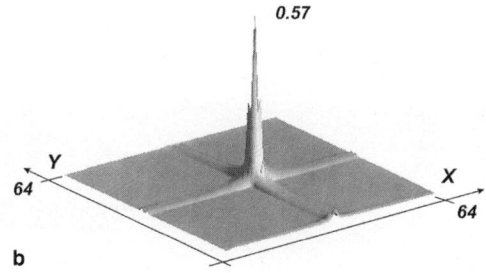

b

$V = 25$ cm/s, ES=1.0 ms

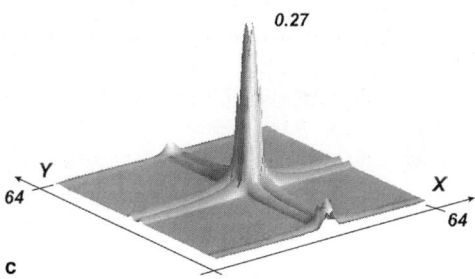

c

$V = 25$ cm/s, ES=1.5 ms

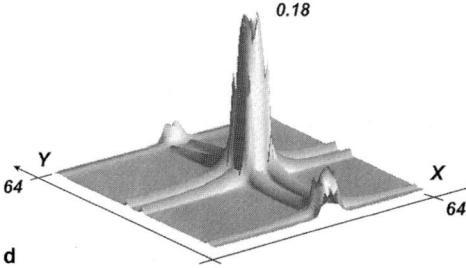

d

Fig. 10a–g. e PSF for a flow velocity of 50 cm/s and an echo spacing of 1.5 ms. **f** Multishot GRE EPI acquiring 16 echoes per RF excitation sharpens the PSF but multiple ghosts appear. **g** Multishot GRE EPI for a 128×128 acquisition. Peak value of each PSF is shown, scaled with respect to the stationary condition. *Ne*, number of echoes acquired for multishot GRE EPI

$V = 50$ cm/s, ES=1.5 ms

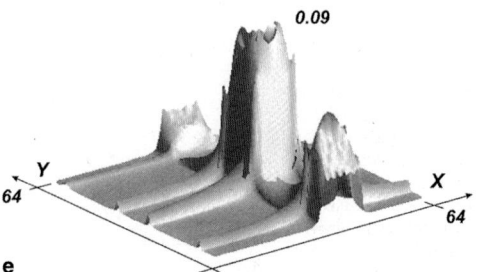

e

$V = 50$ cm/s, ES=1.5 ms , Ne=16

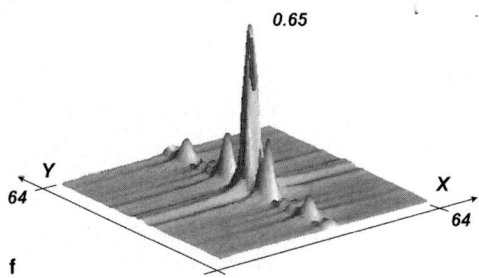

f

$V = 50$ cm/s, ES=1.5 ms, Ne=16

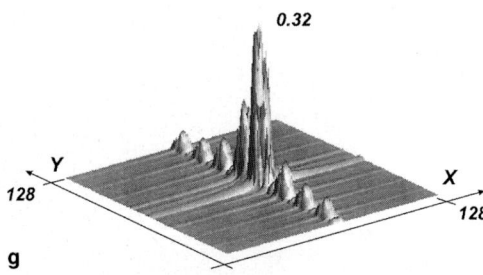

g

Fig. 11a-c. Displacement of flowing spins with velocity components along the slice-selection and frequency-encoding axes. **a** Slice encoded with respect to the flow direction in the tubes. Velocity components existing only along the slice-selection and the frequency-encoding directions with the frequency-encoding direction selected from left to right. **b** 2D blurring. **c** N/2 ghost (*arrow*) and displacement demonstrated after filling with water the surrounding of the flowing tubes. Flowing spins are shifted outside the tube lumen, indicative of the displacement occurring between the center of the RF excitation and the effective TE at the center of k-space. In this flow phantom setup displacement from velocity components along the frequency-encoding cannot be separated from those arising from those along the slice-select direction. A 5-mm section was acquired in 64 ms using a fully velocity compensated GRE EPI scan, 128×128 matrix, TE=15 ms (k-space center after 22% of raw data acquired), FOV=250 mm, echo spacing of 500 μs, and a sinusoidal readout waveform. Figure 6b depicts the stationary condition

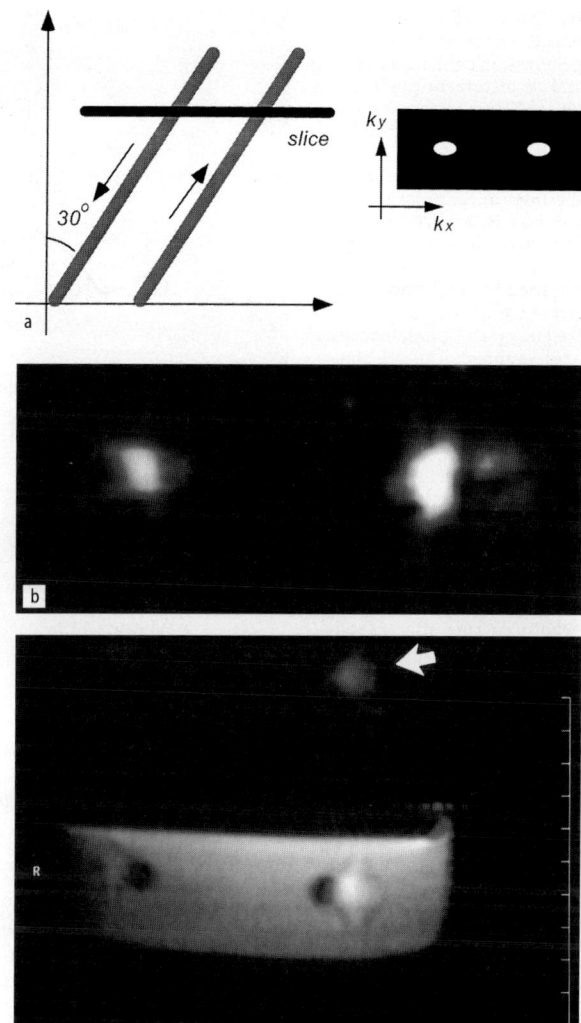

Fig. 12a–d. Single-shot EPI images of the abdominal aorta demonstrating the 2D blurring and displacement predicted in Figs. 10 and 11 for various phases during the cardiac for single-shot GRE EPI. The cardiac phase correspond to late diastole (**a**), peak systole (**b**), 100 ms (**c**), and 200 ms (**d**) after peak systole. The same region as in Fig. 7 was acquired with identical acquisition parameters but with the frequency and phase-encoding axes swapped. The 2D blurring can be seen in comparison to the parabolic displacement noted in Fig. 7d. Acquisition parameters considered a 60×256 matrix acquisition, TE=14.9 ms, FOV=210×280 mm and an EPI readout time of 48 ms using an echo spacing of 800 μs (250 μs sine ramps with a 300 μs flattop), centerline echo occurring after 22 % of raw data were acquired. Banding over the image accurring from aliasing from the arm

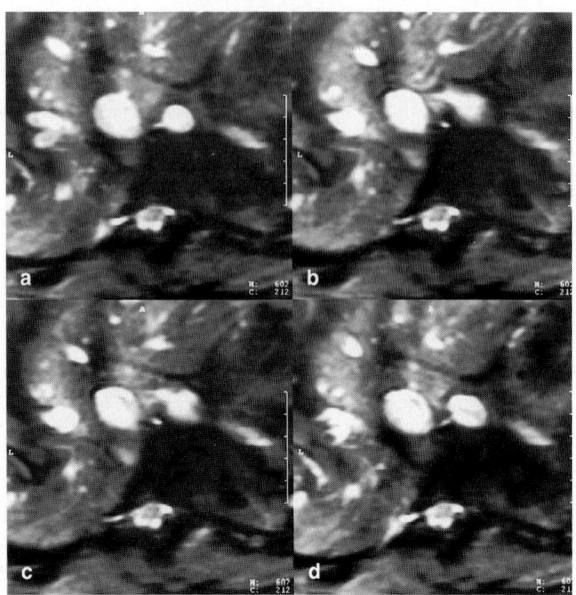

Motion Compensation

Two gradient moment nulling techniques have been applied to the frequency-encoding axis in EPI to compensate either for dephasing and/or ghosting. The first technique proposed nulls the first moment of the centerline echo [7]. This has no effect on the alternation of the first moment from echo to echo and therefore no effect on reducing the N/2 ghost. Another scheme suppresses the N/2 ghost entirely by setting the motion-induced phase difference between even and odd lines to zero. This is achieved with a gradient waveform that eliminates the constant velocity-induced phase on the center of every single echo [2]. The gradient waveform used for this technique is included in the sequence diagram of Fig. 8. This gradient waveform is known as a flyback trajectory [30], for which the echo planar readout becomes unipolar for all the echoes, practically eliminating other sources of N/2 ghost (mismatch between even and odd echoes during time reversal from hardware imperfections and causal response of the receiver filter).

Unfortunately, for the later option there is a time penalty. The time required to sample a given number of lines necessarily becomes longer (the shortest EPI readout is at least twice as long for the same number of echoes), and other motion-induced artifacts can become dominant. Furthermore, the technique cannot eliminate the 2D blurring arising from the continuous change in position at the center of each line, worsening as the readout per echo or the echo train length increases. Higher order motion terms such as acceleration and jerk are not compensated by this echo sampling but do not induce ghosting. Comparatively, the difference between a PSF that samples every echo and one sampling every second echo is similar to those illustrated in Fig. 10b and Fig. 10c using a 0.5-ms and a 1.0-ms interecho spacing but without the N/2 ghost at the edges of the FOV for the latter, a maximum of 0.26 in the PSF and a twofold increase in the readout bandwidth. To save some time a partial flyback trajectory has been proposed that acquires a portion around the center of k-space and the rest using the typical EPI trajectory, effectively eliminating ghosting from low spatial frequency data and consequently most of the N/2 ghost [30].

Multishot EPI

The PSF improves when multishot EPI readouts are used, reducing all the above effects for the single-shot EPI acquisition. Since phase discontinuities occur in the raw data depending on the number of echoes acquired per shot, ghosts also appear along the phase-encoding direction. This can be observed in the simulation results of Fig. 10g,h. Figure 13 demonstrates a cardiac-triggered multishot GRE scan acquired during late diastole and during systole in the abdominal aorta, showing the signal loss and ghosting that appears with flow components oriented mostly along the frequency-encoding direction (cranial-caudal axis).

The sliding window approach discussed previously for flow along the phase-encoding axis does not significantly affect the ghosting generated in multishot EPI with flow along the frequency-encoding direction. Phase discontinuity

Fig. 13a,b. Cardiac triggered multishot GRE EPI acquired in the abdominal aorta at end diastole (**a**) and during peak systole (**b**). Note the intense ghosts appearing on both sides of the aorta during systole with flow directed mainly along the frequency-encoding axis. Ghosting is not present during diastole. Fourteen echoes were used per shot with a total readout window of 15.4 ms, a 140×256 matrix acquisition, TE=8.5 ms, FOV=320 mm, an echo spacing of 1.1 ms (250 µs ramps with a 600 µs flattop) with the echo occurring at the center of k-space. No flow compensation was used along the frequency encoding and phase encoding

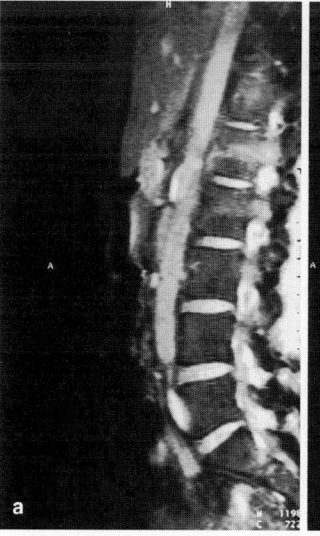
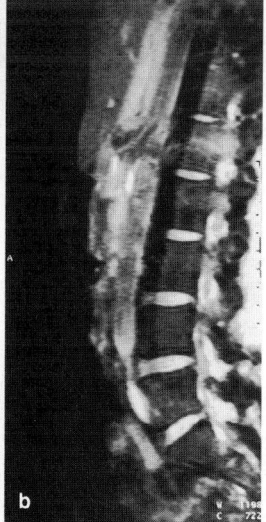

between k-space segments is always present from the same phase difference existing between odd and even echoes. Additionally, the increasing phase differences towards the edges of k-space also contribute to distort the PSF. This phase distribution does not occur for flow along the phase-encoding axis since the phase induced in each line is constant for all frequency-encoding points of each echo reading. In contrast to ghosts from flow parallel to the phase-encoding axis, the location of flow ghosts may not be equidistant, such as demonstrated in the simulation results of Fig. 10g,h. The only chance to suppress ghosting is to use the sliding window approach and the multishot EPI readout using the flyback trajectory of Fig. 7.

In Vivo Visualization of Flow Effects Using Subtraction and Multishot EPI Readouts

Subtraction techniques make it possible to observe flow effects directly in single-shot and multishot GRE EPI sequences in vivo because stationary material can be completely suppressed.

One convenient setup that does not require the acquisition of a subtraction mask during stationary conditions is blood tagging. Figure 14 demonstrates a case in the abdominal aorta acquired during peak systolic flow using a bolus tracking technique based on selective tagging (see "Subtraction with Selective Blood Tagging"). A thin slab of tissue and blood is tagged upstream on alternate readouts of the multishot EPI and subtracted prior to image reconstruction. The flow effects can be effectively monitored throughout the entire cardiac cycle.

Fig. 14a–c. Results in the abdominal aorta during systole showing flow effects along the frequency and phase-encoding axis with a multishot GRE EPI readout. **a** Scout image demonstrates the abdominal region evaluated and depicting and angulation of 18° for the descending aorta from the z axis. A 10-mm band was tagged perpendicular to the upper descending aorta on alternate heart beats 160 ms after the QRS ms and was read 40 ms later, approximately at peak systole. Subtraction of tagged and untagged images yields the movement of blood alone.

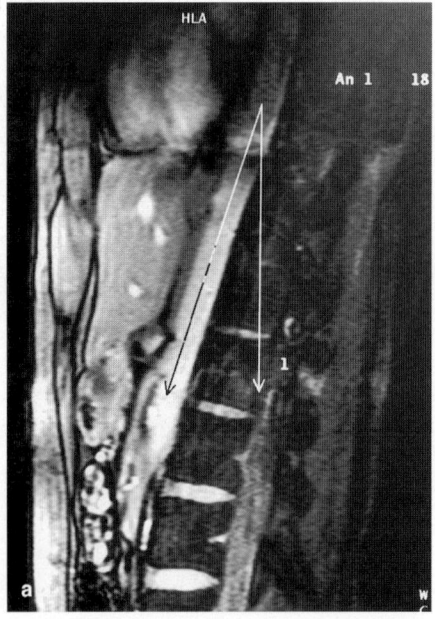

Fig. 14a–c. b Acquisition with the frequency-encoding direction parallel to the z axis (cranial-caudal direction) demonstrates ghosting along the phase-encoding axis. **c** Phase-encoding direction parallel to the z axis demonstrates ghosting propagating in the same direction. While the separation between the ghosts from the tagged bolus is constant for flow along the phase-encoding axis [ghost separation=FOV/(number of shots)], ghost induced for flow parallel to the frequency-encoding axis is not. Tagged blood displaced approximately 5 cm from tagged stationary spins (see **b,c**) and including TE=7 ms for this acquisition, the flow velocity is approximately 100 cm/s. Note that the bolus widens in **b** while it lengthens in **c**. The acquisition was performed during a single breath-hold using a 14-echo multishot EPI readout without the sliding window approach, TE=7 ms (asymmetric echo at 1/3 of the k-space matrix), 140×256 matrix, echo spacing of 1.28 ms, and FOV=400 mm. Tagging was performed using an 18-ms hyperbolic secant inversion pulse

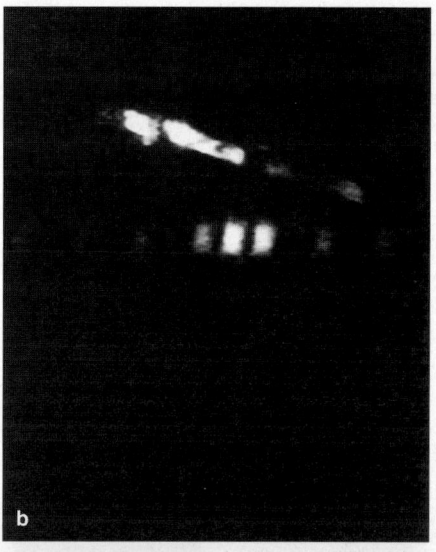

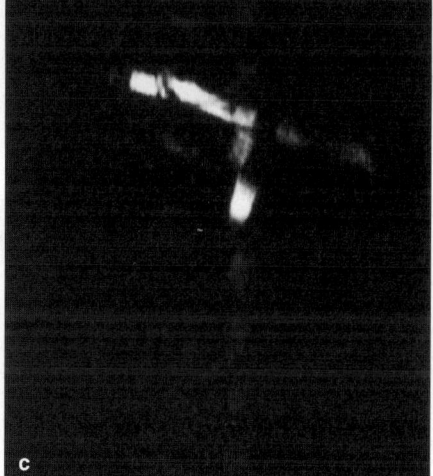

The tagging and substraction technique is also effective for determining flow velocities with very short acquisition times. Using multishot EPI in a bolus tracking configuration (cardiac imaging/multiphase) it is possible to achieve high temporal resolution and small blurring of the tagged bolus. Saturation effects are also reduced compared to other possible readout schemes (e.g., multishot segmented turboFLASH sequences).

Fig. 15. Simulation of oblique flow with single-shot EPI. PSF for a flow velocity of 50 cm/s at 45° from both-encoding axes. Flow component along the frequency encoding induces the N/2 ghost and 2D blurring while the flow component along the phase encoding produces further PSF broadening. Simulation performed for a 64×64 matrix, echo spacing of 0.5 ms, and FOV=240 mm

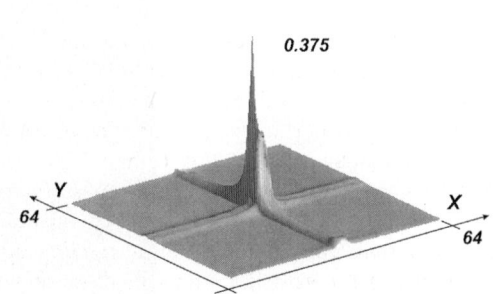

$V = 50 \ cm/s, \ ES=0.5 \ ms$

0.375

Y

X

64

64

Fig. 16a–c. Oblique flow with single-shot GRE EPI. **a** Coronal section of the phantom with flow tubes placed obliquely 30° from the sagittal towards the transverse axis acquired with stationary fluid. **b** With a flow mean velocity of 40 cm/s displacement and blurring are noted. **c** With a mean flow velocity of 95 cm/s the typical flow void and sharp enhancement observed in conventional MRA at high velocities are apparent. Flow-compensated single-shot EPI with flow compensation in all axes, 4-mm section thickness, TE=14.9 ms, 51.2 ms EPI train length with a 64×256 matrix, FOV=160×320 mm, four averages, echo spacing of 800 μs (250-μs ramps with a 300-μs flattop), centerline echo occurring after 22% of raw data were acquired

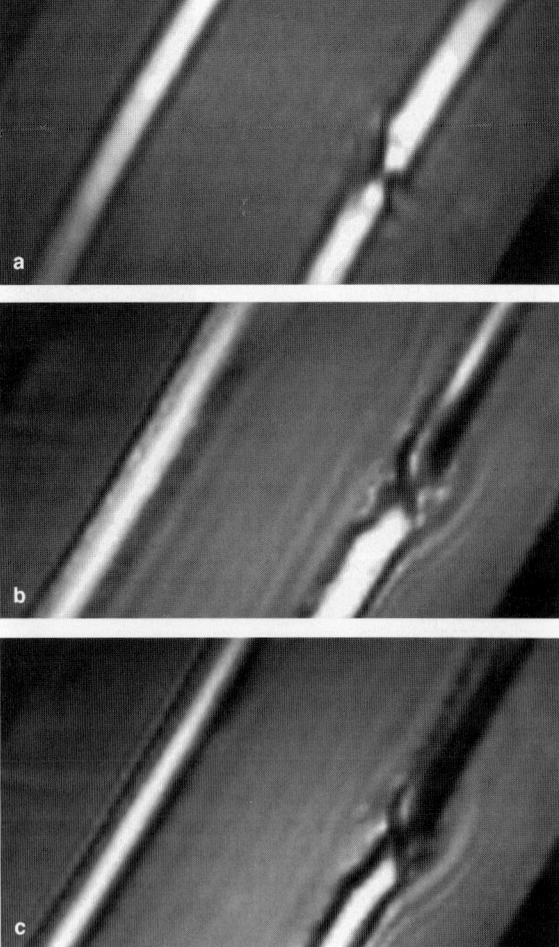

Oblique Flow

As in conventional MRA, oblique displacement artifacts occur in single-shot and multishot EPI when flow components exist along both the frequency- and phase-encoding axes. Conventional MRA displays a distinct misregistration since the encoding times along the frequency- and phase-encoding axes are clearly defined by the time course between the RF and TE and between the center of the phase-encoding pulse and TE, respectively. When laminar flow is present, the signal from more rapidly flowing spins bunch on one side, and their signals add up with the signal from that of slower moving spins. While enhancement occurs on one side of the vessel, a signal void appears on the opposite side as a consequence of this displacement.

The behavior for oblique flow in single-shot EPI combines all artifacts discussed above for each encoding axis. This is manifested in the PSF illustrated in Fig. 15, assuming the same flow velocity components along both the frequency- and phase-encoding axes. The PSF shows distinctively the 2D blurring and N/2 ghost from the velocity component along the frequency-encoding direction, with the broadening from flow along the phase-encoding direction superimposed. Figure 16 demonstrates these flow effects on the flow phantom with the flowing tubes positioned obliquely with similar flow components along both encoding axes.

Practical Observations

Flow effects may be exacerbated in single-shot and multishot EPI readouts depending on circumstances. These readouts may have potential applications especially if the following considerations are taken into account so that artifacts are maximally reduced.

- Flow components along the slice-select direction produce the same flow effects as in conventional MRA sequences. Thus, keeping a short RF excitation and motion compensation helps to minimize dephasing in stenotic regions when imaging is performed perpendicular to the vessel axis.
- Phase variations occurring from line to line in single-shot EPI are small, and ghosting is not present. Thus, pulsation artifacts and signal cancellation from phase variations between phase-encoding lines are not present, such as in conventional imaging.
- To minimize signal dephasing it is sufficient in most physiological circumstances to keep short effective TEs with asymmetric sampling of k-space along the phase-encoding direction and to use the shortest echo spacing possible that permits the desired FOV. To achieve short effective TEs it is more likely that a high degree of asymmetry is used to keep the center of k-space closer to the RF excitation rather than improving hardware performance. In this case partial Fourier reconstructions are necessary to sharpen image detail.
- Flow compensation is not necessary along the frequency-encoding direction. Even echoes are inherently flow compensated while odd echoes have a very small but constant phase shift. N/2 ghosting is likely to occur only at very

high velocities (depending on echo spacing) and usually appears outside the region of interest (unless a rectangular FOV is used).

- Whenever possible, triggering should be used in regions with high flow pulsation. Data should then be acquired during mid or late diastole. This has proven sufficient to minimize displacement and other flow effects under physiological conditions, making it competitive with conventional GRE scans when speed is required.
- For multishot EPI flow compensation should be used along all imaging axes, especially when using lower bandwidth readouts.
- A qualitative evaluation of the flow properties of multishot EPI sequences using first-moment nulling with their counterpart in conventional angiographic sequences demonstrates similar results with respect to flow dephasing in stenotic regions when the effective echo time and the length of the echoplanar readout are comparable to those of the conventional GRE readout.
- The addition of ghosting with high flow velocity components along the frequency-encoding axis is unavoidable for multishot EPI scans. However, with flow along the phase-encoding direction the results can improve significantly when a sliding window approach is implemented. Under physiological conditions flow sequences using a small number of echoes per interleaf (three to eight) with a short effective TE (e.g., with a 50 % echo asymmetry) and readout bandwidths greater than 900 Hz/pixel have proven robust with respect to ghosting and signal loss from dephasing.

Echo-Planar Imaging Angiography

The visualization of the vascular tree noninvasively using MRA has been possible thanks to the sensitivity of the MR signal to the presence of motion. MRA is still considered an experimental tool and continues to be one of the most active research areas in MRI.

With the recent addition of higher gradient strengths with shorter rise times in commercial systems, many of the current deficiencies of conventional MRA techniques, such as the signal loss in stenotic regions and displacement artifacts, can be largely offset by using shorter TE and increased spatial resolution [31]. This hardware enhancement has also opened the doors to faster MRA using imaging encoding strategies based on EPI, making it possible to perform a vascular study in a matter of seconds in regions of the body where conventional techniques would fail due to excessive motion artifacts.

EPI MRA Techniques

Although flow artifacts do occur, as noted in previous sections, single-shot and multishot EPI have been shown to have a potential value for ultrafast MRA [32, 33] and flow quantification [17, 18].

Several techniques that are commonly used in conventional MRA can be adapted for EPI MRA. Since the main advantage of EPI is its speed, it enables further optimization in flow contrast while permitting angiograms free of motion artifacts (due to respiratory motion blurring), particularly in the abdominal and thoracic regions, locations in which conventional MRA could be severely compromised by time constraints.

Figure 17 presents a general classification of MRA techniques that can be used similarly for EPI and multishot EPI scans. These categories include MRA techniques based on TOF effects [34, 35] and those relying on the contrast obtainable using the phase of the MR signal to depict moving blood, as in phase-contrast MRA [36–38].

TOF MRA includes techniques such as saturation recovery, inversion recovery, and more recently rephased-dephased magnitude subtraction, selective blood tagging using selective inversion recovery (SIR) [39, 40] and signal targeting with alternating radio frequency (STAR) [41] with magnitude and complex subtraction, among others. Of these methods, the saturation recovery technique was the one initially investigated to generate the first single-shot EPI MRA [10]. Although the so-called "black-blood" techniques also form part of the TOF classification, only techniques providing a positive blood/tissue contrast have been explored with EPI. This may in part be because the fat suppression pulse generally applied to eliminate chemical shift artifacts along the phase-encoding direction does not permit the visualization of many vessels which are surrounded by fat, such as the renal and coronary arteries. Bright fat is therefore required for vessel visualization in black-blood MRA techniques.

Phase-contrast MRA has been employed using a complex or phase subtraction after sensitizing the phase of moving spins to velocity. However, its initial application to EPI was geared more towards the noninvasive measurements of velocity and flow in vessels perpendicular to the plane of section [17, 18].

Other MRA techniques using some magnetic properties of blood and not the motion itself can be exploited to produce vascular contrast. These take advantage of the higher proton density and longer T2 of blood as well as its immunity to magnetization transfer (MT) irradiation [42–44] in comparison to surrounding tissues. These properties of blood have been utilized in conjunction with conventional TOF techniques to provide an additional enhancement of the blood signal with respect to the surrounding background.

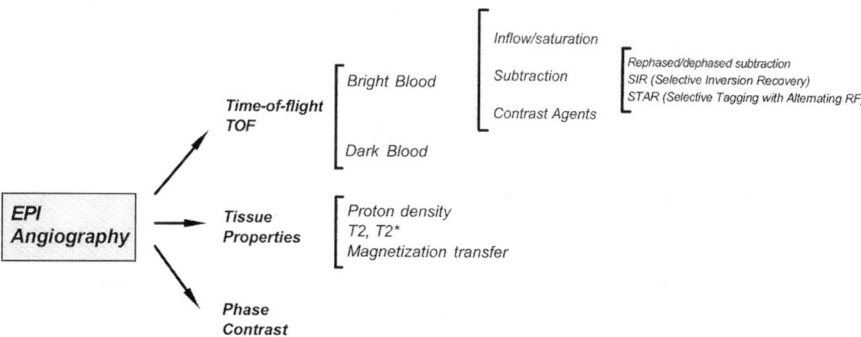

Fig. 17. EPI MRA genealogy

Maximum-intensity projections (MIP) and multiplanar reconstructions (MPR) are commonly used to visualize the angiographic data. These image-postprocessing techniques allow the vascular tree to be viewed from any desired angle and a particular vessel to be examined along any arbitrary cut.

Conventional MRA using EPI Hardware

A system with higher gradient amplitudes and slew rates can be used to improve current MRA protocols in two different ways (Fig. 18). Because higher readout gradients can be used during the echo readout, the acquisition bandwidth can be increased accordingly to sample the echo as quickly as possible. In this case the TE and the field echo (FE) can be made extremely short (Fig. 18a), thus minimizing sensitivity to flow dephasing and displacement. FE indicates the time that it takes to generate an echo once gradients start to be applied along the frequency-encoding axis. Higher readout bandwidths are necessary to reduce the FE/TE ratio, and S/N ratio is decreased by the inverse of the square root of the readout bandwidth.

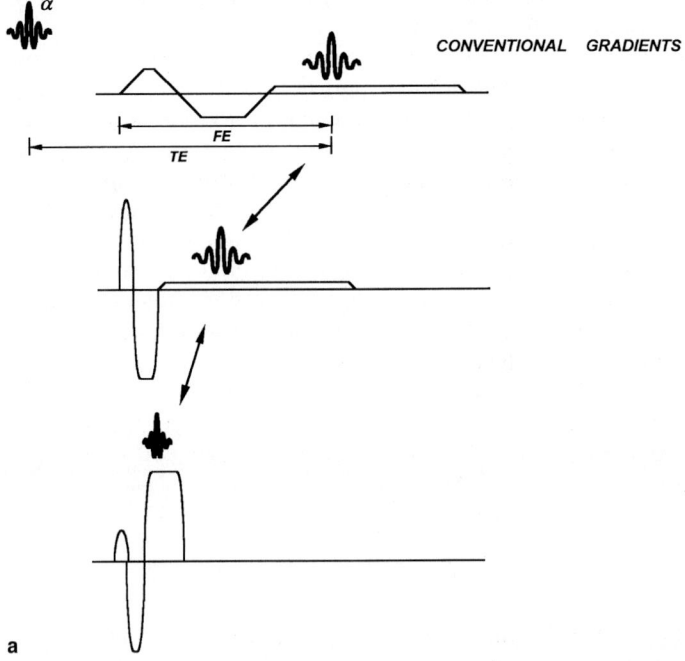

Fig. 18a. Higher gradients and shorter rise times can be used to shorten TE and FE by using sequences with higher acquisition bandwidth and smaller flow sensitivity (a) or design sequences with longer TE/FE with much lower acquisition bandwidths and similar flow sensitivity to conventional MRA sequences to improve S/N (b). *FE*, the time that it takes to obtain an echo once the frequency-encoding gradient is applied

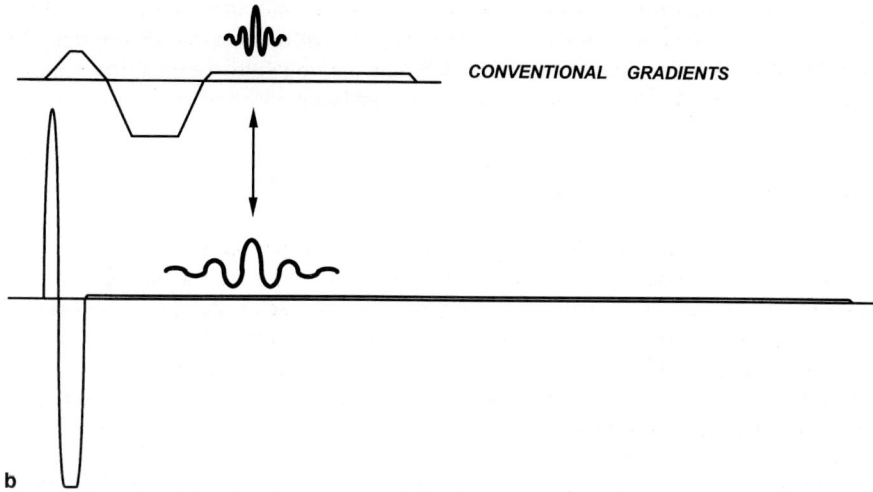

Fig. 18b. Higher gradients and shorter rise times can be used to shorten TE and FE by using sequences with higher acquisition bandwidth and smaller flow sensitivity (**a**) or design sequences with longer TE/FE with much lower acquisition bandwidths and similar flow sensitivity to conventional MRA sequences with a clear improvement in S/N (**b**). *FE*, the time that it takes to obtain an echo once the frequency-encoding gradient is applied

On the other hand, if a trade-off between FE time and increased flow sensitivity can be tolerated, longer readout times can be used (Fig. 18b), resulting in lower acquisition bandwidths to improve S/N. This gain in S/N can be further employed to decrease the FOV to gain resolution. This is possible because the motion-compensating gradients can be applied rapidly prior to the readout window. However, a phase term that evolves quadratically with time, $1/2gGVt^2$, acts as a complex filter along the readout axis and leads to a loss in resolution in the reconstructed image [8] (see "Flow effects along phase-encoding axis point spread function"). Since the phase errors induced by this term are larger towards the end of the readout window because of the quadratic dependence on time, a greater filtering effect is observed for lower bandwidth acquisitions. This is essentially the blurring that occurs for flow along the phase-encoding direction in single-shot EPI readouts.

Mechanisms of Angiographic Contrast in Time-of-Flight EPI MRA

Because blood moves continuously, leading to complete spoiling of the transverse magnetization, the signal strength for moving blood is proportional only to the longitudinal magnetization recovered between successive RF excitations (assuming a steady-state condition). Thus for a GRE EPI sequence repeated with a finite TR the signal from blood remaining within the imaging volume is equivalent to that of a fast low flip angle-shot (FLASH) acquisition [45].

In TOF acquisitions stationary tissues reach an equilibrium condition after several RF excitations. This is a steady-state condition that has been referred to as spin saturation. Fully magnetized blood moving into the imaging volume can replace previously excited blood spins, yielding the known wash-in effect that represents the main contrast mechanism behind TOF acquisitions. Saturation can be experienced by blood as well, particularly in a 3D experiment, when blood may be continuously excited during the time it remains in the imaging volume [46].

Considering pluglike flow through a vessel perpendicular to the imaging volume with a constant velocity V_f, the number of RF excitation pulses, N_{rf}, that a single spin can experience at some location d in the imaging volume from the point of entrances is determined by:

$$N_{rf} = integer\ part\ of\ [d/V_f TR] \tag{11}$$

The signal for blood, $SM(N_{rf})$, at location d is determined by:

$$SB(N_{rf}) = M_o sin(a)[M_s + (1-M_s)r^{Nrf-1}]e^{-TE/T2*} \tag{12}$$

where a represents the flip angle, $E1 = e^{-TR/TI}$, $r = E1\ cos\ \alpha$, $M_s = (1-E1)/(1-r)$, and M_o the proton density of blood. The signal intensity from flowing material is a function of the percentage of moving spins that enter the imaging volume and the number of RF excitations that it receives in relation to the repetition time and flip angle applied. For a flowing spin observing only a single RF excitation, a 90° RF excitation yields the maximum signal possible. When blood experiences an increasing number of RF excitations, the signal from blood saturates, in which case the optimum signal for a particular TR is given by the Ernst angle, a_E [46], with:

$$a_E = cos^{-1}(E1) \tag{13}$$

For a given flow velocity the flow enhancement along a vessel is more uniform with longer TRs, resulting from a reduction in the number of RF excitations that blood observes. Similarly, higher flow velocities produce the same effect with a fixed TR. Nevertheless, flow contrast is greater in the latter condition because stationary tissue becomes increasingly saturated with shorter TRs. With low flow velocities and short TR, lower flip angles must be applied to reduce saturation. This is particularly important for multishot GRE EPI acquisitions where TR decreases when a small number of echoes per interleaf are encoded.

2D and 3D TOF EPI

Single-Shot 2D EPI Readouts

Saturation Recovery. High contrast between blood and stationary tissue can develop after the application of a 90° presaturation pulse over the slice of interest some time prior to the single-shot GRE EPI acquisition. The presaturation helps reduce the signal from stationary material and hence permits good flow contrast from unsaturated blood entering the slice of interest during the presaturation event and imaging. The approach is useful particularly for flow entering perpendicular to the imaging slice. The delay time between the presaturation and the imaging pulse should be set such that blood sees only the single RF excitation that is used to read the signal. This scheme is effective when flow velocities are high.

Inversion Recovery. Nearly complete background suppression and maximum flow contrast is possible using a selective inversion recovery (IR) GRE EPI sequence. The technique uses a slice-selective inversion pulse instead of a presaturation over the slice of interest to further suppress the background tissue. An inversion time (TI) is usually chosen so that the stationary tissue is completely nulled while enough time is allowed for fresh blood to enter the region of interest. Slowly moving blood greatly benefits from this approach because it allows longer inflow times, resulting in greater background signal reduction and flow contrast.

Fat Suppression Only. Because a chemical shift selective fat saturation is routinely used with EPI to reduce shifting of the fat signal over tissues of interest, the visualization of vessels that are surrounded by fat is improved. Figure 19 demonstrates an oblique view of the right coronary artery acquired with single-shot GRE EPI. Because the right coronary is embedded in fat, the 90° presaturation pulse and blood inflow are not necessary to produce the vascular contrast.

Fig. 19. A 48-ms, single-shot, oblique GRE EPI scan demonstrating the right coronary artery of a healthy volunteer acquired during mid-late diastole. The solely use of chemical fat saturation improves the visualization of the vessel. A 4-mm slice thickness was selected with a 96×128 matrix, FOV 200×270 mm, TE=16 ms without flow compensation and the center of k-space acquired after 31% of the raw data matrix were acquired, echo spacing of 0.5 ms, sinusoidal readout. Surface coil acquisition

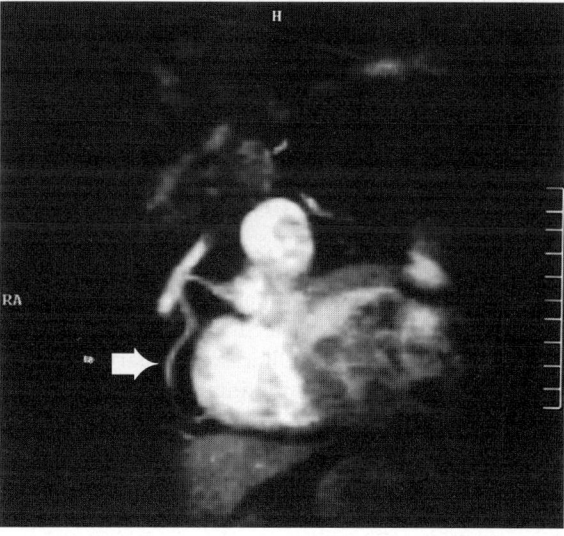

Averaging

The S/N ratio can be improved by averaging multiple excitations. Although this acquisition scheme defies the single-shot concept, the application of several RF excitations with short TR can lead to a substantial saturation of the background tissue while permitting high flow signal to develop, similar to conventional 2D TOF MRA [47]. This technique was initially demonstrated in the first TOF angiograms with GRE EPI [10]. With GRE EPI longer TRs and larger flip angles can be used than with conventional 2D MRA sequences, thus improving the wash-in effects with slower flow while suppressing background tissue signal.

Averaging can be carried out either in the raw data or in the image domain. The choice of one or the other method is especially important when averaging short TR EPI scans in the presence of pulsatile flow. The complex addition of flow signals acquired at different points in the cardiac cycle may generate unwanted signal cancellation and produce signal voids in vessels. Averaging the magnitude images, instead, improves vessel homogeneity [48]. Nonetheless, blurring and displacement artifacts from flow always affect each vessel differently, depending on flow velocity and direction with respect to the plane of section. Although there is a small sacrifice in the S/N ratio of the final image, the addition of magnitude images is more beneficial when cardiac synchronization is not employed during data acquisition.

Vessel Selectivity

The signal from arteries or veins can be eliminated selectively by using a traveling saturation band positioned on either side of the imaging section. The timing and thickness of the traveling presaturation are critical in obtaining a consistent saturation with a single-shot scan. The considerations are similar to those when a presaturation or a selective inversion pulse is used over the slice of interest to suppress the stationary tissue, as noted above. When multiple images are acquired, or when averaging is used, the application of multiple RF excitations creates a steady state in the signal of the undesired blood components, and shorter delays may be used between the traveling saturation band and the corresponding imaging slice. The thickness of the traveling saturation band must be adjusted accordingly so that for a particular TR unwanted blood remains saturated before entering the imaging section.

Improving Vessel Contrast

Selective Water Excitation. A chemical shift selective fat saturation scheme is always applied to eliminate fat superimposing over tissues of interest [49, 50]. This is accomplished by applying a frequency selective, spatially nonselective RF excitation. One of two suppression schemes are generally used: (a) the application of a gaussian pulse centered on the fat frequency (usually several ms long), or (b) a binomial excitation with short "hard" RF pulses (1-1, 1-2-1, 1-3-3-1 excitation schemes, with underlined indicating a 180° phase rotation). With a typical binomial excitation the separation between the RF pulses is given by one-half the time that fat takes to precess 360°, approximately 2.37 ms at 1.5T. This is followed immediately by strong gradient spoiling before data acquisition to eliminate the transverse magnetization of the excited fat spins.

In regions with poor magnetic homogeneity the nonselective fat saturation scheme can disturb the signal from water spins far away from the imaging volume and therefore lead to water rather than fat suppression. This is often observed when imaging the descending aorta and renal arteries. Blood saturation is likely to occur in the thorax, and blood does not recover its full magnetization before it reaches the region of interest, hence delivering poor flow contrast even with transverse 2D scans. Using a spectral-spatial excitation [51–53] can dramatically improve results. With the spectral-spatial excitation, only water spins within the slice excited provide signal, leaving the signal from fat untouched. After shimming in the volume of interest water saturation should be minimal.

Another advantage of a spectral-spatial excitation is that it can be more effective in suppressing the remnant chemical shift observed in single-shot EPI images than with any other techniques. Fat recovers some of its signal between the application of the nonselective chemical shift fat suppression pulse and that of the excitation pulse, time which is completely eliminated using the spectral-spatial excitation.

Magnetization Transfer. Improved vessel contrast is also possible by incorporating MT pulses during the quiescent periods between RF excitations so that the background tissue signal is further suppressed, especially when longer TRs are selected (or a proton density weighted scan is performed) [42–44]. MT pulses can be used when imaging the liver vessels or vessels surrounded by muscle. Both muscle and liver exhibit a large MT effect.

Long TE. Additionally, longer TEs can help improve the angiographic contrast by taking advantage of the longer T2* of blood. However, magnetic susceptibility signal loss and displacement artifacts may preclude the usage of long TEs.

Single-Shot 3D EPI Readouts

General Features of 3D TOF EPI MRA. As in conventional 3D TOF MRA sequences, thinner slices provide robustness by reducing the signal loss from magnetic susceptibility differences and permit the reconstruction of a complex vessel geometry in any desired orientation using MPR or MIP. The flow sensitivity is similar to that in its 2D counterpart. However, 3D scans use multiple RF excitations to encode all the sections prescribed, making the flow contrast mechanism similar to that of a conventional 3D TOF sequence.

The signal of inflowing blood is spatially dependent across the volume as the number of RF excitations experienced by blood increases while within the imaging volume (see Eqs. 11, 12). Flip angles lower than 90° are used to account for the saturation effect, and in general the optimizations described above for con-

Fig. 20. 3D TOF EPI MRA of the liver analyzed with curved MPR. *Left*, the setting for the curved cuts; *right*, the resulting 5-mm slices reconstructed along the middle hepatic and portal veins, respectively. Thirty-two 2.5-mm sections were acquired without cardiac triggering in a single 20-s breath-hold using TR/TE=230/14 ms, 51.4 ms readout window, α=25°, 64×256 matrix with FOV=190×380 mm matrix, and three averages to improve S/N. Body coil requisition

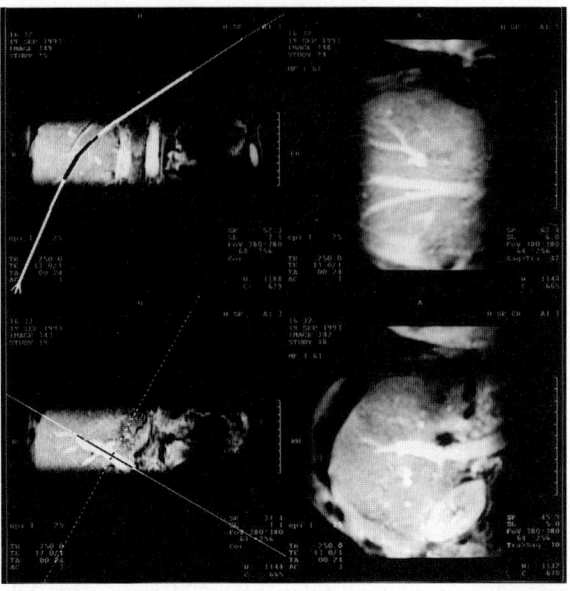

ventional 3D TOF MRA also apply here. MT pulses and specially shaped RF profiles such as tilted optimized nonsaturating excitation (TONE) [54, 55], variable-angle uniform signal excitation (VUSE) [56], and nonlinear excitation profiles [57] can be incorporated to increase the flow contrast by reducing blood saturation. Figure 20 demonstrates a curved plane reformat along two major venous structures in the liver acquired with a velocity compensated 3D GRE EPI acquisition. Figure 21 illustrates the complete liver vasculature processed with volume rendering and acquired using the same scheme as in Fig. 20 but including MT pulses to increase the contrast between the vasculature and liver. Another example in the renal arteries is shown in Fig. 22. All the examples shown were acquired without cardiac triggering and signal averaging.

Potential Artifacts. With 3D acquisitions the potential for motion artifacts is higher than in 2D methods. The slice select phase-encoding process introduces additional artifacts that propagate along the slice-selection direction when any intensity or phase variations in the MR signal arise from changes in the flow velocity between RF excitations. These artifacts are reflected as ghosting, blurring, and occasionally signal loss when untriggered acquisitions without averaging are used. For this reason the flow conditions during each EPI readout must remain constant; otherwise the imaging parameters and the sequence structure should account for the variations in order to reduce the spurious modulations in the MR signal.

Problems can be partially reduced without sacrificing imaging time by monitoring the cardiac signal and consequently reordering the slice-selection phase-encoding table in a manner similar to respiratory ordered phase encoding [58].

Fig. 21a,b. Volume rendering of the liver vasculature from a 3D TOF EPI MRA. **a** A transverse projection. **b** A 45° transverse to coronal view. Thirty-two 2.5-mm sections were acquired without cardiac triggering in a single 24-s breath-hold using TR/TE=250/14 ms, 51.4-ms readout window, α=30°, 64×256 matrix with FOV=190×380 mm matrix, and three averages. MT pulses were applied to enhance the contrast between liver and vascular signal. Remnant signal from fat can be noted at the bottom of the liver in **a** from incomplete fat suppression

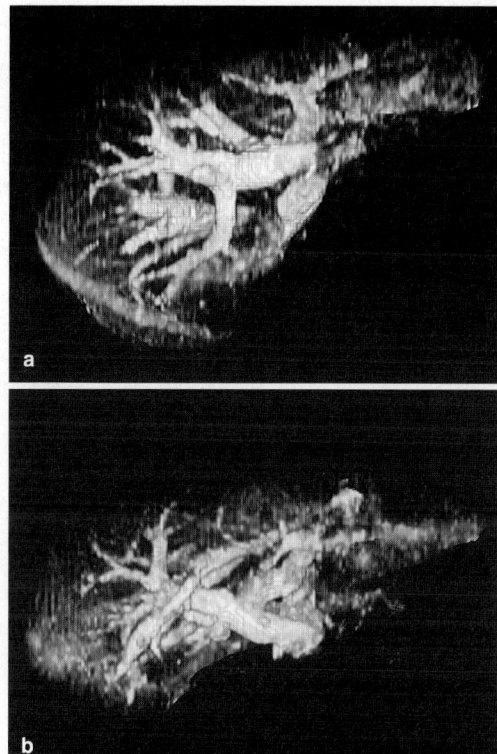

Fig. 22. Curved MPR cut demonstrating the aorta and the take-off of the renal arteries from a data set acquired using a 3D GRE EPI acquisition on a healthy subject. Three right renal arteries are seen. For the 3D GRE EPI acquisition 32 2.2-mm sections were acquired without cardiac triggering in a single 20-s breath-hold using TR/TE=210/14 ms, 51.4-ms readout window, α=30°, 64×256 matrix with FOV=190×380 mm matrix, and three averages

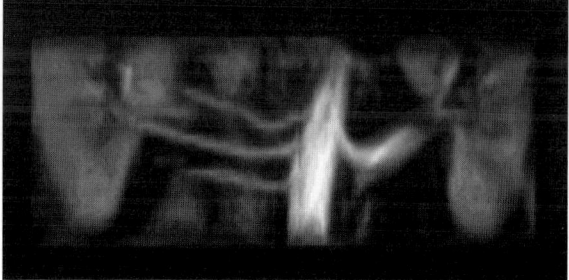

This can effectively reduce the phase cancellations that may arise during periods of positive and negative acceleration despite the presence of blurring and spin displacement. Reasonable results may be achieved without cardiac monitoring, such as illustrated in Figs. 20–22.

Multishot EPI MRA

General Considerations

Multishot EPI overcomes the resolution barrier in single-shot EPI and yet maintains flow effects comparable to those in conventional MRA techniques. However, several points must be taken into account so that the appropriate choice of imaging parameters is made to minimize flow artifacts and other effects that are related to the signal evolution during the multishot EPI readout. These include:

- The signal for each RF excitation must remain constant for all interleaves so that ghosting does not appear from amplitude modulations. This is important for single slice 2D multishot EPI scans when the interleaves are performed in rapid succession with sequential interleaved encoding and short TRs (when the signal from all tissues within the imaging is still evolving towards a steady-state magnetization) [59]. In the limit of very short TRs low flip angles must be used.
- In principle an incremental flip angle series could be employed so that the same signal strength is generated for each excitation when using very short TRs [60]. The simplest approach uses two shots with a 45°–90° flip angle combination (yielding 0.707 of the total signal for each excitation at infinite T1 and TR~o). An incremental flip angle series can be calculated only for a specific T1 relaxation. This means that ghosting can appear if the T1 from one tissue differs considerably from that chosen for the calculation. Even flow perpendicular to the plane of section must be taken into account. Taking the two-shot case, complete inflow between excitations can generate a clear N/2 ghost.
- Flow velocity must remain fairly constant for the acquisition of each k-space segment. Even when the signal for each interleaf is the same, velocity variations between interleaves can introduce additional phase shifts that result in ghosting artifacts from vascular structures. This is the case when short TRs are used between interleaves and the data are acquired over a period that encompasses both systole and diastole. Triggering each interleaf at a specific phase of the cardiac cycle minimizes signal amplitude and phase changes at the expense of imaging time. Imaging can also be performed during a large portion of diastole.
- The echo spacing and number of echoes per RF excitation should be a function of the flow velocities in the specific region under evaluation so that flow displacement and blurring are small. Although the approach may not be robust for quantifying stenotic regions, the greater speed than in conventional techniques permits a large volume to be acquired within a reasonable time in cases in which imaging time is an important consideration.
- With a small number of echoes encoded per interleaf and a short RF excitation, flow compensation is seldom necessary, especially when asymmetric echoes are used along the phase-encoding direction (effectively providing a shorter TE, similar to conventional MRA along the frequency-encoding axis), and the signal is acquired with high readout bandwidths. Partial Fourier

reconstruction techniques may be employed to obtain the full resolution when asymmetric sampling is used [24].

- A 3D setup permits the data acquisition process to be managed more effectively with respect to the course of magnetization when short TRs are selected. 3D multishot EPI is robust only when one direction is segmented using an EPI readout.
- Although a small number of echoes per interleaf reduces the effects of flow and susceptibility artifacts, spatial resolution, speed, and sensitivity to flow and field inhomogeneities need to be investigated for particular vascular regions. This allows enough flexibility in the choice of imaging parameters that the best flow contrast may be obtained.

3D TOF Multishot EPI MRA

Assuming a fixed acquisition time, for example, a short breath-hold, TR can be balanced with the number of echoes per interleaf and the volume coverage. A smaller number of echoes per interleaf translates into shorter TRs, and conversely a larger number of echoes permits longer TRs. The issues of blood saturation are identical to those discussed for conventional 3D TOF MRA. Thus with short TRs blood saturates at a faster rate within the imaging volume, and lower flip angles are required to counteract the effect.

Figure 23 illustrates a 3D multishot acquisition. k-space segmentation is performed along the in-plane phase-encoding direction and chemical shift artifacts consequently appear in this encoding direction. The chemical shift is greater as the number of echoes per RF excitation increases with a fixed readout bandwidth. Longer TRs can be accommodated that can contribute to enhancing the flow contrast at the expense of increased chemical shift and flow artifacts. Therefore a chemical selective fat saturation or spectral spatial water excitation pulses should be applied.

Figure 24 illustrates a 3D multishot EPI acquisition in the thorax acquired over the right lung in the sagittal plane. The 3D multishot acquisition permits

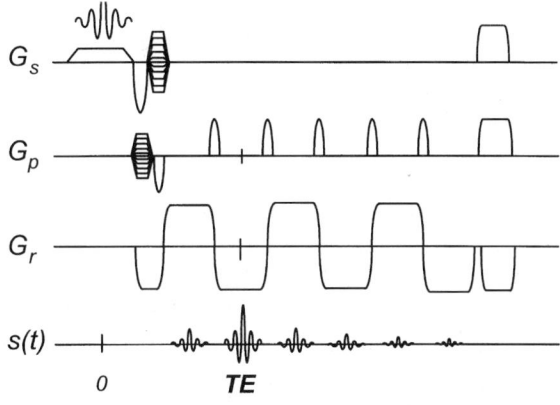

Fig. 23. 3D multishot GRE EPI sequence diagram. For each RF excitation six echoes are acquired (Ne=6). Segmentation is performed along the in-plane phase-encoding direction. In this diagram an asymmetric echo is formed on the second readout window to minimize TE and flow effects. After the EPI readout spoilers are applied. α, *RF excitation angle; Gr,* readout gradient; *Gp,* in-plane phase encoding gradient; *Gs,* section select gradient; s(t), signal

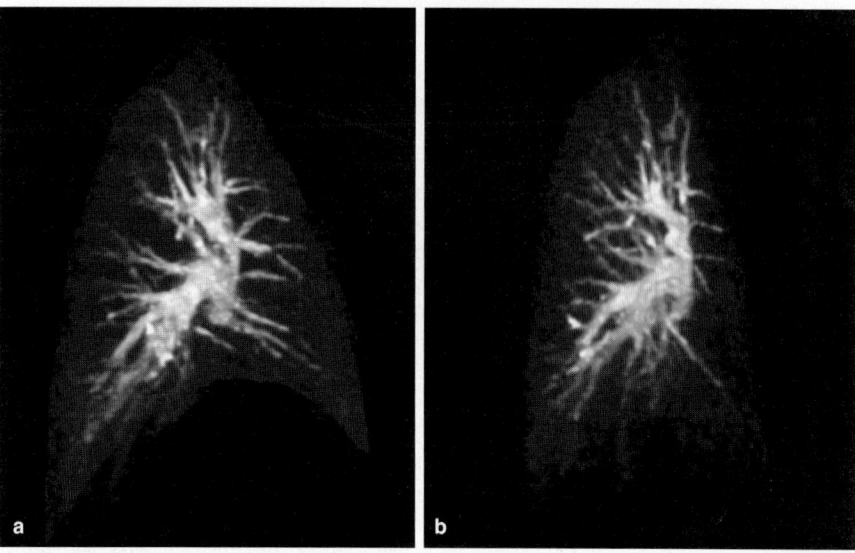

Fig. 24. Sagittal (a) and sagittal to coronal (b) MIP reformation from a multishot 3D EPI acquisition acquired in the sagittal plane over the right lung in 8 s. For each interleaf six echoes were encoded with TR/TE=7.9/3.0 ms, α=7°, 110-mm slab thickness, 64 partitions, 96×256 matrix, FOV=180×350 mm, echo spacing of 1 ms (250-μs ramps with a 500-μs flattop), centerline echo occurring on the 2nd readout of the EPI train. Fat suppression pulses were not applied, and the body coil was used for signal reception

complete isotropic coverage of one lung in a single breath-hold of 8 s. By keeping the effective TE short by using asymmetric echoes along the in-plane phase-encoding direction, signal loss from magnetic susceptibility dephasing between vessels and air in the lungs can be minimized. This makes it possible to visualize the pulmonary vasculature out to the lung periphery (within the limits of the S/N, depending on the receiver coil used). Additional time savings are possible by using partial Fourier scanning, even in the thorax, whenever short TEs are used in conjunction with small voxels. The S/N loss with partial Fourier can be overcome by using longer TRs or by doubling the scanning volume if the breath-hold time is kept the same.

Even shorter TEs, in the order of 1–2 ms, can be obtained by a centrically ordered approach. For this scheme, the phase encoding starts from the center of k-space and acquires both positive and negative quadrants in two separate interleaves [28]. It must be kept in mind that flow and field inhomogeneity phase changes have opposite signs, especially when a large number of echoes are used during the EPI readout. It is preferable to use partial Fourier scanning to achieve the same TEs and keep scanning along the segmentation direction with the same gradient polarity (phase-encoding blips with the same sign) if a large number of echoes per shot (or low bandwidth readouts) are used.

Magnetization-Prepared Acquisitions

Short TRs are inevitable when short breath-hold scans, large number of sections, reasonably high in-plane resolution and a small number of echoes per interleaf are required to minimize both sensitivity to flow and susceptibility artifacts (e.g., scanning in the lungs, see Fig. 24). Short TRs saturate the blood signal (unless low flip angles are applied). The addition of MT pulses, saturation bands, or fat suppression prior to every readout to improve the flow contrast is time consuming, and their application can be even longer than the EPI readout itself and hence double or triple the scanning time.

To counteract this limitation magnetization-prepared (MP) acquisitions can be used to provide a greater flexibility for the effective management of the flow contrast. This is performed by sharing the desired contrast encoded during an MP period (which includes the above options and others, explained below) between several lines of k-space. The contrast characteristics and properties that the MP provides over the acquired data (contrast and filtering effects over k-space) have been validated for ultrafast T1- and T2-weighted imaging with turboFLASH techniques [61–67]. The extension to multishot EPI enables the same potential for encoding more data to help achieve a short acquisition time, large coverage, and improved contrast.

The application of MP to 2D multishot EPI using short TR is feasible; however, the resulting images tend to demonstrate ghosting artifacts that arise from the magnetization course throughout the subsequent RF excitations after the MP process. Several points are made in this respect under "General Considerations" in the sec-

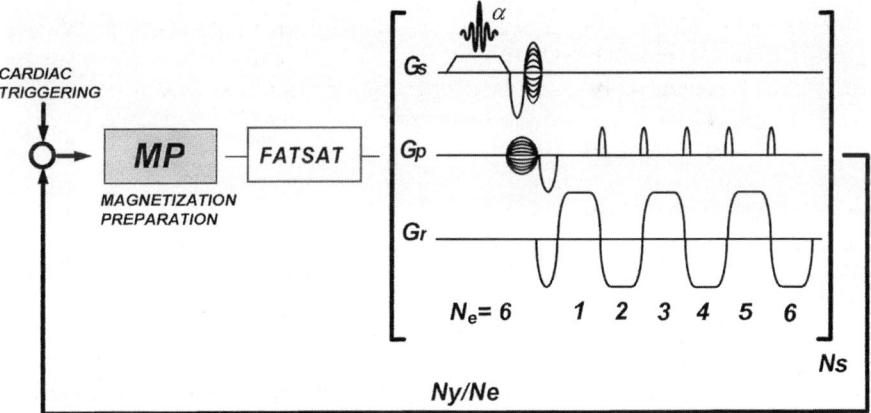

Fig. 25. MP 3D multishot GRE EPI sequence. A magnetization preparation followed by a chemical fat saturation 1-3-3-1 pulse (or other fat suppression scheme) is included prior to data acquisition to generate the desired contrast. With every heartbeat all the partitions are encoded, and a multishot EPI readout is applied, generating several echoes per RF excitation which are phase-encoded independently using an interleaved trajectory along the in-plane phase-encoding direction. Here six echoes are acquired per RF excitation (Ne=6). *a, RF excitation angle; Gr,* readout gradient; *Gp,* in-plane phase encoding gradient; *Gs,* section select gradient; *Ny,* number of in-plane phase-encoding lines; *Ns,* number of sections (partitions); *Ne,* number of echoes; *Ny/Ne,* number of cardiac periods necessary to encode the image

tion "Multishot EPI MRA," and these apply even more so here because of the large change that the longitudinal magnetization may experience throughout the acquisition. Thus, as pointed out above, MP acquisitions are more suitable for 3D multishot EPI because it enables to freely design a k-space trajectory that produces a smooth signal course along both phase-encoding directions [4].

A diagram of a MP 3D multishot GRE EPI scan is illustrated in Fig. 25. A convenient scheme involves the acquisition of all the section-selection phase-encoding steps (partitions) following the MP period. Thus for each partition-encoding step several echoes are interleaved along the in-plane phase-encoding direction. With this setup the course of the signal along the partition direction is smooth, and the partitions can be acquired sequentially or centrally depending on the

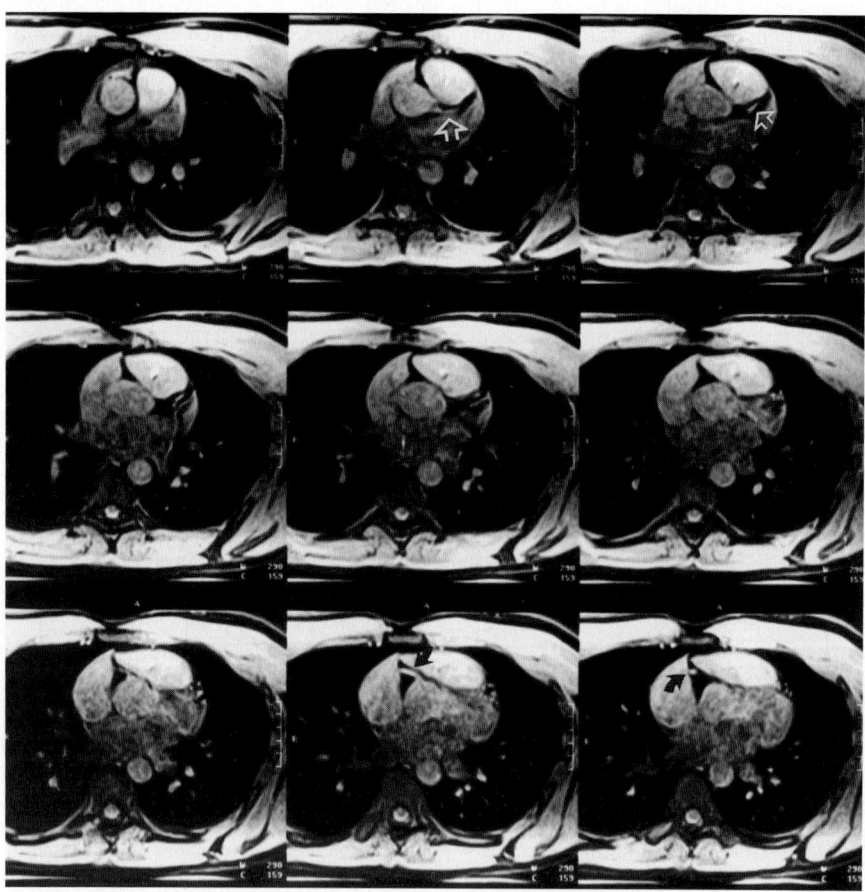

Fig. 26. Nine slices from a 16-partition data set acquired using only a single chemical fat saturation pulse prior to data acquisition (proton density weighted). The origins of the right descending and the left main coronary arteries are depicted (*arrows*). Sixteen 3-mm sections, TR/TE=8.6/3.2 ms, α=16°, Ne=6, 126×256 matrix, FOV=250×340 mm, sequential partition encoding, readout bandwidth of 940 Hz/pixel, acquisition in mid-late diastole with a trigger delay of 650 ms. Data were acquired in 21 heartbeats (23 s) using a phased array body coil

number of partitions selected and the contrast generated by the MP scheme. Another approach reverses the role of each phase encoding, i.e., performs the segmentation along the partition direction and lets the magnetization vary smoothly along the in-plane phase-encoding direction. The acquisition can be triggered so that the data are acquired during the diastolic phase to minimize signal dephasing and other flow effects in regions of stenosis and increased flow velocities. This has been succesfully used to image the cardiac muscle with large volume coverage in a single or multiple short breath-holds [4].

Several magnetization preparations may be used to produce the vessel contrast. These include those that exploit the inherent properties of blood (larger proton density, longer T2, and smaller MT effect) or others that rely on the blood motion itself.

Fat saturation (Proton density). In many cases the sole use of a chemical selective fat saturation has been not only to reduce chemical shift artifacts but also to suppress the surrounding fat that appears around some vessels, such as seen in the coronary and renal arteries. Several partitions demonstrating the branching off of the left and right coronary arteries are illustrated in Fig. 26.

Fig. 27a,b. Two 4-mm slices from a 16-partition data set acquired using a T2 preparation with an effective echo time of 48 ms. The right coronary artery is shown (*arrows*). Trigger delay of 550 ms to the T2 preparation stage (effective delay of 600 ms), T2 preparation using a RF spacing of 4 ms, TR/TE=8.0/3.0 ms, α=13°, 126×256 matrix with FOV=250×340 mm, Ne=6, a readout bandwidth of 1220 Hz/pixel, sequential partition encoding. The images were acquired in 21 heartbeats (23 s) using a phased-array body coil

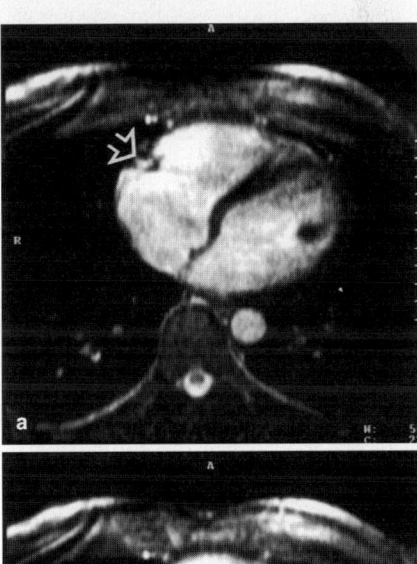

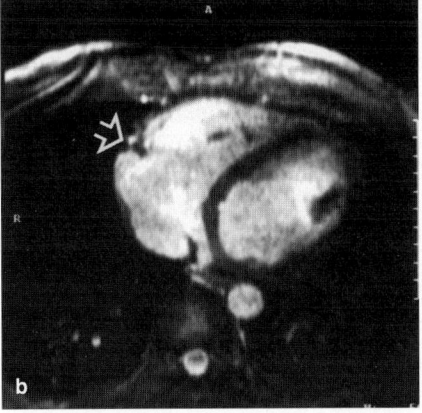

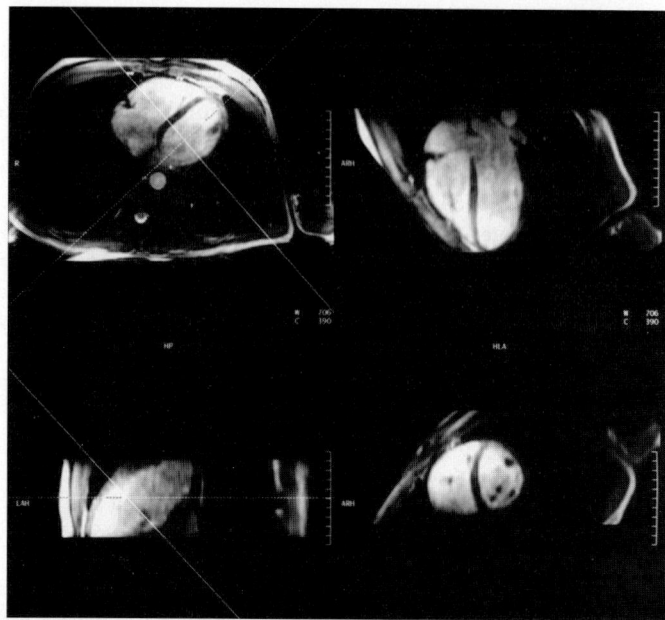

Fig. 28. MPR from a cardiac volume acquired in a single breath-hold using a T2-weighted preparation. T2 preparation with an effective echo time of 48 ms using an RF spacing of 4 ms. Sixteen 6-mm sections with a trigger delay of 550 ms to the T2 preparation stage, TR/TE=9.6/4.2 ms, =14°, 126×256 matrix with FOV=250×340 mm, Ne=6, a readout bandwidth of 940 Hz/pixel, sequential partition encoding. The images were acquired in 21 heartbeats (23 s) using a phased-array body coil

T2 Preparation. This preparation can be used to enhance the longer T2 of blood. A nonselective 90° $_x$–[180° $_y$]$_N$–270°$_x$ –360°$_{-x}$ driven equilibrium T2-weighted preparation (or similar) can be applied [70]. In this way flow independent contrast can develop, and this makes it possible to image blood in regions with slow motion (such as in the peripheral vessels) [66, 67]. One particular application includes enhancing the contrast between the blood pool and the myocardium (Fig. 27) to better visualize the coronary arteries. Similarly, the heart chambers may be evaluated using multiplanar reformats along the short and long axis views, such as depicted in Fig. 28.

Magnetization Transfer Preparation. Similar contrast can be obtained, such as in the T2 prepared case using MT pulses. An initial long MT irradiation should be applied prior to data acquisition to build the MT contrast. Additional irradiation must be employed during the period between data acquisition windows to maintain low signal from tissues with high MT attenuation.

IR Preparation. Vascular contrast can be enhanced with the application of a slice-selective inversion pulse over the imaging volume (see "Single-Shot 2D EPI Readouts"). By setting the inversion time to null the signal from surrounding stationary tissue, inflowing blood can be visualized with high contrast.

Subtraction Techniques

To further increase the contrast between blood and stationary tissues, strategies involving the subtraction of images that differ only in the signal from flowing material have been used. Subtraction techniques are advantageous as they permit the following: (a) Theoretically complete stationary signal suppression with improved visualization of small vessels. (b) Coverage of an entire vascular territory using thicker sections (projection angiography), thus reducing scanning time. (c) Subtractions can be performed either in the magnitude or in the complex domains, the choice depending on S/N and quality of the stationary tissue suppression. Magnitude subtraction introduces a small penalty in S/N but can be more robust whenever hardware imperfections are present. (d) Their results are convenient for EPI readouts because the full strength of the EPI system may be used to provide the smallest FOV that is possible without aliasing problems, especially when the flow information is confined to a small region of interest. (e) Because aliasing does not occur from stationary material, a rectangular FOV enables the EPI readout to be considerably shortened (down to 16–20 ms), helping to reduce flow effects extensively while maintaining adequate spatial resolution.

Magnitude Rephased-Dephased Subtraction

A subtraction of two magnitude images in which flowing spins are encoded with different flow sensitivities can yield an angiogram with good background suppression [68]. A rephased image is formed by using first moment compensation along all the gradient axes. A flow-dephased image is generated with the application of strong velocity-encoding gradients prior to the EPI readout. The velocity-sensitizing gradients can be applied simultaneously to increase dephasing and to maintain short TEs. A small drawback exists in that flowing blood with velocity components that are colinear to the plane defined by the velocity-encoding gradients may not be affected significantly. If a plug velocity profile is present across a voxel, the dephasing applied may be ineffective, yielding inconsistent signal suppression from flowing components (e.g., veins). Systolic acquisitions should be avoided, since blurring and displacement artifacts with single-shot EPI readouts cannot be tolerated. Both flow-rephased and flow-dephased images are subtracted as magnitude images to yield only signal from vascular structures.

The signal for stationary tissue for both images must be the same to obtain a good subtraction. Thus both slices should be acquired either when the magnetization from all tissues has recovered completely between the two shots or by using a saturation pulse over the slice of interest and including a delay interval prior to imaging. In the former the signal of blood is proportional to its proton density (no TOF dependence), and vessels in the plane of section or through plane appear isointense after the subtraction. The saturation-recovery technique is effective whenever cardiac synchronization is employed because of variations in the heart rate. In this case TOF effects are reduced when the time after the application of the saturation is long.

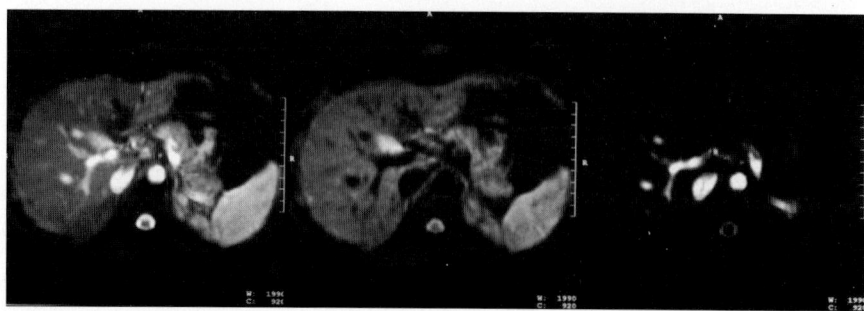

Fig. 29. A single slice rephased-dephased subtraction angiogram at the level of the portal vein. Each image was acquired with a single-shot GRE EPI readout of 64 ms. A 4-mm slice thickness was selected with a 128×128 matrix, FOV=350 mm, echo spacing of 500 µs with a sinusoidal readout waveform. Images were acquired in middle to late diastole and triggered on every heartbeat. The slice was presaturated with a 90° RF excitation to assure the same magnetization for stationary tissues (heatrate independent imaging). The bipolar dephasing gradient had an amplitude of 25 mT/m and a 10-ms duration, applied simultaneously along all imaging axes

Figure 29 illustrates a single slice at the level of the portal vein using a single-shot GRE EPI readout with the saturation-recovery setup with the application of the saturation slice at the QRS and imaging during middle to late diastole. Although flow effects are reduced during diastolic acquisitions, the size of the flow-encoding gradients must increase and can somewhat lengthen TE and induce image distortions from eddy currents. Possible mismatch may be present in the subtracted image.

Signal differences in blood arise from TOF effects only when the two images are acquired with a finite TR, as for a 2D acquisition using the saturation-recovery concept or a 3D acquisition in which TOF effects dominate the signal differences between inflowing blood and blood remaining in the imaging volume. A low flip angle should then be used for 3D scans so that blood signal becomes more homogeneous.

Subtraction with Selective Blood Tagging

Several techniques have been reported that use a combination of blood tagging and TOF effects to produce an angiogram with a high degree of background suppression [3, 40, 41, 69–73]. In principle these techniques depict the vascular signal in a way analogous to X-ray digital subtraction angiography. The initial implementation of these techniques using multishot turboFLASH [40, 41, 69, 71] has recently been extended to single-shot and multishot EPI readouts to decrease data acquisition times or obtain higher in-plane resolution and coverage [3, 72, 73].

The STAR/SIR Concept. The basic idea of STAR [41] and SIR [39, 40, 69] is to perform a subtraction between two data sets that are identical except for the longitudinal magnetization of inflowing arterial or venous spins that have been previously tagged.

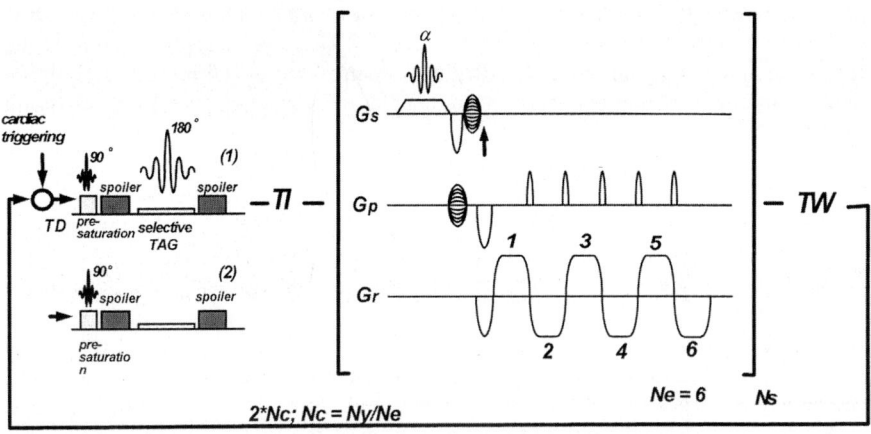

Fig. 30. Timing diagram and gradient pulse events for the 3D STAR technique using multishot GRE EPI readouts. A selective inversion pulse tags a bolus of blood on alternate readouts. A presaturation slab applied over the imaging volume for every readout prior to the application of the tagging pulse is used to reduce signal variations in stationary tissue. The inversion time (TI) corresponds to the time between the tag and the first RF applied during the readout. A complex subtraction between tagged (*1*) and untagged (*2*) acquisitions provides only signal from blood that has moved during TI to the volume of interest. Gradient timing and amplitudes are kept identical for *1* and *2* to reduce eddy currents that may introduce inhomogeneous subtraction of stationary material. With untriggered acquisitions a recovery time is incorporated before tagging to enable unsaturated blood to move into the tagging region. α, RF excitation angle; Gr, readout gradient; Gp, in-plane phase encoding gradient; Gs, section select gradient; Ny, number of in-plane phase-encoding lines; Ns, number of sections; Ne, number of echoes; Nc, number of cardiac periods encoded for a single, unsubtracted image ($=Ny/Ne$); TD, trigger delay; TW, recovery time

Blood tagging can be accomplished either by using a selective saturation or an inversion RF pulse over inflowing blood. Another tagging technique is based on the nonselective excitation of moving spins by using a flow-sensitive MP process that affects only the spins that move along the direction of the velocity-sensitizing gradients [71]. Additional presaturation pulses can be applied over the volume of interest prior to tagging to reset the magnetization of stationary material and ensure that its signal recovery is the same at each of the readouts, especially when cardiac triggering is used during the acquisition.

Signal encoding can be performed with any known k-space trajectory. Figure 30 depicts a 3D implementation of STAR/SIR using multishot EPI. With the 3D implementation illustrated, once each presaturation and tagging event is completed, all the 3D section select phase-encoding steps and part of the in-plane phase-encoding lines (corresponding to the echoes acquired per RF excitation) are acquired after the tagged spins have moved into the region of interest. When cardiac triggering is not employed, a recovery time is included prior to the next tagging/presaturation event to allow for freshly magnetized blood to enter the tagging region. The acquisition strategy for encoding k-space is similar to that of the MP acquisitions (see "Magnetization Prepared Acquisitions"); thus ensuring a smooth variation of the magnetization along all encoding axes.

Signal Strength for STAR/SIR with Single-Shot and Multishot EPI Readouts. During alternate acquisitions a single 180° adiabatic RF pulse is applied to invert the inflowing spins. The signal for STAR/SIR is determined by taking the magnitude of the complex subtraction between the tagged and untagged condition for blood to yield:

$$S_{STAR}(N_{rf}) = 2M_o sin(a)E_{TI}r^{Nrf-1}e^{-TE/T2^*} \tag{14}$$

as a function of N_{rf}, the number of RF pulses experienced by the tagged spin during the acquisition, and with *TI* referring to the inflow time, $E_{TI}=e^{-TI/T1}$, $E1=e^{-TI/T1}$, $r=E1\ cos\ \alpha$, and M_o the proton density of blood. This formula is applicable for segmented turboFLASH and multishot EPI readouts. As the number of RF pulses experienced by blood increases, the effect of the tag fades out as the signal approaches zero in the limit of a high number of excitations. Conversely, the choice of larger flip angles makes the signal converge more rapidly to zero.

For *TI=0*, the signal from STAR is maximum at the first RF pulse applied during the readout and is equal to *2M_osin(α)*. For long inflow times between the tag

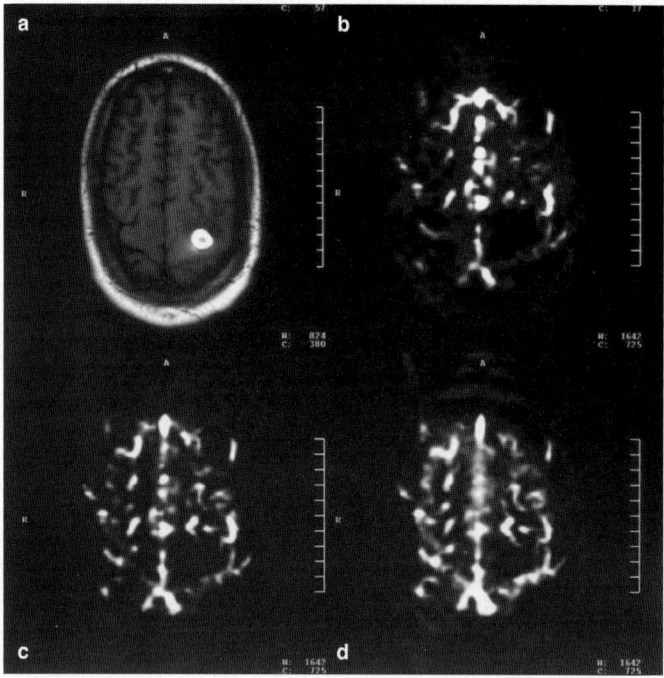

Fig. 31a–d. Qualitative perfusion brain scan using EPI STAR on a patient with a necrotic tumor in the left parietal lobe. **a** T1-weighted scan demonstrates strong paramagnetic enhancement in the tumor center. **b–d** EPI STAR demonstrates an abnormal perfusion pattern surrounding the tumor, slowly enhancing as the inflow time TI increases. The corresponding TIs are: **b** TI=400 ms; **c** TI=700 ms; **d** TI=950 ms. Blood was tagged at the base of the brain with a slab thickness of 110 mm. Sixteen acquisitions were performed for each inflow delay. A 5-mm-thick slice was excited and read with a 64-ms sinusoidal EPI readout, an echo spacing of 500 µs, TE=18 ms, 128×128 matrix, FOV=250 mm (Courtesy of Jochen Gaa, University Hospital Mannheim, Mannheim, Germany)

and the start of data acquisition the subtracted signal approaches zero with complete loss of signal from tagged spins. Magnitude subtraction can be used when the inflow time is selected longer than the inversion time for blood.

For EPI STAR a single RF excitation is applied, and the signal defined in Eq. 14 reduces to:

$$S_{STAR}(1) = 2M_o sin(a)E_{TI}e^{-TE/T2^*} \tag{15}$$

and using a 90° excitation it becomes:

$$S_{EPISTAR} = 2M_o E_{TI}e^{-TE/T2^*} \tag{16}$$

Clinical Applications of STAR in the Head. EPI STAR has been used clinically to demonstrate tissue perfusion patterns in the brain qualitatively without the use of contrast agents. This technique has the potential to detect abnormal tumor vascularity [72] and ischemic regions in stroke. Moreover, EPI STAR has also been utilized to localize the site of brain activation in functional imaging studies [73]. Although the signal at different inflow times depends on the T1 relaxation of blood, extensive lengths of the vessels may be filled by tagged protons.

Abnormal brain perfusion is demonstrated in Fig. 31 in a patient with a brain tumor in the left occipital territory. The lack of signal enhancement around the tumor for any value of the inflow delay indicates the poor vascularity of the region, subsequently confirmed using a bolus injection of Gd-DTPA and dynamic scanning with a T2*-weighted GRE EPI scan.

Rapid angiograms can also be generated in the head with 3D STAR using multishot GRE EPI without cardiac triggering. This technique is useful for screening

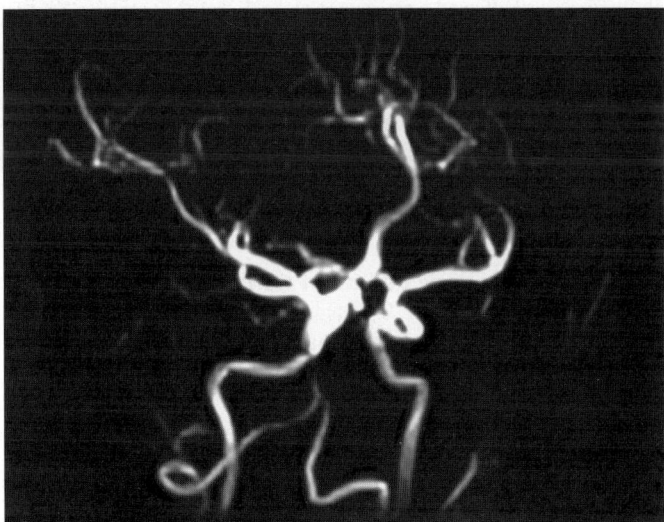

Fig. 32. MIP of the entire head of a healthy subject using 3D STAR and multishot GRE EPI readouts. Three overlapped slabs, each 48 mm thick and encoding 32 1.5-mm thin sections in 44 s, were acquired with 128×256 matrix, FOV=195×260 mm, TR/TE=9.8/3.3 ms, Ne=6, α=16°, TW=400 ms TI=300 ms, readout bandwidth of 1220 Hz/pixel. No cardiac triggering used

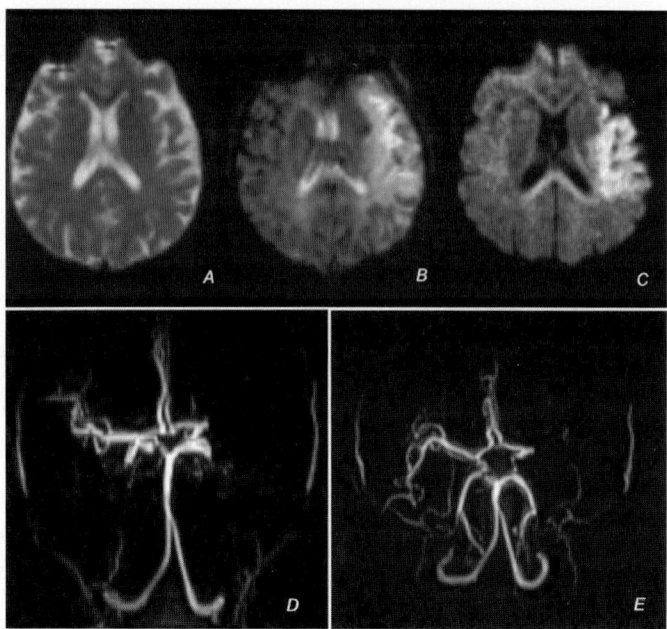

Fig. 33A–E. Patient with an early stroke of approximately 3 h localized in the left side of the brain.
A 2D single-shot SE EPI scan performed at the level of the stroke shows no signs of abnormal
tissue intensity. **B** Perfusion scan performed with single-shot GRE EPI with TE=40 ms at the
same level using a quick bolus injection of Gd-DTPA shows a regions of increased intensity
(lower perfusion) that is correlated with the territory of the left intracranial artery. **C** Diffusion-weighted single-shot SE EPI with b=1200 s^2/mm demonstrates a region with higher signal
intensity indicating a lower diffusion coefficient. Note in **B** that the perfusion defect occurs over
a larger region than that of the stroke, indicating brain tissue that may be affected at later time.
D–E Two MIPs demonstrating a complete occlusion of the left intracranial artery. Furthermore,
there is a complete occlusion of both carotid arteries. The rapid angiogram was generated with
3D STAR with a multishot GRE EPI readout. Two 64-mm-thick slabs covering the neck and the
intracranial circulation were acquired, 32 partitions per slab, 128×256 matrix,
FOV=170×260 mm, TR/TE=9.8/3.3 ms, Ne=6, α=16°, TI=300 ms, TW=400 ms, readout bandwidth of 1220 Hz/pixel. No cardiac triggering used (Courtesy of Steven Warach, Beth Israel
Hospital, Boston, USA)

patients with stroke to minimize evaluation time when used in conjunction with
diffusion-weighted and perfusion EPI scans. Figure 32 demonstrates a MIP of
the entire brain of a healthy subject using a multi-slab acquisition with 3D
STAR. Scanning time for the entire head can be kept under 3 min with isotropic
voxels and good flow sensitivity in regions such as the carotid siphon, without
the use of cardiac triggering (two faint ghosts close to the vessel have been
noted in the intracranial branches when portions run parallel to the frequency-encoding axis, similar to Fig. 14b). Figure 33 presents an example
acquired in a patient with an acute stroke in which an entire EPI protocol including diffusion, perfusion, a turboSE protocol, and a STAR 3D scan was possible
under 15 min.

Clinical Applications of STAR in the Lower Abdomen. Subtraction angiograms covering large regions of interest can be generated in several seconds. These can serve as quick localizers for a large vascular territory so that they may be used to guide a more detailed evaluation using higher resolution angiographic techniques in a vascular region of interest.

Angiography in the abdomen is always hampered by ghosting and blurring from motion artifacts, especially when 3D scanning is performed. Ultrashort TR 3D FLASH sequences (TR ~2-4 ms) using EPI hardware have recently been used in conjunction with contrast agents to cover the abdominal vascular region in a single breath-hold. Alternatively, good-quality renal angiograms can be obtained for screening purposes, for example, in a large population of healthy individuals (renal donors) [74] using STAR acquisitions without the need for contrast agents.

Obtaining maximum flow contrast with STAR for renal angiography requires that triggering be used so that tagging occurs exactly prior to systole and acquisition during diastole so that all tagged spins are injected into the region of interest. This permits renal angiograms with minimal flow effects even with single-shot EPI readouts. Figure 34 illustrates a thick transverse projection of the renal vasculature acquired with EPI STAR. Positively, EPI STAR acquired in two heartbeats shows comparable image quality as STAR acquired with a multishot turboFLASH readout module acquired in ten heartbeats.

Multishot EPI permits the acquisition of a 3D STAR renal angiogram in a single breath-hold [3]. Figure 35 demonstrates several MIP reconstructions of the renal arteries.

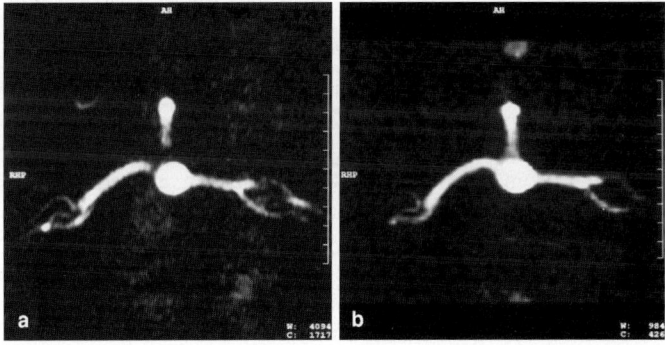

Fig. 34a,b. 2D renal angiogram using EPI STAR. **a** The renal arteries are demonstrated with a STAR technique using a multishot turboFLASH readout encoding 21 lines per segment, with a FOV=225×300 mm and a 105×256 matrix. A 25-mm inversion tag was applied along the aorta on alternate excitations prior to systole (TD=200 ms) and read with a 300 ms inflow delay. Imaging time was 10 heartbeats with a section thickness of 20 mm, sufficient to encompass the entire length of both renal arteries. **b** EPI STAR renal angiogram acquired in two heartbeats using a 64×128 matrix, 32-ms readout time, with FOV=150×300 mm. Note the similarity between the two scans. In both cases the signal readout was performed during diastole to reduce flow artifacts (Courtesy of Robert Edelman, Beth Israel Hospital, Boston, USA)

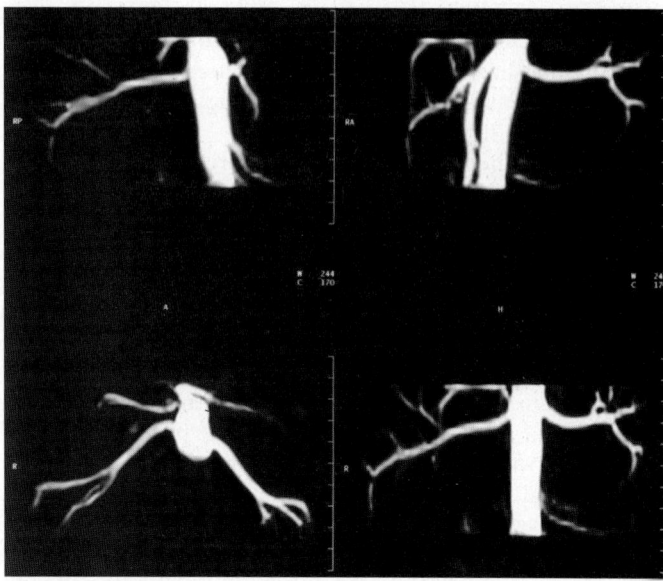

Fig. 35. MIP views of the renal arteries acquired with multishot GRE EPI 3D STAR. A 64-mm thick volume was encoded with 32 2.0-mm thin section using a 66×256 matrix, FOV=170×340 mm, TR/TE=9.8/3.3 ms, Ne=6, α=16°, TD=170 ms, TI=270 ms, readout bandwidth of 940 Hz/pixel. The aorta was tagged sagittally using a 35-mm-thick inversion slab. Imaging time was 25 s, a total of 23 heartbeats, using the posterior channels of a body phased-array coil

Phase-Contrast EPI Angiography

The phase of moving spins provides another possibility for imaging blood vessels. Phase-contrast MRA techniques utilize the additional phase shift induced on the MR signal from moving spin to produce an angiogram [36, 37, 38]. To obtain an angiogram a complex subtraction is performed between two velocity-sensitized images using a bipolar gradient structure prior to the signal readout that changes polarity between the two images. To obtain maximum flow contrast for a specific flow velocity the velocity-encoding gradients are set such that a π phase difference exists for the moving spins between the two images. Although four images are usually acquired to reconstruct an angiogram that presents flow components in all directions [38], two images can be acquired in which the direction of the bipolar gradient is chosen so that flow components perpendicular to the plane of interest defined by the magnetic gradient field are observed.

When using single-shot EPI, complete background suppression is possible only when both images have the same signal for stationary tissues for each RF excitation. This means that the acquisition must occur during steady-state conditions or when each image is acquired while all spins are fully magnetized. When cardiac triggering is employed to reduce the flow effects in single-shot

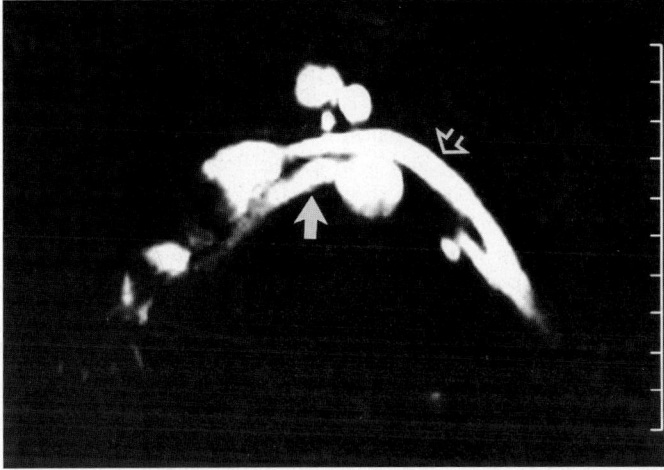

Fig. 36. 2D phase contrast single-shot EPI of the renal vessels. The right renal artery (*solid arrow*) and the left renal vein (*open arrow*) are shown. A bipolar gradient encoding a 40 cm/s velocity along the vector (1, 1, 1) was used to provide the flow contrast. A 15-mm-thick section was read with a 64×256 matrix, 51.2-ms readout time, TE=16 ms, FOV=140×280 mm, and four averages. The acquisition was cardiac triggered to diastole. To eliminate variations in the signal from stationary tissues the imaging volume was presaturated at each QRS complex. Body coil acquisition

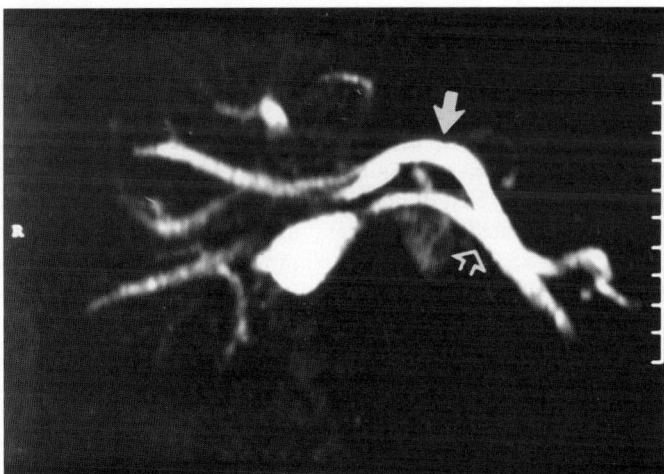

Fig. 37. 3D multishot phase contrast EPI acquisition in the abdominal region. An axial MIP created from 16 4-mm slices encoded transversely covered a 64-mm thick volume in the lower abdomen. *Open arrow*, left renal vein; *large arrow*, the splenic vein. A saturation was applied over the heart to eliminate the signal from arterial components. A 126×256 matrix was acquired with FOV=260×340 mm, TR/TE=22/9 ms, Ne=6, α=10°, readout bandwidth of 1220 Hz/pixel. Cardiac triggering was not used, assuming a fairly constant flow velocity in veins. Acquisition time was 16 s using the body coil for signal reception

EPI, the signal variation from stationary components can be reset at the occurrence of each QRS complex by presaturating the plane of section. This maneuver effectively eliminates the differences in the signal recovery between excitations induced by changes in the cardiac period. Figure 36 presents an example using a 2D PC EPI acquisition in the renal arteries acquired in two shots using cardiac triggering and setting the flow sensitivity using a bipolar gradient of equal intensity in all three imaging axes [sensitizing blood with flow components along the vector (1, 1, 1)]. Conversely, using a multishot 3D PC EPI to cover a larger volume in a single breath-hold, Fig. 37 demonstrates vascular structures in the lower abdomen encasing part of the renal and splenic veins using the same velocity sensitization as above. When vessels are oriented along a particular direction, the acquisition of two images sensitized along the direction of flow is sufficient to obtain good vascular anatomy.

Conclusions

Although MRA sequences using single-shot EPI readouts are sensitive to motion occurring on the scale of the data-acquisition window, they demonstrate sufficient immunity to flow artifacts that they may be used as an initial and rapid angiographic guide in many vascular regions in the body.

FOV limitations, flow effects, and susceptibility artifacts in single-shot EPI scans can be largely avoided by using multishot EPI acquisitions. Multishot EPI further increases the robustness of fast angiography by reducing flow displacement and blurring. However, there is a limit to the benefits of multishot EPI acquisitions that depend on the relationship between the flow velocities with respect to the length of the acquisition window, number of lines acquired per interleaf, and echo spacing. The best results are achieved in both single-shot and multishot EPI acquisitions with the shortest echo time and echo spacing that meet imaging goals, dictated mainly by the minimum FOV that is used and the flow velocities encountered in a particular vascular territory. Angiographic results are best if the data are acquired during diastole, when acceleration and associated displacement artifacts from flow components in the plane of section can be minimized. Shimming should always be performed prior to image acquisition so that the quality of the results is more consistent between studies.

In general the choice of angiographic technique is determined by the vascular territory to be imaged and the specific difficulties encountered. Results may be considered of good image quality for single-shot EPI in the brain and lower abdomen and pelvis. Multishot EPI can be used more extensively even in the thorax for imaging the pulmonary and coronary vessels. However, coverage, speed, and resolution must be carefully weighted to obtain the maximum benefits from older, more robust approaches. This should be considered, for example, when imaging in the abdomen. Enhancement of blood contrast in many instances requires preparing the magnetization of the imaged slice so that a specific contrast develops. This can be comparable to the time for imaging with turboFLASH, or conventional, ultrashort TR acquisitions. It must also be taken into account that ultrashort TE techniques can acquire images at any given time in the cardiac cycle, while it is better to restrict the use of EPI with highly pulsatile flow to data acquisition during diastole using cardiac synchronization.

References

1. Butts K, Riederer ST (1992) Analysis of flow effects in echo-planar imaging. J Magn Reson Imaging 2(3):288–293
2. Duerk JL, Simonetti OP (1991) Theoretical aspects of motion sensitivity and compensation in echo-planar imaging. J Magn Reson Imaging 1(6):643–650
3. Wielopolski PA, Adamis MK, Prasad P, Gaa J, Edelman RR (1995) Breath-hold 3D STAR MR Angiography of the renal arteries using segmented echo planar readouts. J Magn Reson Med 33:432–438
4. Wielopolski PA, Manning WJ, Edelman RR (1995) Breath-hold volumetric imaging of the heart using magnetization prepared 3D segmented echo planar imaging. J Magn Reson Imaging 4:403–409
5. Edelman RR, Mattle HP, Wallner B et al (1990) Extracranial carotid arteries: evaluation with "black blood" MR angiography. Radiology 177:45–50
6. Nishimura DG, Irarrazabal P, Meyer CH (1995) A velocity k-space analysis of flow effect in echo-planar and spiral imaging. Magn Reson Medicine 33:549–556
7. Weiskoff RM, Crawley AP, Wedeen V (1990) Flow sensitivity and flow compensation in instant imaging In: Book of abstracts: Society of Magnetic Resonance in Medicine, p 398
8. Haacke EM, Lenz GW (1987) Improving image quality in the presence of motion using rephasing gradients. Am J Roentgenol 148:1251–125
9. Duerk JL, Pattany PM (1989) Analysis of imaging axes significance in motion artifact suppression technique (MAST): MRI of turbulent flow and motion. Magn. Reson Imaging 7(3): 251–263
10. Crawley AP, Cohen MS, Yucel EK et al (1992) Single-shot magnetic resonance imaging: applications to angiography. Cardiovasc Intervent Radiol 15:32–42
11. Simonetti OP, Wielopolski P, Duerk JL (1994) Experimental evaluation of flow effects in echo-planar imaging. In: Book of abstracts: Society of Magnetic Resonance, Society of Magnetic Resonance, San Francisco, p 460
12. Edelman RR, Wielopolski PA, Simonetti L, Li W, Schmitt FX (1993) Coronary artery MR angiography with a prototype whole-body echo planar imaging system. J Magn Reson Imaging 3:58
13. McKinnon GC (1994) Interleaved echo planar phase contrast angiography. Magn Reson Med 31:682–685
14. Wildermuth S, Debatin JF, Huisman TAG, Leung DA, McKinnon GC (1995) 3D phase contrast EPI MR angiography of the carotid arteries. J Comput Assist Tomogr 19(6):871–878
15. Leung DA, Debatin JF, Holtz D, Wildermuth S, Schopke WD, McKinnon GC (1995) 3D-PC echoplanar MR-angiography of the trifurcation vessels in the lower extremities. Eur Radiol [Suppl] 5:S25
16. Holtz DJ, Debatin JF, Unterweger M, Wildermuth S, Leung DA, von Schulthess GK (1994) Phase-contrast evaluation of venous flow-augmentation: effect on ultrafast MR-venography of the calf. In: Book of abstracts: Society of Magnetic Resonance, San Francisco, p 957
17. Firmin DN, Klipstein RH, Hounsfield GL, Paley MP, Longmore DB (1989) Echo-planar high-resolution flow velocity mapping. Magn Reson Med 12:316–327
18. Guilfoyle DN, Gibbs P, Ordidge RJ, Mansfield P (1991) Real-time flow measurements using echo-planar imaging. Magn Reson Med 18:1–8
19. McKinnon GC, Debatin JF, Wetter DR, von Schultess GK (1994) Interleaved echo planar flow quantification. Magn Reson Med 32:263–267
20. Weeden VJ, Wendt RE, Jerosh-Herold M (1989) Motional phase artifacts in Fourier transform MRI. Magn Reson Med 11:114
21. Hurst GC, Hua J, Simonetti OP, Duerk JL (1992) Signal-to-noise, resolution, an bias function analysis of asymmetric sampling with zero padded FT reconstruction. Magn Reson Med 27(2):247–269
22. Margosian P, Schmitt F, Purdy D (1986) Faster MR imaging: imaging with half the data. Health Care Instrum 1:195–197

23. Fischer H, Schmitt FX, Barfuss H, Bruder H (1988) Half Fourier echo planar imaging at 2 tesla. In: Book of abstracts: Society of Magnetic Resonance in Medicine, p 972
24. Haacke EM, Lindskog E, Lin W (1991) Partial-Fourier imaging: a fast, iterative, POCS technique capable of local phase recovery. J Magn Reson 126–145
25. Nishimura DG, Jackson JI, Pauly JM (1991) On the nature and reduction of the displacement artifact in flow images. Magn Reson Med 22:481–492
26. Meyer C, Hu B, Nishimura D, Macovski A (1992) Fast spiral coronary artery imaging. Magn Reson Med 28:202–213
27. Luk Pat GT, Nishimura DG (1994) Reducing flow artifacts in echo-planar imaging. In: Book of abstracts: Society of Magnetic Resonance, p 473
28. Laub G, Deimling M, Petsch R (1994) Segmented volume imaging with multi-echo gradient echo sequences. In: Book of abstracts: Society of Magnetic Resonance, p 468
29. Feinberg DA, Turner R, Jakab PD, von Kienlen M (1990) Echo-planar imaging with asymmetric gradient modulation and inner-volume selection. Magn Reson Med 13:162–169
30. Luk Pat GT, Meyer CH, Pauly JM, Nishimura DG (1997) Reducing flow artifacts in echo-planar imaging. Magn Reson Med 37(3):436–447
31. Wielopolski P, Zisk J, Patel M et al (1993) Evaluation of ultrashort echo time MR angiography with a whole body echo-planar imager. In: Book of abstracts: Society of Magnetic Resonance in Medicine, San Francisco, p 384
32. Goldberg MA, Yucel EK, Saini S, Hahn PF, Kaufman JA, Cohen MS (1993) MR angiography of the portal and hepatic venous systems: preliminary experience with echo planar imaging. AJR 160:35–40
33. Cohen M, Goldberg M, Yucel E (1992) Ultra-fast MR angiographic methods. In: Book of abstracts: Society of Magnetic Resonance in Medicine, p 2804
34. Edelman RR (1993) Magnetic resonance angiography: an overview. Invest Radiol 28 [Suppl 4]:S43–46
35. Nishimura DG (1990) Time-of-flight angiography. Magn Reson Med 14:194–201
36. Dumoulin CL, Souza SP, Walker MF, Wagle W (1989): Three-dimensional phase contrast angiography. Magn Reson Med 9:139–149
37. Dumoulin CL, Souza SP, Darrow RD et al (1991) Simultaneous acquisition of phase-contrast angiograms and stationary-tissue images with Hadamard encoding of flow-induced phase shifts. J Magn Reson Imaging 1:399–404
38. Hausmann R, Lewin JS, Laub G (1991) Phase-contrast MR angiography with reduced acquisition time: new concepts in sequence design. J Magn Reson Imaging 1:415–422
39. Nishimura DG, Macovski A, Jackson JI, Hu RS, Stevick CA, Axel L (1988) Magnetic resonance by selective inversion recovery using a compact gradient echo sequence. Magn Reson Med 8:96–103
40. Wang SJ, Hu BS, Macovski A, Nishimura DG (1991) Fast angiography using selective inversion recovery. Magn Reson Med 18:417–423
41. Edelman RR, Siewert B, Adamis M, Gaa J, Laub G, Wielopolski P (1994) Signal targeting with alternating radiofrequency (STAR): application to MR angiography. Magn Reson Med 31:233–238
42. Balaban RS, Ceckler TL (1992) Magnetization transfer contrast in magnetic resonance imaging. Magn Reson Q 2:116–137
43. Wolff SD, Balaban RS (1994) Magnetization transfer imaging: practical aspects and clinical applications. Radiology 192:593–599
44. Edelman R, Ahn S, Chien D et al (1992) Improved time-of-flight MR angiography of the brain with magnetization transfer contrast. Radiology 184:395–399
45. Frahm J, Haase A, Matthaei D (1986) Rapid NMR imaging of dynamic processes using the FLASH technique. Magn Reson Med 3:321–327
46. Haacke EM, Masaryk TJ, Wielopolski P et al (1990) Optimizing blood vessel contrast in fast three-dimensional magnetic resonance imaging. Magn Reson Med 14:202–221
47. Keller P, Drayer B, Fram E et al (1989) MR angiography with two-dimensional acquisition and three-dimensional display. Radiology 173(2):527–532
48. Weeden V, Crawley A, Weisskoff R et al (1990) Real time MR imaging of structured fluid flow. In: Book of abstracts: Society of Magnetic Resonance in Medicine, p 164
49. Joseph PM (1985) A spin echo chemical shift MR imaging technique. J Comput Assist Tomogr 9(4):651–658
50. Dumoulin CL (1985) A Method for Chemical Shift Imaging. Magn Reson Med 2:583
51. Meyer CH, Pauly JM, Macovski A, Nishimura DG (1990) Simultaneous spatial and spectral selective excitation. Magn Reson Med 15:287–304

52. Thomason DM, Purdy DE, Finn JP (1994) Fast spectrally selective excitation in 3D gradient echo imaging. J Magn Reson Imaging 4:56

53. Thomasson DM, Moore JR, Purdy DE, Finn JP (1994) Minimum-time spatial-spectral pulses using a phase modulated 1-1 binomial pulse design. In: Book of abstracts: Society of Magnetic Resonance in Medicine, p 120

54. Purdy D, Cadena G, Laub G (1992) The design of variable flip angle slab selection pulses for improved 3-D MR angiography. In: Book of abstracts: Society of Magnetic Resonance in Medicine, p 882

55. Nägele T, Klose U, Grodd W, Petersen D, Tintera J (1994) The effects of linearly increasing flip angles on 3D inflow MR angiography. Magn Res Med 31:561–566

56. Priatna A, Paschal C (1995) Variable-angle uniform signal excitation (VUSE) for three-dimensional time-of-flight MR angiography. J Magn Reson Imaging 4:421–427

57. Nägele T, Klose U, Grodd W, NŸysslin F, Voigt K (1995) Nonlinear excitation profiles for three-dimensional inflow MR angiography. J Magn Reson Imaging 4:416–420

58. Bailes DR, Gilderdale DJ, Bydder GM et al (1985) Respiratory ordered phase encoding (ROPE): a method for reducing motion artifacts in MR imaging. J Comput Assist Tomogr 9(4):835–838

59. McKinnon GC (1993) Ultrafast interleaved gradient-echo-planar imaging on a standard scanner. Magn Reson Med 30:609–616

60. Stehling MK (1992) Improved signal in "snapshot" FLASH by variable flip angles. Magn Reson Imaging 10(1)165–167

61. Haase A (1990) Snapshot FLASH MRI: application to T1, T2, and chemical-shift imaging. Magn Reson Med 13:77–89

62. Matthaei D, Haase A, Henrich D, Duehmke E (1992) Fast inversion recovery T1 contrast and chemical shift contrast in high-resolution snapshot FLASH MR images. Magn Reson Imaging 10(1)1–6

63. Bampton AE, Riederer SJ, Korin HW (1992) Centric phase-encoding order in three-dimensional MP-RAGE sequences: application to abdominal imaging. J Magn Reson Imaging 2:3, 327–334

64. Deichmann R, Adolf H, Noth U, Morrissey S, Schwarzbauer C, Haase A (1995) Fast T2-mapping with snapshot flash imaging. Magn Reson Imaging 13:4, 633–639

65. Li D, Haacke EM, Mugler III JP, Berr S. Brookeman JR, Hutton MC (1994) Three-dimensional time-of-flight MR angiography using selective inversion recovery RAGE with fat saturation and ECG-triggering: application to renal arteries. Magn Reson Med 31:414–422

66. Brittain JH, Hu BS, Wright GA, Meyer CH, Macovski A, Nishimura DG, (1995) Coronary angiography with magnetization-prepared T2 contrast. Magn Reson Med 33(5)689–696

67. Buttain JH, Olcott EW, Szuba A, Gold GE, Wright GA, Iranrazabal P, Nishimura DG (1997) Three-dimensional flow independent peripheral angiography. Magn Reson Med 38(3):343–354

68. Axel L, Morton D (1987) MR flow imaging by velocity-compensated/uncompensated difference images. J Comput Assist Tomogr 11:31–34

69. Nishimura DG, Macovski A, Pauly JM (1988) Considerations of magnetic resonance angiography by selective inversion recovery. Magn Reson Med 7:472–484

70. Dixon WT, Du LN, Faul DD, Gado M, Rossnick S (1987) Projection angiograms of blood labeled by adiabatic fast passage. Magn Reson Med 4:193–202

71. Korosec FR, Grist TM, Polzin JA, Weber DM, Mistretta CA (1993) MR angiography using velocity-selective preparation pulses and segmented gradient echo acquisition. Magn Reson Med 30:704–714

72. Gaa J, Warach S, Wen P, Thangaraj V, Wielopolski P, Edelman RR (1996) Noninvasive perfusion imaging of human brain tumors with EPISTAR. Eur Radiol 6:518–522

73. Edelman RR, Siewert B, Darby DG, Thangaraj V, Nobre AC, Mesulam MM, Warach S (1994) Qualitative mapping of cerebral blood flow and functional localization with echo-planar MR imaging and signal targeting with alternating radio-frequency. Radiology 192:513–520

74. Adamis MK, Gaa J, Edelman RR (1994) STAR (signal targeting with alternating radio-frequency) renal artery imaging. J Magn Reson Imaging 4:S22

CHAPTER 9

Diffusion Imaging with Echo-Planar Imaging

R. Turner

What Is Diffusion?

By diffusion we mean the random, thermally activated motion of particles from site to site, often given the name of Brownian motion, after its first observer. This may be self-diffusion, as in the case of a pure liquid in which we may conceptually label one of the molecules and follow its motion over the course of time, or diffusion of one type of particle among others, such as the movement of hydrogen atoms through certain types of metal, the movement of small dust particles through still water, or the diffusion of water molecules through cell membranes. In solids self-diffusion is extremely slow because the energy barriers separating atomic sites are considerably greater than the thermal energy available, $3kT/2$ per molecule.

If means can be devised in which the average displacement over time of molecules in a given environment can be measured, much information can clearly be obtained about the nature of that environment. For a pure liquid Einstein showed that this displacement r is related to the elapsed time t and a diffusion coefficient D by the relationship:

$$\bar{r} = \sqrt{6Dt} \tag{1}$$

This follows from the diffusion equation for the concentration c of the labeled molecules:

$$\frac{dc}{dt} - DV^2c = 0 \tag{2}$$

which in turn derives from Fick's first law relating the molecular flux to the concentration gradient.

Why Is Diffusion Important in Biological Tissue?

Tissue can be alive only within a relatively narrow temperature range, from about 273 K to 315 K, when many components of tissue are in a liquid or liquid-crystalline state, or in water solution. In consequence, diffusion plays a large part in the transport of enzymes, metabolic substrates, and metabolites. It is crucial for water, comprising 60 %–95 % of tissue by volume, to be in the liquid state, so that it can serve as a carrier for biochemical compounds and as a participant in many reactions. Tissue is very inhomogeneous on a microscopic level: the membranes forming cell boundaries and organelles present obstacles to the movement of water and other molecules which are highly characteristic of tissue type, as is seen below. The measurement of water mobility can probe this local environment.

Thus it can be predicted that mapping of water molecular mobility, which can be characterized by an apparent diffusion coefficient (ADC) [1, 2], will give useful information regarding tissue type and tissue pathology. Many examples are provided elsewhere in this volume.

Methods of Measuring Diffusion

The simplest and earliest method for measuring the diffusion of one substance in another is to use a tracer [3], which can be injected into the sample at one point and assayed over time at another point in space, giving a measure of the diffusion coefficient if active transport does not occur. In animal models the technique of microdialysis has provided fascinating insights into transport of biochemical compounds. If a measure of self-diffusion, for instance, water in water, is required, radioisotopes may be employed as the tracer.

Another technique is that of quasielastic neutron scattering [4], in which slow neutrons are used to probe the velocity distribution of water molecules. Accurate values of the diffusion coefficient for very small molecular displacements may be obtained by such methods, which make a useful complement to the more macroscopic but less invasive techniques on which we focus here, based on magnetic resonance (MR).

The Effect of Diffusion on the MR Signal

Consider a water sample in an MR imaging (MRI) scanner, of static field B_0. If a linear magnetic field gradient G_x is applied during the free induction decay following a radiofrequency (RF) excitation pulse, the precession frequency ω of a proton in the sample depends on its x coordinate:

$$\omega = \gamma(B_0 + G_x x) \tag{3}$$

Now suppose a particular proton, as part of its water molecule, moves diffusively through the sample with a displacement in the x direction, given by $\xi(t) = \xi_0 + \delta(t)$, where ξ_0 is the mean position of the proton. After a time T the phase angle ϕ accumulated in the rotating frame by the proton spin is:

$$\phi = \int_0^T \omega \, dt = \gamma \int_0^T G_X \, \xi(t) \, dt = \gamma \int_0^T G_X \, (\xi_0 + \delta(t)) \, dt \tag{4}$$

If the gradient direction is now reversed for an additional time T (Fig. 1), the net phase angle accumulated is:

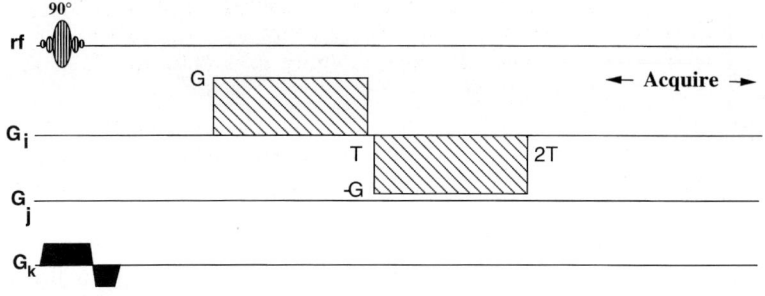

slice selection gradients   diffusion gradients

Fig. 1. Bipolar diffusion-weighting gradient pulses

$$\phi = \gamma\, G_X \left(\int_0^T \delta(t)\, dt - \int_T^{2T} \delta(t)\, dt \right) \tag{5}$$

Clearly, if the protons did not move, this phase accumulation would be zero, and all the proton spins in the sample would be brought back into phase at time 2T. However, the protons do diffuse, and it is easy to see that the residual phase angle gives a measure of the extent of this movement (Fig. 2). The amplitude S(t) of the free induction decay at time 2T is given by:

$$S(2T) = \int_V \rho(r)\, \exp\left(i\phi(r, 2T)\right)\, d^3r \tag{6}$$

where $\rho(r)$ is the proton density.

If the protons follow a true random walk, obeying the diffusion equation (Eq. 2), this can be rewritten [1, 2, 5]:

$$S(2T) = S(0)\, \exp(-bD) \tag{7}$$

where:

Fig. 2. Evolution of the phase in the transverse plane of static spins and spins moving with constant velocity, experiencing the diffusion gradients of Fig. 1. Note that moving spins are not refocused (phase = 0) at the same time as static spins, and that the degree of phase offset at t = TE depends on velocity

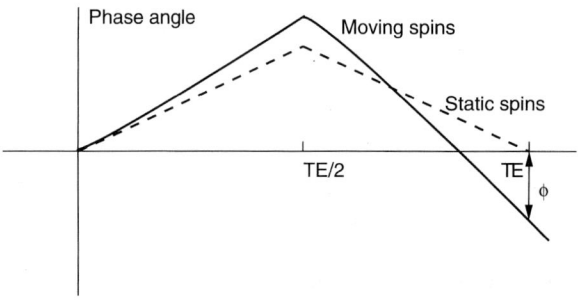

$$b = \int_0^{2T} |k(t)|^2 \, dt \tag{8}$$

$$k(t) = \gamma \int_0^t G(t') \, dt' \tag{9}$$

G(t) describes all of the gradients applied during the time 2T between the RF excitation pulse and the formation of the gradient echo, and S(0) is the amplitude of the free induction decay just after the RF excitation pulse.

Equation 7 describes a pure attenuation of the MR signal, such that a plot of ln[S(2T)/S(0)] against the gradient factor b gives a straight line of slope –D. The usual way of determining the diffusion coefficient by MR consists of measuring S(2T) for a range of values of G, keeping the gradient pulse duration and separation fixed. For pure liquids it is also feasible to keep G fixed and to vary T, but this method does not give a linear plot of ln[S(2T)/S(0)] versus b for systems with microscopic inhomogeneity. For the gradient configuration shown in Fig. 1, the gradient factor b is:

$$b = 2\gamma^2 \, T^3 \, G^2/3 \tag{10}$$

neglecting the finite gradient rise time. This shows the characteristic quadratic dependence on G, and the strong dependence on the duration of the diffusion gradients.

More frequently the spin-echo version of this experiment is used [5], in which the first gradient lobe is followed by a 180° refocusing pulse and then another gradient lobe with the same polarity, amplitude, and duration as the first (Fig. 3). If the gradients are on for a duration T for each lobe, and the onset of each is separated by a time τ, the b factor becomes:

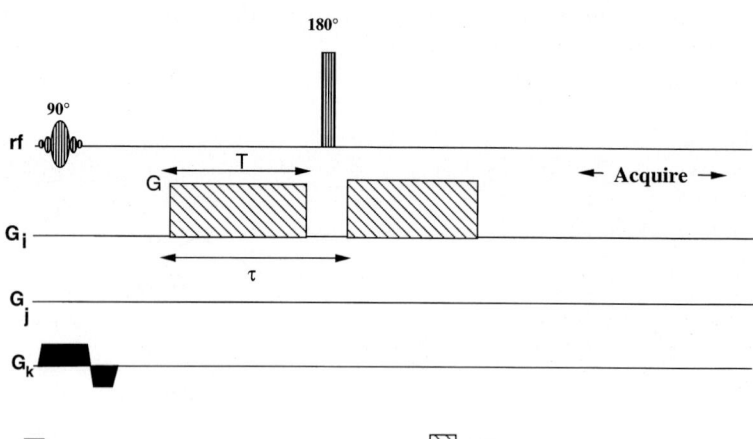

Fig. 3. Stejskal-Tanner gradient pulses in a spin-echo sequence

$$b = \gamma^2 \ G^2 \ T^2 \ (\tau - T/3) \tag{11}$$

The same expression is appropriate for the gradient-echo case of Fig. 1 if the two gradient lobes are separated in time. For $T \ll \tau$ the situation arises in which a short gradient pulse dephases the spin magnetization, the molecules freely diffuse for a time τ, and then the second gradient pulse refocuses the spin magnetization, giving a signal diminished by the degree to which diffusion has moved the spins away from their original positions. In this case the time τ can be viewed as a *diffusion time*, the time during which the molecular motion is sampled. In the general case it is less easy to define a diffusion time since the spin dephasing is taking place more slowly, while the molecules are diffusing.

This type of approach has been used for many years to measure diffusion and self-diffusion coefficients.

Restricted and Hindered Diffusion

Typically the diffusion coefficient of water measured in tissue at body temperature is about $1 \times 10^{-5} \ cm^2 \ s^{-1}$, perhaps one-third of what it would be in pure water. This already suggests that the 10%–20% nonaqueous content of tissue presents considerable hindrance to the free mobility of water. Use of the Einstein relation (Eq. 1) shows that a water molecule takes less than 4 ms to diffuse to the boundary of a 10-µm-diameter cell from its center. There are many reasons to suppose (see other chapters of this volume) that the cell membrane, composed of a bilamellar sheet of phospholipids and embedded proteins, acts as a partial barrier to water diffusion. Thus an MR experiment in which the diffusion time is longer than, say, 5 ms, would be sensitive to the effects of the effects of the cell boundary. In practice it is difficult to perform experiments with shorter diffusion times because (see Eq. 11) very large, rapidly switched gradients are then needed to provide large enough b factors to give accurately measurable attenuation. Such powerful gradients are not usually available on commercial MR systems.

More usually experiments are performed with diffusion times longer than 10 ms, and the value of D just quoted refers to such measurements. It is entirely possible that for very short diffusion times the effective value of D increases to close to its pure water value [4]. If the cell boundary is impermeable to water, as in the case of yeast cells [6] and plant cells [7], it is correct to speak of *restricted* diffusion. In this case the apparent value of the diffusion coefficient decreases monotonically as the diffusion time is increased. If, as in most animal cells, the membrane allows some water flux, it is better to describe the diffusion as *hindered*. Here the diffusion coefficient tends to an asymptote for long diffusion times, corresponding to the hindrance to water mobility presented by the membranes.

Diffusion Imaging by MRI

In order to form a map of the spatial variation of the ADC in an object it is only necessary to apply the diffusion-weighting gradients at appropriate points in an MRI sequence. The technique of diffusion imaging was pioneered by Bushell [8] and Le Bihan [1, 2], who used a standard spin-echo sequence, inserting equal gradient pulses on either side of the 180° refocusing pulse (Fig. 3). Such a sequence gives an image with greater loss of intensity in regions of relatively higher ADC, the effect increasing with larger gradient values. A series of such images with different gradient strengths provides enough information to allow the computation of a diffusion image, showing the spatial variation of ADC as varying image intensity. This can give valuable information in a number of clinical contexts, such as stroke and brain tumors, because it is inherently different from images weighted by the relaxation times T1 and T2. The ADC, expressing water mobility in tissue, is a more fundamental physical parameter which is independent of the assumptions leading to the Bloch equation and of the MR frequency used.

Images showing information about spatial variations of the diffusion coefficient can be presented in several ways. The simplest is simply to show the raw image resulting from the application of large diffusion gradients [30]. Here regions with low diffusion coefficients appear anomalously bright, as in the case of brain infarcts within a few hours of the ischemic insult. More quantitative images of the ADC can be created by evaluating:

$$\frac{ADC(x, y)}{b} = -\ln \frac{S(x, y, G)}{S(x, y, 0)} \tag{12}$$

for each pixel, after acquiring only two images, without and with a diffusion gradient G applied, and displaying the "diffusion image" with an appropriate gray scale so that dark regions have a low ADC and vice versa.

Diffusion maps which are more accurate still can be generated if more than two values of diffusion gradient are used. With a fast MRI acquisition, such as echo-planar imaging (EPI), as many as 16 different values of G, corresponding to 16 values of b, can be obtained in less than a minute. The attenuation with increasing b of each pixel in the resulting images may then be fitted to the exponential decay of Eq. 7, using the nonlinear least-squares Levenberg-Marquardt algorithm [9] to extract the important variable ADC. This may then be displayed as an image as before.

Motion Artifact

Early work [1, 2] using the conventional spin-echo intravoxel incoherent motion (IVIM) technique at low field (0.5 T) gave satisfactory images, but work at higher fields was marred [10, 11] by the pervasiveness of motion artifact. In conventional multi-pulse imaging, even without diffusion gradients, motion artifact arises when the object or part of the object is displaced by a distance Δx, say, between successive acquisition cycles. The subsequent echo is phase modulated by the function exp(ikΔx), where k is the phase-space coordinate, and so there is a discontinuity between this and the previous echo. Once the complete data set is collected, and the two-dimensional Fourier transform performed to produce an image, such a discontinuity manifests itself as the familiar ghost artifact distributed in the phase-encode direction seen in many images. Since the magnitude of the discontinuity depends on k (a first-order effect), the power in the ghost images is large only in the case of gross motion such as in major vessels, the chest wall during breathing, and the heart.

However, the situation is much worse when the large gradients used in diffusion imaging are applied. The signal then depends on the velocity of coherent and incoherent flows within the object, as well as its displacement. For no artifact to appear *all* of these variables must be the same at each echo acquisition. Cardiac gating is of some benefit, especially in brain imaging, but noncyclic changes in blood flow and perfusion, CSF flow, and involuntary patient motion often cause unreliable results. The phase factor introduced by a variation of velocity of Δv between successive echoes is now of the form $\exp(i\gamma G\Delta v\, t^2)$, where t is the time during which the diffusion gradients are applied (Fig. 2). There is a discontinuity at all values of k (a zeroth-order effect), and the ghost images can have a large enough amplitude to make calculation of the diffusion image meaningless. This has been found to be the case even in so static an organ as the brain. The low amplitude pulsations of the brain tissue and CSF [12] are large enough to give uninterpretable or highly misleading results. While some recent progress has been made using so-called turbo-FLASH techniques [13], in which a diffusion-weighted "spin-preparation module" is followed by a very rapid series of low flip-angle RF pulses with gradient-echo image acquisition, the signal-to-noise ration is poor, and the contrast arises from a complex mixture of T1, T2, and diffusion contributions.

A much more rapid method for gathering diffusion-weighted images is therefore desirable. In 1986 Turner [14] suggested that EPI, the snapshot MRI technique developed by Mansfield [15], could be equipped with diffusion gradients and form the basis of a motion artifact-free method of diffusion imaging. The first EPI diffusion-weighted images were shown by Avram and Crooks [16]. With EPI the entire set of echoes to be Fourier-transformed to form an image is collected in a single acquisition period of 25–100 ms. No discontinuity can possibly arise between successive data points, and hence there can be no motion-derived ghosting. Even if there were motion as large as several voxel widths during this short acquisition, only blurring and banding of the image would be likely to result. Such velocities are not normally encountered in the brain.

Echo-Planar Diffusion Imaging Sequences

EPI may be sensitized to flow and diffusion in precisely the same way as conventional spin-echo or gradient-echo imaging sequences. For a spin-echo sequence a pair of diffusion gradient pulses of the same polarity may be placed on either side of the refocusing 180° pulse, or if a gradient-echo sequence is desired, a bipolar pair of gradients may be placed before signal acquisition (Fig. 1).

The major problems involved in implementing diffusion EPI stem from the same causes; the shortness in tissue of the transverse relaxation time T2 and the inhomogeneity-related dephasing time T2*. If too long a time elapses between the excitation of the spin system and the acquisition of data, no signal remains to be observed. Thus the large excursions of the trajectory in k space needed in order to provide reasonable resolution must be traversed very rapidly, typically in 50–100 ms; thus large, rapidly switched gradients must be provided. Furthermore, the diffusion gradients must be of short duration, less than 40 ms per lobe, say. Given typical tissue values for D of $0.5–1.0 \times 10^{-3}$ mm^{-2} s^{-1}, this implies that gradient strengths of at least 10 mT/m are desirable for this gradient too, if a significant diffusion-related signal attenuation is to be obtained.

Both of the IVIM EPI sequences described above have been successfully implemented on 1.5-T whole-body gradient-echo Signa scanners [17a, b], a Siemens 1.5-T prototype scanner [18], and 2.0- and 4.7-T medium-bore gradient-echo chemical shift imaging systems [19, 20]. Most studies described in this volume were performed at 64×64 or 64×128 resolution. Other work [21] has been performed using a gradient-echo Signa system retrofitted with fast imaging gradients and acquisition hardware (Advanced NMR Systems, Woburn, Mass.).

An essential precaution is to obtain the best shim possible with the magnet used. EPI image quality depends critically on good field homogeneity (see Chap. 2, this volume).

Whole-Body Implementation

Normal commercial whole-body gradient hardware gives gradients up to 10 mT/m, but the switching time of 0.5–1.0 ms is far too slow to allow the 64 or more gradient switches to be made in the time available before the signal decays. Switching time of 400 ms or less is required for EPI to be feasible, and a maximum gradient strength of about 20 mT/m is needed to achieve an in-plane resolution of 2.5×2.5 mm.

These stringent gradient requirements may be met by using the existing gradient coils while increasing the number or power of the gradient current amplifiers so that a larger current is made available, along with a higher maximum voltage to raise the current faster to its desired value. This is the strategy currently employed by Mansfield [22], and in commercial implementations of EPI for whole-body imaging. The alternative is to build a small special-purpose gradient coil which fits over the head, which can be designed to give much greater efficiency and smaller inductance than standard whole-body gradient coils. In this case no additional gradient power supplies are required. Besides the work of Turner, the principal proponent of this approach has been the laboratory of Hyde [23].

Using the target field coil design method [24] a z-gradient coil with 20 cm diameter volume of linear gradient, with 100 µH inductance and 40 mT m^{-1} (100 A)$^{-1}$ efficiency can be designed. Such coils can be compact enough to fit round the head in such a way that the shoulders are barely touching the end, yet the entire brain can be imaged without distortion. Transverse gradient coils which have such excellent specifications are not feasible [25], but reasonably compact designs of about half this efficiency for the same inductance have been built [26, 27].

It is possible to build an RF coil inside the gradient coil former, but great care must be taken to reduce coupling between the gradient coil and the RF coil. Preferably, if space permits, the RF coil should be equipped with a copper shield, broken up using capacitors in order to obviate eddy currents induced by gradient coil switching. Such a shield may be conveniently made by placing overlapping strips of copper foil alternately on the inside and outside of a very thin plastic film, the film itself acting as the dielectric forming the required capacitors. If an RF shield cannot be fitted, it is possible to reduce coupling by judicious placement of pieces of copper foil, screening the gradient wires themselves from the RF fields. These should be tuned to create an antiresonance mode in the gradient coils, thus preventing inductive coupling to the RF coil. A simple four-element RF saddle coil can be used, with a balanced capacitive-match feed, and also equipped with copper foil guard rings to avoid excessive RF electric fields within it, which in the presence of a patient's head causes detuning, reduction in Q, and unacceptable power deposition.

The reliability of IVIM EPI sequences should be established using experiments on water-containing phantoms. A bottle containing undoped water can be imaged with varying diffusion gradients. The signal from a given region of interest is plotted against gradient b factor [4] and should agree with the theoretical predictions, with a value of the diffusion constant close to that found by the majority of workers [1, 2].

Studies in Human Brain

Diffusion EPI has been successfully carried out on both volunteers and patients using a gradient-echo Signa 1.5-T imaging system and the small head coil described above. The rate of switching of the current in this coil was restricted so that a maximum rate of magnetic field variation of 16 T/m was experienced by the subject, well below the maximum specified in guidelines of the United States Food and Drug Administration. No nonauditory sensory effects were reported by any subject. The acoustical noise generated during switching was sufficiently loud that all subjects wore earplugs for comfort.

Typically a series of 8 or 16 images of a single slice was collected, with different diffusion gradient strengths. A repetition time of 4 s was used. Each imaging shot was usually preceded by a phase reference shot with the phase-encode gradient switched off, which was used to correct the echo spacing and hence to avoid the "Nyquist ghost" artifact which otherwise appears half-way across the field of view (FOV) from the image (see Chap. 3, this volume). Even with the highest diffusion gradient used, 38 mT/m for a duration of 20 ms per lobe, no motion artifact could be seen on the image. Images were normally obtained using the spin-echo MBEST [22] sequence, echo time TE 100 ms, 16 cm FOV, 10-mm slice thickness, 64×64 pixel matrix. With no diffusion weighting the single-shot signal-to-noise ratio in gray matter was about 50. The image contrast

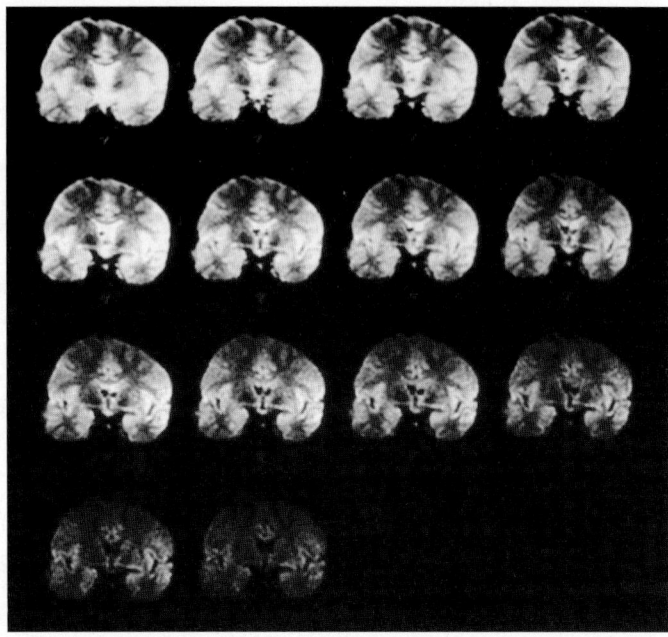

Fig. 4. Set of 14 diffusion-weighted 64×64 coronal EPI images of volunteer head. FOV = 16 cm, slice thickness = 10 mm, TE = 100 ms, TR = 4 s, total acquisition time per image = 50 ms. The diffusion gradient duration was 20 ms/lobe, and the maximum gradient used was 38 mT/m

was dominated by tissue T2 variations, as shown in Fig. 4. Gray and white matter could be clearly distinguished, and the anisotropy of the diffusion coefficient in white matter [17, 28, 29] was easily observable, the intensity from fibers running perpendicular to the diffusion gradient decreasing more slowly than that of fibers parallel to the gradient.

These results have been reproduced in several laboratories, and other chapters of this volume provide details of useful applications of the techniques described.

Hardware Requirements for Diffusion Imaging

In order to obtain good quality diffusion-weighted images, from which quantitative measures of ADC may be obtained, it is vital to have good RF stability and high-quality gradient hardware. Eddy currents, which can cause gradients to persist several milliseconds longer than they should, can be avoided by the use of a local gradient coil, as described above, or by active shielding of the gradient coil, both of which minimize the fringe fields leading to eddy current formation. Eddy current compensation, in which the gradient coil current is adjusted to cancel out some of the lingering gradient fields, is helpful, but because of the nonuniform character of these lingering fields both in time and space, it is best applied as an adjunct. With MRI scanners designed for EPI operation this generally does not present a problem since for that sequence it is necessary to have large, rapidly switchable gradients.

In some commercial MRI scanners the gradient fields are linear only within a rather small volume, in order to reduce the gradient current driver power requirements, and hence cost. Since the error in the calculated diffusion coefficient varies as the square of the gradient, quite large inaccuracies may result. The alternatives are either to obtain accurate gradient field plots, allowing appropriate corrections to be made, or to install gradient coils with better specifications.

Application of Diffusion Imaging

There are now two areas in which diffusion EPI is proving to be the technique of choice. These are evaluation of ischemic stroke at the hyperacute and acute stages, and mapping of fiber tract directions in brain white matter.

It has been shown by many workers [30] that within 5 min of loss of blood flow to a region of brain tissue the membrane pumps become depleted of energy and cease functioning. Thus there is no longer any counter to the osmotic pressure between the dilute extracellular fluid and the osmolyte-rich cytoplasm. The result is a movement of water from the extracellular space (about 10%–20% of the total tissue volume) to within the cells. The cells swell to a point at which the membranes of adjacent cells can be in close contact, separated only by their respective coatings of glycocalyx. This affects water mobility in tissue in two ways. The first relates to extracellular motion. Water does not easily cross the cell membrane, and thus for it to travel far in the tissue it must do so by way of the extracellular space. If this space is obliterated by cell swelling, water mobility is inevitably reduced. Model calculations [31] suggest that another mechanism is also important. The cytoplasm is crowded with organelles and large molecules of various kinds, which impede the movement of water molecules considerably. When there is cell swelling, a larger proportion of water molecules experience this more hindered environment, again reducing the ADC.

What observations in animal models and recently in humans have shown is that this reduction in ADC is very easily observable using diffusion-weighted MRI within 5 min of the onset of ischemia, far sooner than with any other imaging technique. The ischemic region is clearly demarcated, with a visible boundary presumably corresponding to the threshold of cerebral perfusion allowing normal metabolic functioning of the membrane pumps. Furthermore, if the ischemic is maintained, the ADC value in the ischemic region continues to evolve in time, decreasing further for several hours, then returning to baseline, and finally rising above baseline as the cells, starved of nutrients, necrose, and disintegrate [32]. It is only at this stage that other imaging techniques such as conventional T2-weighted MRI and computed tomography can visualize the ischemic lesion.

The ability to visualize the extent, and by reference to the change in ADC, the severity of the ischemic insult, at a very early stage of stroke, gives an unprecedented opportunity for effective stroke therapy. However, a crucial element in the

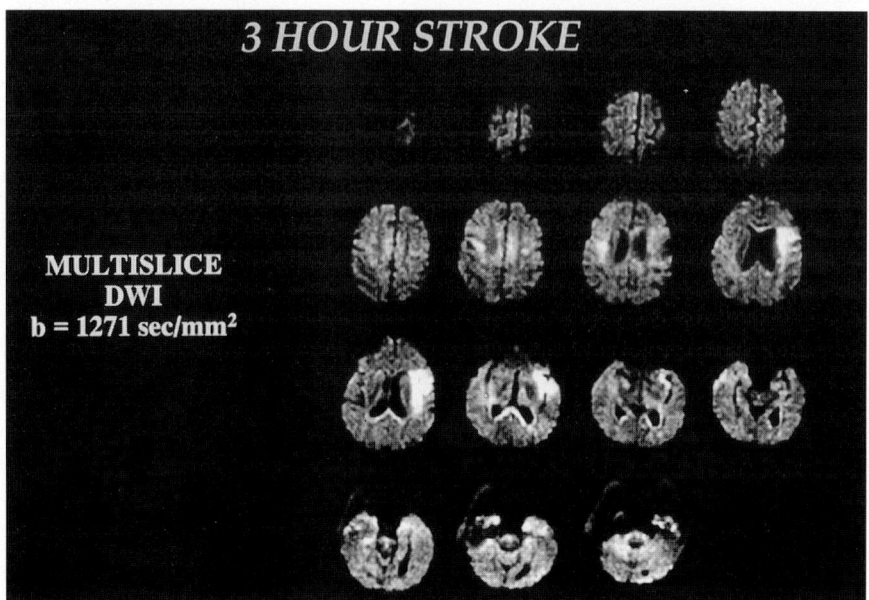

Fig. 5. Diffusion-weighted echo-planar images of the brain of a patient in acute stroke. Note the hyperintense regions showing reduced water mobility associated with cell swelling. (Provided by S. Warach, Harvard Medical School)

potential success of this approach is the use of rapid, artifact-free MRI diffusion imaging techniques. Stroke patients may be in poor condition and cannot tolerate long imaging times. Head motion may be difficult to prevent. Scanning of the entire brain is most desirable to ensure that no ischemic areas have been missed. The only technique capable of fulfilling these requirements is diffusion-weighted EPI. In the hands of Warach [33] (Fig. 5) and Sorenson [34] the technique has now been used for more than 100 cases of stroke, with excellent results. The efficacy of neuroprotective and anticoagulant drug therapy can be directly and rapidly assessed [35].

A further development of diffusion-weighted EPI arose from the observation that diffusion of water in white matter is highly aniotropic, as we have pointed out. The cell membrane and the myelin sheath surrounding an axon represent quite significant barriers to water molecules, which can move much more easily along the axonal lumen and in the extracellular space along the axon direction. In cases such as these it is best to write the generalized diffusion coefficient as a tensor D [36] where now Fick's law must be rewritten:

$$J = -D \, \nabla c$$

where J is the current of the diffusing molecules (in this case water). The six independent elements of D can be determined in principle at any point in the brain with seven MRI experiments, with diffusion gradients placed in turn along six different directions. With this information it is possible [36] to determine the direction of greatest water mobility, which corresponds naturally to the mean direction of the white matter fibers lying within the volume of interest.

Conclusions

Single-shot EPI enables precise, reproducible measurements of diffusion coefficients of human brain tissue in vivo, without confusing motion artifacts. The implications for effective and timely evaluation of hyperacute stroke [18, 30] in humans are considerable since an entire imaging session need take no more than 5 min. For further research work the rapidity and ease of acquiring images of adequate quality facilitate far more detailed analyses of the attenuation curve than heretofore.

References

1. Le Bihan D, Breton E (1985) Imagerie de diffusion in-vivo par resonance magnetique. CR Acad Sci [II] 15:1109–1112
2. Le Bihan D, Breton E, Lallemand D, Grenier P, Cabanis E, Laval-Jeantet M (1986) MR imaging of intravoxel incoherent motions: application to diffusion and perfusion in neurologic disorders. Radiology 161:401–407
3. Jost W (1960) Diffusion in solids, liquids, gases. Academic, New York
4. Hazlewood CF, Rorschach HE, Lin C (1991) Diffusion of water in tissues and MRI. Magn Reson Med 19:214–216
5. Stejskal EO, Tanner JE (1964) Spin diffusion measurements: spin echoes in the presence of a time-dependent field gradient. J Chem Phys 42:288–292
6. Corey DG, Garroway AN (1990) Measurement of translational displacement probabilities by NMR: an indicator of compartmentation. Magn Reson Med 14:435–444
7. Von Meerwall E, Ferguson RD (1981) Interpreting pulsed-gradient spin-echo diffusion experiments with permeable membranes. J Chem Phys 74:6956–6959
8. Taylor DG, Bushell MC (1985) The spatial mapping of translational diffusion coefficients by the NMR imaging technique. Phys Med Biol 30:345–349
9. Le Bihan D, Turner R, Moonen CTW, Pekar J (1991) Imaging of diffusion and microcirculation with gradient sensitization: design, strategy and significance. J Magn Reson Imaging 1:7–28
10. Merboldt KD, Bruhn H, Frahm J, Gyngell ML, Hänicke W, Diemling M (1989) MRI of 'diffusion' in the human brain: new results using a modified CE-FAST sequence. Magn Reson Med 9:423–429
11. Chenevert TL, Brunberg JA, Schielke GP (1989) Quantitative improvement of in vivo tissue perfusion and diffusion imaging. In: Book of abstracts: Society of Magnetic Resonance in Medicine 1989. Berkeley, Society of Magnetic Resonance in Medicine, 1989, p 62
12. Poncelet B, Wedeen VJ, Cohen MS, Weisskoff RM, Brady TJ (1991) Brain motion measurement with EPI. In: Book of abstracts, Society of Magnetic Resonance in Medicine 1991. Berkeley: Society of Magnetic Resonance in Medicine, 1991, p 855
13. Deimling M, Mueller E, Laub G (1990) Diffusion weighted imaging with turbo-FLASH. In: Book of abstracts: Society of Magnetic Resonance in Medicine 1990. Berkeley: Society of Magnetic Resonance in Medicine. 1990, p 387
14. Turner R (1988) Perfusion studies and fast imaging. In: Rescigno A, Boicelli A (eds) Cerebral blood flow. Plenum, New York, pp 245–258
15. Mansfield P (1977) Multi-planar image formation using NMR spin echoes. J Phys C 10:L55–L58
16. Avram HE, Crooks LE (1988) Effect of self-diffusion on echo-planar imaging. In: Book of abstracts: Society of Magnetic Resonance in Medicine 1988. Berkeley: Society of Magnetic Resonance in Medicine, 1988, p 980

17a. Turner R, Maier J, Vavrek R, Le Bihan D (1989) EPI diffusion imaging of the brain at 1.5 tesla without motion artifact using a localized head gradient coil. In: Book of abstracts: Society of Magnetic Resonance in Medicine 1989. Berkeley: Society of Magnetic Resonance in Medicine, 1989, WIP, p 1123

17b. Turner R, Le Bihan D, Maier J, Vavrek R, Hedges LK, Pekar J (1990) Echo-planar imaging of intra-voxel incoherent motion. Radiology 177:407–414

18. Warach S, Wielopolski P, Edelman RR (1993) Identification and characterization of the ischemic penumbra of acute human stroke using echo-planar diffusion and perfusion imaging. In: Book of abstracts, Society of Magnetic Resonance in Medicine 1993. Berkeley, Society of Magnetic Resonance in Medicine, 1993, p 249

19. Turner R (1989) Single shot imaging at 4.7 tesla. Relaxation times, GE NMR Instrum. Newslett 6:4–6

20. Turner R, Le Bihan D (1990) Single-shot diffusion imaging at 2.0 tesla. J Magn Reson 86:445–452

21. McKinstry RC, Weisskopf RM, Cohen MS, Vevea JM, Kwong KK, Rzedzian RR, Brady TJ, Rosen BR (1990) Diffusion-weighted Imaging of the Brain using EPI. In: Book of abstracts: Society for Magnetic Resonance Imaging, WIP, p 5

22. Howseman AM, Stehling MK, Chapman B, Coxon R, Turner R, Ordidge RJ, Cawley MG, Glover P, Mansfield P, Coupland RE (1988) Improvements in snapshot nuclear magnetic resonance imaging. Br J Radiol 61:822–828

23. Wong EC, Bandettini PA, Hyde JS (1992) Echo-planar imaging of the human brain using a three axis local gradient coil. In: Book of abstracts, Society of Magnetic Resonance in Medicine 1992. Berkeley, Society of Magnetic Resonance in Medicine, 1992, p 105

24. Turner R (1986) A target field approach for optimal coil design. J Phys D 19:L147–L151

25 Turner R (1988) Minimum inductance coils. J Phys E 21:948–952

26. Wong EC, Jesmanowicz A, Hyde JS (1991) Coil optimization for MRI by conjugate gradient descent. Magn Reson Med 21:39–48

27. Turner R (1993) Gradient coil design: a review of methods. Magn Reson Imaging 11:903–20

28. Moseley ME, Cohen Y, Mintorovitch J, Chileuitt L, Shimizu H, Kucharczyk J, Wendland MF, Weinstein PR (1990) Early detection of regional cerebral ischemia in cats: comparison of diffusion- and T2-weighted MRI and spectroscopy. Magn Reson Med 14:330–346

29. Chenevert TL, Brunberg JA, Pipe JG (1990) Anisotropic diffusion in human white matter: demonstration with MR techniques in vivo. Radiology 177:401–405

30. Moseley ME, Kucharczyk J, Mintorovitch J et al (1990) Diffusion-weighted MR imaging of acute stroke: correlation with T2-weighted and magnetic susceptibility-enhanced MR imaging in cats. AJNR 11:423–429

31. Szafer A, Zhong J, Gore JC (1995) Theoretical model for water diffusion in tissues. Magn Reson Med 33:697–712

32. Helpern JA, Dereski MO, Knight RA, Ordidge RJ, Chopp M, Qing ZX (1993) Histopathological correlations of nuclear magnetic resonance imaging parameters in experimental cerebral ischemia. Magn Reson Imaging 11:241–246

33. Warach S, Gaa J, Siewert B, Wielopolski P, Edelman RR (1995) Acute human stroke studied by whole brain planar diffusion-weighted magnetic resonance imaging. Ann Neurol 37:231–241

34. Sorensen AG, Buonanno FS, Schwamm L, Lev MH, Huang-Hellinger FR et al (1995) Diffusion and perfusion weighted MR imaging in the clinical diagnosis of acute stroke. Proceedings, Third Meeting of the Society of Magnetic Resonance, p 81

35. Lo EH, Matsumoto K, Pierce AR, Garrido L, Luttinger D (1994) Pharmacological reversal of acute changes in diffusion-weighted magnetic resonance imaging in focal cerebral ischemia. J Cereb Blood Flow Meta 14:597–603

36. Basser PJ, Mattiello J, Le Bihan D (1994) MR diffusion tensor spectroscopy and imaging. Biophys J 66:259–267

37. Moseley ME, Kucharczyk J, Mintorovitch J et al (1990) Diffusion-weighted MR imaging of acute stroke: correlation with T2-weighted and magnetic susceptibility-enhanced MR imaging in cats. AJNR 11:423–429

CHAPTER 10

Echo-Planar Imaging of the Abdomen

P. Reimer and R. Ladebeck

Introduction

Magnetic resonance imaging (MRI) of the abdomen has been of limited clinical value because of long examination times, motion artifacts, and lack of suitable contrast agents [1–7]. Echo-planar MRI (EPI) and its derivatives have been developed to provide ultrafast imaging capability thus eliminating motion-related volume-averaging and phase-encoding artifacts (Fig. 1) combined with the acquisition of purely T2-weighted images using single-excitation techniques (TR = ∞) [8–19]. Major disadvantages in the past have been the need for specifically designed systems, suboptimal resolution (64×64 or 64×128), narrow magnet bores, limited multi-slice capability, and restricted slice orientation [20–23]. Limitations due to poor signal-to-noise ratio (SNR) have encouraged a trend from low-field MR systems to middle- or high-field MR systems [1, 10, 20, 24–26]. EPI is currently being prepared for installation into clinical MR systems by various manufactures [1, 9, 20, 24] because recent technical advances provide multi-slice capability, almost free-slice orientation, anatomical resolution, and sufficient SNR values [1, 27, 28]. EPI and its derivatives can be performed on conventional scanners, and a wide spectrum of pulse sequences is available [14, 15, 17–19, 29]. The purpose of this chapter is to describe the potential clinical applications of abdominal EPI.

Fig. 1a–c. Motion reduction with EPI. Conventional MR images and EPI in a patient with ascites at 1.5 T (GE Signa and ANMR Hyperscan, Wilmington, Mass.). **a** T1-weighted SE images (TR/TE/NAQ 250/20/4).

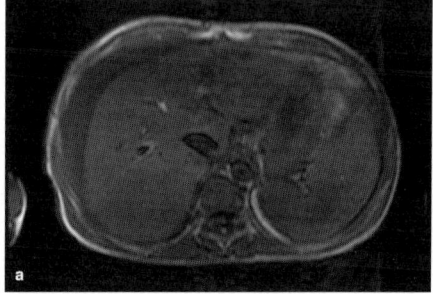

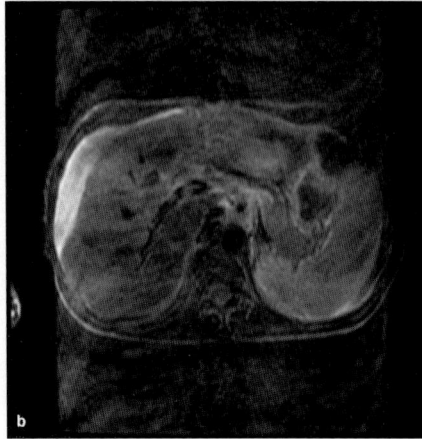

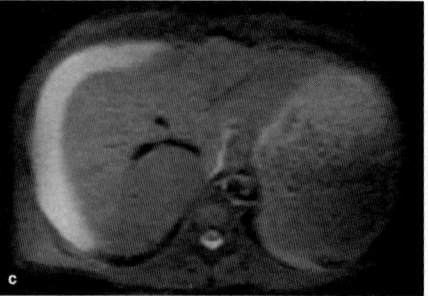

Fig. 1a–c. (continued) **b** Conventional T2-weighted SE images (2200/100/4). **c** Single-excitation T2-weighted SE EPI (∞/26/1). These images demonstrate reduction in motion artifacts caused by ascites on EPI compared to conventional MRI

Imaging Parameters for Abdominal EPI

Technical parameters in EPI are more complex than those of conventional MRI. Therefore, the effect of various operator-defined parameters on image quality in EPI of the abdomen must be discussed. Clinical EPI imaging requires careful attention to the choice of imaging parameters.

Breath Holding

EPI facilitates breath-held examinations of the entire abdomen within 5–10 s. However, various techniques are available, such as single-excitation acquisitions with high temporal but limited spatial resolution (128×128 matrix) and segmented techniques with reduced temporal but improved spatial resolution (128×256, 256×256, or 128×512 matrix) [30], and therefore the potential benefit of breath-hold versus non-breath-hold images must be clarified. Significant improvements in resolution, as for rapid spin echo (RARE), turbo-spin echo, fast spin echo, and turbo-gradient spin echo (GRASE) imaging techniques [14, 15, 19, 31] with a 256–512×512–1024 matrix, are unlikely to be feasible since high-resolution EPI techniques suffer from low SNR [19, 32].

The lack of breath holding has little effect on image degradation for single-excitation images, supporting the notion that EPI is fast enough to eliminate motion-induced signal loss and artifacts (Fig. 2). However, breath-hold single-excitation EPI is required to avoid skips in anatomical coverage and to obtain a defined slice position. For segmented k space techniques such as mosaic scanning breath holding is required additionally to achieve the full signal for data acquired in the same plane to and maintain image quality.

Because two-excitation images are blurred and grainy when acquired during breathing, this technique is unlikely to be applied in patients unable to maintain adequate breath holding (Fig. 2). When single- and two-excitation images are

Fig. 2a,b. Effect of breath
holding in abdominal EPI at
1.5 T (ANMR Hyperscan).
a Liver SNR shown (mean±SD)
for breath-held (*bh*) and non-
breath-held (*nbh*) acquisitions.
Liver SNR decreases significantly ($p<0.05$) on non-
breath-held acquisitions when
a two-excitation technique is
applied.

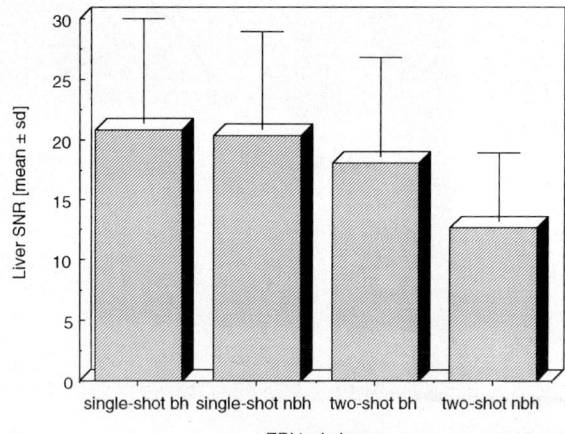

a   EPI techniques

b Comparison between
single-excitation SE
(TR ∞, TE 26 ms) –
breath-hold (*upper left*)
and non-breath-hold
(*lower left*) – and two-
excitation SE (TR 6 s,
TE 26 ms) – breath-
hold (*upper right*) and
non-breath-hold (*lower
right*) – abdominal
EPI images show that
only two-excitation
images are blurred
when acquired during
breathing

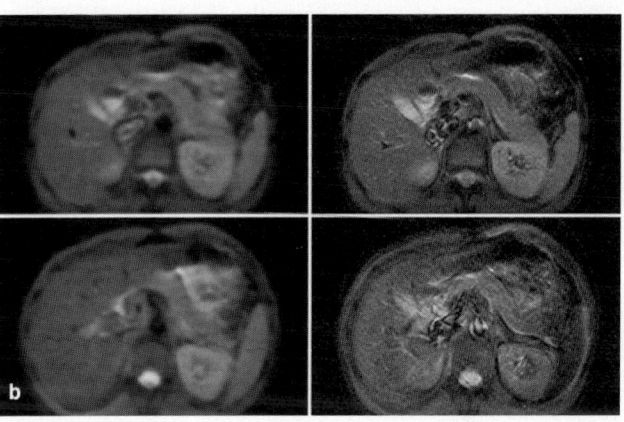

acquired with the same 128×256 acquisition matrix, SNR in single-excitation
images is higher than in two-excitation images. This unequivocally demonstrates
the superiority of single-excitation techniques in avoiding losses in SNR due to
motion between successive excitations [32].

Slice Thickness

Incremental reduction in slice thickness of EPI images results in significantly
lower SNR in abdominal organs than does the next thicker slice. Qualitatively,
images become unacceptable when slice thickness is reduced below 6–7 mm
using the body coil (Fig. 3). Since freezing motion is a major advantage of single-excitation EPI, signal averaging from multiple acquisitions at a given plane
which would compensate for loss in SNR at thinner slices may not be advantageous except perhaps in combination with perfect breath holding [32].

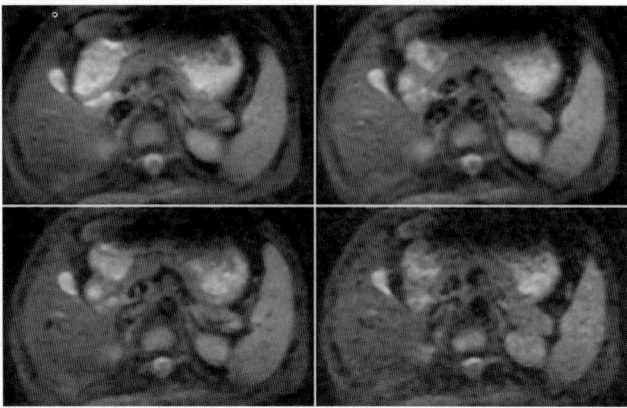

Fig. 3. Effect of slice thickness on image quality. EPI at 1.5 T (ANMR Hyperscan). Single-excitation SE (TR ∞, TE 26 ms) abdominal EPI with decreasing slice thickness from 10 mm (*upper left*), 8 mm (*upper right*), 6 mm (*lower left*), and 4 mm (*lower right*) with a constant interslice gap of 50 %. SNR of parenchymatous abdominal organs (liver, spleen, pancreas, and kidney) decreases substantially with decreasing slice thickness, and image quality appears nondiagnostic below a slice thickness of 6 mm

K Space

The effect of changes in raw data or k space coverage [1] on SNR is important in understanding the drawbacks of decreasing the k space coverage which is required to shorten TE time. Increasing the k space coverage is intended to increase SNR due to the extended acquisition period. The SNR is proportional to the square root of the imaging time (k space fraction) if the MR data are distributed evenly in k space. Smaller imaging features should show greater SNR

Fig. 4a,b. Effect of k space coverage on SNR of abdominal organs. EPI at 1.5 T (ANMR Hyperscan). **a** SNR (mean-±SD) of abdominal organs decreases with decreasing k space coverage, which is required to obtain images with shorter echo time.

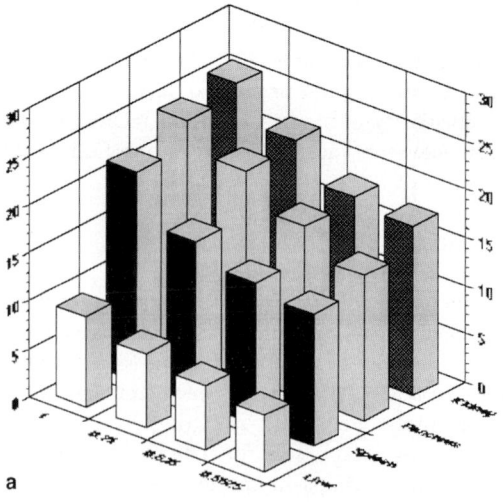

a

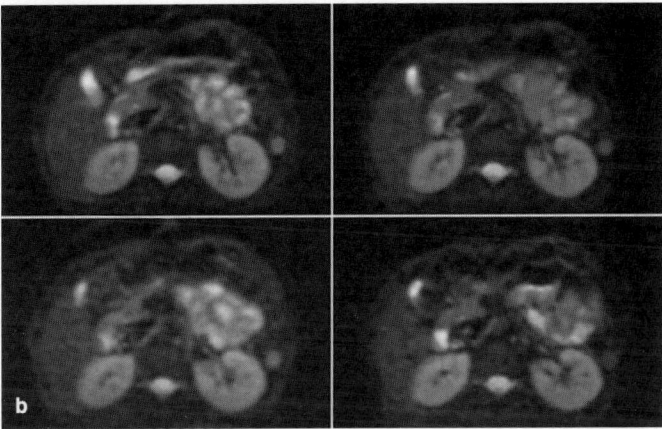

Fig. 4a,b. b Single-excitation SE (TR ∞, TE 73 ms) abdominal EPI with decreasing k space coverage from full k space coverage (*upper left*), 75 % (*upper right*), 63 % (*lower left*), and 57 % (*lower right*) show decreasing image quality with decreasing k space coverage going along with decreasing SNR

advantage as coverage is increased. The acquisition of EPI images with full k space coverage is desirable from a SNR point of view; however, a TE minimum of 73 ms is inappropriate for abdominal EPI. Therefore, k space coverage is adjusted to a smaller TE time, with the drawback of decreasing SNR (Fig. 4). Thus to further optimize image quality the maximum k space coverage at a given TE should be exploited. Automatic adjustment of the maximum k space coverage possible at a given echo time should be implemented in clinical EPI systems as a standard feature.

Contiguous Imaging

Contiguous imaging is feasible as a clinical tool without decrease in SNR due to cross-talk at scan times or a breath-hold of longer than 12 s (Fig. 5). This should be considered whenever a decrease in TR is required to shorten the time for breath-hold in patients, or when T1-weighted images are obtained. In a multi-slice acquisition the odd-numbered images are obtained in the first half of the duration of scan time and hence they have an infinite TR. However, the even-numbered images are obtained in the second half of the scan time and may have a noninfinite effective TR due to interslice cross-talk. The time between excitation of adjacent slices is approximately breath-hold/2 (assuming the images are spaced evenly over the breath-hold). As a result of cross-talk effects tissues with long T1 times may show a significant decrease in SI in the even-numbered images in comparison to odd numbered images when breath-holds of under 10–12 s are used.

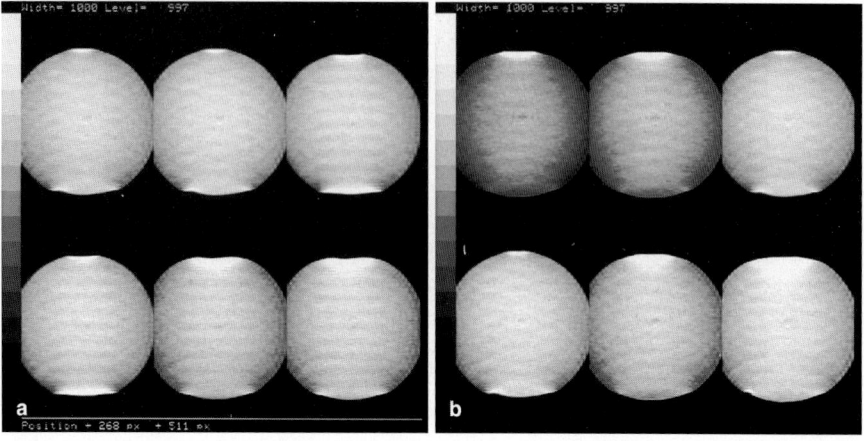

Fig. 5a,b. Contiguous imaging: effect of TR on cross-talk effects. Signal intensity behavior of two adjacent slices (first and second slices in a multi-slice slab) in a water phantom is shown for increasing TR time. **a** Odd-numbered slices: *upper left row,* TR times of 4, 6, and 8 s; *lower row,* TR times of 10, 12, and 14 s. **b** Even-numbered slices: *upper left row,* TR times of 4, 6, and 8 s; *lower row,* TR times of 10, 12, and 14 s. Note that SI increases gradually on the even-numbered slice with increasing TR times

Hepatic EPI

MRI techniques have been advocated for screening of focal liver lesions [33]. However, "portal" computed tomography (CT) and dynamic contrast-enhanced CT have been reported to be equal or superior to present conventional MR techniques for the detection of focal liver lesions [34–37]. Various fast (turbo-FLASH, turbo-spin echo, fast spin echo) and ultrafast MRI techniques (EPI, GRASE, turbo-gradient spin echo) have been introduced to overcome the limitations of conventional MRI of the abdomen [1, 9, 12, 14, 15, 18, 19, 24, 31, 38, 39].

EPI Pulse Sequence Options

The array of pulse sequence options available for EPI are similar to that of conventional MRI [36, 40–44]. EPI can be performed with the following techniques: spin echo (SE; T2-weighted, proton density weighted, partial saturation T1-weighted), inversion recovery (IR; T1-weighted), and gradient echo (GE; T1, T2, and T2* weighted).

Signal intensity behavior of the liver has been investigated comparing conventional MRI and T1 and T2-weighted EPI techniques [45, 46]. With varying TE one observes on SE images differences in tissue signal intensity related to T2 decay. Similarly, variation of TI time produces T1-related effects on IR images. Within any given set of T2-weighted sequences an increase in TE results in decreased SNR (Fig. 6). The single-excitation technique with a 128×128 acquisition matrix shows significantly higher SNR than the two-excitation technique with a 128×256 acquisition matrix ($p<0.05$). On T1-weighted images the short TI (100 ms) and long TI (800 ms) IR sequences have a significantly ($p<0.05$) higher SNR than with an inversion time of 380 ms near the null point of the liver (Fig. 6).

Quantitative data (Fig. 6) also demonstrate that single-excitation T2-weighted EPI with short TE has a significantly higher liver SNR than two-excitation T2-weighted, single-excitation T1-weighted EPI, and conventional SE techniques ($p<0.05$). Multi-slice two-excitation techniques require a breath-hold of about 12 s, making them more susceptible to spatial misregistration. However, there is a tradeoff between anatomical resolution and SNR. When the matrix size is increased from 128×128 to 256×128, the SNR is expected to decrease as a result of the two-fold reduction in voxel volume. Although the expected decrease in SNR is only $\sqrt{2}$, experimental data demonstrate somewhat lower SNR, presumably as a consequence of abdominal motion between excitations.

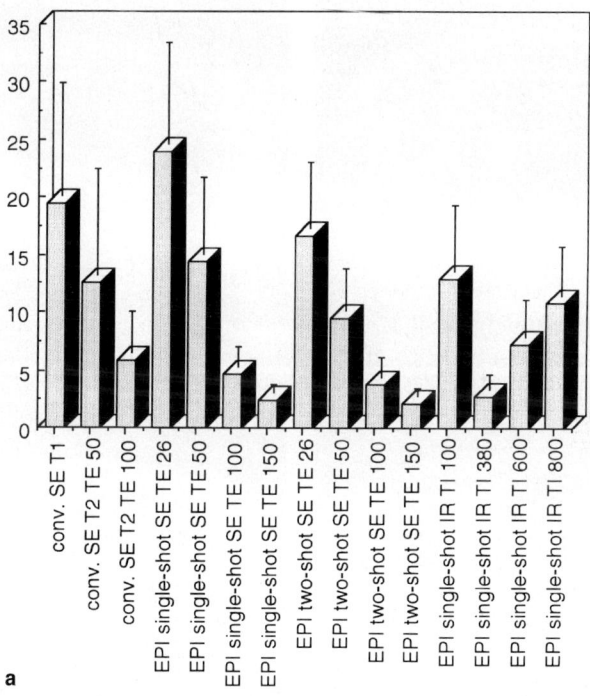

a

Fig. 6a–f. Hepatic EPI: SNR and image quality. **a** Liver SNR for T1- and T2-weighted conventional MR and EPI. Liver SNR of SE single-excitation T2-weighted EPI is higher than conventional MRI and comparable for T2-weighted SE two-excitation EPI. SNR of single-excitation IR EPI depends on the inversion-time (lowest SNR near null point of the liver at TI 380).

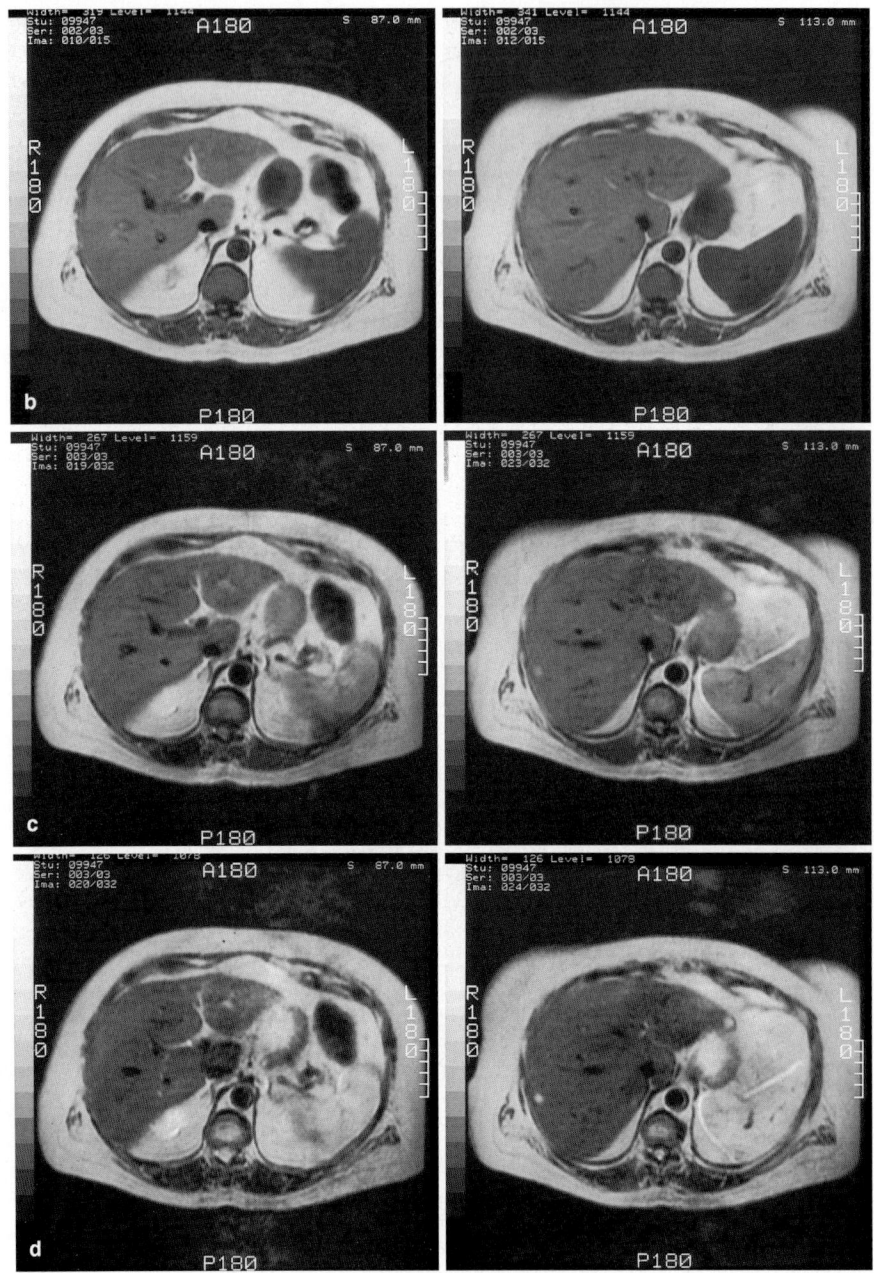

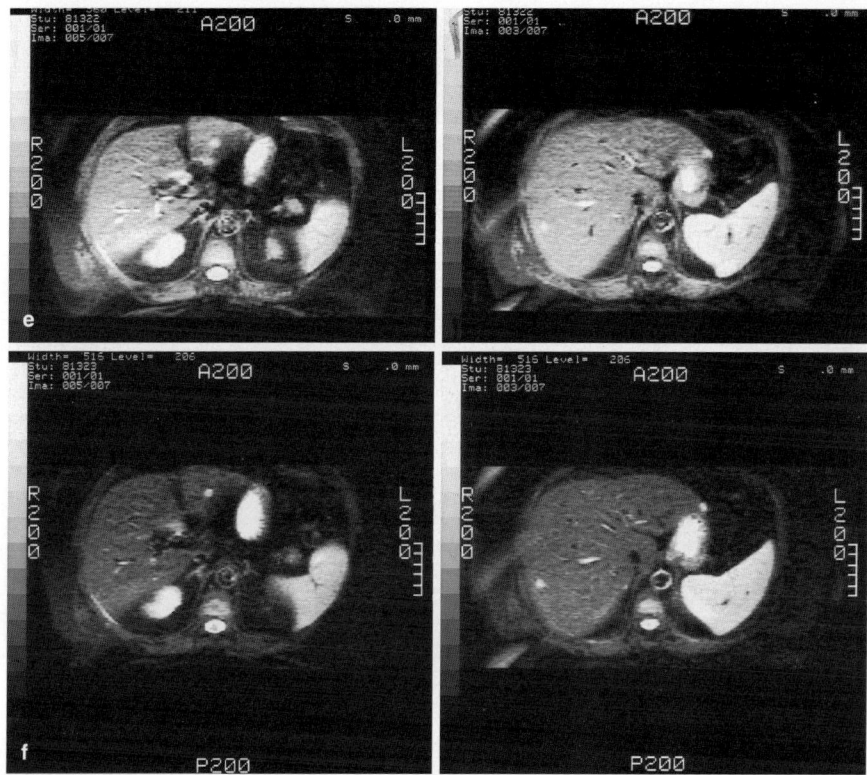

Fig. 6a–f. (continued) **b–f** Hepatic EPI and conventional MR images in a patient with multiple metastases: EPI at 1.5 T (GE Signa and ANMR Hyperscan). **b** Two adjacent conventional T1-weighted SE images (TR/TE/NAQ 250/20/4). **c,d** Conventional T2-weighted SE images (**c** 2200/50/2; **d** 2200/100/4). **e,f** Single-excitation T2-weighted SE EPI (**e**, ∞/26/1; **f**, ∞/50/1). Liver metastases in both liver lobes are identified readily on EPI with comparable liver SNR and superior tumor-liver contrast

Since hepatic SNRs are similar to those in conventional MRI, all prerequisites are available to apply this technique to the detection and characterization of focal hepatic lesions. These might be detected and identified based upon the difference in their signal behavior and good tissue contrast (Fig. 7), as has previously been demonstrated in hepatic MR [12, 47]. IR techniques nulling the signal from normal liver (Fig. 7) may be advantageous for lesion detection [48], despite their limited SNR, because focal lesions have different null points and therefore appear hyperintense at this TI [48].

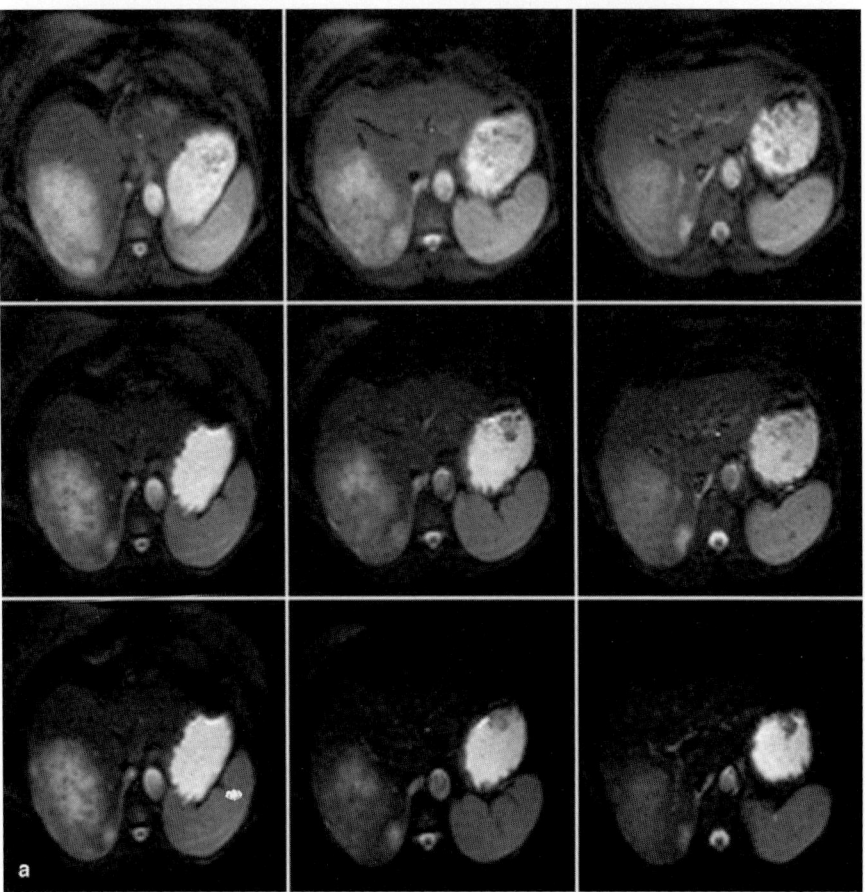

Fig. 7a,b. Image contrast at 1.0 T. Adjacent images of a patient with primary cholangiocarcinoma imaged at 1.0 T (Siemens, Erlangen). **a** Single-excitation T2-weighted SE EPI: *upper row,* TE 35 ms; *middle row,* TE 70 ms; *lower row,* TE 100 ms. **b** Single-excitation T1-weighted IR EPI (TE 35 ms): *upper row,* TI 100 ms; *middle row,* TI 300 ms. Liver signal decreases with increasing TE on SE images and is low near the null point of the liver with a TI time of 300 ms on IR images showing high tumor-liver contrast

Detection of Focal Liver Lesions

Contrast-enhanced dynamic CT and conventional MRI are currently the imaging modalities of choice for detecting focal liver lesions. Therefore the performance of EPI must be compared to these two modalities.

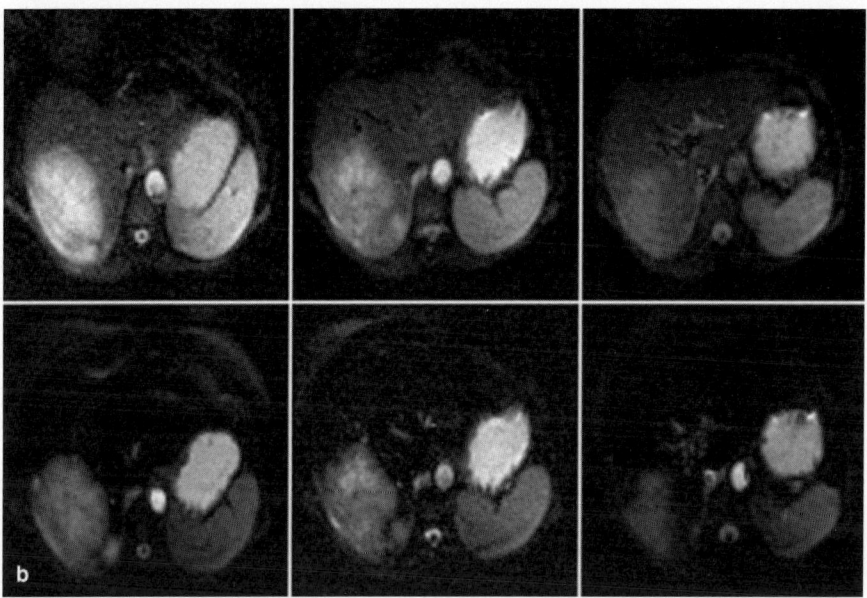

b

Contrast-Enhanced Dynamic CT

Detectability of focal lesions with EPI has also been compared to that with dynamic contrast-enhanced CT [49]. Patients were examined preoperatively, and imaging results were compared to those from surgery and pathology. In this study CT was performed on state-of-the art CT scanners using standard technical parameters. EPI was performed on an experimental 1.0-T system (Siemens, Erlangen) using fat-suppressed single-excitation spin-echo (TR = ∞, TE 35/70/100 ms) and single-excitation IR techniques (TR = ∞, TE 35 ms, TI 100/300 ms). All images were obtained in suspended expiration, and patients were instructed to breathe in a sequential, reproducible pattern between scans. K space was covered by a sinusoidal resonant read gradient together with a constant phase gradient [50].

Single-shot SE with a TE of 70 ms showed the best lesion detectability as measured by the area under the receiver-operating characteristic (ROC) curve [49]. The tendency towards EPI techniques was obvious (Fig. 8); however, the difference between ROC values of contrast-enhanced CT and T2-weighted single-excitation EPI with an echo-time of 70 ms was not statistically significant ($p<0.1$). Among EPI techniques the IR sequence with a TI of 300 ms to null liver showed high lesion liver contrast, but all reviewers have reported problems assessing liver size and anatomy [49]. These results are encouraging since optimized CT techniques were used as an imaging gold standard for comparison. Future technical developments in EPI are likely further to improve image quality and therefore diagnostic performance.

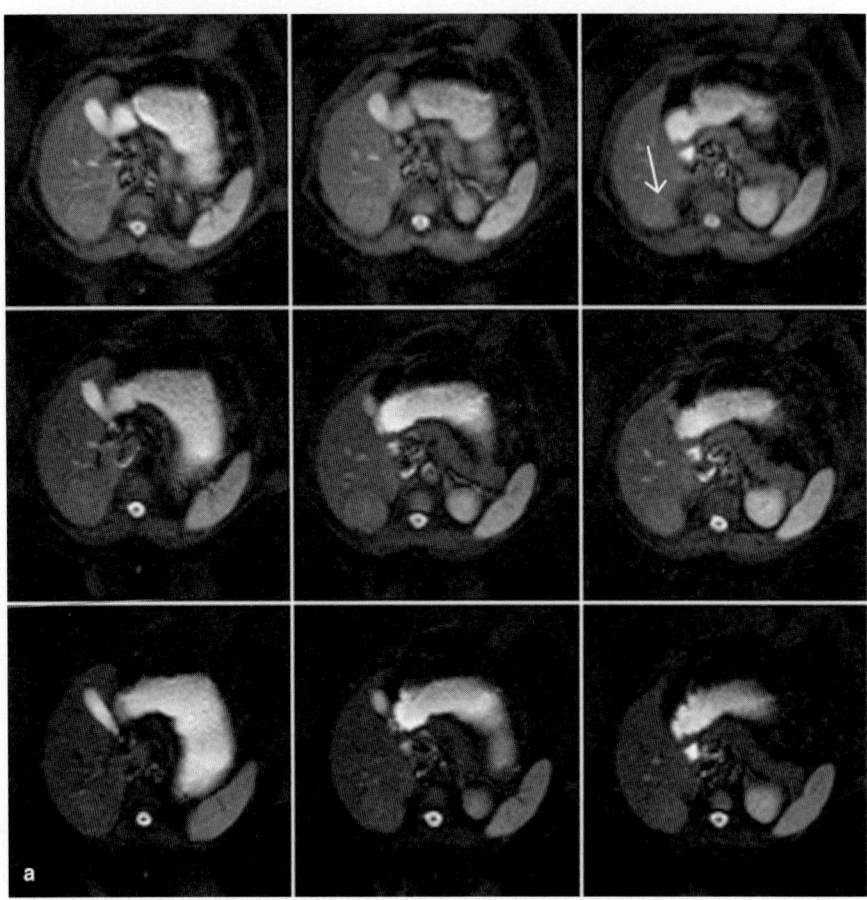

Fig. 8a–d. EPI versus CT. Adjacent images of a patient with FNH imaged at 1.0 T (Siemens, Erlangen). **a** Single-excitation T2-weighted SE EPI: *upper row*, TE 35 ms; *middle row*, TE 70 ms; *lower row*, TE 100 ms. **b** Single-excitation T1-weighted IR EPI: *upper row*, TI 100 ms; *middle row*, TI 300 ms. **c,d** CT scans (Somatom Plus, Siemens) showing the lesion on unenhanced (**c**) and contrast-enhanced images (**d**). EPI shows comparable tumor-liver contrast as CT demonstrating comparable detectability of focal liver lesions with EPI

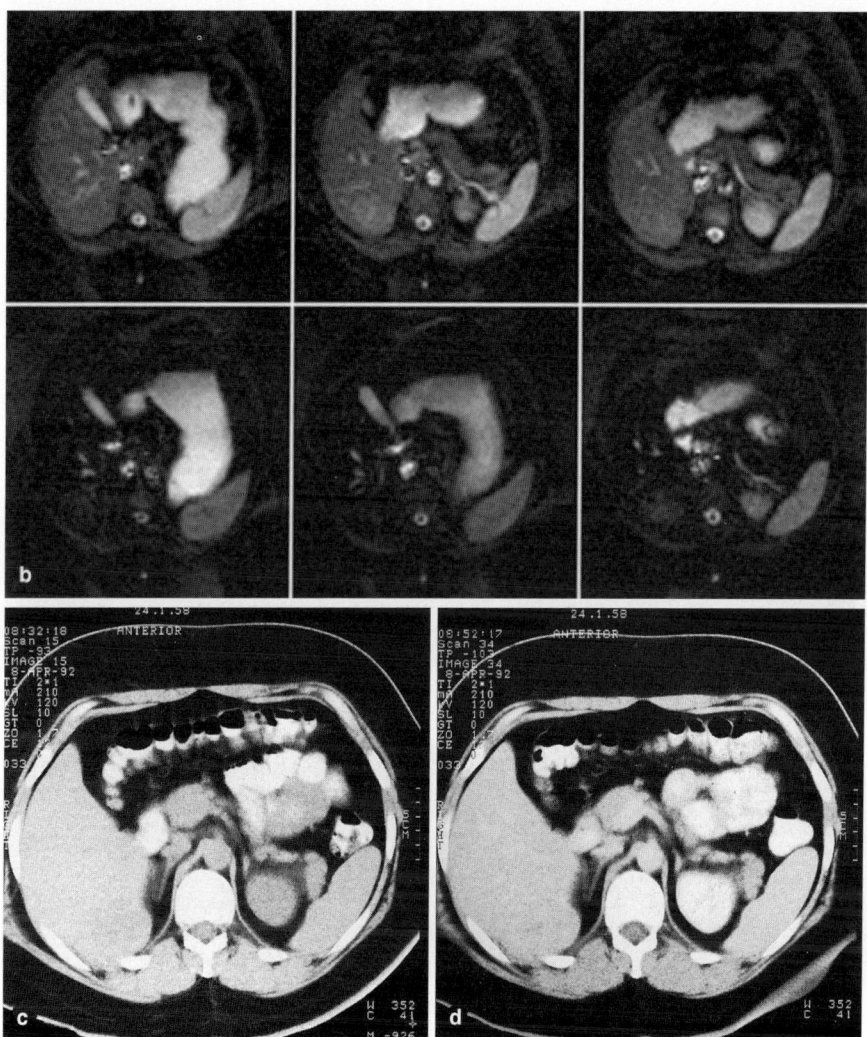

Quantitative Analysis Compared to Conventional MRI

Detection of focal liver lesions on a commercially available 1.5-T system has been compared to conventional MRI based on quantitative analysis [45, 46]. T2-weighted single-excitation SE techniques at TE of 50 and 100 ms and T1-weighted IR techniques with TI of 100 and 380 ms a provide significantly ($p<0.05$) higher tumor-liver contrast-to-noise ratio (CNR) than conventional SE pulse sequences (Table 1; Figs. 9–11). Two-excitation SE images are inferior to single-excitation images at comparable TE [45]. Different relaxation times of cysts, hemangiomas, and metastases lead to differences in tumor-liver CNR (Table 1). Cysts show the

Table 1. CNR of focal liver lesions with conventional MRI and EPI in 35 patients (7 cysts, 13 hemangiomas, 15 metastases) for all pulse sequences

Sequences	Cysts	Hemangiomas	Metastases	Total
Conventional MRI				
SE T1 250/20/4	−10.1±4.9	−5.1±5.5	−5.3±4.6	−6.4±5.4
SE T2 2500/50/1	7.9±6.9	9.6±11.1	4.0±2.5	6.9±7.7
SE T2 2500/100/1	13.8±7.6	12.6±9.9	6.0±2.8	10.8±7.9
EPI				
Single-excitation T2				
SE TE 26 ms	27.2±17.4	20.7±5.9	10.4±6.3	17.5±11.8
SE TE 50 ms	32.4±21.8	27.1±7.3	12.9±6.6	21.8±14.3
SE TE 100 ms	39.9±25.3	26.7±8.2	10.3±7.4	22.6±18.0
SE TE 150 ms	35.5±20.1	24.4±7.6	5.7±5.0	18.9±16.3
Two-excitation T2				
SE TE 26 ms	12.9±4.0	12.8±3.6	6.0±4.2	10.4±5.0
SE TE 50 ms	19.8±5.7	18.6±8.1	6.7±3.5	14.6±8.4
SE TE 100 ms	22.3±8.1	20.3±7.5	5.9±3.5	16.1±9.8
SE TE 150 ms	18.2±8.9	15.7±3.4	4.2±2.2	14.2±7.8
Single-excitation T1				
IR TI 100 ms	29.3±22.5	21.5±5.0	7.2±4.2	16.6±12.8
IR TI 380 ms	32.0±22.5	24.7±5.0	8.4±5.2	21.0±14.5
IR TI 600 ms	25.3±23.7	7.7±3.1	−1.3±4.4	6.9±13.4
IR TI 800 ms	13.3±20.2	−4.2±5.5	−5.4±3.8	−2.1±10.2

Highest CNR is achieved with the T2-weighted single-excitation technique at echo times of 50–100 ms.

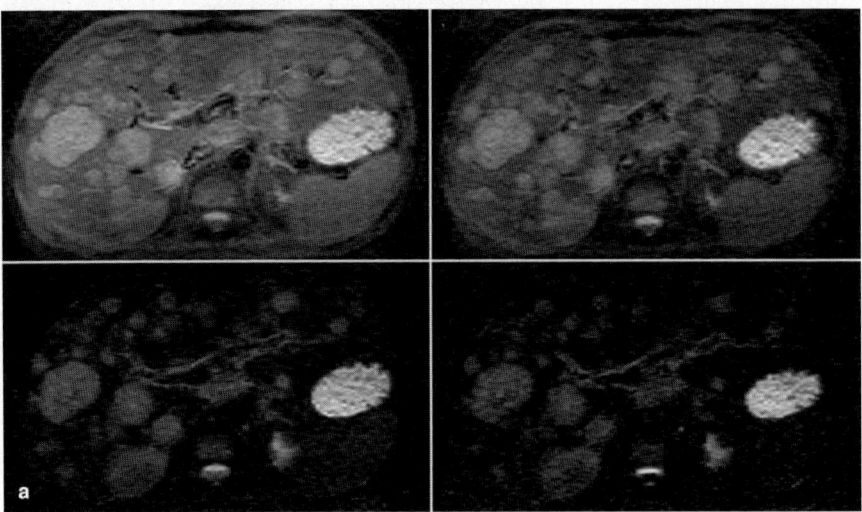

Fig. 9a–d. EPI of liver metastases. EPI at 1.5 T (ANMR Hyperscan). **a** Single-excitation T2-weighted SE EPI of a patient with multiple liver metastases at different TE times: *upper left,* TE 26 ms; *upper right,* TE 50 ms; *lower left,* TE 100 ms; *lower right,* TE 150 ms. **b** Two-excitation (TR 6 s) T2-weighted SE EPI of a patient with multiple liver metastases at different TE times: *upper left,* TE 26 ms; *upper right,* TE 50 ms; *lower left,* TE 100 ms; *lower right,* TE 150 ms. **c** Single-excitation T1-weighted IR (TE 26 ms) EPI of a patient with multiple liver metastases at different TI times: *upper left,* TI 100 ms; *upper right,* TI 380 ms; *lower left,* TI 600 ms; *lower right,* TI 800 ms.

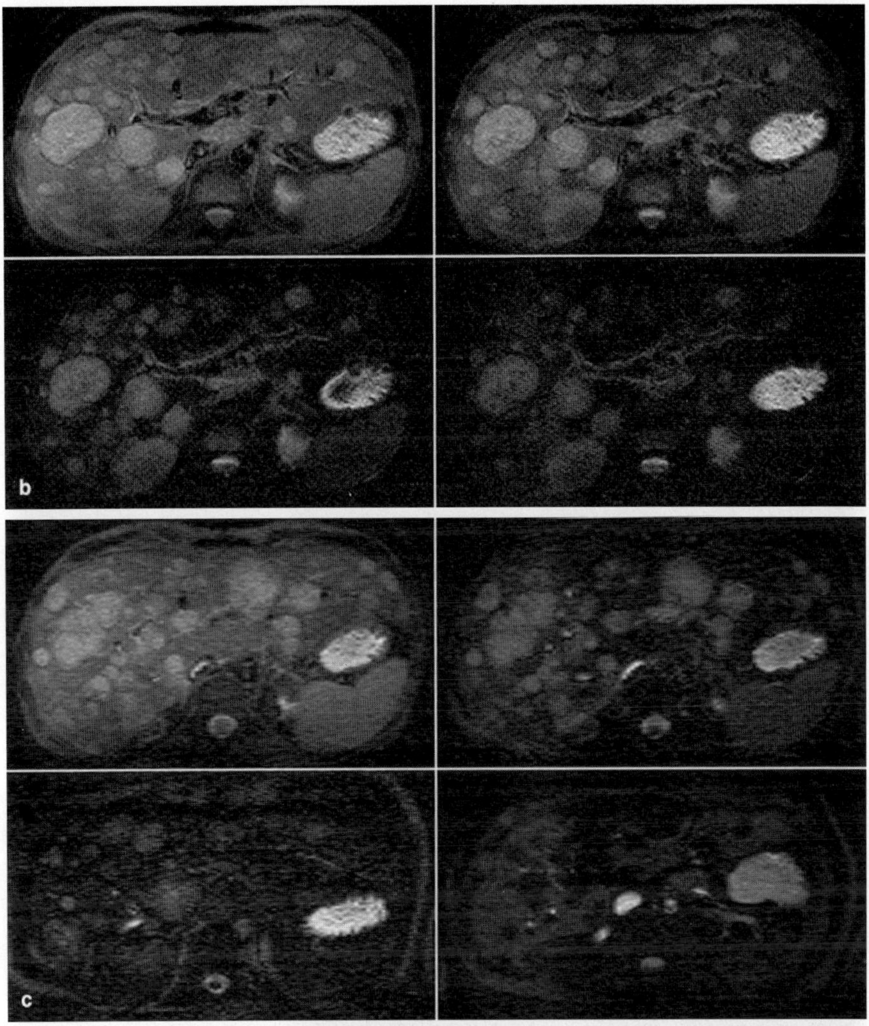

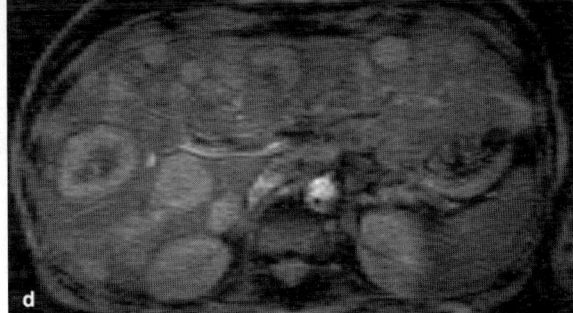

Fig. 9a–d. d Single-excitation T2*-weighted GE EPI of a patient with multiple liver metastases (TE 20 ms). Metastases show highest tumor-liver contrast on SE images with TE times of 50 ms and on IR images near the null point of the liver. Lesion signal intensity decreases rapidly at increasing TE times. GE EPI demonstrates lower tumor-liver contrast than SE or IR techniques

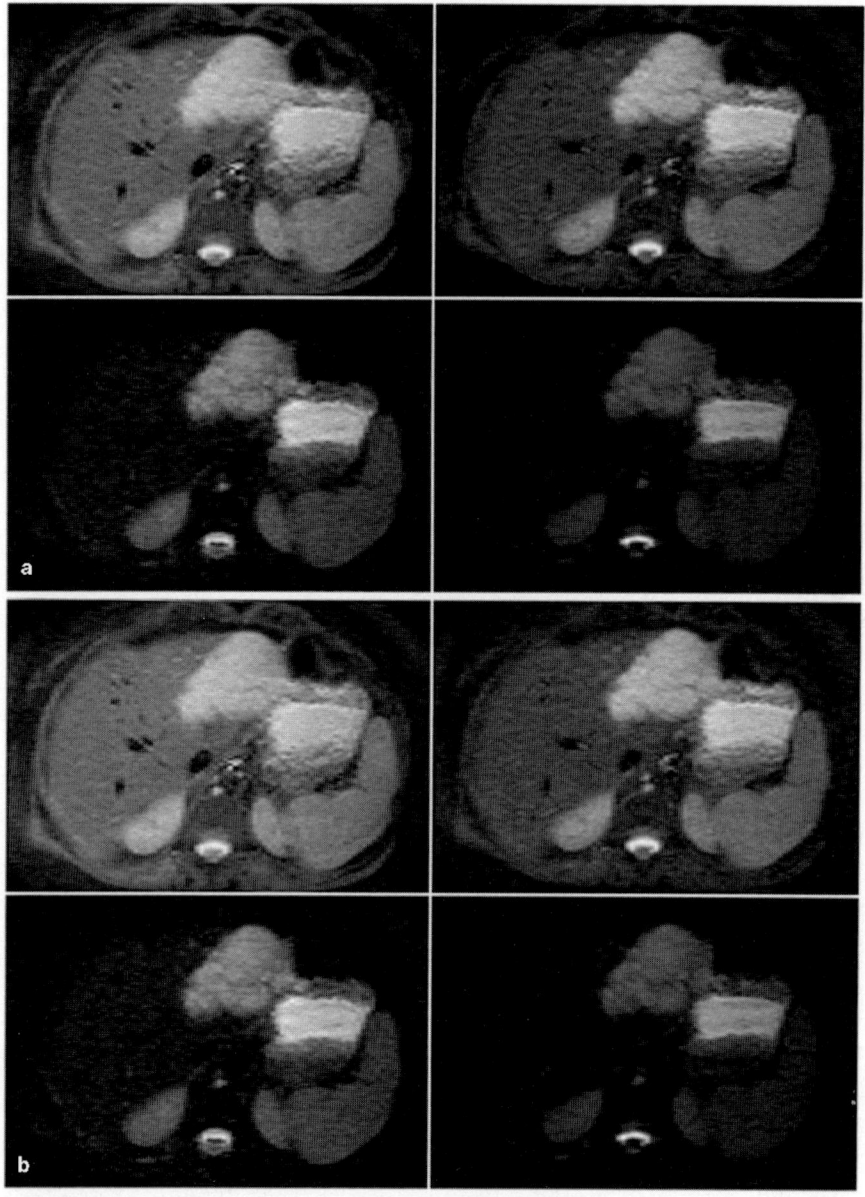

highest CNR at TE of 100 ms while hemangiomas and metastases demonstrate
the highest CNR at a shorter TE of 50 ms (Figs. 9–11) [46]. T1-weighted IR
images at the null point of the liver yield high CNR but are often difficult to
interpret because of transition from lung to liver and from liver to extrahepatic
abdominal and retroperitoneal structures due to fat suppression [45].

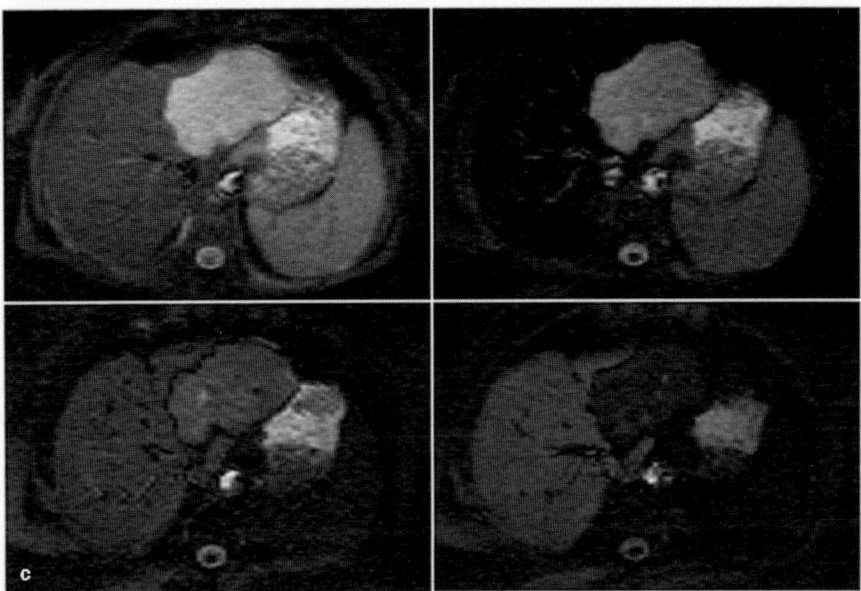

Fig. 10a–c. EPI of liver hemangioma. EPI at 1.5 T (ANMR Hyperscan). **a** Single-excitation T2-weighted SE EPI of a patient with hemangioma in the left liver lobe at different TE times: *upper left*, TE 26 ms; *upper right*, TE 50 ms; *lower left*, TE 100 ms; *lower right*, TE 150 ms. **b** Two-excitation (TR 6 s) T2-weighted SE EPI of a patient with hemangioma in the left liver lobe at different TE times: *upper left*, TE 26 ms; *upper right*, TE 50 ms; *lower left*, TE 100 ms; *lower right*, TE 150 ms. **c** Single-excitation T1-weighted IR (TE 26 ms) EPI of a patient hemangioma in the left liver lobe at different TI times: *upper left*, TI 100 ms; *upper right*, TI 380 ms; *lower left*, TI 600 ms; *lower right*, TI 800 ms. Hemangioma shows highest tumor-liver contrast on SE images with TE times of 50 and 100 ms and on IR images near the null point of the liver. Signal intensity of the lesion decreases slowly at increasing TE times

Another drawback of EPI IR techniques is that the duration of scan time per image is longer than for single-excitation SE images since the inversion time must be added to the scan time of a single-excitation SE image. Since high SNR and high CNR are both important in MRI, single-excitation techniques are preferable for routine imaging of the liver. It is necessary to collect images at a variety of TEs: shorter TE scans yield higher SNR but limited CNR, whereas long TE images have improved CNR at the cost of reduced SNR. Further studies are currently underway comparing the detection of focal liver lesions by novel conventional MRI techniques and spiral CT techniques in patients scheduled for liver surgery.

The development and implementation of various hybrid EPI techniques on conventional MR systems has been described in preliminary reports [14, 19, 29, 51, 52]. Current implementation of one such technique at 1.0 T (Fig. 12) allows coverage of the upper abdomen in two sets of T2-weighted acquisitions with a 192×256 matrix in approximately 20 s with high tumor-liver contrast and good image quality [14, 19]. Clinical studies are underway at various insti-

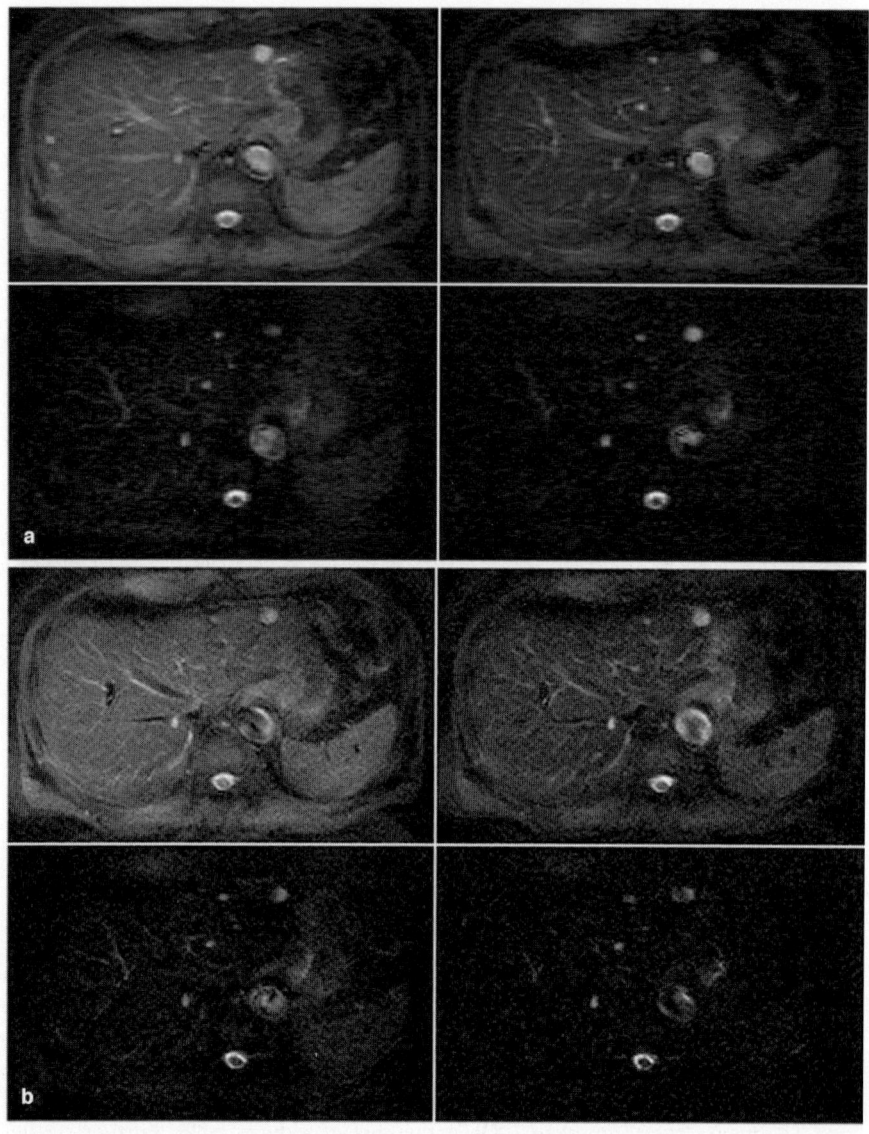

tutions and on various scanners evaluating the diagnostic utility of hybrid EPI techniques for abdominal MRI and specifically for detection of focal liver lesions. Whether the loss of small objects that is encountered with EPI and its hybrid versions affects detectability of lesions with short TE must also be clarified within these studies [53].

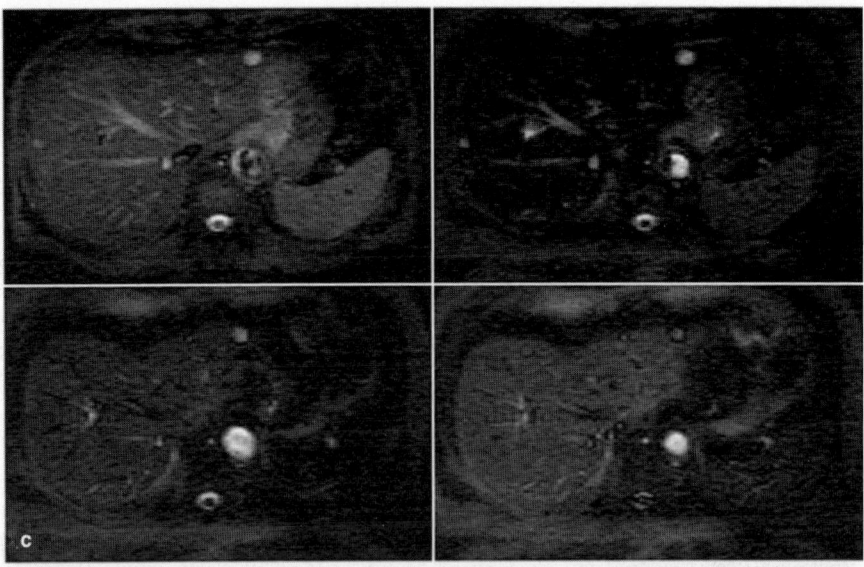

Fig. 11a–c. EPI of liver cysts. EPI at 1.5 T (ANMR Hyperscan). **a** Single-excitation T2-weighted SE EPI of a patient with multiple liver cysts at different TE times: *upper left*, TE 26 ms; *upper right*, TE 50 ms; *lower left*, TE 100 ms; *lower right*, TE 150 ms. **b** Two-excitation (TR 6 s) T2-weighted SE EPI of a patient with multiple liver cysts at different TE times: *upper left*, TE 26 ms; *upper right*, TE 50 ms; *lower left*, TE 100 ms; *lower right*, TE 150 ms. **c** Single-excitation T1-weighted IR (TE 26 ms) EPI of a patient with multiple liver cysts at different TI times: *upper left*, TI 100 ms; *upper right*, TI 380 ms; *lower left*, TI 600 ms; *lower right*, TI 800 ms. Lesions are best seen on SE images with long TE times displaying high signal intensity or IR images near the null point of the liver. Signal intensity of the lesion decreases only slightly at increasing TE times

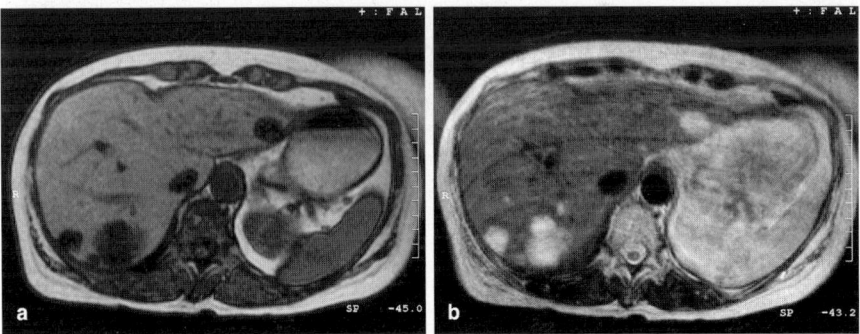

Fig. 12a–f. Hybrid EPI on a conventional MR system. MR images of a patient with liver metastases from malignant melanoma imaged with conventional and hybrid EPI techniques (1.0-T Magnetom Impact, 15 mT gradient coil, Siemens, Erlangen). **a** T1-weighted FLASH: TR 112 ms, TE 5 ms, matrix 160×256, acquisition time (TA) 17 s for 5 slices, flip angle (FA) 70°. **b** T2-weighted turbo-SE: TR 4000 ms, TE 90 ms, matrix 252×256, acquisition time (TA) 4.56 min for 21 slices.

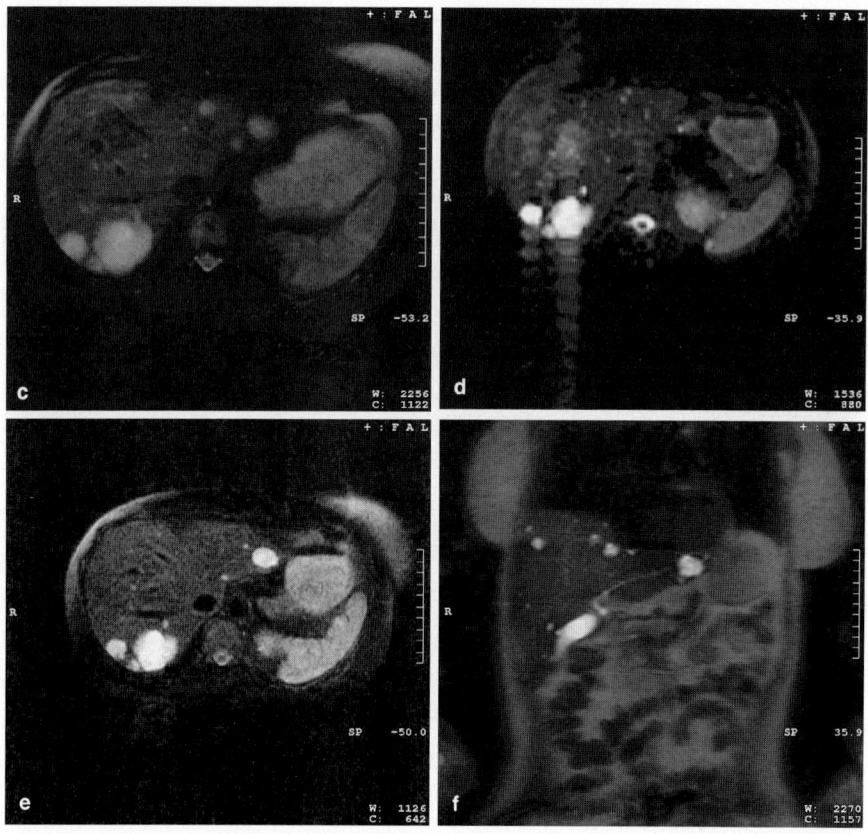

Fig. 12a–f. (continued) **c** T2-weighted "fat-saturated" turbo-SE: TR 2500 ms, TE 98 ms, matrix 250×256, acquisition time (TA) 4.16 min for 21 slices. **d** T2-weighted turbo-gradient SE: TR 2400 ms, TE 120 ms, matrix 198×256, acquisition time (TA) 16 s for 11 slices. **e** T2-weighted single-shot turbo-gradient SE: TR 400 ms, TE 78 ms, matrix 115×128, acquisition time (TA) 6 s for 21 slices. **f** T2-weighted single-shot turbo-SE with half-Fourier acquisition (HASTE): TR 10.9 ms, TE 87 ms, matrix 128×256, acquisition time (TA) 15 s for 11 slices. Tumor conspicuity estimated by tumor-liver contrast and image quality is best with T2-weighted turbo-gradient SE and T2-weighted single-shot turbo-SE with half-Fourier acquisition (HASTE)

Characterization of Focal Liver Lesions

Characterization of focal liver lesions is important because autopsy series have shown a high prevalence of benign liver tumors [54, 55]. Tissue characterization with conventional MRI has been difficult because of substantial overlap in the qualitative characteristics and image-derived measurements of solid and nonsolid tumors [56–59]. EPI offers certain advantages for lesion characterization because of the elimination of motion-related volume averaging and phase-encoding artifacts combined with the acquisition of purely T2-weighted images using single-excitation techniques (TR = ∞) [58]. Thus EPI-derived T2 times promise greater accuracy than those derived from conventional imaging (Figs. 9–11).

In a preliminary study on an experimental 2.0-T scanner EPI discriminated between metastases and hemangiomas based on T2-weighted images [22, 60]. This concept has been extended by Goldberg on a 1.5-T clinical EPI scanner with the calculation of both T1 and T2 values based on fat-suppressed single-excitation IR and SE images in 45 patients with confirmed focal liver lesions [59].

T1 relaxation times as derived by fitting a magnetization recovery curve to the measured signal intensities from IR acquisitions with four different inversion times were not reliable for tissue characterization of liver lesions. The mean T1 was 1004±234 ms for solid lesions, 1337±216 ms for hemangiomas, and 3143±1392 ms for cysts. Six hemangiomas had overlapping T1 times with the standard deviation of solid lesions [59].

T2 relaxation times calculated on the basis of a linear regression analysis of a plot of the natural logarithm of signal intensity versus echo time for each of four SE acquisitions were useful in discriminating metastases from hemangiomas based on a threshold of 116 ms. The mean T2 was 80±18 ms for solid lesions, 178±40 ms for hemangiomas, and 517±429 ms for cysts [59]. The distinction between solid and nonsolid lesions, however, does not reliably distinguish benign from malignant in general since malignant lesions can be cystic as well. The distinction between benign from malignant based on the 116-ms threshold was possible in 93 % of patients [59].

Similar results were obtained in another study comparing single-excitation and two-excitation T2-weighted SE acquisitions. Figure 13 demonstrates that two-excitation T2-weighted techniques show comparable thresholds as single-excitation techniques [61].

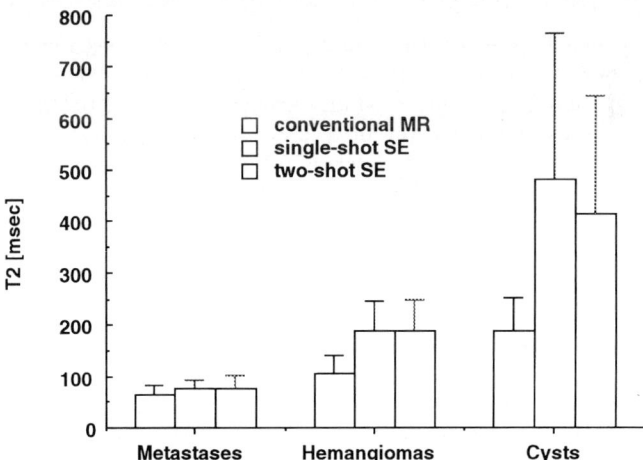

Fig. 13. Liver lesion characterization with EPI. T2 relaxation times calculated on the basis of linear regression for single-excitation EPI, two-excitation EPI, and conventional MRI. EPI shows no overlap in T2 times of metastases and hemangiomas in this study. Single-excitation and two-excitation T2-weighted EPI techniques show comparable thresholds for discrimination of metastases and hemangiomas

These encouraging results do not overcome the need for qualitative assessment of lesions, and a small overlap in T2 times of solid and nonsolid lesions is likely to remain. MR contrast agents are likely to play an increasingly important role in tissue characterization, potentially in combination with EPI depicting dynamic contrast behavior of focal liver lesions [62, 63].

Extrahepatic EPI

Conventional MRI has been of limited value in extrahepatic sites [64]. The principal reasons for this are phase-encoding artifacts secondary to gross physiological motion [65, 66] and the lack of suitable bowel contrast agents [2]. However, published reports so far have been limited to general descriptions of potential bowel contrast agents for EPI and [67, 68] pancreatic EPI [69]. A study compared conventional and EPI pulse sequences qualitatively and quantitatively at 1.5 T for pancreatic examinations. In all cases the EPI technique produced diagnostic-quality images, free of motion artifacts. With dark retroperitoneal fat (due to fat suppression) and usually bright bowel lumen (high water content), these images had a CT-like appearance. Overall image quality varied somewhat among patients, with reduced efficiency in fat suppression apparent especially in the larger subjects. The intrapancreatic segment of the common bile duct was visible in 32/36 normal patients as a high signal intensity structure, and portions of the pancreatic duct could be identified as a high signal intensity structure in 8/36 normal subjects [69].

In 72 % of patients without bowel lumen enhancement, independently of the imaging technique, the entire pancreas could be identified completely and distinguished from adjoining bowel. This is best explained by intrinsic bowel secretions which appeared hyperintense on IR and SE EPI. The entire pancreas (head, body, and tail) was identified in all patients with bowel lumen enhancement by an oral aqueous CT contrast agent. The difference between bowel-enhanced and bowel-unenhanced study groups was statistically significant ($p<0.05$). The oral administration of a high signal intensity bowel contrast agent improved the distinction of pancreas from adjoining bowel and enhanced intraluminal SNR by an average factor of 10–15 [69]. Long T2 aqueous gastrointestinal contrast media may well serve as bowel enhancement agents in EPI. Increased signal in the bowel lumen contributes noise to a conventional image because the bowel moves during image acquisition [70]. However, the time required for EPI acquisition is extremely short compared to that of all gross physiological motion. High intraluminal bowel signal is therefore achieved without a reduction in overall image quality [69].

Quantitative image analysis has shown that the single-excitation SE sequence with a short TE of 26 provides the highest ($p<0.05$) pancreatic SNR (Fig. 14), as has been shown for hepatic EPI. The single-excitation technique showed significantly higher SNR than the two-excitation technique ($p<0.05$; Fig. 14). On T1-weighted images, the short TI (100 ms) and long TI (800 ms) IR sequences had a significantly ($p<0.05$) higher SNR than the sequence with an inversion time of 380 ms (which was chosen to minimize or eliminate signal from pancreas

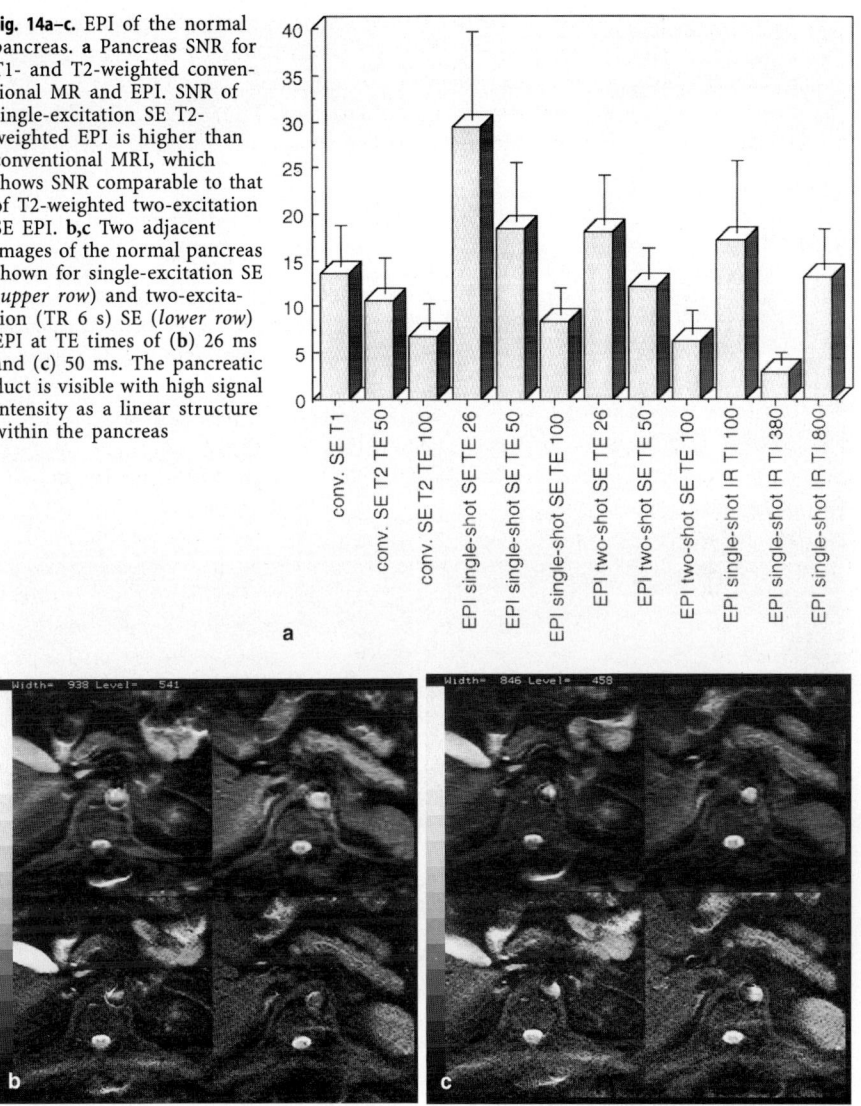

Fig. 14a–c. EPI of the normal pancreas. **a** Pancreas SNR for T1- and T2-weighted conventional MR and EPI. SNR of single-excitation SE T2-weighted EPI is higher than conventional MRI, which shows SNR comparable to that of T2-weighted two-excitation SE EPI. **b,c** Two adjacent images of the normal pancreas shown for single-excitation SE (*upper row*) and two-excitation (TR 6 s) SE (*lower row*) EPI at TE times of (**b**) 26 ms and (**c**) 50 ms. The pancreatic duct is visible with high signal intensity as a linear structure within the pancreas

and liver; Fig. 10) [47, 69]. EPI is generally believed to be limited by low SNRs [1, 22, 68]. However, EPI of the pancreas provides excellent SNR, probably because motion noise is suppressed by the short acquisition time. Therefore pancreatic SNR actually exceeded SNR in our conventional T2-weighted images and in those reported in the literature [71, 72].

Preliminary studies in patients with pancreatic disease and bowel enhancement have demonstrated that diseased areas or lesions are visible based on their different signal intensity relative to normal pancreas (Fig. 15). Tumor tissue

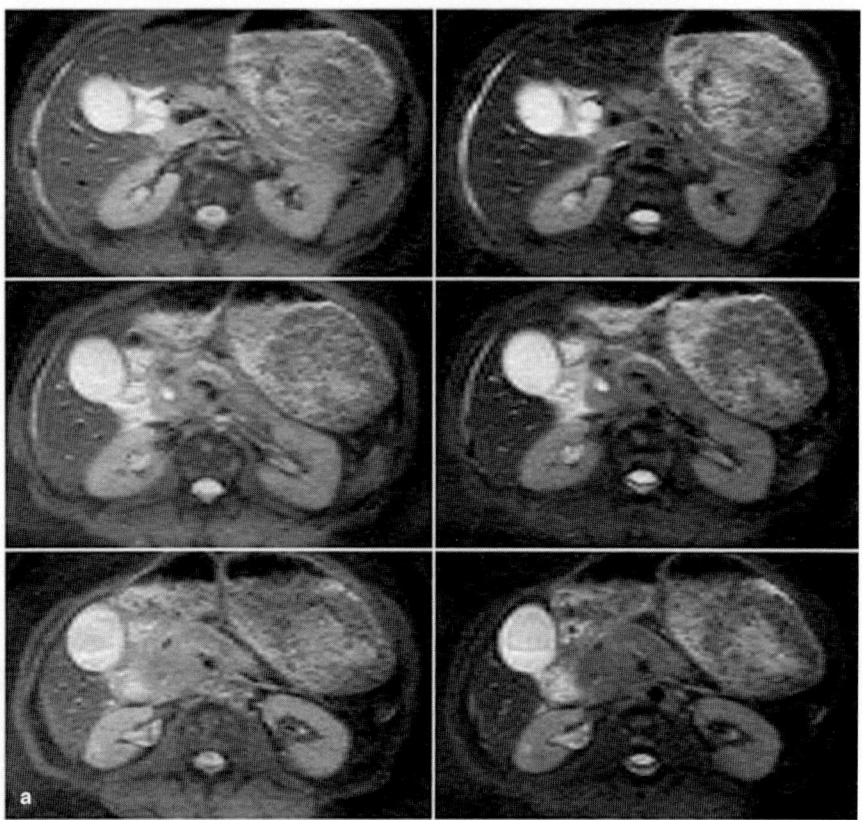

Fig. 15a-c. EPI in pancreatic disease. EPI at 1.5 T (ANMR Hyperscan). **a** Three adjacent slices of a single-excitation T2-weighted SE EPI examination in a patient with acute pancreatitis (*left column*, TE 26 ms; *right column*, TE 50 ms). Enlargement of the pancreas with dilation of the pancreatic duct is shown.

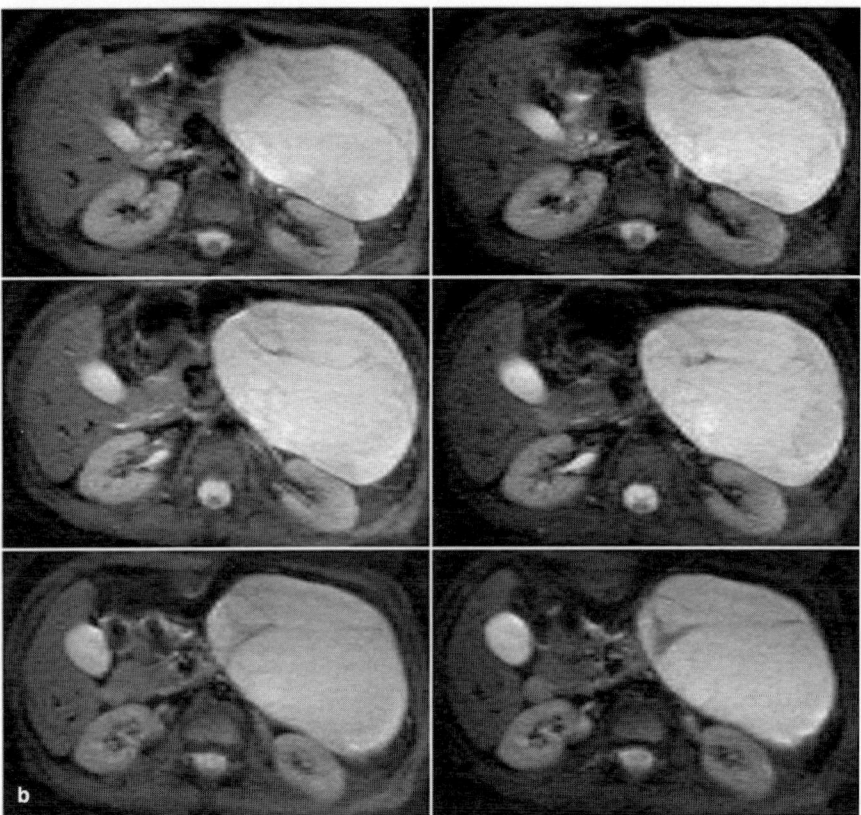

Fig. 15a–c. b Three adjacent slices of a single-excitation T2-weighted SE EPI examination in a patient with mucinous cystadenoma of the pancreas (*left column*, TE 26 ms; *right column*, TE 50 ms). The cystic lesion is seen with high signal intensity on EPI.

and areas of pancreatitis demonstrated higher signal intensity than normal pancreas. The diseased areas were also identified by morphological changes such as a dilated common bile duct, dilated pancreatic duct, mesenteric stranding, and pancreatic contour deformity. EPI studies are currrently evaluating tumor detectability with positive and negative oral contrast agents. Clinical utility of EPI for the diagnostic work-up of pancreatic disease must be assessed in comparison to current CT and MR techniques [73].

Other extrahepatic organs have been examined in unpublished preliminary studies demonstrating the potential applications of abdominal EPI [23, 74]. EPI may be applied to examine the spleen, adrenal glands (Fig. 16), kidneys, major abdominal vessels, and abdominal and retroperitoneal lymphadenopathy (Fig. 17).

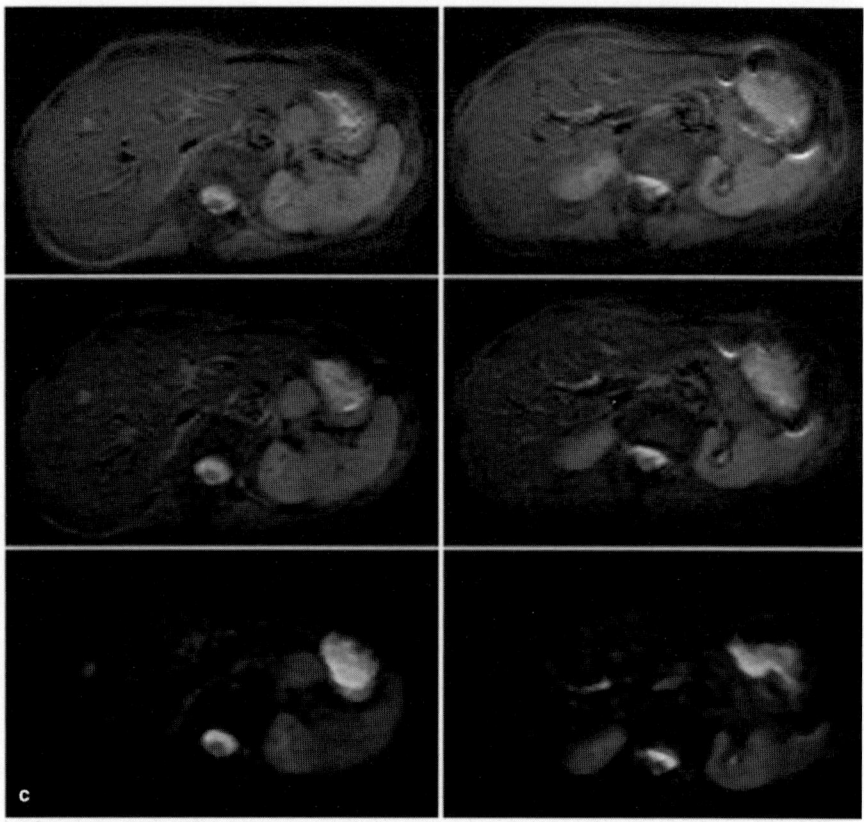

Fig. 15a–c. (continued) c Two adjacent slices of a single-excitation T2-weighted SE EPI examination in a patient with adenocarcinoma of the pancreas and liver metastases (*upper row*, TE 26 ms; *middle row*, TE 50 ms; *lower row*, TE 100 ms). Pancreatic carcinoma is seen behind the stomach with a liver lesion in the right liver lobe

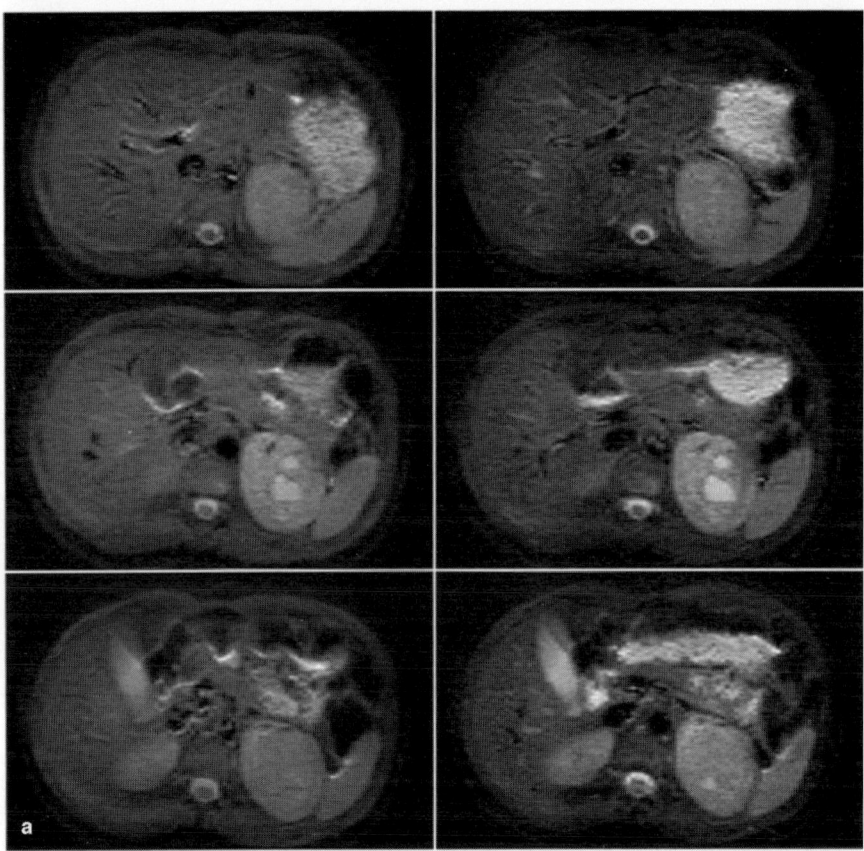

Fig. 16a–c. EPI of the adrenal glands. EPI at 1.5 T (ANMR Hyperscan). a Three adjacent slices of a single-excitation T2-weighted SE EPI examination in a patient with pheochromocytoma (*left column*, TE 26 ms; *right column*, TE 50 ms).

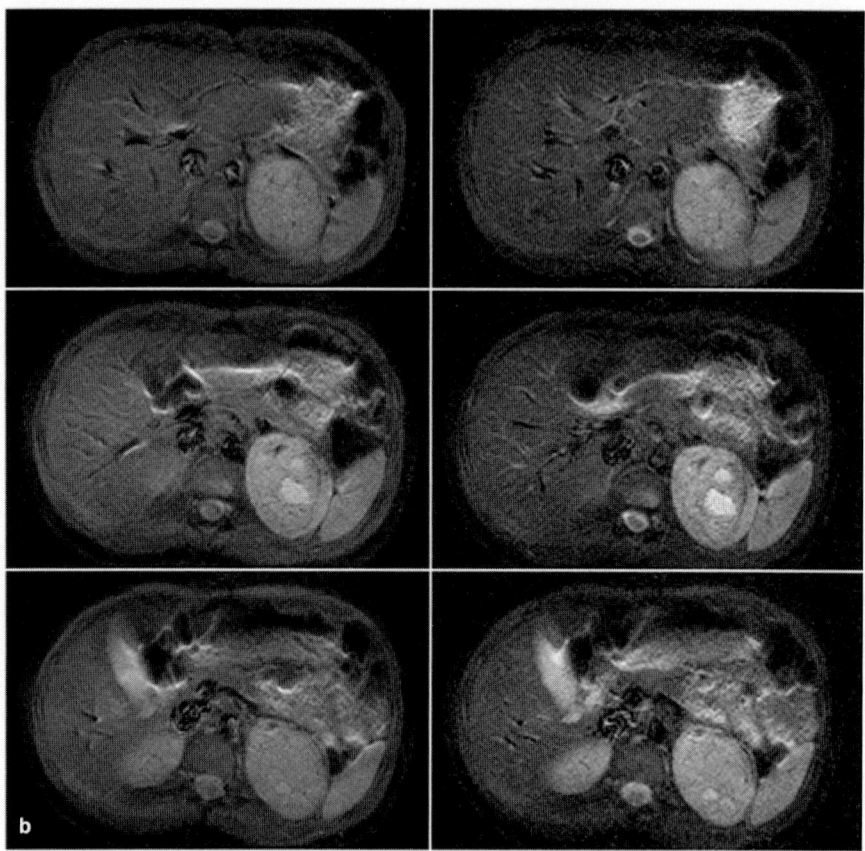

Fig. 16a–c. (continued) **b** Three adjacent slices of a two-excitation (TR 6 s) T2-weighted SE EPI examination in a patient with pheochromocytoma (*left column,* TE 26 ms; *right column,* TE 50 ms).

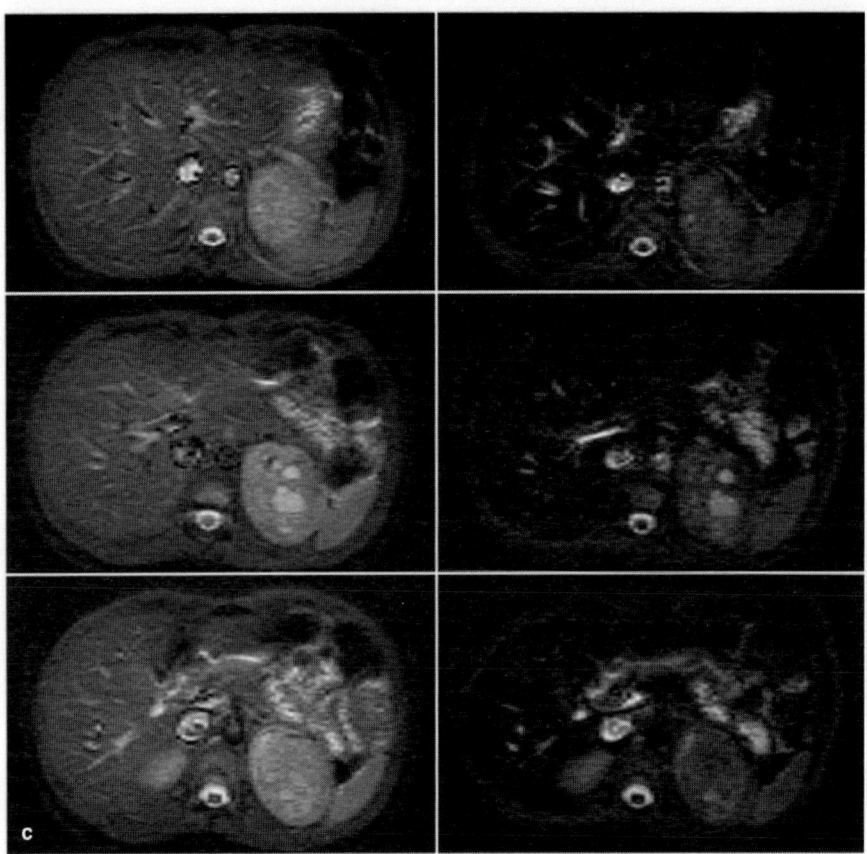

Fig. 16a–c. c Three adjacent slices of a single-excitation T1-weighted IR (TE 26 ms) EPI examination in a patient with pheochromocytoma (*left column,* TE 26 ms; *right column,* TE 50 ms). The lesion is seen with inhomogeneous high signal intensity on all acquisitions and lower SNR on two-excitation images

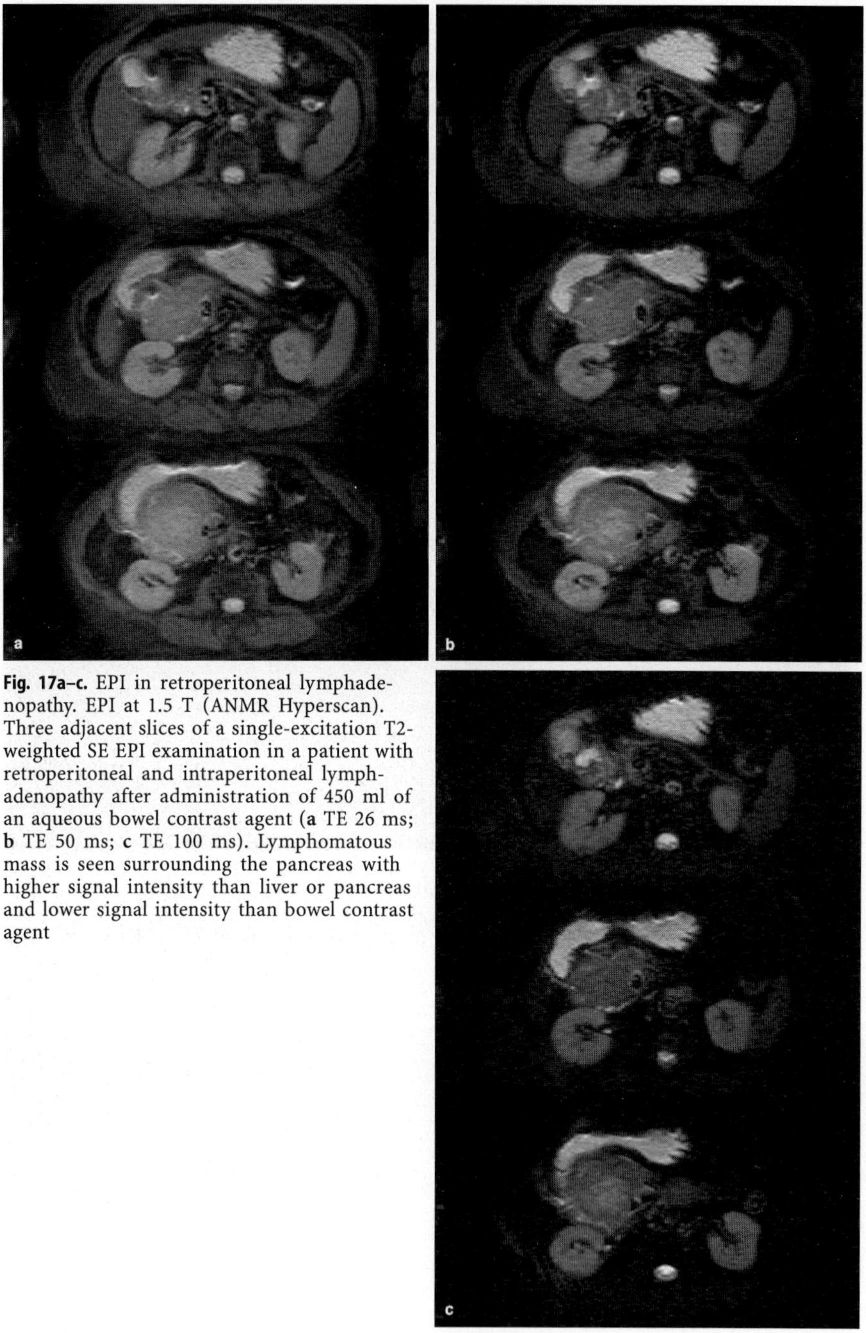

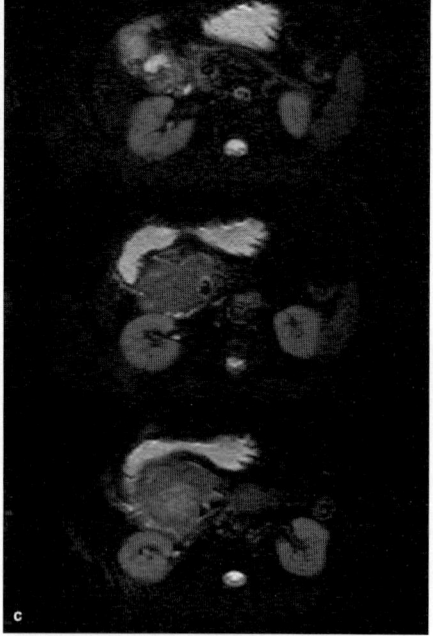

Fig. 17a–c. EPI in retroperitoneal lymphadenopathy. EPI at 1.5 T (ANMR Hyperscan).
Three adjacent slices of a single-excitation T2-
weighted SE EPI examination in a patient with
retroperitoneal and intraperitoneal lymphadenopathy after administration of 450 ml of
an aqueous bowel contrast agent (**a** TE 26 ms;
b TE 50 ms; **c** TE 100 ms). Lymphomatous
mass is seen surrounding the pancreas with
higher signal intensity than liver or pancreas
and lower signal intensity than bowel contrast
agent

EPI MRA

Flow-related effects in EPI have been analyzed previously [75]. MR angiograms of the major abdominal vessels can be obtained, and a unique feature is the temporal resolution that is achieved. Diagnostic-quality EPI angiograms of the hepatic and portal venous systems have been presented by Goldberg et al. [76] (Fig. 18). This study compared a GE echo-planar time-of-flight MR angiography technique to conventional MR angiography [76, 77]. While noise was lower with the conventional technique, vessel-to-liver signal intensity ratios were higher with EPI, and qualitative scores were comparable in EPI and conventional MR angiography. Noise is also increased when maximum intensity projections are used since these maximize not only vascular signal but also noise. The reduced number of breath-holds required increases patients' tolerance. EPI angiography has also been performed in preliminary studies by using phase-based EPI techniques [78, 79].

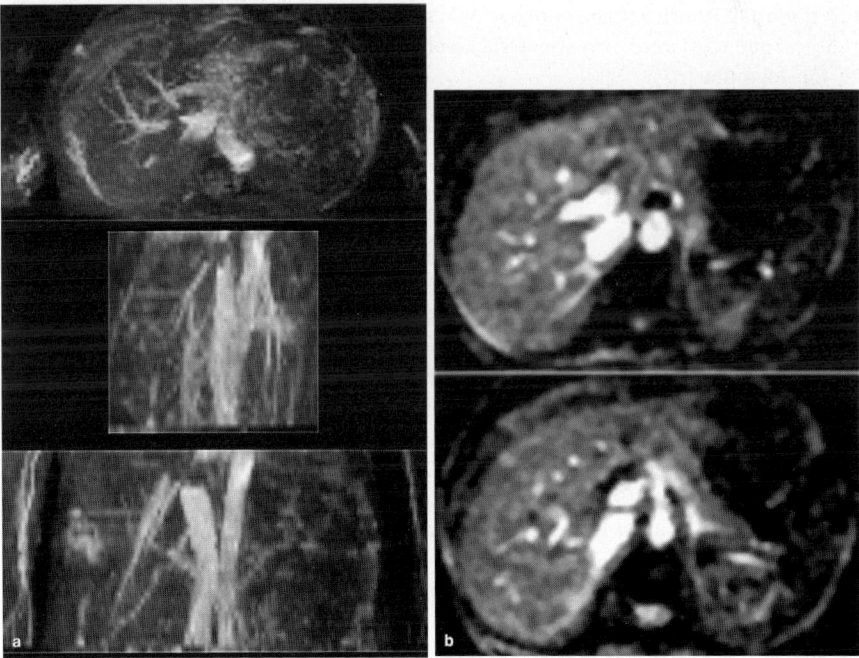

Fig. 18a,b. Abdominal and hepatic EPI-MRA. **a** Maximum intensity projection of an abdominal EPI MRA data set reconstructed from a single breath-held single-excitation GE acquisition showing major abdominal vessels with low resolution due to the limited 128×128 acquisition matrix. (Courtesy of Mark S. Cohen, Massachusetts General Hospital) **b** Two slices through the liver of a breath-held single-excitation GE EPI MR angiography dataset displaying high vessel-liver contrast but low resolution due to the restricted acquisition matrix. (Courtesy of Sanjay Saini and Mark A. Goldberg, Massachusetts General Hospital; see also [76])

Contrast Agents

Extracellular Agents

Rapid scanning is critical when extracellular contrast agents such as gadolinium-based compounds are used for examination of the liver [80–82]. The effect of paramagnetic contrast agents on MR images is complex and has been shown to yield either positive or negative tissue enhancement depending upon tissue concentration and pulse sequence [83–85].

Preclinical Studies

Among the approved extracellular contrast agents only gadopentetate dimeglumine has been tested for EPI of the abdomen [62, 82]. The effect of various concentrations of gadopentetate dimeglumine and pulse sequences on liver signal intensity has been evaluated in an experimental study [86]. Dynamic EPI was performed before and following bolus administration of gadopentetate dimeglumine: 0.05, 0.1, and 0.2 mmol/kg bodyweight; the clinically recommended dose is 0.1 mmol/kg (Berlex Laboratories, Wayne, N.J.). Fat-suppressed SE, IR, and GE pulse sequences were investigated. Liver enhancement was calculated according to the formula [87]:

$$\text{Liver enhancement} = SI_{postinjection}/SI_{preinjection}$$

Hence liver enhancement values less than 1 represent liver signal increase postcontrast, and liver enhancement values greater than 1 represent liver signal loss postcontrast.

The current clinically recommended dose of 0.1 mmol/kg gadopentetate dimeglumine enhanced MR EPI obtained during the perfusion phase can yield either positive (due to increased T1 relaxation rates) or negative (due to susceptibility increased T2 relaxation rates) liver enhancement depending upon the choice of pulse sequence and its timing parameters (Figs. 19–22). The best pulse sequence to demonstrate T1 effects is an IR technique, while susceptibility effects are seen best with a T2*-weighted GR technique. Utilizing T1-weighted techniques at the current clinical dose of 0.1 mmol/kg, a 20% peak increase is observed at the SE pulse sequence (Fig. 19) and 250% at the IR pulse sequence (Fig. 20), lasting for more than 30 s and 100 s, respectively. T2-weighted techniques generate a decrease in liver SI of 20% at the SE pulse sequence (Fig. 21) and of more than 30% at the GE pulse sequence with a duration of more than 20 s and 10 s, respectively (Fig. 22).

The observed T2 effects were present on T1-weighted images at higher doses. When the T1-weighted SE technique was used, liver SI did not increase when the clinical dose was doubled (Fig. 19). This was even more pronounced with the IR technique, with which liver SI began to decrease when the dose was increased from 0.05 to 0.1 mmol/kg (Fig. 20). The diminished increase in liver SI at increasing doses can best be explained by susceptibility effects at these dose levels given the somewhat long TE times used for the T1-weighted imaging

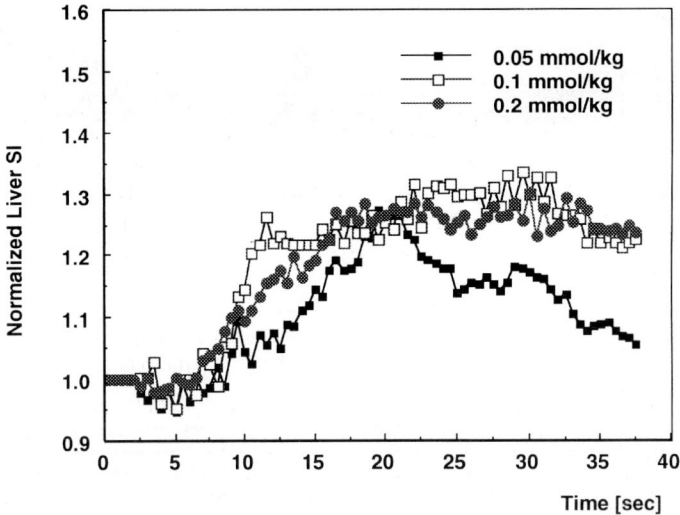

Fig. 19. Dynamic T1-weighted SE EPI. Dynamic single-excitation T1-weighted SE EPI (TR 500 ms, TE 20 ms, flip angle 90°) before and following intravenous injection of 0.05, 0.1, and 0.2 mmol/kg gadopentetate dimeglumine, showing no further increase in signal intensity at 0.2 mmol/kg

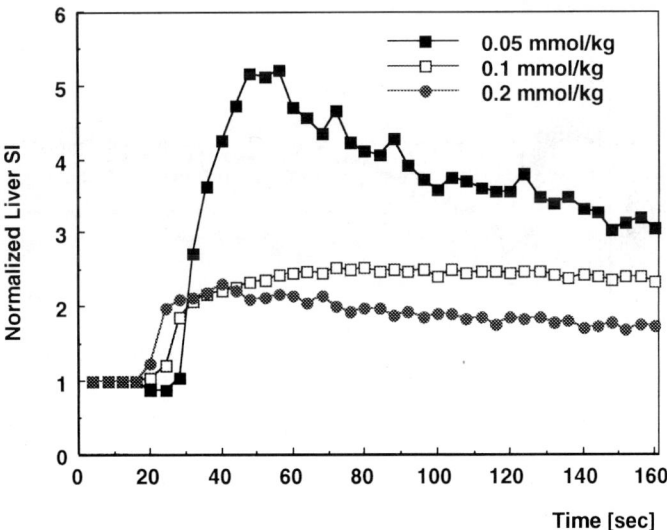

Fig. 20. Dynamic T1-weighted IR EPI. Dynamic single-excitation T1-weighted IR EPI (TR 500 ms, TE 20 ms, TI, 370 ms, flip angle 90°) before and following intravenous injection of 0.05, 0.1, and 0.2 mmol/kg gadopentetate dimeglumine, showing highest signal intensity at 0.05 mmol/kg and decreasing signal intensity with increasing dose

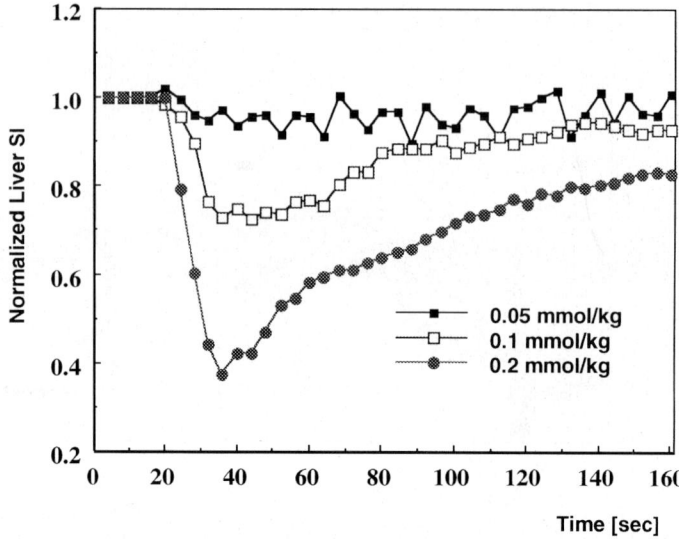

Fig. 21. Dynamic T2-weighted SE EPI. Dynamic single-excitation T2-weighted SE EPI (TR 4000 ms, TE 40 ms, flip angle 90°) before and following intravenous injection of 0.05, 0.1, and 0.2 mmol/kg gadopentetate dimeglumine, showing decreasing signal intensity with increasing dose

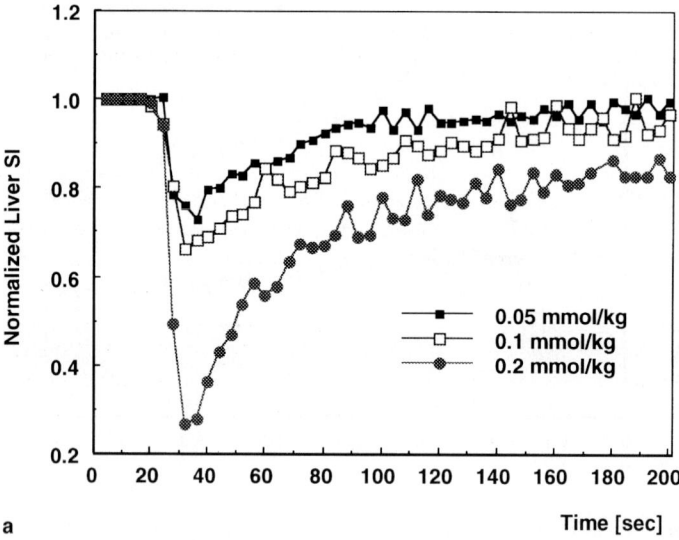

Fig. 22a,b. Dynamic T2*-weighted GE EPI. **a** Dynamic single-excitation T2*-weighted GE EPI (TR 4000 ms, TE 40 ms, flip angle 10°) before and following intravenous injection of 0.05, 0.1, and 0.2 mmol/kg bodyweight gadopentetate dimeglumine, showing even more pronounced decrease in signal intensity with increasing dose.

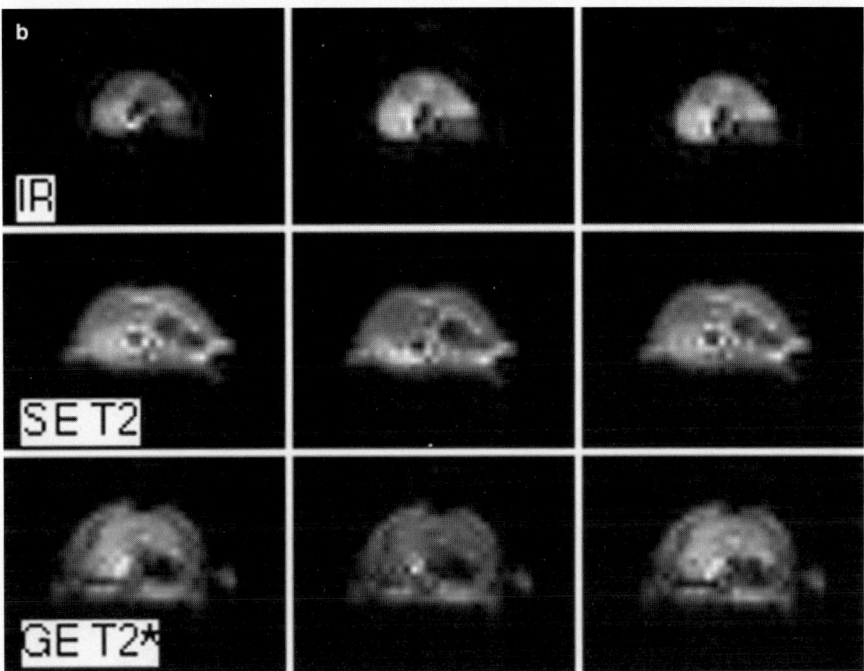

Fig. 22a,b. b Dynamic single-excitation gadopentetate dimeglumine enhanced EPI (*upper row,* IR; *middle row,* SE T2; *lower row,* GE T2*) before (*left column*), during peak enhancement (*middle column*), and during equilibrium (*right column*) following intravenous injection of clinical dose of 0.1 mmol/kg. Liver signal intensity increases using T1-weighted IR EPI and decreases using T2 and T2*-weighted SE and GE EPI

experiments. The signal in all of the MR pulse sequences is affected to varying degrees by T1, T2, and T2* changes, and no single sequence can successfully deconvolve these effects from one another. The mechanism of transverse relaxation enhancement by gadopentetate dimeglumine is presumably its generation of local magnetic field inhomogeneities seen best on GE scans, and indeed the larger signal intensity changes seen in GE studies reflect this presumption. Gadopentetate dimeglumine in high doses also shows T2 relaxation effects which are diffusion mediated [83]. Our results show that liver SI increases at low doses due to T1 shortening of liver (Fig. 20).

Clinical Studies

Clinical studies are now underway assessing the role of clinical gadopentetate dimeglumine enhanced EPI for lesion characterization using IR techniques [63]. Prior to injection of the contrast agent the null point of the lesion is identified in a series of acquisitions with incrementally increasing TI. When the null point is identified, gadopentetate dimeglumine is administered by bolus injection, and the tumor perfusion is monitored (Fig. 23) [63], allowing depiction of specific tumoral enhancement or perfusion patterns [62]. In principle, tissues with T1 times different from the null point may enhance positively (if tissue T1 time is less than the null point) or negatively (if tissue T1 time is greater than null point). Since the T1 of most liver tumors exceeds that of liver, their SI would be expected to increase, while that of liver decreases. These strategies have also been exploited with turbo-Flash rapid MRI techniques [88].

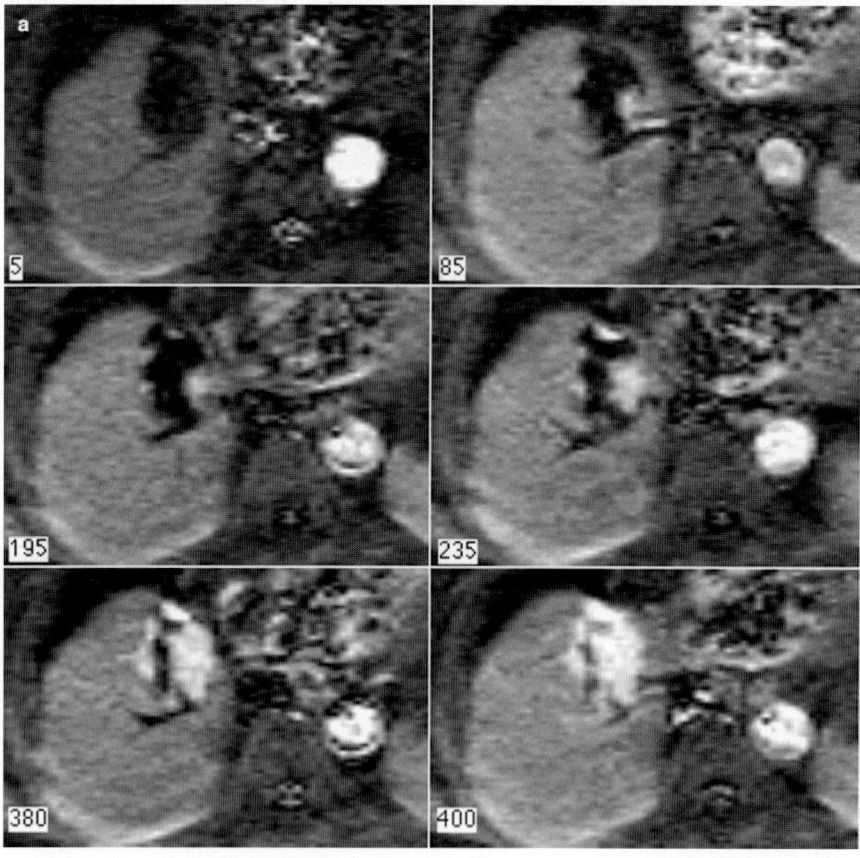

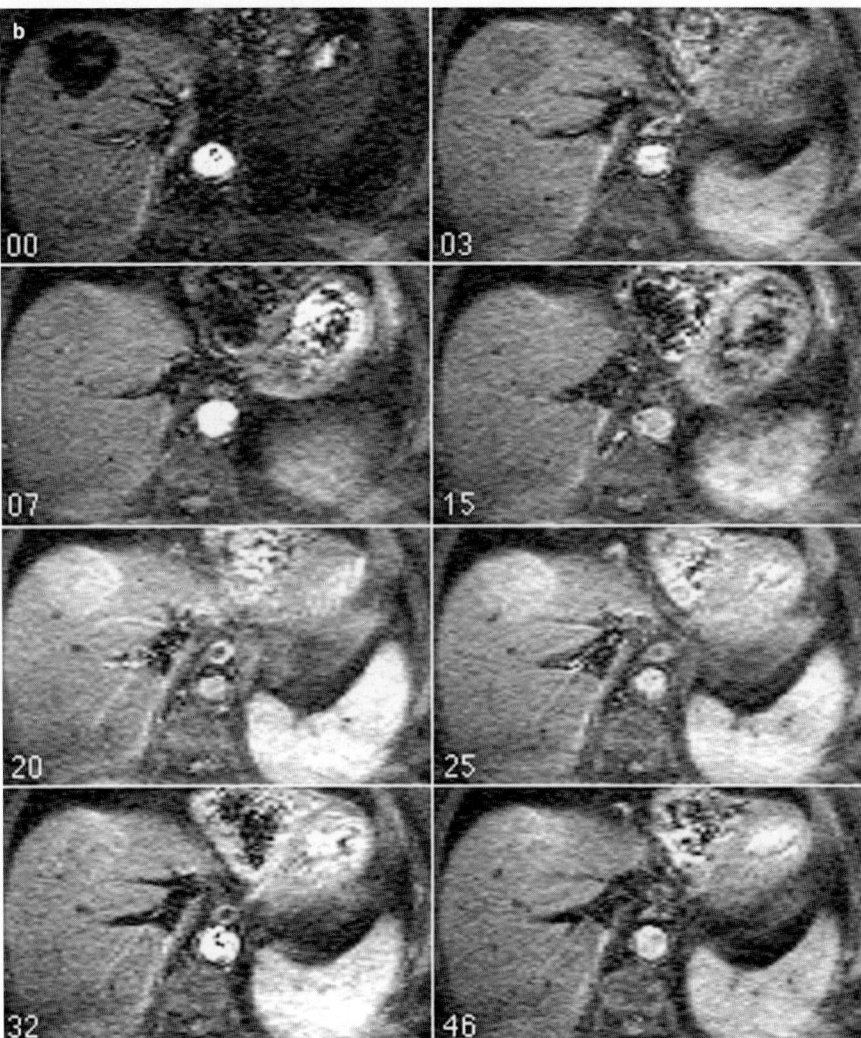

Fig. 23a,b. Dynamic contrast-enhanced EPI of focal liver lesions with gadopentetate dimeglumine. EPI at 1.5 T (ANMR Hyperscan). **a** Six images of a dynamic contrast-enhanced single-excitation EPI study in a patient with hemangioma (IR TE 26 ms and TI 800 ms) showing characteristic slow peripheral contrast filling of the lesion. (Courtesy of Sanjay Saini, Massachusetts General Hospital, see also [63]) **b** Eight images of dynamic contrast-enhanced single-excitation EPI study in a patient with colon carcinoma metastases (IR TE 26 ms and TI 800 ms) showing characteristic early filling of the lesion with rapid contrast equilibrium of the lesion with normal liver. (Courtesy of Sanjay Saini, Massachusetts General Hospital, see also [63])

Intracellular Agents

A spectrum of preclinical MR contrast agents with intracellular distribution is currently under investigation (Fig. 24). These agents include hepatobiliary agents, blood pool agents, conventional superparamagnetic iron oxides, immunospecific agents, and receptor-directed agents [6, 89–91]. Dynamic liver signal intensity changes induced by iron oxide preparations have been studied with EPI [92]. The different liver SI curves of hepatocyte receptor agents and RES agents studied demonstrate that we might be able visualize different uptake mechanisms of MR contrast agents with EPI.

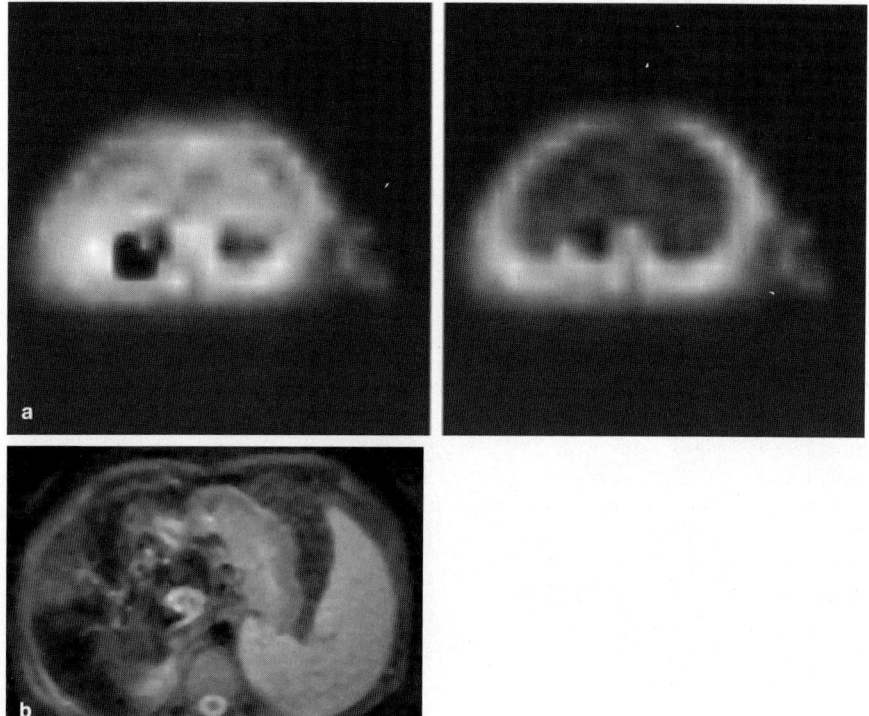

Fig. 24a,b. Superparamagnetic iron oxide enhanced EPI. EPI at 1.5 T (ANMR Hyperscan). **a** Single-excitation T2-weighted SE EPI of a rat before and 10 min following intravenous administration of 10 µmol/kg ASF-MION showing decreased hepatic signal following administration of the contrast agent. **b** Single-excitation T2-weighted SE EPI (TE 26 ms) in a patient with hemochromatosis and liver metastases from colon carcinoma. Note high tumor-liver contrast due the signal decrease in normal liver signal

Oral Contrast Agents

The elimination of motion artifacts with EPI offers an encouraging way to evaluate the entire abdomen. The need for gastrointestinal contrast agents is obvious, as has been shown with the abdominal application of CT [93, 94]. Both the elimination of motion artifacts and the administration of suited gastrointestinal contrast agents are prerequisites for the development of a strategy for abdominal MRI in a clinical setting. Requirements for a gastrointestinal agent suited for EPI are shared with CT. The agent should distend bowel loops uniformly and small bowel transit should be complete within 30–60 min. Contrast material should also maintain constant signal in the bowel lumen throughout the entire small and large bowel [67].

Water as a simple contrast agent has been described first for use in EPI [68] but has several disadvantages. Because of low osmolarity it is absorbed readily from the gastrointestinal tract and therefore large volumes must be administered for adequate marking of bowel loops. The low viscosity leads to substantial variations in bowel distention from loop to loop, and even in the same bowel segment within seconds [67, 68]. Clinical studies are currently evaluating the administration and distribution of aqueous gastrointestinal contrast media for EPI. It remains to be investigated whether dedicated contrast agents must be developed, or whether these already approved aqueous oral contrast agents may be used [2, 6, 7].

Bowel Lumen Signal Enhancement

Bowel lumen signal enhancement has been shown to improve differentiation of abdominal organs from adjoining bowel [69, 95, 96].

Following the oral administration of aqueous barium sulfate preparations fluid-filled bowel loops are distended and display high bowel lumen SI while fatty retroperitoneal and mesenteric structures are of low signal intensity (Figs. 25, 26). The mean score for bowel lumen "enhancement" increased from 2.3 (1 = poor bowel lumen enhancement, 2 = fair bowel lumen enhancement, 3 = good lumen enhancement, 4 = excellent lumen enhancement) on precontrast images to 3.0 on postcontrast images. Bowel enhancement improved the differentiation of abdominal organs from adjoining bowel (Figs. 25, 26).

Approved aqueous gastrointestinal CT contrast agents containing barium sulfate and gastrografin are applicable for abdominal EPI [67, 97]. Fat-suppressed EPI techniques provide bright bowel lumen enhancement due to T2 weighting and a dark retroperitoneum (Fig. 25), exhibiting contrast behavior similar to CT [67]. Therefore with iron oxide based oral contrast agents the entire abdomen demonstrates low signal intensity with almost no contrast between bowel loops and surrounding mesentery. Due to the short data acquisition time physiological motion does not degrade EPI, and because the technique is inherently T2-weighted, intraluminal fluid renders the bowel hyperintense. Alternatively, flavored isotonic saline, exhibiting the same relaxation time and SI characteristics with the additional advantage of being isoosmolar may be used [98].

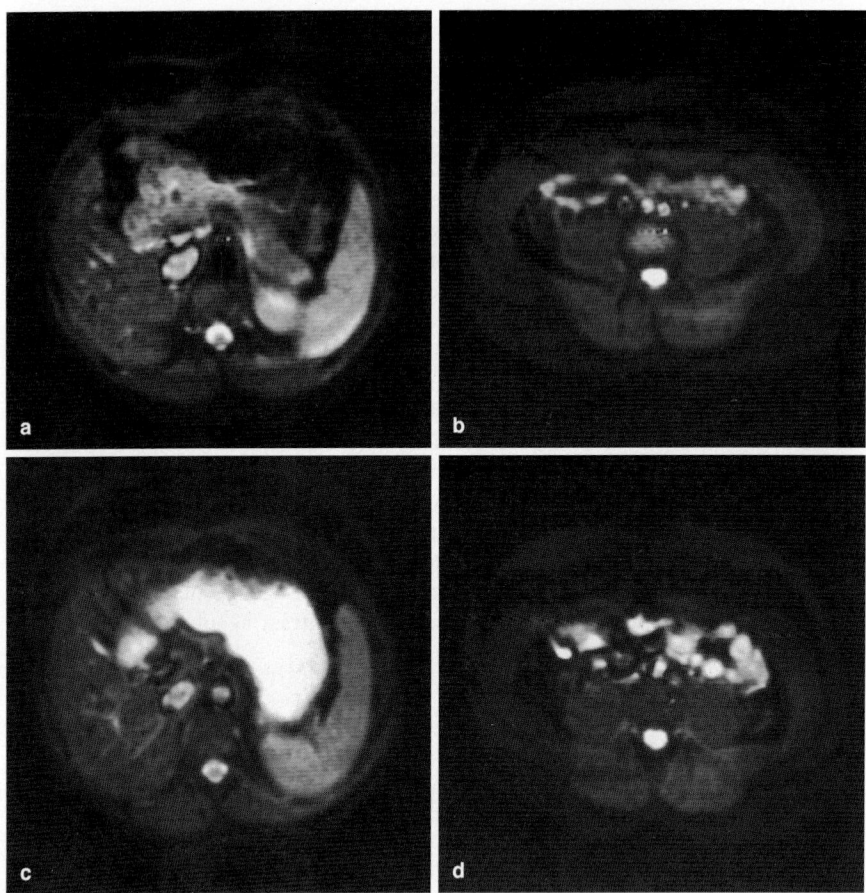

Fig. 25a–d. Bowel enhancement and reduction in susceptibility artifacts following administration of an oral contrast agent. EPI (SE: TR ∞, TE 35 ms) before (**a** upper abdomen; **b** lower abdomen) and following (**c** upper abdomen; **d** lower abdomen) oral administration of 1000 ml of an aqueous barium sulfate suspension on adjacent images (1.0-T, Siemens, Erlangen). Bowel marking is achieved by intraluminal signal enhancement reducing susceptibility artifacts surrounding the gas filled bowel loops on precontrast images

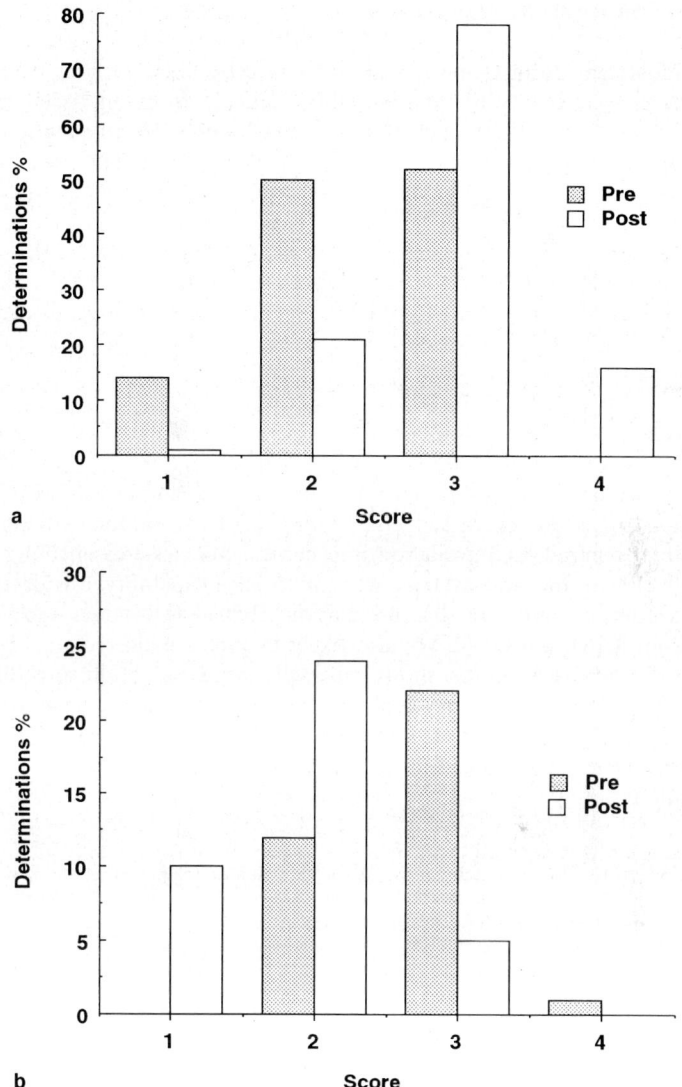

Fig. 26. a Presence or absence of bowel lumen "filling" on pre- and postcontrast EPI (*x-axis*) and pooled determinations of readers (*y-axis*). Administration of the oral contrast agent increased bowel filling and thus bowel lumen signal enhancement. **b** Presence or absence of susceptibility artifacts on pre- and postcontrast EPI (*x-axis*) and pooled determinations of readers (y-axis). Administration of the oral contrast agent decreased susceptibility artifacts

Reduction of Susceptibility Artifacts

Another important point is the reduction in susceptibility artifacts from air-tissue interfaces (Figs. 25, 26). Susceptibility artifacts from air-tissue interfaces (gas-filled bowel versus liver, spleen, or pancreas) which are frequently observed on precontrast images are reduced on postcontrast images. The mean score for the presence of susceptibility artifacts increased from 1.9 on precontrast images (see above) to 2.4 on postcontrast images (Figs. 25, 26).

Susceptibility artifacts from air-tissue interfaces such as between the gas filled stomach and left liver lobe in the upper abdomen are reduced with oral administration of barium sulfate based preparation, resulting in an overall decrease in spatial distortions [98].

Perspective

EPI offers certain solutions to current problems in abdominal MRI because examination times are decreased and motion artifacts eliminated. EPI is currently being prepared for installation into clinical MR systems enabling conventional and EPI on the same systems with multi-slice capability, a wide spectrum of pulse sequences, and free slice orientation. Hybrid techniques such as those derived from RARE or GRASE are also likely to play a major role in abdominal MRI [14]. Preliminary results show impressive time reduction and diagnostic performance (Fig. 21). The development of suitable contrast agents will also play a critical role in the clinical improvement of MRI techniques [6, 99]. Future studies must clarify the clinical utility of abdominal EPI competing with current CT and MR techniques.

Acknowledgements. I am indebted to my former colleagues from the Department of Radiology at the Massachusetts General, especially at the MGH NMR Center, for many helpful comments and continuing support: Sanjay Saini, Mark S. Cohen, Robert M. Weisskoff, Ken Kwong, Peter F. Hahn, Mark A. Goldberg, Bruce R. Rosen, and Thomas J. Brady.

References

1. Cohen MS, Weisskoff RM (1991) Ultra-fast imaging. Magn Reson Imaging 9:1–37
2. Saini S, Modic MT, Hamm B, Hahn PF (1991) Advances in contrast-enhanced MR imaging. AJR 156:235–254
3. Mitchell DG, Vinitski S, Saponaro S, Tasciyan T, Burk DL, Rifkin MD (1991) Liver and pancreas: improved spin-echo T1 contrast by shorter echo time and fat suppression at 1.5T. Radiology 178:67–71
4. Mitchell DG (1991) Rapid-acquisition spin-echo MR imaging of the liver: a critical view. Radiology 179:609–612
5. Mirowitz SA, Lee JKT (1991) Optimizing MR imaging of the abdomen: the case for rapid acquisition spin-echo MR imaging. Radiology 179:612–614
6. Brasch RC (1992) New directions in the development of MR imaging contrast media. Radiology 183:1–11
7. Patten RM, Moss AA, Fenton TA, Elliot S (1992) OMR, a positive bowel contrast agent for abdominal and pelvic MR imaging: safety and imaging characteristics. JMRI 2:25–34
8. Mansfield P, Maudsley AA (1977) Planar spin imaging by NMR. J Magn Reson 27:101–107

9. Pykett IL, Rzedzian RR (1987) Instant images of the body by magnetic resonance. Magn Reson Med 5:563–571
10. Stehling MJ, Charnley RM, Blamire AM et al (1990) Ultrafast magnetic resonance scanning of the liver with echo-planar imaging. Br J Radiol 63:430
11. Haase A (1990) Snapshot FLASH MRI: application to T1, T2, and chemical-shift imaging. Magn Reson Med 13:77–89
12. Edelman RR, Wallner B, Singer A, Atkinson DJ, Saini S (1990) Segmented turboFlash: method for breath-hold MR imaging of the liver with flexible contrast. Radiology 177:515–521
13. Mirowitz SA, Lee JKT, Brown JJ, Eilenberg SS, Heiken JP, Perman WH (1990) Rapid acquisition spin-echo (RASE) MR imaging: a new technique for reduction of artifacts and acquisition time. Radiology 175:131–135
14. Feinberg D, Oshio K (1991) GRASE (gradient- and spin-echo) MR imaging: new fast clinical imaging technique. Radiology 181:280–293
15. Oshio K, Feinberg D (1991) GRASE (gradient- and spin-echo): a novel fast MR imaging technique. Magn Reson Med 20:344–349
16. Wehrli FW (1991) Fast-scan magnetic resonance: principles and applications. Raven Press, New York
17. Melki PS, Jolesz FA, Mulkern RV (1992) Partial RF echo-planar imaging with the FAISE method II. Contrast equivalence with spin-echo-sequences. Magn Reson Med 26:342–354
18. Melki PS, Jolesz FA, Mulkern RV (1992) Partial RF echo-planar imaging with the FAISE method I. Experimental and theoretical assessment of artifact. Magn Reson Med 26:328–341
19. Kiefer B, Hausmann R (1993) Turbo-gradient-spin echo: technique, implementation and comparison to turbo-spin-echo-imaging. 8th European congress of radiology, Vienna, p 186
20. Rzedzian RR, Pykett IL (1987) Instant images of the body by magnetic resonance. Magn Reson Med 5:563–571
21. Crooks LE, Arakawa M, Hylton NM et al (1988) Echo-planar pediatric imager. Radiology 166:157–163
22. Saini S, Stark DD, Rzedzian RR et al (1989) Forty-millisecond MR imaging of the abdomen at 2.0 T. Radiology 173:111–116
23. Stehling MJ, Howseman AM, Ordidge RJ et al (1989) Whole-body echo-planar MR imaging at 0.5 T. Radiology 170:257–263
24. Mansfield P (1977) Multi-planar image formation using NMR spin echoes. J Phys (Solid State Phys) C10:L55–58
25. Ordidge RJ, Howseman A, Coxon R et al (1989) Snapshot imaging at 0.5 T using echo-planar techniques. Magn Reson Med 10:227–240
26. Mansfield P, Coxon R, Glover P, Bowtell R (1993) High resolution echo-planar imaging at 3.0 T. SMRM, 12th annual meeting, New York, p 480
27. Fahrzaneh F, Riederer SJ (1988) Hybrid imaging with use of gradient-recalled echoes (abstract). Radiology 169 (P):379
28. Weisskoff RM, Cohen MS, Rzedzian RR (1993) Nonaxial whole-body instant imaging. Magn Reson Med 29:796–803
29. Butts K, Riederer SJ, Ehman RL, Felmlee JP, Grimm RC (1993) Echo-planar imaging of the liver with a standard MR imaging system. Radiology 189:259–264
30. Feinberg D, Hale JD, Watts JC, Kauffman L, Mark A (1986) Halving MR imaging time by conjugation: demonstration at 3.5 kG. Radiology 161:527–531
31. Hennig J, Nauerth A, Friedburg H (1986) RARE imaging: a fast method for clinical MR. Magn Reson Med 3:823–833
32. Reimer P, Saini S, Hahn PF, Brady TJ, Cohen MS (1994) Clinical application of abdominal echoplanar imaging: Optimization using a retrofitted EPI system. JCAT 18:673–679
33. Stark DD, Wittenberg J, Butch RJ, Ferrucci JT (1987) Hepatic metastases: randomized, controlled comparison of detection with MR imaging and CT. Radiology 165:399–406
34. Nelson RC, Chezmar JL, Sugarbaker PH, Bernardino ME (1989) Hepatic tumors: comparison of CT during arterial portography, delayed CT, and MR imaging for preoperative evaluation. Radiology 172:27–34
35. Heiken JP, Weyman PJ, Lee JKT et al (1989) Detection of focal hepatic masses: prospective evaluation with CT, delayed CT, CT during arterial portography, and MR imaging. Radiology 171:47–51
36. Rummeny EJ, Wernecke K, Saini S et al (1992) Comparison between high-field-strength MR imaging and CT for screening of hepatic metastases: a receiver operating characteristics analysis. Radiology 182:879–886

37. Nelson RC, Thompson GH, Chezmar JL, Harned II RK, Fernandez MP (1992) CT during arterial portography: diagnostic pitfalls. Radiographics 12:705–718
38. Oshio K, Jolesz FA (1993) Fast MRI by creating multiple spin echoes in a CPMG sequence. Magn Reson Med 30:251–255
39. Jakob PM, Haase A (1992) Scan time reduction in snapshot FLASH MRI. Magn Reson Med 24:391–396
40. Semelka RC, Simm FC, Recht M, Deimling M, Lenz G, Laub GA (1991) T1-weighted sequences for MR imaging of the liver: comparison of three techniques for single-breath whole-volume acquisition at 1.0 and 1.5 T. Radiology 180:629–635
41. Butts RK, Farzaneh F, Riederer SJ, Rydberg JN, Grimm RC (1991) T2-weighted spin-echo pulse with variable repetition and echo times for reduction of MR image acquisition time. Radiology 180:551–556
42. Holsinger-Bampton AE, Riederer SJ, Campeau NG, Ehman RL, Johnson CD (1991) T1-weighted snapshot gradient-echo MR imaging of the abdomen. Radiology 181:25–32
43. Semelka RC, Shoenut P, Kroeker MA et al (1992) Focal liver disease: comparison of dynamic contrast-enhanced CT and T2-weighted fat suppressed, FLASH, and dynamic gadolinium-enhanced MR imaging at 1.5 T. Radiology 184:687–694
44. Pauly J, Spielman D, Macovski A (1993) Echo-planar spin-echo and inversion pulses. Magn Reson Med 29:776–782
45. Saini S, Hahn PF, Reimer P, Nadeau KA, Cohen MS, Mueller PR (1991) Ultrafast MR Imaging of the liver: analysis of pulse sequence performance. Society of Magnetic Resonance in Medicine, 10th annual scientific meeting and exhibition, San Francisco, USA, p 24
46. Reimer P, Saini S, Hahn PF, Cohen MS, Brady TJ (1993) Klinische Anwendung der echoplanaren MR-Tomographie in der Detektion fokaler Leberläsionen: Ergebnisse einer quantitativen Untersuchung. RÖFO 159:16–21
47. Stehling MJ, Ordidge RJ, Coxon R, Mansfield P (1990) Inversion-recovery echo planar imaging (IR-EPI) at 0.5 T. Magn Reson Med 13:514–517
48. Bydder GM, Young IR (1985) MR Imaging: clinical use of the inversion recovery sequence. JCAT 9:659–675
49. Reimer P, Ladebeck R, Rummney EJ, Repp H, Peters PE, Schmitt F (1994) Detection of focal liver lesions with EPI: preliminary clinical results with CT comparison. MRM 32:733–737
50. Bruder H, Fischer H, Reinfelder H-E, Schmitt F (1992) Image reconstruction for echo-planar imaging with nonequidistant k-space sampling. Magn Reson Med 23:311–323
51. Bampton AEH, Riederer SJ (1992) Improved efficiency in 2DFT magnetization-prepared rapid gradient echo imaging: application to abdominal imaging. Magn Reson Med 25:195–203
52. Ortendahl AD, Kaufman L, Kramer DM (1992) Analysis of hybrid imaging techniques. Magn Reson Med 26:155–173
53. Constable RT, Gore JC (1992) The loss of small objects in variable TE imaging: implications for FSE, RARE, and EPI. Magn Reson Med 28:9–24
54. Karhunen PJ (1986) Benign hepatic tumours and tumour like conditions in men. J Clin Pathol 39:183–189
55. Wittenberg J, Stark DD, Forman BH et al (1988) Differentiation of hepatic metastases from hepatic hemangiomas and cysts by using MR imaging. AJR 151:79–84
56. Ohtomo K, Itai Y, Furui S, Yashiro N, Yoshikawa K, Iio M (1985) Hepatic tumors: differentiation by transverse relaxation time (T2) of magnetic resonance imaging. Radiology 155:421–423
57. Egglin TK, Rummeny EJ, Stark DD, Wittenberg J, Saini S, Ferrucci JT (1990) Hepatic tumors: quantitative tissue characterization with MR imaging. Radiology 155:55–59
58. Itoh K, Saini S, Hahn PF, Inam N, Ferrucci JT (1990) Differentiation between small hemangiomas and metastases on MR images: importance of size-specific quantitative criteria. AJR 155:61–66
59. Goldberg MA, Hahn PF, Saini S et al (1993) Value of T1 and T2 relaxation times from echo-planar MR imaging in the characterization of focal hepatic lesions. AJR 160:1011–1017
60. Goldberg MA, Hahn PF, Saini S, Egglin TK, Mueller PR (1991) Differentiation between hemangiomas and metastases of the liver with ultrafast MR imaging: preliminary results with T2 calculations. AJR 157:727–730
61. Reimer P, Saini S, Tombach B et al (1996) Echoplanar imaging (EPI) des Abdomens. Radiologe (in press)
62. Hamm B, Fischer E, Taupitz M (1990) Differentiation of hepatic hemangiomas from metastases by dynamic contrast-enhanced MR imaging. J Comput Assist Tomogr 14:205–216

63. Saini S, Hahn PF, Cohen MS, Reimer P, Campbell T, Brady TJ (1993) Dynamic gadolinium-enhanced echo-planar MR Imaging of the liver. RSNA, Chicago, p 116
64. Chezmar JL, Rumancik WM, Megibow AJ, Hulnik DH, Nelson RC, Bernardino ME (1988) Liver and abdominal screening in patients with cancer: CT versus MR imaging. Radiology 168:43–47
65. Ehman RL, McNamara MT, Brasch RC, Felmlee JP, Gray JE, Higgins CB (1986) Influence of physiologic motion on the appearance of MR images. Radiology 159:777–782
66. Henkelman RM, Bronskill MJ (1987) Artifacts in magnetic resonance imaging. Rev Magn Reson Med 2:1–126
67. Hahn PF, Saini S, Cohen MS, Goldberg M, Reimer P, Mueller PR (1992) An aqueous gastro-intestinal contrast agent for use in echo-planar MR imaging. Magn Reson Med 25:380–383
68. Stehling MJ, Evans DF, Lamont G et al (1989) Gastrointestinal tract: dynamic MR studies with echo-planar imaging. Radiology 171:41–46
69. Reimer P, Saini S, Hahn PF, Mueller PR, Brady TJ, Cohen MS (1992) Techniques for high-resolution echoplanar MR imaging of the pancreas. Radiology 182:175–179
70. Hahn PF, Stark DD, Lewis JM et al (1989) First clinical trial of a new superparamagnetic iron oxide for use as an oral superparamagnetic contrast agent in MR imaging. Radiology 175:695–700
71. Tscholakoff D, Hricak H, Thoeni R, Winkler ML, Margulis AR (1987) MR imaging in the diagnosis of pancreatic disease. AJR 148:703–709
72. Steiner E, Stark DD, Hahn PF et al (1989) Imaging of pancreatic neoplasms: comparison of MR and CT. AJR 151:487–491
73. Semelka RC, Ascher SM (1993) MR imaging of the pancreas. Radiology 188:593–602
74. Müller MF, Prasad PV, Siewert B et al (1993) Abdominal diffusion mapping using a whole body echo planar system. 12th annual meeting, New York, p 45
75. Butts RK, Riederer SJ (1992) Analysis of flow effects in echo-planar imaging. JMRI 2:285
76. Goldberg MA, Yucel EK, Saini S, Hahn PF, Kaufman JA, Cohen MS (1993) MR angiography of the portal and hepatic venous systems: preliminary experience with echoplanar Imaging. AJR 160:35–40
77. Crawley AM, Cohen MS, Yucel EK, Poncelet B, Brady TJ (1991) Single-shot magnetic resonance imaging: applications to angiography. Cardiovasc Intervent Radiol 15:32–42
78. Firmin D, Klipstein R, Hounsfield G, Paley M, Longmore D (1989) Echo planar high resolution flow velocity mapping. Magn Reson Med 12:316–327
79. Feinberg D, Jakab P (1990) Tissue perfusion in humans studied by Fourier velocity distribution, line scan, and echo planar imaging. Magn Reson Med 16:280–293
80. Saini S, Stark DD, Brady TJ, Wittenberg J, Ferrucci JT (1986) Dynamic spin-echo MRI of liver cancer using gadolinium-DTPA: animal investigation. AJR 147:357–362
81. Hamm B, Wolf KJ, Felix R (1987) Conventional and rapid MR imaging of the liver with GD-DTPA. Radiology 164:313–320
82. Edelman RR, Siegel JB, Singer A, Dupuis K, Longmaid HE (1989) Dynamic MR imaging of the liver with Gd-DTPA: initial clinical results. AJR 153:1213–1219
83. Villringer A, Rosen BR, Belliveau JW et al (1988) Dynamic imaging with lanthanide chelates in normal brain: contrast due to magnetic susceptibility effects. Magn Reson Med 6:164–174
84. Fisel CR, Ackerman JL, Buxton RB et al (1991) MR contrast due to microscopically hetero-geneous magnetic susceptibility: numerical simulations and applications to cerebral physiol-ogy. Magn Res Med 17:336–347
85. White DL, Aicher KP, Tzika AA, Kucharzyk J, Engelstad BL, Moseley ME (1992) Iron-dextran as a magnetic susceptibility contrast agent: flow-related contrast effects in the T2-weighted spin-echo MRI of normal rat and cat brain. Mag Reson Med 24:14–28
86. Reimer P, Saini S, Kwong KK, Cohen MS, Weissleder R, Brady TJ (1994) Dynamic gadopen-tetate dimeglumine enhanced echoplanar MR Imaging of the liver: effect of pulse sequence and dose on liver enhancement. JMRI 4:1–5
87. Greif WL, Buxton R, Lauffer RB, Saini S, Vincent AC (1985) Optimization of pulse sequences for imaging of hepato-biliary contrast agents. Radiology 157:461–466
88. Rummeny EJ, Stober U, Adolph J et al (1991) turbo-FLASH MR imaging: perfusion patterns of hepatic tumors. ARRS, Boston May 1991, p 203
89. Weissleder R, Elizondo G, Wittenberg J, Rabito C, Bengele HH, Josephson L (1990) Ultra-small superparamagnetic iron oxide (USPIO): characterization of a new class of MR contrast agents. Radiology 175:489–493
90. Lauffer RB, Vincent AC, Padmanabhan S et al (1987) Hepatobiliary MR contrast agents: 5-substituted Iron-EHPG derivatives. Magn Res Med 4:582–590

91. Reimer P, Weissleder R, Lee AS, Wittenberg J, Brady TJ (1990) Receptor imaging: application to MR imaging of liver cancer. Radiology 177:729–734
92. Reimer P, Kwong KK, Weisskoff R, Cohen MS, Brady TJ, Weissleder R (1992) Dynamic signal changes in liver with superparamagnetic MR contrast agents. JMRI 2:177–181
93. Moss AA, Kressel HY, Korobkin M, Goldberg HI, Rohlfing BM, Brasch RC (1978) The effect of gastrografin and glucagon on CT scanning of the pancreas: a blind clinical trial. Radiology 126:711
94. Hahn PF, Stark DD, Saini S, Lewis JM, Wittenberg J, Ferrucci JT (1987) Ferrite particles for bowel contrast in MR imaging: design issues and feasibility studies. Radiology 164:37–41
95. Laniado M, Kornmesser W, Hamm B, Clauss W, Weinmann HJ, Felix R (1988) MR imaging of the gastrointestinal tract: value of GD-DTPA. AJR 150:817–821
96. Kaminsky S, Laniado M, Gogoll M et al (1991) Gadopentate dimeglumine as a bowel contrast agent: Safety and efficacy. Radiology 178:503–508
97. Ros PR, Steinman RM, Torres GM et al (1991) The value of barium as a gastrointestinal contrast agent in MR imaging: a comparison study in normal volunteers. AJR 157:761–767
98. Reimer P, Schmitt F, Ralf Ladebeck R, Graessner J, Schaffer B (1993) Evaluation of potential gastrointestinal contrast agents for echoplanar MR imaging. EJR 3:487–492
99. Weissleder R, Bogdanov A, Papisov M (1992) Drug targeting in magnetic resonance imaging. Magn Reson Q 8:55–63

CHAPTER 11

Abdominal Diffusion Imaging Using Echo-Planar Imaging

M. F. Müller and P. V. Prasad

Introduction

The most significant advantage of echo planar imaging (EPI) is the ability to provide "snapshot" images devoid of any motion artifacts [1, 2]. Susceptibility to motion artifacts was the prime reason for conventional magnetic resonance (MR) imaging to be restricted primarily to imaging the brain. However, with the evolution of several ultrafast imaging techniques [1, 3] this restriction has been lifted. Cardiac and abdominal MR imaging have become routine examinations.

In the brain one area of study that has attracted immense attention in recent years is diffusion imaging. The effects of molecular diffusion on MR spin echoes were first studied several decades ago [4, 5]. Diffusion is the process of thermally induced random molecular motion. The apparent diffusion coefficient (ADC) is used as a measure of diffusion in biological systems because the measured diffusion coefficient may depend on factors such as temperature, perfusion, and Brownian motion [6–8]. MR is the only method available today to evaluate the molecular diffusion process in vivo in a noninvasive fashion. Many technical problems, most relating to physiological motion, influence the diffusion measurements [8, 9]. Thus in vivo diffusion imaging to date [8, 9] has been limited primarily to the brain. Diffusion imaging in the evaluation of stroke shows changes much earlier than conventional relaxation parameters [10, 11]. Also, since molecular diffusion is very sensitive to microscopic tissue makeup, it has immense potential in tissue characterization. Anisotropic diffusion imaging is useful in mapping the orientation of myelin fibers in the white matter, being greater along than across axons [12, 13]. However, because a diffusion imaging sequence is made to be sensitive to microscopic motion, conventional MR image acquisition methods suffered from severe motion artifacts [14]. Thus, the ability to perform EPI is highly desirable for carrying out routine diffusion imaging even in the brain. For more details refer to Chap. 16.

EPI was originally devised in 1977 by Mansfield [15], but it has become a research tool in only very few laboratories around the world. This is due to several critical demands of EPI on MR scanner hardware [2]. With several improvements in the hardware over the years the availability of commercial MR scanners with EPI capability has slowly become a reality.

This chapter demonstrates the way in which in vivo diffusion measurements can be obtained for the abdominal organs using a sequence based on a stimulated echo excitation and echo planar readout (STEAM EPI). Using this sequence, we provide some of our preliminary experience with a prototype MR scanner with EPI capability to perform diffusion imaging of the liver, spleen, kidney, and erector trunci muscle in healthy volunteers and in patients with various pathologies of the liver. This opens up a new arena because diffusion serves as a new contrast mechanism in addition to the conventional proton density and relaxation parameters. The combined information could lead to better tissue characterization.

The kidney is a particularly interesting organ to study by diffusion imaging because of its high blood flow and water transport functions. In the kidneys' structure and function are closely linked [16, 17]. The functional unit of the kidney is the nephron, composed of cells that are uniquely suited to perform specific transport functions (passive, facilitated, active). In addition, concentrating mechanisms by countercurrent multiplication in the loop of Henle are involved. These factors could have a substantial influence on the ADC values of various regions of the kidneys. Moreover, alterations in water mobility can be expected to occur in various disease states of the kidneys. To evaluate several physiological and anatomical factors that influence the in vivo ADC measurements of the kidneys we performed examinations in healthy subjects and in a pig model. Factors that were studied included renal perfusion, hydration state, ureteral occlusion, and the effect of diffusion gradient orientation.

Patients and Methods

Methods

All examinations were performed using a 1.5-T whole-body imager (Siemens Medical Systems, Erlangen, Germany) with EPI capabilities. We designed a pulse sequence combining a STEAM type of excitation with an EPI readout expressly to perform diffusion imaging in the abdomen (Fig. 1). The first two 90° pulses for the STEAM excitation were nonselective. A short 2- or 3-ms diffusion gradient pulse with gradient strengths up to 28 mT/m was applied along the slice select direction between the two nonselective 90° pulses. A third slice-selective 90° pulse followed by a balancing diffusion gradient pulse was applied after a long diffusion interval (Δ in Fig. 1). This was followed with an EPI readout with a typical data acquisition times for a 128×128 matrix of 64 ms. Images were acquired within a breath-hold interval to avoid respiratory motion. The sequence was amenable to cardiac gating. Under these conditions diffusion weighting depends on the time interval between the diffusion gradient pulses, which varies with the subject's heart rate. Diffusion sensitivity is governed by the gradient factor $b = \gamma^2 G^2 \delta^2 (\Delta - \delta/3)$, where γ is the gyromagnetic ratio, G and δ are the strength and duration of the diffusion gradient pulse, and Δ is the separation between the diffusion gradient pulses. The range of maximum b values was 328–454 s/mm^2 for a range of RR intervals 650–900 ms.

As a control, diffusion coefficients were measured using water and agar gel phantoms.

Subjects

Human Studies

The subjects consisted of 33 normal volunteers (17 women, 16 men) aged 19–37 years (mean 28 years). Additionally, we examined 9 patients (5 women, 4 men) aged 49–70 years (mean 62 years) who had been referred for evaluation of liver lesions (liver cyst $n = 3$, liver hemangioma $n = 3$, liver cirrhosis $n = 2$, hepatocellular carcinoma $n = 1$, and liver metastases $n = 1$). Cysts and hemangiomas were confirmed by typical imaging findings using ultrasound, computed tomography, or MR imaging. The hepatocellular carcinoma and cirrhosis cases were biopsy confirmed. All patients had been evaluated previously with ultrasound ($n = 8$) and/or computed tomography ($n = 3$) and MR imaging ($n = 3$). For studies of the effect of hydration state 18 normal volunteers (8 women, 10 men) aged 19–37 years (mean 28 years) were imaged both dehydrated (12 h fasting) and hydrated (1 h after drinking 20 ml water per kilogram BW). Five volunteers were reexamined on separate days to determine the reproducibility of measurements. The states of dehydration and hydration were confirmed by examining urine osmolality. For studies of diffusional anisotropy we studied 10 healthy volunteers (5 women, 5 men) aged 21–32 years (mean 27 years). In these subjects the hydration state was not monitored.

Animal Studies

A porcine model was used in accordance with the hospital Animal Studies Committee. The cardiovascular and renal systems of swine are more similar to humans than are those of other species such as dog [18], rat, and sheep [19]. In addition, the porcine kidney is similar to the human in that it has predominantly short-looped nephrons, in contrast to the dog which has long-looped nephrons [20].

Seven Yorkshire pigs (mean weight 41 kg) were studied. Renal artery stenosis was produced in seven pigs and ureteral obstruction in four pigs. When performed in the same animal, the right ureteral occlusion study was carried out after completion of the left renal artery stenosis studies. In some animals an acute osmotic diuresis ($n = 4$) was induced with mannitol (50 ml 20% solution in 10–15 min intravenous infusion; $n = 2$) or furosemide (20 mg in 2 ml NaCl intravenous injection; $n = 2$). This was performed before ($n = 2$) or after ($n = 2$) completion of the left renal artery stenosis studies.

The animals were well hydrated by infusing saline through an ear vein during the surgery and the MR study. On the day of study the pigs were anesthetized with intramuscular ketamine (10 mg/kg BW) and then with intravenous α-chlorolose (3.2 g) and urethane (20 g) in 100 ml normal saline, 60 ml given initially and 10–15 ml every 45–60 min as needed. The animals were intubated and mechanically ventilated. Central venous access was then obtained, and electrocardiographic leads were attached. An arterial line was placed for pressure and blood gas monitoring, and a central venous line was placed for fluid administration. Median laparotomy was performed under general anesthesia. Saline-filled balloon occluders (In Vivo Metric, Healsburg, Calif., USA) were used to induce arterial stenosis or ureteral occlusion. For the renal artery stenosis model a 5-mm occluder was applied around the surgically exposed proximal left renal artery; for the ureteral occlusion model a 12-mm occluder was applied around the proximal right ureter. The balloon was secured by tying sutures through the eyelets. Saline was injected into the tubing with a syringe, thereby inflating the diaphragm and stenosing or occluding the vessel or ureter. To deflate the diaphragm the saline was withdrawn. A single renal artery was surgically verified to ensure an optimal effect of renal artery stenosis on the kidney. An MR-compatible ultrasound volume flow probe (Transonic Systems, Ithaca, N.Y., USA) placed distal to the occluder was used to monitor the degree of flow deficit. Urine output was monitored with a Foley catheter placed in the bladder.

The animal was transferred fully anesthetized to the MR imaging system where it was connected to a ventilator, and the arterial line signal was wired to the trigger channel. A special panel in the wall of the magnet room allowed passage of the signal lines shielded from noise. Animals were anesthetized, intubated, and mechanically ventilated for imaging so that data were acquired without body motion. A remote switch connected to the ventilator allowed breath holding during the MR acquisition. Pancuronium HCl was administered by continuous infusion to ensure the absence of self-ventilatory efforts.

Sets of three or four images with different b values were acquired at 3-s intervals within a breath hold which typically lasted for 16 s (Fig. 1). Each image set was repeated three times in separate breath holds and the data was combined for analysis. The imaging parameters for the STEAM EPI diffusion-weighted

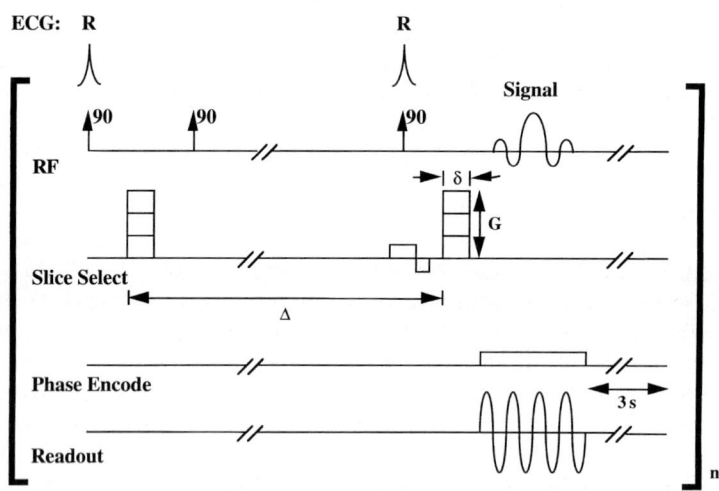

Fig. 1. STEAM EPI diffusion pulse sequence. The pulse sequence is repeated three or four times (*n* = 3 or 4) within a breath-hold, using different gradient strength values for the diffusion gradient pulse and a 3-s equilibrium time between repetitions. When used with cardiac gating the first and the third radiofrequency pulses are gated to two sequential R waves

sequences were as follows: $\Delta = 770$ ms, TE $= 18$ ms, field of view $= 300–400 \times 300–400$ mm, matrix $= 128 \times 128$, slice thickness $= 8$ mm, and number of acquisitions $= 1$. All the image acquisitions within a breath-hold were preceded by a dummy scan to avoid TR inconsistency between the first and the subsequent acquisitions within a breath-hold. We typically acquired images with eight different b values over two breath-hold periods. The b values within each of the breath-holds were interleaved, for example, 176, 57, 22, 8 s/mm^2 in one breath-hold and 395, 89, 32, 2 s/mm^2 in another. The order of the b values within a breath-hold, whether ascending or descending, did not make a difference in the volunteer studies. In patients we found it desirable to use the descending order, as this theoretically minimized any possible motion occurring towards the end of the breath-hold. In one subject the STEAM EPI sequence was synchronized to the cardiac cycle to determine the influence of vascular pulsation. For this purpose the diffusion gradients were applied at the same delay after the R wave in successive cardiac cycles using prospective electrocardiographic gating.

For evaluating anisotropic diffusion in the kidneys scout gradient-echo images (TR/TE/flip angle $= 30/10$ ms/30°) were obtained along the true anatomical transverse, sagittal, and coronal orientations of the kidney. A series of diffusion images were then acquired with the diffusion-sensitizing gradient (and hence the direction of diffusion sensitivity) oriented along each of these directions (cephalocaudad, anteroposterior, and medial-lateral for true transverse, sagittal, and coronal diffusion gradient orientations), and the directional ADCs were calculated (ADC_{tra}, ADC_{sag}, ADC_{cor}). The regions of interest (ROIs) were positioned for these measurements separately over the dorsal and lateral medulla and over the cortex and interseptal cortex. Images were always obtained at the level of the midpole of the kidney in an axial orientation, irrespective of the orientation of the diffusion-sensitizing gradient. Only four b values were usually obtained for studies of diffusional anisotropy: 198, 138, 88, and 8 s/mm^2. For these images a circularly polarized 18-cm flat surface coil positioned posteriorly was used as receiver for maximal signal-to-noise; for studies of hydration state the body coil was used as receiver.

Data Analysis

The diffusion coefficients were determined by a linear regression analysis of the ln(signal intensity) vs. diffusion-sensitizing gradient factor (b) (Fig. 2). This analysis was performed by using ROI placed on different organs or pathologies or on different locations (cortex, interseptal cortex, medulla) within the kidney (anisotropic diffusion studies), and on a pixel by pixel basis resulting in calculated diffusion maps (Fig. 3). All quantitative diffusion measurements reported here were made using ROI analysis. We preferred ROI analysis over calculation of diffusion maps as misregistration artifacts occurred when images from different breath-holds were combined.

ADC measurements for the hydrated and dehydrated states were analyzed statistically by means of a paired t test. Analysis of variance was used to examine the effect of location (peripheral cortex, interseptal cortex, and medulla) and

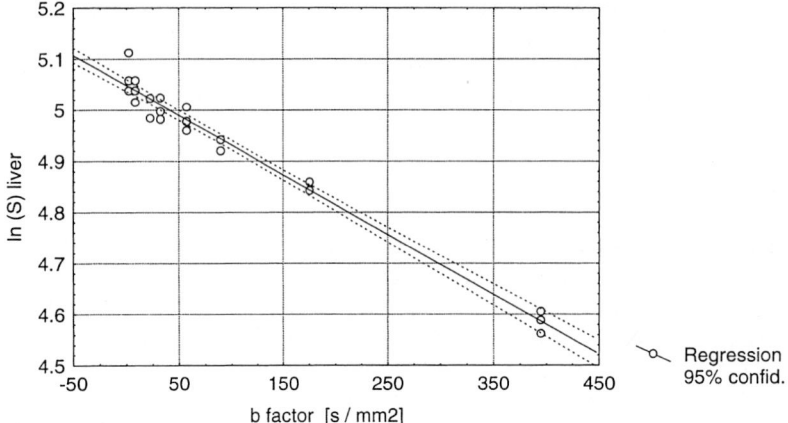

Fig. 2. ADC [ln(signal intensity of liver) vs. b factors] in a patient with liver cirrhosis. Data were acquired in six breath-holds (total eight b values)

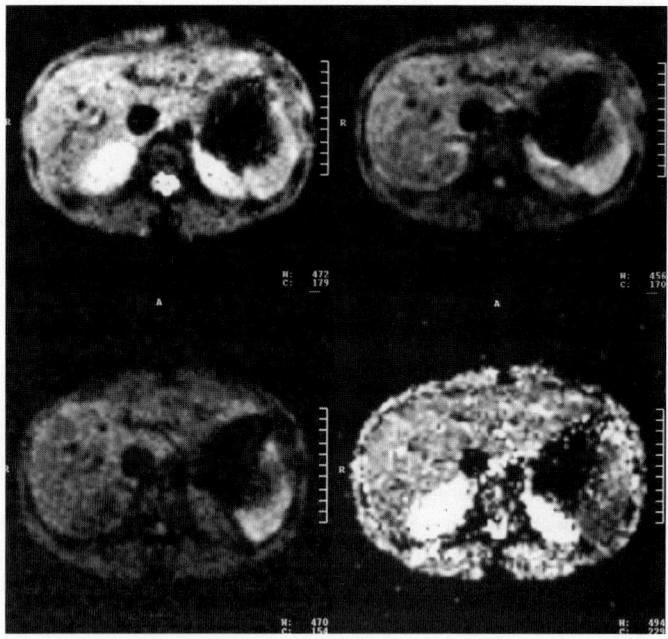

Fig. 3. Three different diffusion-weighted images in the same STEAM EPI sequence [b factors: 2 (*upper left*), 175 (*upper right*), 394 s/mm^2 (*lower left*)] of the abdomen in a normal volunteer and their diffusion map (*lower right*) with distinctive ADC values for liver, spleen, muscle, and kidneys

direction of diffusion sensitivity (three orthogonal components) with respect to the true sagittal, coronal, and transverse axes of the kidney, using an additive model based on a comparison of means weighted by locus [21]. A p value less than 0.05 was considered statistically significant.

Results

Phantom Diffusion Studies

Homogeneous diffusion images of the phantoms were obtained. The diffusion coefficients at room temperature (20 °C) for water (Fig. 4) and agar gel (1 % by weight) were calculated as 2.27×10^{-3} mm^{-2} s^{-1} and 2.34×10^{-3} mm^{-2} s^{-1}, respectively. These are consistent with values reported in the literature [22, 23]. The diffusion coefficient is temperature sensitive, varying 2.4 % per degree Celsius [7]. The expected diffusion coefficient of water at body temperature (37 °C) is 3.24×10^{-3} mm^{-1}/s^{-1}.

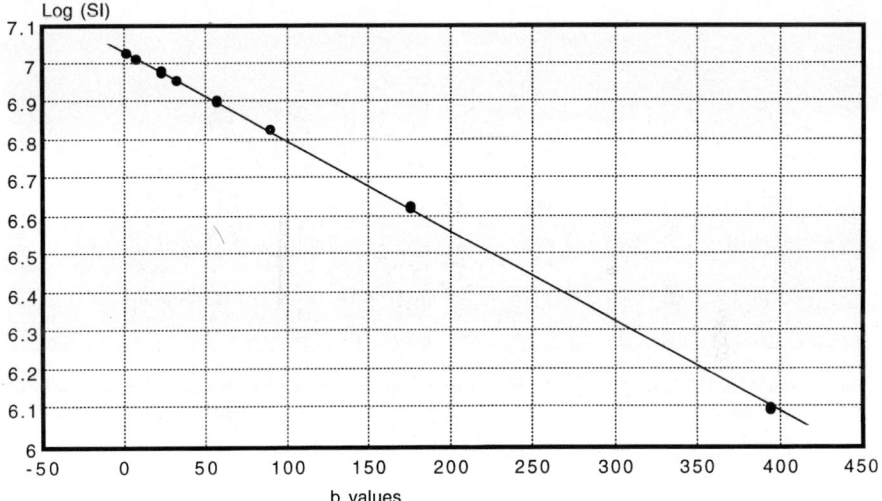

Fig. 4. Linear regression of a water phantom. Data were acquired with two sequences, each repeated three times (total eight b values). Correlation: $r = -0.9999$, $p < 0.00001$

Volunteers

The various diffusion values obtained for liver, spleen, and muscle were consistent among the volunteers studied and distinct from organ to organ. The measured ADC values were as follows: liver, 1.39 ± 0.16; spleen, 0.95 ± 0.15; erector trunci muscle, 1.99 ± 0.16; kidney, $3.54 \pm 0.47 \times 10^{-3}$ mm^2/s (Table 1, Fig. 3). The standard deviations shown here represent the intersubject variability.

Table 1. Results

Organ	ADC	Pathology	ADC $(\text{mm}^2 \text{ s}^{-1} \text{ } 10^{-3})$
Liver	1.39±0.16	Liver cysts	3.9–5.3
Spleen	0.95±0.15	Liver hemangiomas	2–2.8
Muscle	1.99±0.16	Liver metastases	1.2
Kidney	3.54±0.47	Hepatocellular Ca	1.7
		Liver cirrhosis	0.9–1.2

Our initial approach (in two volunteers) was to use cardiac gating along with breath-hold acquisitions to minimize misregistration and motion artifacts. Due to the dependence of the diffusion sensitivity of the sequence on the individual's heart rate we subsequently obtained diffusion-weighted images without cardiac gating using a constant of 770 ms. We found no substantial degradation of the diffusion-weighted image quality and no significant difference in the calculated diffusion values in the organs of interest except for the left lobe of the liver. When the Δ was made much shorter, for example, 200 ms, motion artifacts were substantially increased (Fig. 5).

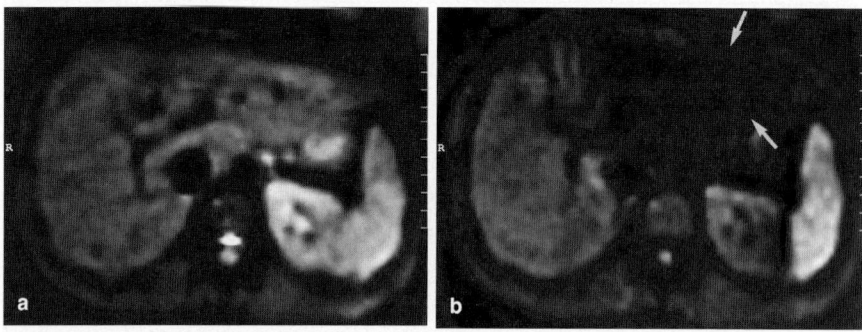

Fig. 5. Comparison of EKG-triggered acquisition (**a**) vs. untriggered acquisition (**b**). Without cardiac gating (**b**) there is gross signal loss in the left lobe of the liver (*arrows*) and the ADC is overestimated due to propagation of cardiac motion. However, the left lobe signal loss was generally much less severe in most cases

Patients

The diffusion measurements in the various hepatic pathologies (nine patients, ten lesions) were different from normal liver. The ranges (Table 1) were as follows: liver cysts ($n = 3$), 3.9–5.3; liver hemangiomas ($n = 3$), 2.0–2.8; liver metastases from an islet cell tumor ($n = 1$), 1.2; hepatocellular carcinoma ($n = 1$), 1.7; liver cirrhosis ($n = 2$), $0.9–1.2\times10^{-3} \text{ mm}^{-2} \text{ s}^{-1}$. In the one patient with an 8-cm hepatocellular carcinoma and underlying cirrhosis and portal hypertension the diffusion coefficients were measured at 1.71, 0.98, and $0.67\times10^{-3} \text{ m}^{-2} \text{ s}^{-1}$ for the tumor, the underlying liver parenchyma, and the spleen, respectively (Figs. 6, 7).

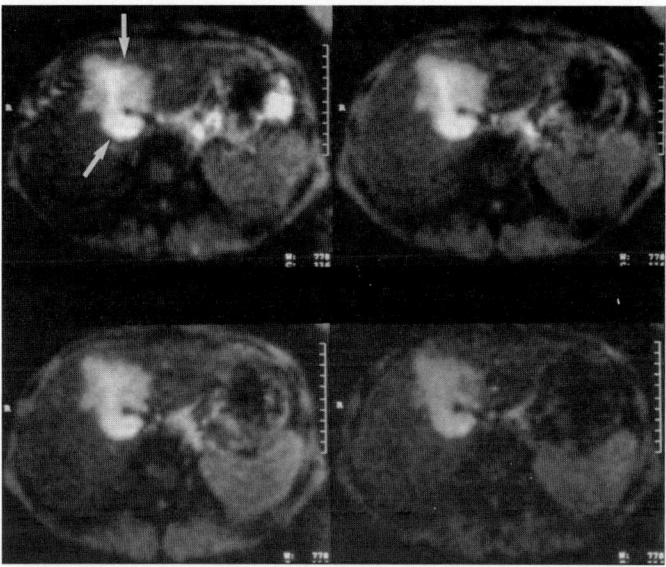

Fig. 6. Hepatocellular carcinoma (*arrows*). Four different diffusion-weighted images in the same STEAM EPI sequence [b factors: 8 (*upper left*), 22 (*upper right*), 57 (*lower left*), 175 s/mm² (*lower right*)]

Fig. 7. Diffusion map with hepatocellular carcinoma (*arrows*) in cirrhotic liver

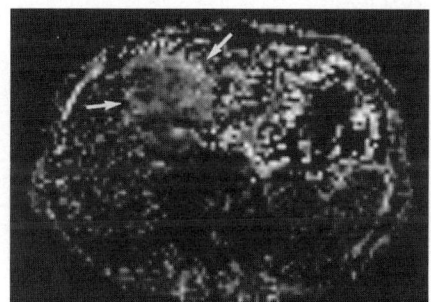

Diffusional Anisotropy. Figure 8 presents an example of an ADC measurement for a z-axis diffusion-sensitizing gradient orientation. Correlation coefficients for ln(signal intensity) vs. b value were in excess of 0.95. The direction of the diffusion gradient (Table 2) and location strongly affected the ADC ($p<0.002$, 99.8 % confidence, and $p<0.001$, 99.9 % confidence, respectively). The ADC was higher in the medulla than in the cortex ($p = 0.006$). As shown in Fig. 9, the ADC was strongly directional, having a pronounced radial component with respect to the collecting system. In one subject in whom the diffusion imaging sequence was cardiac gated ADC measurements acquired during systole (delays after R wave = 200–400 ms) and diastole (delay after R wave = 0 ms) were similar.

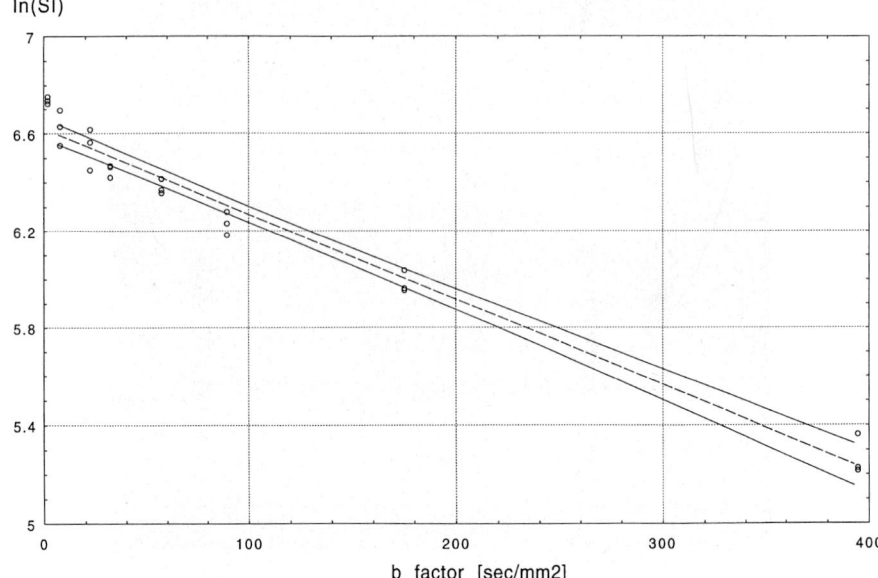

ln(SI)

b factor [sec/mm2]

Fig. 8. ADC [absolute value of the slope of the natural log of signal intensity (*SI*) of kidney vs. b factor] in a normal volunteer with the diffusion gradient oriented along the z-direction (long axis of magnet). The data for eight b values was acquired in two breath-holds; the measurements were repeated three times. ADC $= 3.6 \times 10^{-3}$ mm^2/s ($r = -0.99$, $p<0.0001$); *solid line*, regression at 95 % confidence level

Table 2. Comparison of directional ADC measurements ($\times 10^{-3}$ mm^{-2} s^{-1} for the dorsal (DM) and lateral medulla (LM), dorsal (DC) and lateral cortex (LC), and dorsal (DISC) and lateral interseptal cortex (LISC)

	DM	LM	DC	LC	DISC	LISC
ADC$_{sag}$	5.8±0.5	5.0±0.5	4.9±0.3	3.8±0.3	4.4±0.3	3.4±0.3
ADC$_{cor}$	5.1±0.6	6.0±0.5	3.7±0.3	5.1±0.3	3.3±0.3	4.5±0.3
ADC$_{tra}$	4.5±0.5	4.3±0.5	3.4±0.2	3.5±0.3	3.7±0.4	3.8±0.4

Fig. 9a–d. Diffusional anisotropy. **a–c** Four different diffusion-weighted images in the same STEAM EPI sequence [b factors: 8 (*upper left*), 88 (*upper right*), 138 (*lower left*), and 198 s/mm^2 (*lower right*)] obtained at the level of the midpole of the right kidney in a normal volunteer. True sagittal (**a**), coronal (**b**), and transverse (**c**) orientations of the diffusion-sensitizing gradient with respect to the orientation of the kidney. Note the different signal loss for each of the orientations of the diffusion-sensitizing gradient. **d** Corresponding anatomic image with corticomedullary differentiation (*upper left*) obtained in the same section as the diffusion-weighted images (**a–c**). *Upper right*, diffusion-sensitivity was along the true sagittal (anteroposterior) direction; *lower left*, diffusion-sensitivity was along the true coronal (medial-lateral) direction; *lower right*, diffusion-sensitivity was along the true transverse (cephalocaudad) direction. Higher signal intensity represents more diffusion; *each color* corresponds to a particular directional component of the ADC. The diffusion in the medulla is higher than in the cortex. The highest component of diffusion in the medulla is observed in a radial direction from the collecting system of the kidney

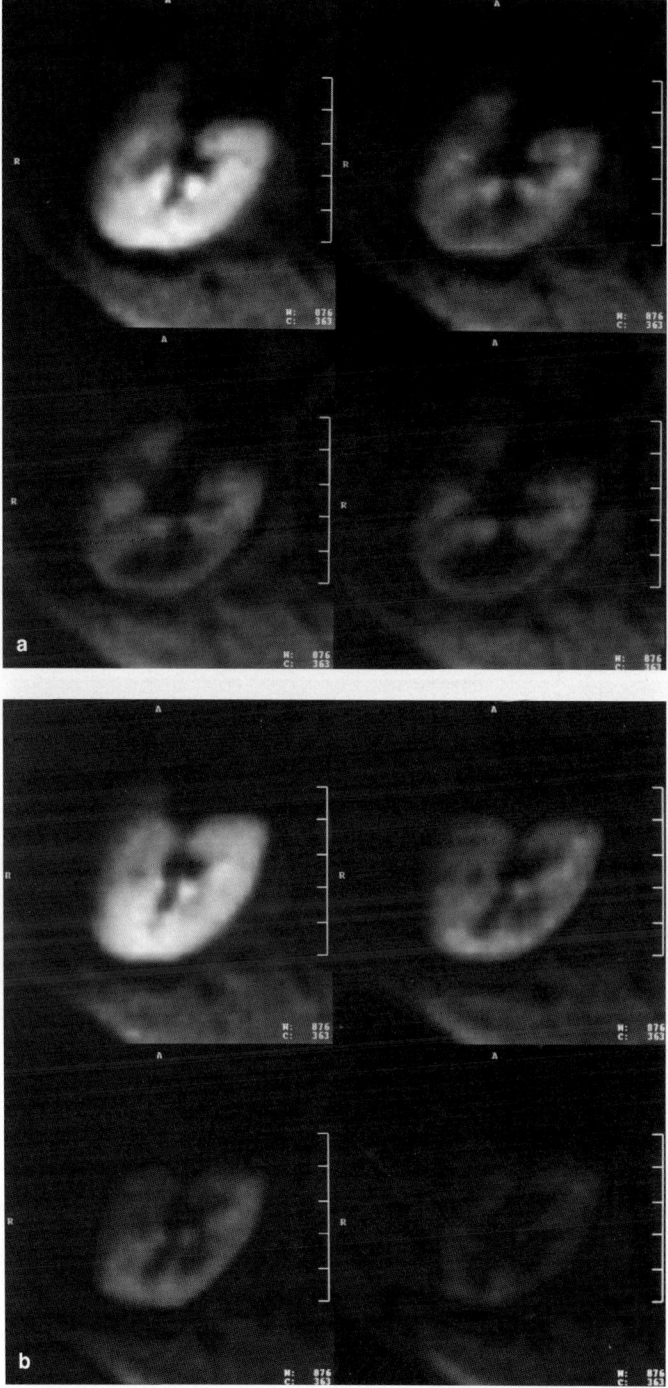

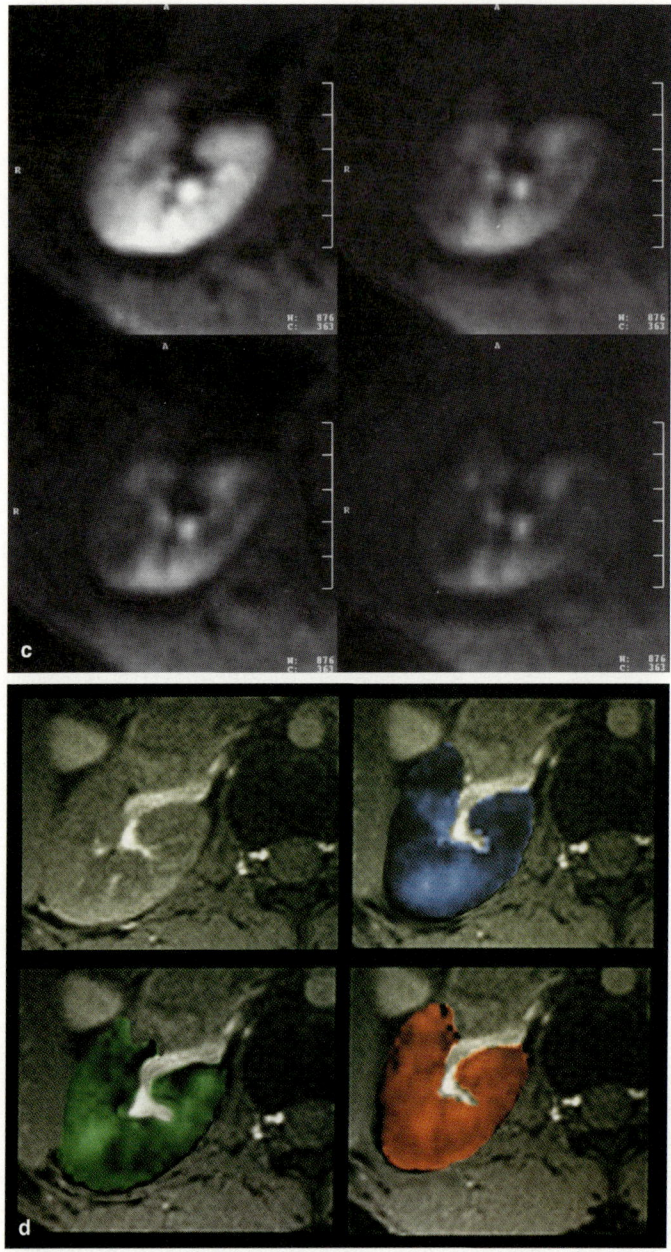

Fig. 9a–d. (*continued*)

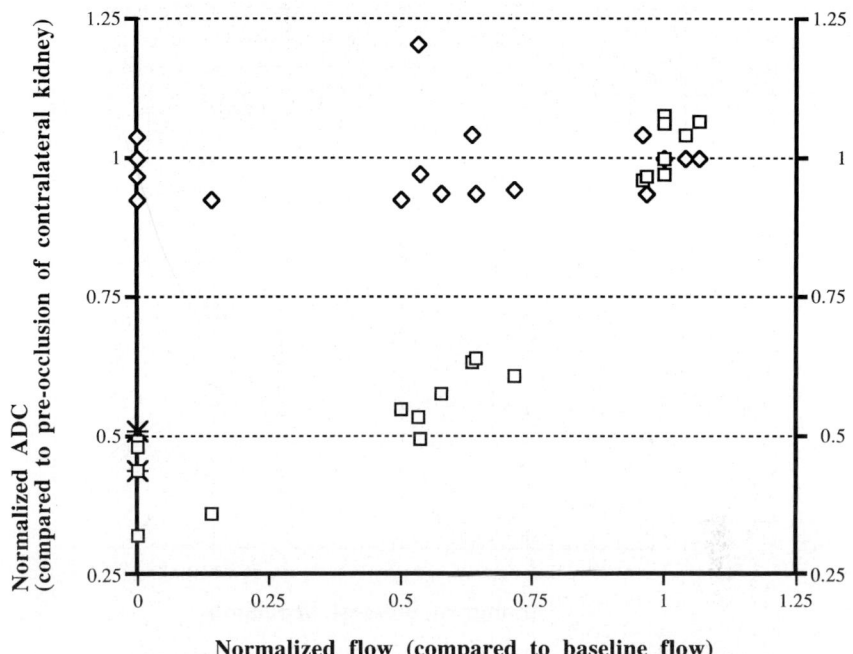
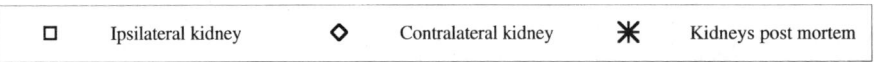

| □ | Ipsilateral kidney | ◇ | Contralateral kidney | ✳ | Kidneys post mortem |

Fig. 10. ADC of the ipsilateral and contralateral kidney before, during, and after graded stenosis of the renal artery ($n = 7$) as a function of blood flow. There is a flow-dependent decrease in the ADC values with progressive stenosis of the ipsilateral kidney; the ADC values of the contralateral kidney do not change. The ADC values at full occlusion are similar to those obtained immediately after death

Renal Artery Stenosis. Figure 10 depicts the pooled data from seven animals, showing the variation of ADC as a function of blood flow to the kidney. In the kidney supplied by the stenosed vessel the ADC decreased, with progressive stenosis with a nearly 50% reduction at full occlusion. The contralateral kidney showed no significant change during or after the acute stenosis or occlusion, as also shown in Fig. 10. The ADC values at full occlusion were similar to the values obtained postmortem.

Ureteral Occlusion. ADC measurements obtained 1 h after ureteral occlusion showed a decrease in the ipsilateral kidney and a small increase in the contralateral kidney. Figure 11 presents the pooled data from the four animals.

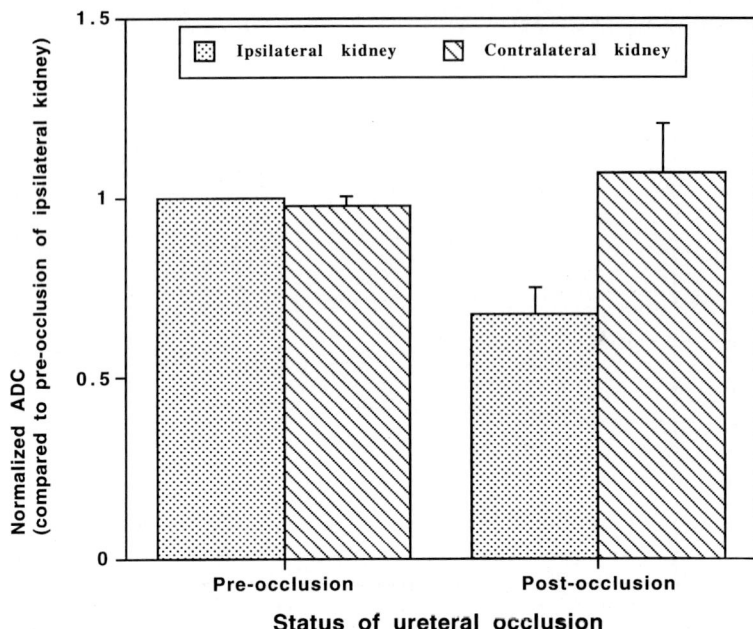

Fig. 11. Dependence of ADC measurements on the ureteral obstruction. The ADC of the ipsilateral kidney decreases after ureteral occlusion, whereas the ADC of the contralateral kidney increases

Diuresis. In the four animals that underwent diuresis we found no significant difference in the measured ADC, although the urine flow increased several-fold (from mean 2.4 to 26 ml/min).

Hydration State. Paired t test analysis showed a significant increase of the apparent diffusion coefficient from the dehydrated to the hydrated state ($p<0.0001$). There was no significant difference between the left and right kidneys. The ADC in the dehydrated state was $2.9\pm0.1\times10^{-3}$ mm^{-2} s^{-1}, which increased in the rehydrated state to $3.6\pm0.1\times10^{-3}$ mm^{-2}s^{-1} (Fig. 12). In each case dehydration and hydration was confirmed by examining urine osmolality (dehydrated 856 ± 23, hydrated 130 ± 7 mosm/l; $p = 0.0001$). In the five volunteers in whom the examination was repeated the ADCs were reproducible, with no significant difference.

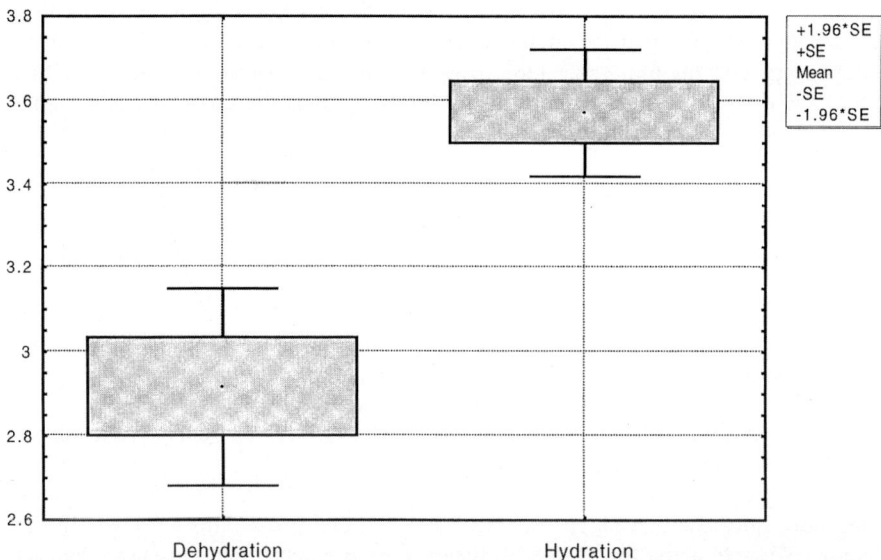

Fig. 12. Box and whisker plot of the ADCs of 18 healthy volunteers from dehydration to hydration. The ADC in the dehydrated state was $2.9\pm0.1\times10^{-3}$ mm²/s which increased in the rehydrated state to $3.6\pm0.1\times10^{-3}$ mm²/s

Discussion

Previous reports on diffusion MR imaging [4, 5, 7–9, 11, 22, 24–26] have described diffusion measurements either in vivo in the brain or ex vivo in models or phantoms. Abdominal diffusion studies in vivo have not hitherto been possible, primarily due to motion artifacts. With the evolution of EPI the entire set of echoes necessary to form an image can now be collected within a single acquisition period, thus reducing motion artifacts during the acquisition. For this study we used a STEAM type preparation with spatially nonselective radiofrequency pulses and an EPI readout. Additionally, the data was acquired during a breath-hold period.

Our results in normal volunteers indicate that the measured diffusion coefficients are different in each of the abdominal organs studied, and from our preliminary data in patients we observed differences in the measured diffusion coefficients under various pathological conditions.

The ADCs of the kidneys were much higher than those of other organs that we have studied, exceeding even the ADC of water at body temperature; the values also showed a wide scatter among the volunteers. The high ADC of the kidney may related to its high perfusion, high water content (about 83%, higher than any other organ [27]), and the presence of transport and concentrating mechanisms (filtration, resorption, secretion, concentration gradients, and electrical potential differences) that are unique to the kidneys and influence the water mobility. The kidneys receive about 25 % of the cardiac output although they constitute only about 0.5 % of the total body weight, representing perfusion of more than 400 ml min^{-1} g^{-1} [28]. However, one can infer from our data that the ADC does not represent perfusion directly because the medulla has a higher ADC than the cortex, despite the several-fold higher perfusion of the latter region.

Nonetheless the ADC depends strongly on perfusion, as shown in the porcine renal artery stenosis model. The ADCs of the kidney approached those of other organs when the renal artery was totally occluded. Moreover, in the two cases in which we obtained postmortem data within minutes after death the ADCs were similar to those obtained with renal artery occlusion. In the brain intracellular edema is generally believed to account for the drop in ADC with ischemia. This hypothesis is less likely to explain the changes that we have observed in the kidney since even moderate stenoses caused decreases in the ADC. It seems more likely that the dependence of ADC on perfusion reflects flow-dependent effects on water transport mechanisms.

Large increases in urine production with pharmacologically induced diuresis did not significantly change the renal ADC, thereby discounting a significant contribution of urine flow to the diffusion measurement. Acute ureteral obstruction causes a transient increase in blood flow to the kidney, followed by progressive vasoconstriction and a decrease in glomerular filtration rate [29, 30]. Our data obtained with unilateral ureteral obstruction showed a drop in ADC ipsilaterally and an increase contralaterally, possibly reflecting changes in functional status. However, studies of more chronic ureteral occlusion and concomitant blood flow and functional monitoring would be needed to evaluate this further.

Hydration state had a significant effect on the ADC. The greater intersubject variance in our ADC measurements ($3.5 \pm 0.5 \times 10^{-3}$ m^{-2} s^{-1}) than in those from other abdominal organs could be partly attributed to the differences in the hydration status of each volunteer or to kidney orientation because of the presence of anisotropic diffusion. The increase in ADC with rehydration could be due to an increase in water content, increased plasma volume and glomerular filtration rate, or an increase in osmotically driven water movements within the kidney [31].

There was a marked degree of diffusional anisotropy within the renal medulla and to a lesser extent in the cortex. That there is a pronounced directional component of diffusion with respect to the collecting system may be related to the radial orientation of the tubules and vasa recta and the different morphology of the interstitium in different parts of the kidney. A direct effect of vascular pulsation cannot be entirely excluded. However, in one subject in whom cardiac gating was used, ADC measurements obtained during systole and diastole were similar.

In the few patients studied we observed different diffusion coefficients in the diseased state than in the normals. In the case of hepatic cysts and hemangiomas the diffusion coefficients were higher than for normal parenchyma. This is to be expected in cysts, as these lesions are comprised of fluid collections in which the water mobility is relatively free. The elevated ADC values (with respect to water at body temperature) are possibly related to the fact that the fluid was still experiencing residual physiological motion during the breath-hold. Conversely, in cirrhotic liver the diffusion coefficients were measured as lower than normal. This may reflect the fibrotic nature of the tissue, with more restricted water mobility. We need to study a larger patient population before drawing any conclusions in this regard.

Since diffusion is a measure of motional freedom and a sensitive parameter characterizing the tissue makeup at the microscopic scale, it is conceivable that diffusion imaging may prove helpful in characterizing the pathology in the liver. Diffusion-weighted imaging also reflects the water balance between intra- and extracellular compartments. This has been shown to have a major impact on detection and monitoring of stroke [11]. Thus diffusion MR imaging may prove of particular interest for the study of ischemia and obstructive disorders of the kidney.

Other factors than water diffusion may affect the ADC. Microscopic and macroscopic susceptibility gradients or bulk motion could artifactually raise the ADC. However, these effects are probably minor given the low intersubject variability. Of interest is the low ADC of spleen, which is unexpected given its high water content, perfusion, and long T2. Further study of the factors determining the spleen's ADC value is needed.

In conclusion, in vivo diffusion measurements in the abdominal organs are now possible using STEAM EPI. The data, although preliminary in nature, suggest that measuring ADCs in vivo can prove helpful in the identification and classification of abdominal disease. The ADC of the kidney is higher than that of other organs due to several factors including high perfusion and water content. The dependence of ADC on perfusion is probably related to flow-dependent functional changes rather than to blood flow directly. The presence of diffusional anisotropy in the renal medulla indicates a dependence on tubular and/or vascular orientation. The capability of in vivo diffusion measurements in the kidney offers a noninvasive means for exploring its functional status and has potential value for the study of renovascular disease, acute tubular necrosis, and other conditions that alter kidney perfusion and function. Although availability of EPI is still limited, it is conceivable that single voxel, volume-localized STEAM sequences could yield similar data on conventional scanners.

References

1. Cohen MS, Weisskopf RM (1991) Ultra-fast imaging. Magn Reson Imaging 9:1–37
2. Stehling MK, Turner R, Mansfield P (1991) Echo-planar imaging: magnetic resonance imaging in a fraction of a second. Science 254:43–50
3. Chien D, Edelman RR (1991) Ultrafast imaging using gradient echoes. Magn Reson Q 7(1):31–56
4. Carr HY, Purcell EM (1954) Effects of diffusion on free precession in nuclear magnetic resonance experiments. Phys Rev 94:630–635
5. Steijskal EO, Tanner JE (1965) Spin diffusion measurements: spin echoes in the presence of a time-dependent field gradient. J Chem Phys 42:288–292
6. Le Bihan D, Breton E, Lallemand D, Grenier P, Cabanis E, Laval JM (1986) MR imaging of intravoxel incoherent motions: application to diffusion and perfusion in neurologic disorders. Radiology 161(2):401–407

7. Le Bihan D, Delannoy J, Levin RL (1989) Temperature mapping with MR imaging of molecular diffusion: application to hyperthermia. Radiology 171(3):853–857
8. Le Bihan D (1991) Molecular diffusion nuclear magnetic resonance imaging. Magn Reson Q 7(1):1–30
9. Turner R, Le BD, Maier J, Vavrek R, Hedges LK, Pekar J (1990) Echo-planar imaging of intravoxel incoherent motion. Radiology 177(2):407–414
10. Moseley ME, Kucharczyk J, Mintorovitch J et al (1990) Diffusion-weighted MR imaging of acute stroke: correlation with T2-weighted and magnetic susceptibility-enhanced MR imaging in cats. AJNR Am J Neuroradiol 11(3):423–429
11. Warach S, Chien D, Li W, Ronthal M, Edelman RR (1992) Fast magnetic resonance diffusion-weighted imaging of acute human stroke [published erratum appears in Neurology 1992, Nov; 42(11):2192]. Neurology 42(9):1717–1723
12. Moseley ME, Cohen Y, Kucharczyk J et al (1990) Diffusion-weighted MR imaging of anisotropic water diffusion in cat central nervous system. Radiology 176(2):439–445
13. Douek P, Turner R, Pekar J, Patronas N, Le Bihan D (1991) MR color mapping of myelin fiber orientation. J Comput Assist Tomogr 15:923–929
14. Prasad PV, Nalcioglu O (1991) A modified pulse sequence for in vivo diffusion imaging with reduced motion artifacts. Magn Reson Med 18(1):116–131
15. Mansfield P (1977) Multi-planar image formation using NMR spin echoes. J Phys C 10:L55–L58
16. Lemley KV, Kriz W (1987) Cycles and separations: the histotopography of the urinary concentrating process. Kidney Int 31:538–548
17. Kriz W, Kaissling B (1992) Structural organization of the mammalian kidney. In: Seldin DW, Giebisch G (eds) The kidney: physiology and pathophysiology, vol 1, 2nd edn. Raven, New York, pp 707–777
18. Powers TA, Lorenz CH, Holburn GE, Price RR (1991) Renal artery stenosis: in vivo perfusion MR imaging. Radiology 178:543–548
19. Terris JM (1986) Swine as a model in renal physiology and nephrology: an overview. In: Tumbleson ME (ed) Swine in biomedical research, vol 3. Plenum, New York, pp 1673–1689
20. Nielsen TW, Maaske CA, Booth NH (1965) Some comparative aspects of porcine renal function. In: Bustad LK, McCellan RO (eds) Swine in biomedical research. Frayn, Seattle, pp 529–536
21. Snedecor GW, Cochran WG (1980) Two-way classifications. In: Snedecor GW, Cochran WG (eds) Statistical methods, 7th edn. Iowa State University Press, Ames, Iowa, pp 255–273
22. Lorenz CH, Pickens DR, Puffer DB, Price RR (1991) Magnetic resonance diffusion/perfusion phantom experiments. Magn Reson Med 19:254–260
23. Wesbey GE, Moseley ME, Ehman RL (1984) Translational molecular self-diffusion in magnetic resonance imaging. I. Effects on observed spin-spin relaxation. Invest Radiol 19(6):484–490
24. Wesbey GE, Moseley ME, Ehman RL (1984) Translational molecular self-diffusion in magnetic resonance imaging. II. Measurement of the self-diffusion coefficient. Invest Radiol 19(6):491–498
25. Le Bihan D, Breton E, Lallemand D, Aubin ML, Vignaud J, Laval-Jeantet M (1988) Separation of diffusion and perfusion in intravoxel incoherent motion MR imaging. Radiology 168(2):497–505
26. Pickens D III, Jolgren DL, Lorenz CH, Creasy JL, Price RR (1992) Magnetic resonance perfusion/diffusion imaging of the excised dog kidney. Invest Radiol 27(4):287–292
27. Laiken ND, Fanestil DD (1990) Physiology of the body fluids. In: West JB (ed) Best and Taylor's physiological basis of medical practice, 12th edn. Williams and Wilkins, Baltimore, pp 406–418
28. Harth O (1980) Nierenfunktion. In: Schmidt RF, Thews G (ed) Physiologie des Menschen, 20th edn. Springer, Berlin Heidelberg New York, pp 668–702
29. Klahr S (1991) New insights into the consequences and mechanisms of renal impairment in obstructive nephropathy. Am J Kidney Dis 18(6):689–699
30. Klahr S, Harris KPG (1992) Obstructive uropathy. In: Seldin DW, Giebisch G (eds) The kidney: physiology and pathophysiology, vol 3. Raven, New York, pp 3327–3369
31. Koushanpour E, Kriz W (1986) Body fluids: turnover rates and dynamics of fluid shifts. In: Koushanpour E, Kriz W (eds) Renal physiology: principles, structure, and function, 2nd edn. Springer, Berlin Heidelberg New York, pp 21–40

CHAPTER 12

Echo-Planar Imaging of the Heart

D. N. Firmin and B. P. Poncelet

Introduction

The initial exploratory studies into the potential use of echo-planar imaging (EPI) to study the heart were carried out by the pioneers of the technique, Mansfield and his group at the University of Nottingham. As early as 1982 Ordidge and colleagues [63] first demonstrated the potential of the method by "freezing" the motion of the heart while imaging the thorax of a rabbit. The work was carried out at a field strength of 0.094 T, acquiring a 32×32 data matrix in 32 ms, and the heart could be seen with varying signals from blood in the cardiac chambers at different times in the cardiac cycle. Only one year later the first clinical findings were reported using the same technique to investigate three young infants with different cardiothoracic diseases [72]. Further clinical development of the same system later allowed more detailed studies enabling rapid assessment of infants with congenital heart disease [8, 9].

Despite the obvious potential there were a number of reasons why the technique developed more slowly than might have been possible, including the technical demands of a system capable of adult cardiac imaging and the greater interest of the manufacturers of magnetic resonance (MR) systems in developing techniques to image in detail other regions of the body. However, later in the 1980s there was a significant advance when Rzedzian and Pykett developed a system working at 1.5 T with an extremely fast resonant gradient drive on one axis, and Mansfield and his colleagues at Nottingham University developed a new system working at 0.5 T. Both groups demonstrated excellent single-shot cardiac images on their respective systems [71, 79]. In the early 1990s interest increased considerably, although the high cost of enabling whole-body EPI has meant that even today there are very few systems around the world capable of applying it.

More conventional MR imaging (MRI) of the heart developed during this period, initially with techniques to image anatomy and later to measure cardiac function [3, 47, 64, 82] and to accurately measure blood flow in and around the cardiac chambers [23, 60, 61, 81] and perfusion through the myocardium around the heart [95]. There has always been an interest in imaging the coronary arteries; however, it was not until the development of more rapid breath-hold techniques that have reduced the problems caused by respiratory motion that imaging these vessels has become more reliable [18, 50, 66]. The importance of applying even faster, EPI techniques to overcome problems of cardiac motion can be seen by studying a set of curves showing the relative temporal changes of

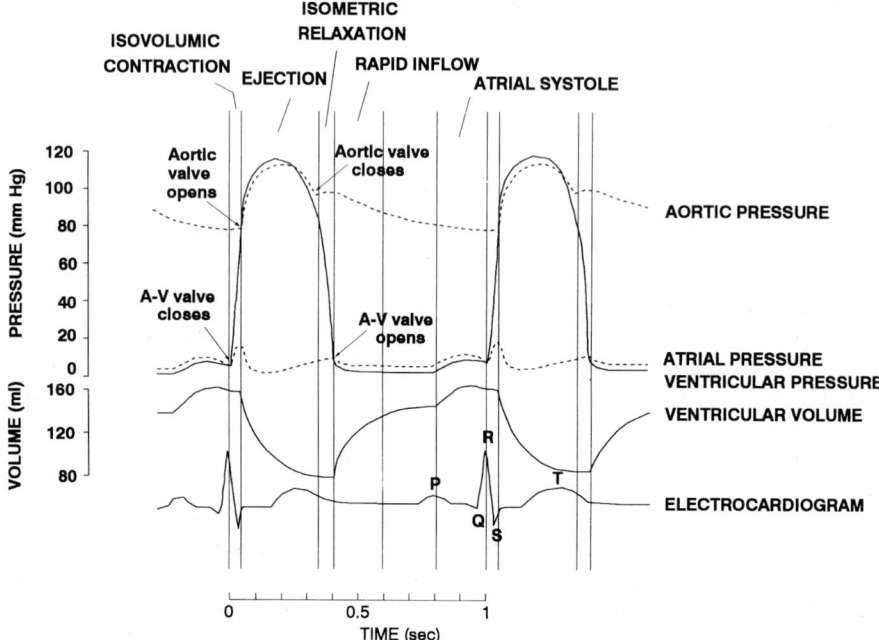

Fig. 1. Plot showing the relationship between cardiac pressures, volumes, and ECG, giving an idea of the typical timings of cardiac motion

pressure and volumes in the heart with relation to the electrocardiogram (Fig. 1). EPI is the only technique capable of acquiring a complete two-dimensional (2D) data set in a time scale that is short enough (<50 ms) to "freeze" the heart's motion at any point of the cardiac cycle. In addition to this, the application of EPI to study the heart allows a cardiac examination to be carried out much more rapidly and also promises to improve our ability to image the coronary arteries throughout the cardiac cycle and study the perfusion of blood through the myocardium. This chapter describes the work been carried out thus far on such applications.

Measurement of Stroke Volume and Cardiac Output

There have been two approaches to the study of cardiac anatomy and functional parameters such stroke volume, cardiac output, and wall motion by MR. In the first a spin-echo sequence is used to give good contrast between the myocardium and the blood, and multiple slices are acquired at one systolic and one diastolic timing of the cardiac cycle so that the area of the cardiac chambers can be measured for each slice and added to give a volume measurement [47]. Although this method has the advantage of enabling accurate volume measurements from any cardiac chamber regardless of shape, it is very time consuming, and the volume of the left ventricle can normally be measured more rapidly by making the assumption that its shape is an ellipsoid [3, 64, 82]. Two oblique orthogonal long-axis views of the chamber imaged at the times of systole and diastole can then be used to give the required measurements to calculate the volume. Both these spin-echo techniques have the disadvantage, however, that an assumption must be made as to the times of systole and diastole, and although a cine gradient-echo technique can be used to address this problem [48], it introduces another problem because the blood/myocardial contrast with such techniques is not as good, with the result that measurement errors are introduced.

The spin-echo EPI technique also produces the best contrast for making anatomical measurements from the images of the heart [11, 21]. The main reasons for this are that the signal from blood is minimal, partly because of the washout of excited spins between the 90° and 180° pulses and also because of the flow-dephasing gradient pulses that can be added either side of the 180° radiofrequency (RF) pulse [17]. These gradient pulses introduce flow-related phase shifts that cancel the signal from flowing blood, and this not only produces good contrast with the other cardiac tissues but also avoids potential problems of artifacts due to blood flowing during the acquisition. Another advantage is that the spin-echo images are less affected by susceptibility variations such as those found between the myocardium and the lung which can cause loss of signal on the gradient-echo version of EPI [17]. The problem of knowing the timings of systole

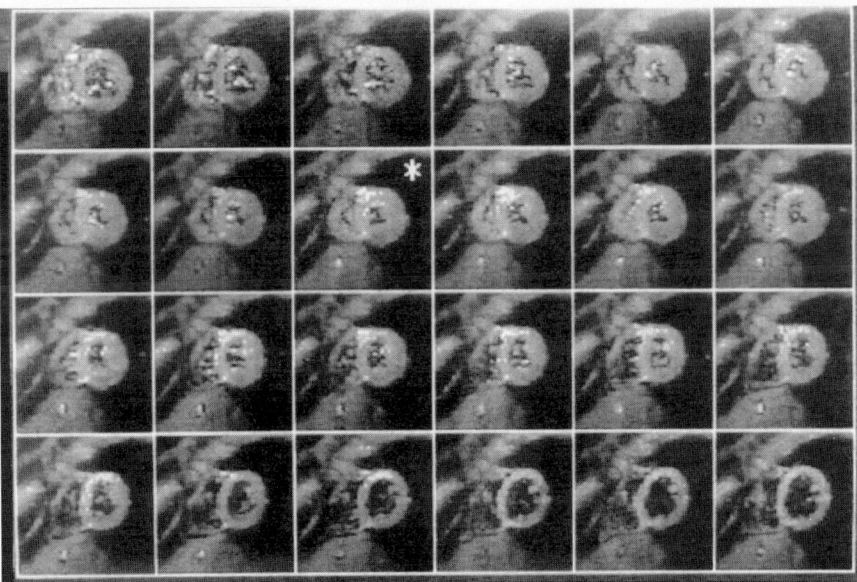

Fig. 2. Example of the progressive-delay series of images obtained at a midventricular section position. One image is acquired per cardiac cycle, with the time relative to the R wave of the ECG incremented by 30 ms between acquisitions. The effect is to show the contraction and relaxation of the ventricles with 30 ms temporal resolution, allowing end systole to be identified within 15 ms. *Asterisk*, image used to define the time of mechanical end systole, in this case 243 ms after the R wave. (Reproduced with permission of SMR from Hunter et al. [35])

and diastole is easily addressed by EPI; acquiring several spin-echo EPI versions of the same slice through the left ventricle but with each successive image acquisition at an increased delay from the R wave of the ECG can easily provide a measure of the relevant timings of the cardiac cycle. Hunter and colleagues [35] used this approach with a series of 56 consecutive images using an R wave delay increment of 30 ms to measure the systolic timing (Fig. 2), while the diastolic timing was taken to be immediately after the R wave of the ECG. The measurements of stroke volume and cardiac output were then made by acquiring a stack of 12 or 14 short-axis images at these times. All the images could be acquired in a breath-hold of 12 or 14 cardiac cycles by rotating through acquiring separated diastolic and systolic slices. The results of this study suggested a similar, if not better, accuracy to that of the more conventional MR methods but with a considerably shorter acquisition time.

The above type of imaging strategy could be useful not only for the measurement of stroke volume and cardiac volume but also for the rapid assessment of cardiac tumours or pericardial cysts and for investigating the various forms of sometimes complex anatomy found with congenital heart disease. This could be particularly important for studying children, in whom motion is often a problem when using other longer acquisition techniques.

Study of Myocardial Perfusion

The study of myocardial perfusion requires an imaging technique that can acquire all the required image data in the order of 1 s or less so that a bolus of contrast can be monitored as it flows through the cardiac muscle. Initial MR studies used gadolinium DTPA as a contrast agent and subsecond fast low-angle shot (FLASH) as an imaging technique with an acquisition time of 300–500 ms, used to image a short-axis slice during the diastolic part of successive cardiac cycles [94]. Gadolinium DTPA has the effect of reducing the T1 of the blood and the T2* of the myocardium that contains the supplying vasculature. The subsecond FLASH sequence, which is relatively insensitive to T1 and T2*, has been applied in conjunction with a preinversion RF pulse prior to the sequence to give T1 weighting. Although this technique is very robust, it does have the problem that only one slice of the myocardium can be imaged without compromising the temporal resolution. Additionally, the technique is not very efficient in terms of signal-to-noise ratio (SNR), thus requiring the use of a high field strength system. Initial investigations using these techniques tended to be rather qualitative, looking at relative signal changes as the bolus of contrast agent flows through the myocardium; however, recent studies by Wilke and colleagues [95] on model-based analysis of myocardial perfusion suggest that some level of quantification will be possible.

With EPI either the T1 or the T2* changes can be monitored [17, 92]. T1-weighted images are achieved by adding a preinversion RF pulse prior to the spin-echo version of the sequence, whereas T2* weighting is intrinsic to the gradient-echo version. The effect of a bolus of contrast flowing through the myocardium is to increase the signal from the T1-weighted sequence and to reduce it from the T2*-weighted one; a poorly perfused region of the myocardium results in a reduction of this signal change. The contrast-to-noise ratio is higher with the spin-echo sequence, and more importantly the change in contrast resulting from a bolus of contrast agent is considerably greater than with the gradient-echo version [17]. Two possible negative points, however, are that the required inversion time appears to be larger, and the flow sensitivity of the spin-echo sequence complicates the analysis if the blood-pool signal time curves are to be used as input functions for model-based analysis of myocardial perfusion [95].

One technical problem is that of oblique imaging because from a clinical standpoint the short-axis view of the left ventricle is the best for studying perfusion. This was an issue in the past because systems tended to have the capability of driving the alternating frequency encoding gradient on only one axis, so that at best only single-oblique imaging could be performed. Although it has been possible to position subjects in such a way as to achieve a short-axis view

Fig. 3. Comparison of T2*-weighted gradient-echo and T1-weighted spin-echo EPI images of a transverse section through the heart of a normal subject. *Above,* gradient-echo image shows a higher blood signal and a low myocardial signal, especially around the apex of the heart where the signal appears to be attenuated due to susceptibility effects. *Below,* spin-echo image shows a low blood signal and high myocardial signal. (Courtesy of Prof. R.R. Edelman)

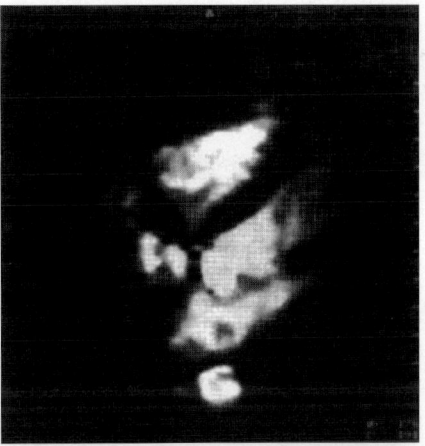
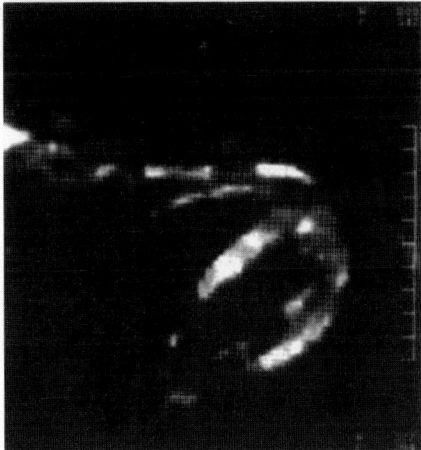

with a single-oblique [35], a double-oblique capability is desirable. This is demanding from technical point of view not only because all the three axes must be capable of driving the alternating frequency encoding gradient, but also as the waveforms are shared between the three axes, the timings must be precisely synchronized.

Much of the work to date has been carried out on animal models, using a small, more efficient set of gradient coils [92]; however, a human study has been reported by Edelman and Li [17] in which the gradient-echo and spin-echo versions of the EPI sequence were compared (Fig. 3). The great advantage of EPI is that with an image acquisition time of the order of 50 ms a number of slices can be acquired within a single cardiac cycle, and therefore the contrast agent bolus can potentially be monitored flowing through a greater volume of the myocardium.

Another approach to studying myocardial ischemia may be to use MR diffusion imaging. Brain ischemia, for example, has been shown to cause a decreased diffusion coefficient, probably as a result of an increased intracellular edema [44]. Motion sensitivity renders the methods used to study the brain unsuitable for the heart; however, Edelman and colleagues [20] have developed a stimulated echo excitation and echo-planar readout (STEAM EPI) sequence to overcome this problem. Figure 4 shows a set of four STEAM EPI images of a transverse section

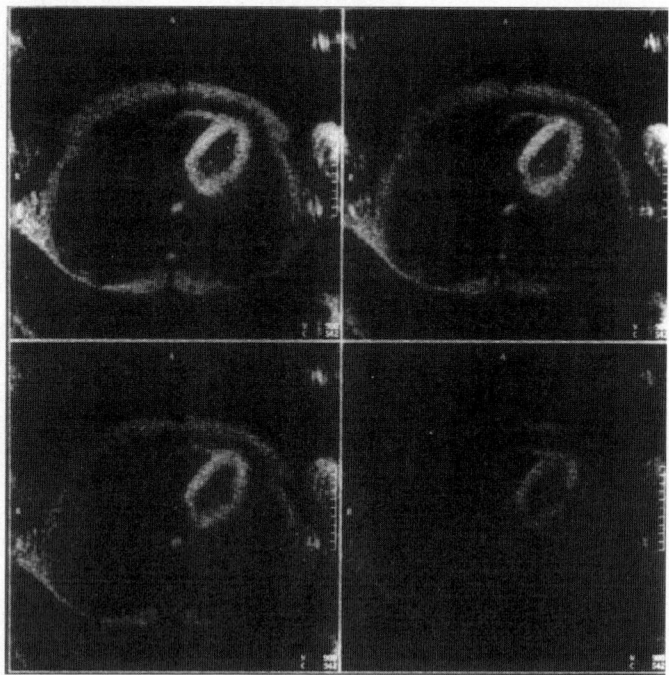

Fig. 4. EPI diffusion-weighted imaging of the normal myocardium. *From top left to bottom right,* the b value was increased (b = 3/12/20/42 s mm^{-2}) to achieve signal attenuation in the myocardium caused by diffusion. (Reproduced with permission from Chapman and Hall [75])

through the heart showing increasing attenuation due to diffusion coinciding with increasing b values. Cardiac diffusion imaging could be useful in the diagnosis and management of patients with diseases involving alterations in water mobility, such as myocarditis, rejection of cardiac transplants, and ischemic heart disease.

Imaging of Cardiac Dynamics

The study of cardiac dynamics has conventionally used gradient-echo sequences with velocity compensation and a low RF flip angle. The sequence, which is either triggered from the R wave of the ECG or gated retrospectively [45, 77], is repeated rapidly with multiple data frames per cardiac cycle requiring an acquisition time of the order of minutes. This type of imaging has allowed measurements of cardiac functional parameters such as regional wall motion throughout the cardiac cycle [48] as well as a qualitative view of blood flow patterns in the cardiac chambers. One area in which this form of qualitative blood flow imaging has been particularly useful is in the study of stenotic and regurgitant cardiac valves; complex and turbulent flow is generated downstream of the valve, and this results in loss of signal on the velocity compensated gradient-echo image [31].

The gradient-echo EPI sequence can be used to acquire a cine set of images, either by acquiring images over several cardiac cycles at a rate of one frame per cycle with an incremental increase in delay between the ECG R wave and each successive acquisition [79] or more rapidly by using a low RF flip angle with repeated acquisitions throughout the cardiac cycle [12]. The characteristics of the sequence are similar to the more conventional technique discussed above. The blood signal is affected similarly by flow types. With rapid repetition of the sequence in-plane or slow flow results in a decreased signal due to saturation; more rapid flow entering the slice has an enhanced signal and complex or turbulent flow results in loss of signal. The sensitivity of the sequence to this signal loss can also be reduced in the same way as for more conventional sequences; velocity compensation can be added [24] and the echo time can be shortened by using asymetric sampling or fractional k space sampling. The SNR is always an issue with cardiac EPI, and Stehling and colleagues [79] used a method of temporal Fourier filtering [13] to increase it. An improvement in SNR of (M/L) was obtained, where M is the number of frames per cycle, and L is the number of Fourier coefficients used. Although the cine aspect of the sequence is useful for assessing dynamic regional wall motion, as with the conventional gradient-echo imaging the contrast between blood and muscle is not as high as with the spin-echo version of the sequence.

From the point of view of cardiac imaging, the relatively poor spatial resolution can introduce limitations in that fine structures within and around the heart, such as valve leaflets, membranous septums, and coronary arteries, are poorly visualized at best. The potential of improving resolution is limited; if more sampling points per echo and more lines of k space are acquired, for example, these tend to extend the total sampling time to a point where there is no improvement as the signal will have completely decayed due to T2*. In the heart this problem is particularly severe because T2 is only about 35 ms and T2* is likely to be considerably shorter. Another problem with the gradient-echo EPI technique is that of uneven signal levels around the heart probably due to local field inhomogeneities because of the differing susceptibilities of surrounding tissues [17]. This problem and that of the limited signal duration due to T2* should be reduced by operating at a lower field strength, and it is possible that the optimum operating field for single-shot cardiac EPI is somewhat lower than the 1.5 T that is most commonly used today.

McKinnon [53] investigated another approach to addressing these problems by developing a hybrid sequence that used a number of reduced flip-angle RF pulses, with a shorter data acquisition consisting of fewer gradient echoes interleaved to give the same k space coverage in a slightly longer time than for the single shot. This means that T2* and susceptibility effects are reduced because the acquisition period after each RF pulse is significantly shortened, and problems relating to chemical shifts and field inhomogeneities are reduced because the speed of k space coverage in the phase blip direction is increased. The other

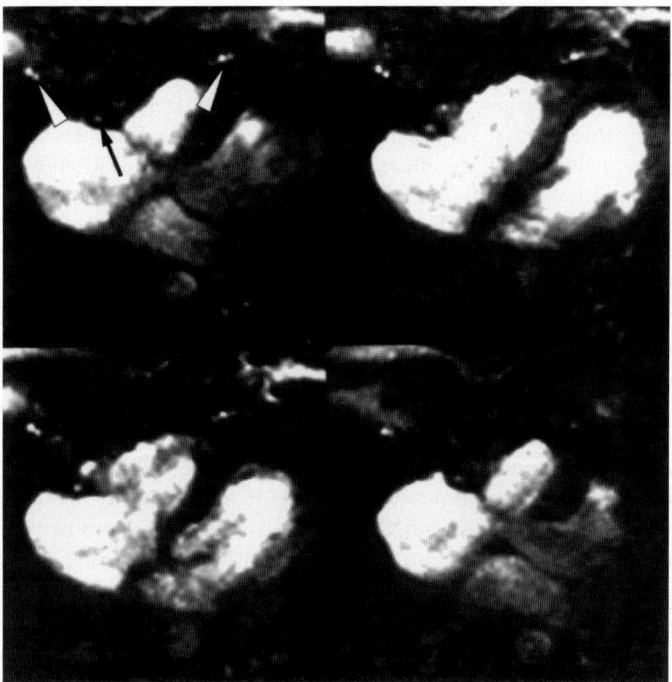

Fig. 5. High-resolution interleaved gradient EPI of the heart. The images were obtained by acquiring each of four interleaves in a nonsequential manner (in a separate heartbeat), collecting a total of 80 k space lines (half k space technique) and thereby producing an in-plane resolution of 0.75×1.5 mm. The atrioventricular leaflets are clearly visible. Even small vessels, such as the internal mammary arteries (*arrowheads*) and right coronary artery (*arrow*) are well depicted. (Reproduced with permission of the SMR from Davis et al. [12])

advantage with this approach is that the effective echo time is shorter, and as with conventional gradient-echo imaging, the shorter the echo time the lower the sensitivity to complex flow is. Additionally, McKinnon reduced the echo time further still by the use of fractional k space sampling. From the same group, Davis and colleagues [12] demonstrated this approach using four inter-leaves to help visualize the cardiac valve leaflets. The most important factor was the increased homogeneity of blood signal in the cardiac chambers, which was due mainly to the reduction in effective echo time from 13 to 3.4 ms; the small increase in acquisition time from 36 to 50 ms, on the other hand, would presumably have a slight negative effect of increased blurring of structures.

These interleaved methods were originally developed to enable EPI to be performed on a conventional scanner. A relatively low-resolution image could be acquired in the order of 100 ms. With high-performance EPI gradients and a similar overall acquisition time, either within one cardiac cycle or split into two or more cardiac cycles, the spatial resolution can be increased as larger areas of k space are covered. In these cases cardiac motion becomes a greater problem, either during the heart cycle or in the latter case from heart beat to heart beat. Davis et al. [12] presented impressive results of images acquired over four heart cycles in which details such as the valve leaflets, the internal mammary arteries, and the right coronary artery were clearly seen (Fig. 5).

Blood Flow Measurement in and Around the Cardiac Chambers

One MRI tool that has been developed and has important implications for the measurement of the function of the heart and blood vessels is that of quantitative blood flow imaging. The various approaches use either the effects of flow on the signal magnitude [88] or the signal phase [22, 61]. Although the different methods have their own advantages and disadvantages for different applications, the great majority of clinical studies have used the method known as phase-velocity mapping [61]. The methods have allowed us to accurately measure volume blood flow [23, 56] and to study the details of flow patterns within the cardiac chambers and great vessels [58]. For clinical diagnosis the method has been used in the assessment of stenotic valves [42], to quantify cardiac shunts [57], and to help unravel complex congenital diseases [32]. The methods also show potential in the measurement of coronary velocity and flow and the assessment of coronary lesions [40, 41].

The requirement to develop methods of EPI flow measurement is not only to increase the speed of the above clinical applications but also to enable physiological studies on the flow response to exercise or drug administration for example. Interleaved conventional and spiral EPI also offer advantages over the subsecond FLASH approaches to coronary flow imaging mainly in terms of reducing the problems of motion because of the shorter acquisition time. It should also be mentioned that the hardware required for EPI is also useful for other rapid gradient-echo techniques. For example, extremely short echo time flow imaging sequences can be developed and used to improve the accuracy of clinical blood flow measurement [25].

Early attempts to measure flow with EPI involved the use of flow-related phase shifts [24, 30]. Firmin and colleagues [24] incorporated the method of phase-velocity mapping into a 16-echo strip-selected EPI technique that was validated both by using flow phantoms and in vivo by comparing the measurement of carotid artery flow with that measured using the conventional phase mapping approaches (Fig. 6). The use of a strip selection method enabled high-resolution EPI to be applied on a conventional scanner, and as blood vessels are normally small, the strip could be offset and orientated to include the vessels. Velocity compensation was included to some extent for all three gradient axes; the slice selection gradient waveform was velocity corrected in the same way as in conventional gradient-echo sequences, the phase-encoding waveform was corrected at the time of the imaging echo (center of k space), and the frequency encoding

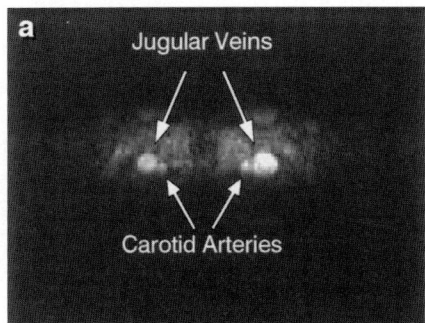
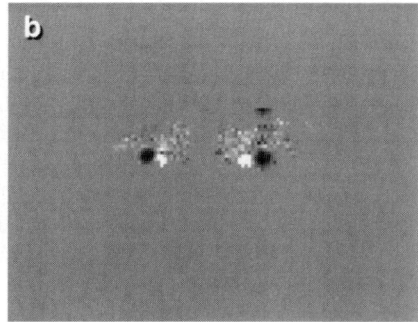

Fig. 6. Magnitude (a) and phase-velocity map (b) reconstructions of EPI data acquired with a strip-selected 16-echo EPI sequence. The strip-selected region includes the carotid arteries (*straight arrows*) and jugular veins (*curved arrows*) which can be seen exhibiting high blood signal on the magnitude image. Flow in the carotid arteries can be seen tending towards white while that in the jugular veins tends toward black with stationary material middle gray on the velocity map. c Comparison of the flow versus time for the right carotid artery of a normal volunteer obtained from EPI velocity images and conventional phase-velocity images. The close comparison between

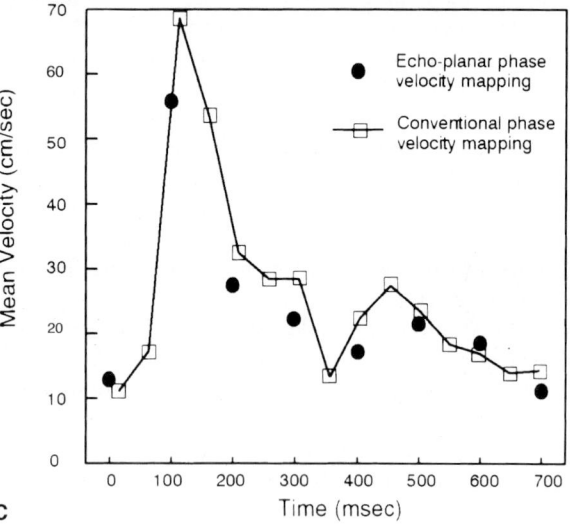

the two plots suggests that EPI velocity measurements are as accurate as the conventional phase-velocity mapping measurements [23]. (Reproduced with permission of Academic Press from Firmin et al. [24])

gradient was corrected on every other echo. The flow sensitivity of the technique was, however, noted as being greater than for more conventional sequences.

The flow sensitivity of EPI is in part due to the relatively long duration of the sequence, and as with more conventional scanning the time from signal excitation to the echo is important in terms of the extent of flow-related signal loss [25]. Analyses have shown that flow in the phase-encoding and frequency-encoding directions are the most important; flow in the former results in blurring while flow in the latter direction can result in Nyquist ghosts due to the induced phase alternation between odd and even echoes [5, 15, 90]. The echo time of the EPI sequence can be reduced by forming an asymmetric imaging echo in the phase blip direction, with the disadvantage that some high spatial frequency information is not acquired, and blurring can therefore occur in the phase-encoding direction. This can be resolved to some extent by applying the principles of conjugate symmetry to the k space data; however, this is not actually valid where velocity-dependent phase shifts are being encoded on the data, such as in the case of phase-velocity mapping. McKinnon and colleagues [54] used this approach, however, in an interleaved EPI technique capable of acquiring a cine flow study in just 4 s; errors were not measurable on the phantom validation studies but would perhaps be expected to be more significant in smaller vessels.

Spiral EPI allows the ultimate reduction in echo time because after slice selection the center of k space (the echo) is the first information to be acquired. For this reason it is relatively insensitive to flow-related signal loss problems [26].

Gated Sequence

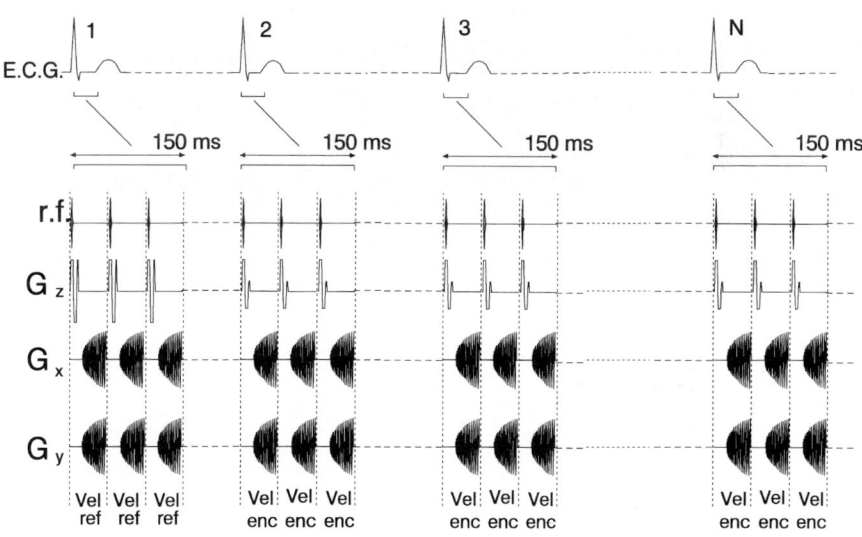

Fig. 7. A cine spiral EPI imaging sequence capable of real-time blood flow measurement over several cardiac cycles. The cine sequence is triggered off the R wave of the ECG. On the first cardiac cycle velocity-compensated images are acquired, followed on subsequent cardiac cycles by velocity encoded images for subtraction

These sequences have, again, been combined with phase-velocity mapping to produce rapid and accurate measurements of flow velocity. Gatehouse and colleagues [27] developed a single-shot sequence that could be repeated at intervals of 50 ms, allowing multiple frames to be acquired per heart cycle (Fig. 7). The 40-ms spiral gradient waveforms enables sampling over 32 cycles of k space that could be reconstructed into a 64×64 matrix image (Fig. 8). The main problem

Fig. 8. Four frames of a cine spiral flow study acquired using the sequence illustrated in Fig. 7. The images are of a transverse slice through the heart and the highest flow velocities can be seen on the systolic frame (*upper right*), in the outflow of the right and left ventricles (*lighter gray*) and in the descending aorta (*DA, darker gray*). *PO,* Pulmonary outflow; *AO,* aortic outflow. (Reproduced with permission of Williams and Wilkins from Gatehouse et al. [27])

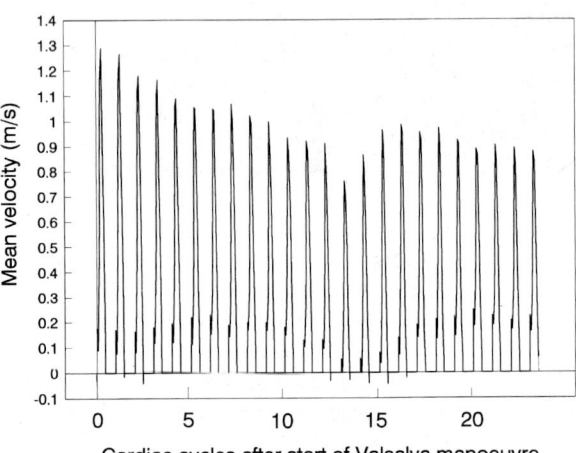

Cardiac cycles after start of Valsalva manoeuvre

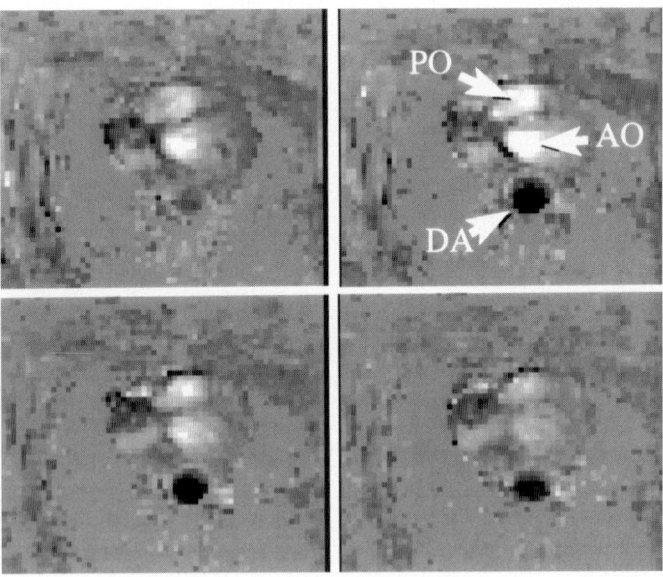

Fig. 9. Real-time measurements of descending aortic blood velocity over 25 cardiac cycles during a Valsalva maneuver. As expected, the blood flow velocity tends to drop as the heart rate increases. (Reproduced with permission of Williams and Wilkins from Gatehouse et al. [27])

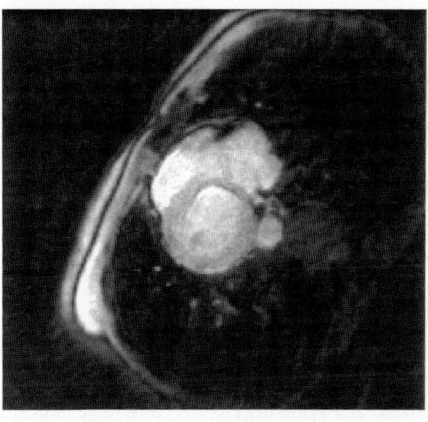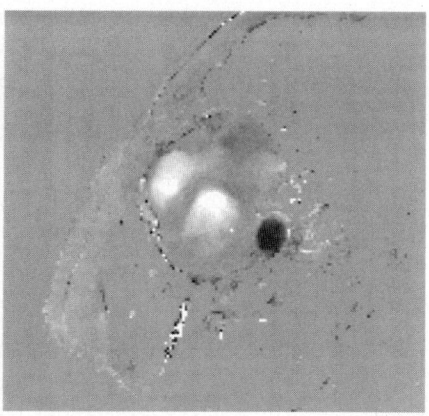

Fig. 10. Magnitude and phase-velocity images of a single frame from a high-resolution interleaved spiral-flow study. The image is of a short-axis slice near to the base of the heart at a systolic timing and shows high flow velocities in the left ventricle (*lighter gray*) and the descending aorta (*darker gray*)

was the sensitivity of the technique to blurring due to field inhomogeneities, requiring that extremely careful shimming was performed. As well as making rapid measurements of cardiac function and assisting in clinical diagnosis, the technique offers great potential in the study of blood flow physiology. For example, the single-shot spiral has been applied to measuring real-time aortic blood flow velocity changes during an application of a Valsalva maneuver (Fig. 9) as well as before, during, and after a period of exercise [59]. If real-time measurements are not essential, the acquisition period can again shortened and interleaved to improve the resolution and reduce the type of errors outlined above (Fig. 10).

Echo-Planar Imaging of the Coronary Arteries

Introduction

For many years there has been considerable interest in imaging the coronary arteries with MR. Although there have been a number of reports in which the main branches have been well visualized using conventional spin-echo and gradient-echo techniques [65], the problems of motion and in particular respiratory motion have meant that these small vessels could not be imaged reliably. For this reason there has been a long-standing interest in the possibility of using EPI to acquire the image data in a short enough period to remove such problems. The first reported use of EPI to image the coronary vessels was by Stehling and colleagues [78]; the images were acquired on a 0.1-T system with an acquisition time of 35 ms and even though the in-plane pixel size was 6 mm, the coronary sinus was clearly seen, as were suggestions of other smaller coronary structures.

Coronary Disease and Diagnostic Techniques

Nonocclusive coronary artery lesions cause symptoms by limiting the increase in flow necessary to offset an increased myocardial oxygen demand. Current methodology for evaluating this decrease in coronary flow reserve relies on either anatomical measurement of coronary lesions (X-ray angiography), or radionuclear examination of tracer distribution or transit in the myocardium [thallium and positron emission tomography (PET) scan]. Although valuable, anatomical measurements of a coronary stenosis (such as percentage of diameter narrowing) are insufficient to fully evaluate its physiological significance [29, 93]. More direct assessment of coronary flow dynamics and flow reserve requires the use of invasive techniques such as intravascular Doppler ultrasound [97] and transesophageal echocardiography [36]. The former technique, combined with X-ray angiography, requires the placement of a probe inside the coronary arteries, adding further risk to an already invasive procedure. The second technique, less invasive, can reach only the proximal coronary branches.

The leading cause of death in the United States and most other industrialized countries, coronary heart disease produces sudden death or myocardial infarction without prior symptoms in 60 % of the patients [38, 49]. Up to 13 % of middle-aged men in the general population have coronary disease, apparently without any symptoms [43]. However, none of the current diagnostic techniques suits the need for large population screening. The high cost and nonnegligible risks of intracoronary catheterization, the limited vascular access of transesophageal echocardiography, and the small number of PET resources make all of them inadequate. There is thus a need for a new noninvasive modality to assess and/or follow coronary artery disease.

MRI of the Coronary Arteries

MRI offers a unique noninvasive alternative approach which could prove useful for both anatomical and functional assessments of coronary disease. In addition to simply depicting the coronary anatomy, the possibility of achieving a functional evaluation of coronary flow dynamics has been driving all past and recent efforts to develop coronary MRI.

However, imaging the coronary arteries is a challenging task. The coronary arteries are difficult targets to track because of their small size, their tortuous course along the myocardium, and their complex cyclic excursions with cardiac and respiratory motions over distances much larger than their lumen size. Most limiting of all, motion, if not compensated, generates blurring and ghosting interferences not only from the coronary vessels themselves but also from the surrounding tissues. The key to succeed in imaging these highly mobile vessels is thus to freeze the motion.

The development of ultrafast MRI has enabled steady progress to be made in coronary imaging by several groups in recent years [7, 16, 18, 46, 55, 85]. Among the various proposed methods the most successful are the segmented turbo-

FLASH [18] and spiral-scan [55] gradient-echo techniques. Each produces a 2D image of the coronary arteries within a single breath-hold, acquiring 16–20 segments or spirals through k space in consecutive heart beats. In order to freeze vessel motion each combines cardiac gating and breath holding and acquires the information exclusively during middiastole, the most quiescent period in the cardiac cycle.

By collecting a 2D image in less then 60 ms, EPI offers a unique way to completely freeze the effect of both cardiac and respiratory motions [10, 51, 71]. EPI holds thus great promise for imaging the coronary vessels. This section presents a series of applications of single-shot EPI both to image the coronary vessels and to measure coronary flow velocity [68]. Using a time-of-flight (TOF) EPI method, we demonstrate the phasic changes of coronary flow through the cardiac cycle and measure transient flow increase induced by physical exercise and pharmacological vasodilation. Finally, we present preliminary clinical results on the difference in coronary flow velocity reserve between angiographically normal and diseased coronary artery [69]. All EPI was carried out on a General Electric Signa 1.5-T system retrofitted by Advanced NMR [10, 71].

Coronary Imaging

Single-Shot Imaging Protocol

The choice of a single-shot EPI imaging protocol must address several aspects of the anatomy of the coronary arteries in order to detect them and maximize contrast with the surrounding tissues.

Preliminary Considerations

The coronary vessels have a tortuous course along the myocardium, oriented in a double-oblique angulation. Visualizing these vessels either in-plane or through-plane requires a flexible orientation capability of the imaging system. Current EPI implementation on our system is limited, however, to single-axis oblique imaging. By rotating the subject inside the magnet in a 30°–45° left anterior oblique right decubitus position, the long axis of his heart can be aligned with the sagittal plane of the magnet. Such configuration enables short-axis and long-axis imaging of the heart [91].

Among the coronary vessels the left anterior descending (LAD) coronary artery constitutes a prime target because of its clinical importance in the left circulation [6, 84]. Running along the interventricular groove, the LAD coronary is oriented mostly in parallel to the long axis of the heart. Short-axis imaging of the heart should thus allow to visualize it in cross-section.

Regardless of the orientation of the vessel, contrast must be developed between blood in the coronary vessels and the surrounding tissues. Signal from the epicardial fat may be suppressed in EPI using a chemical shift selective saturation hard pulse series [89]. Any residual fat signal appears shifted by several pixels (between 7 and 15) away from the heart due to the large chemical shift effects of EPI [10].

Several sources of contrast can be used to separate the coronary vessels from the myocardium wall – T2 relaxation, magnetization transfer, and inflow effects from blood flow. Blood in the coronary arteries, depending on its oxygenation state, has a longer T2 relaxation time (between 100 and 200 ms) than the myocardium (50 ms [2, 96]). Single-shot EPI technique, with its intrinsic T2 weighting, automatically takes advantage of this source of contrast. The use of magnetization transfer off-resonance pulses allows to minimize selectively the signal from the myocardium without affecting the blood [46]. Finally, inflow contrast can be used between blood and myocardium [7, 16, 18, 46, 55, 85]. In the cardiac cycle middiastole represents the most favorable phase for inflow contrast; during this phase cardiac motion is minimal while coronary flow remains high.

Imaging Parameters

EPI of the coronary arteries was performed with a cardiac-gated single-shot gradient-echo pulse sequence [10, 71]. In order to maximize SNR and contrast, minimize flow-related signal loss, and depict the coronary vessels with sufficient spatial resolution we chose the following acquisition parameters: TE of 29 ms, 75%–79% partial k acquisition, flow-compensation along the slice select direction, flip angle of 90°, slice thickness of 10 mm and pixel size of 1.5×3 mm (field of view of 20×40 cm and 128×128 acquisition matrix). The resulting readout time was 48 ms. A fat suppression pulse was applied just prior to the excitation pulse. Signal was recorded with a 5×11 in. rectangular surface RF coil, used not only to improve SNR but also to allow short-axis imaging of the heart without aliasing problems.

Applications of Single-Shot EPI

The real-time imaging capability of EPI is best utilized in coronary imaging to track their motion within and across heart beats and to follow their volumetric course within a single breath-hold. Depending on the number of sampled heart beats, the duration of the breath-hold ranges from 2 to 25 s.

Real-Time Cine Imaging of the Coronary Artery

Unlike any conventional MRI techniques which create composite cine images from data acquired over multiple heart cycles, single-shot EPI allows to detect the coronary vessels and capture their motion through a single cardiac cycle with a temporal resolution of 95 ms per frame (see Fig. 11).

One unique advantage of real-time cine imaging is that it can be performed without any form of electrocardiogram gating. This could be particularly useful,

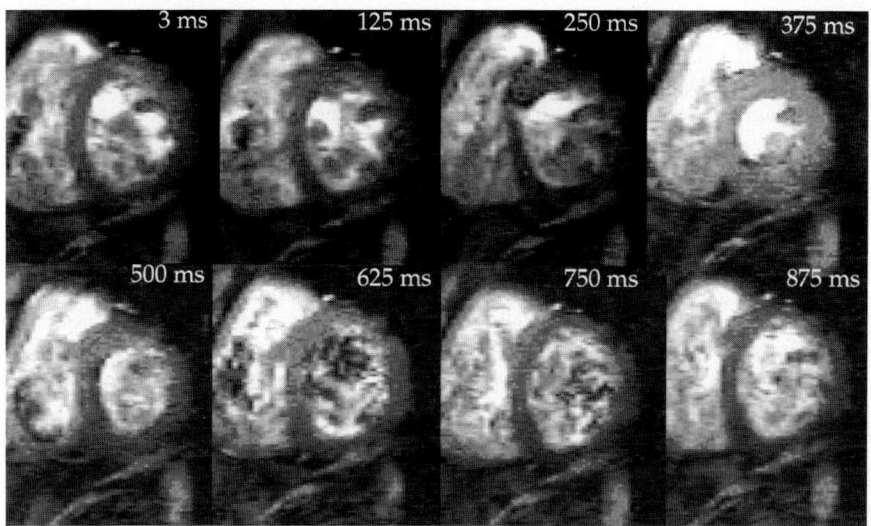

Fig. 11. Real-time cine short-axis imaging of the heart at a level near from its base. The LAD coronary artery is visible throughout the entire cardiac cycle and shows a high contrast with the interventricular groove tissues (epicardial fat and myocardium). A secondary vessel appears as well on most of the frames. Both vessels are moving during the cardiac cycle in response to the complex cyclic motion of the cardiac wall. Coming off the same artery (left main coronary), they draw closer together from frame to frame as a result of the cyclic though-plane translation of the heart

for instance, in patients with arrhythmias and during physical and pharmacological experiments producing transient changes in the subject's heart rate.

Beat-to-Beat Coronary Artery Tracking

Another advantage that real-time single-shot imaging offers is to probe the reproducibility of vessel position across cardiac cycles during a breath-hold. By collecting a series of single-shot gradient-echo images over multiple heart beats, substantial variability in the position of the LAD coronary artery has been detected during long (20 s) or short (10 s) breath-holds, up to 4 pixels (6 mm). Although not observed systematically, this beat-to-beat variability corresponded typically to a progressive drift of the vessel, starting from the beginning of the breath-hold. Such pattern most likely reflects the effect of breath holding on the heart rate regularity. Prone positioning of the subject, although less comfortable, could reduce the influence of the breath-hold by fixing the chest anterior wall.

Multi-Slice Imaging of the Coronary Artery

Complete coverage of the coronary tree with 2D segmented or spiral cardiac-gated imaging techniques, without gaps or overlap, relies on the good reproducibility of breath holding. Alternatively, multi-slice imaging performed within a single breath-hold, using multiple segments per heart beat, is prone to geometrical distortion effects from cardiac motion [14, 34].

Single-shot EPI allows to acquire a stack of contiguous slices in consecutive heart beats, covering the full heart within a single breath-hold (see Fig. 12). With each slice acquired at a fixed phase in the cardiac cycle, only vessel drift from breath holding can distort the volumetric data.

Combining short-axis imaging with relatively thick slices (1 cm) has been ideal to track coronary vessels in cross-sections, such as the LAD coronary artery and other branches of the left coronary vessel, including the circumflex and diagonal branches. Such protocol has, however, proven inadequate to depict the right coronary artery, coursing nearly in parallel in a slice too thick compared to the vessel diameter.

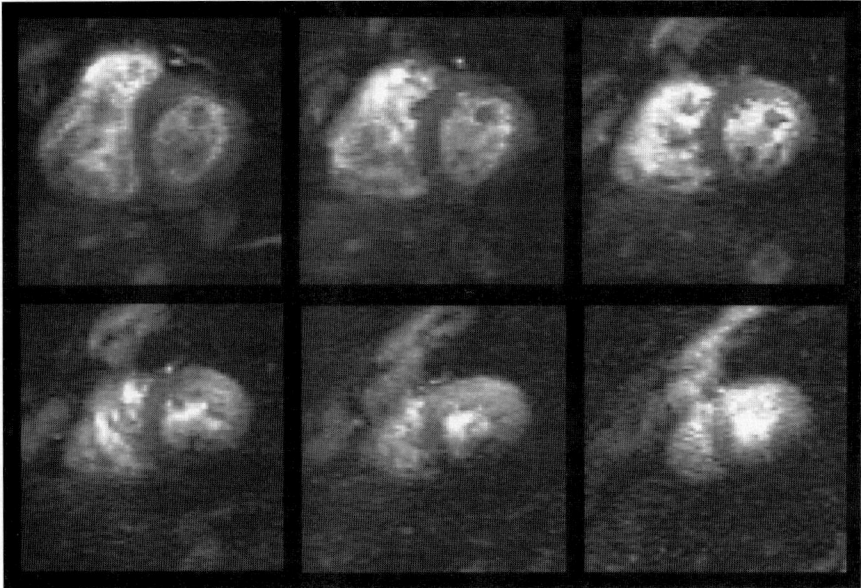

Fig. 12. Multi-slice imaging of the LAD coronary artery in cross- section. Six contiguous slices (1 cm thick) of the heart imaged in a short-axis view from base to apex were collected within a single breath-hold in consecutive heart beats. Acquired in a real-time multi-phase mode, the images shown were obtained in middiastole

Coronary Artery Motion: Single-Shot EPI vs. Multi-Shot Conventional Techniques

Single-shot EPI has uniquely demonstrated two important aspects of the motion of the coronary vessels: the large cyclic movements occurring both in-plane and through-plane which leave only middiastole free of movement and the beat-to-beat drift in the vessel position of a magnitude equal to or greater than its diameter. Both aspects of this motion must be considered when comparing the performances of single-shot EPI with the other imaging techniques. Except for our single-shot EPI, most of the coronary imaging techniques use either 2D multi-shot acquisitions during single or multiple breath-holds [14, 18, 55, 85] or three-dimensional (3D) segmented techniques without breath holding [33, 46]. One of the advantages these multi-shot techniques can offer is a higher spatial resolution. However, one may question the content of anatomical information provided by these techniques.

The readout window in our single-shot acquisition lasts less than 50 ms. The readout window per heart beat in the multi-shot techniques lasts 17.5 ms for 2D spiral scan [55], 104 ms for 2D segmented turbo-FLASH [18], and 270 ms for 3D segmented turbo-FLASH [46]. The 2D spiral-scan acquisition is thus the best at freezing the cardiac motion and tracking the full cyclic motion of the coronary vessels in a cine fashion. The 3D segmented technique, on the other hand, with the longest readout window, is reduced to imaging the coronary vessels during the only quiescent period of the cardiac cycle, middiastole.

In the 2D segmented turbo-FLASH technique k space is covered in an interleaved fashion. Any cyclic motion of the vessel occurring through each segment readout is distributed monotonically across k space and generates image blurring. Any vessel drift from beat to beat, on the other hand, becomes periodic in k space and produces ghosting in the image. In the 2D spiral-scan technique, only beat-to-beat vessel motion can produce image artifacts in the form of streaks. For each technique the control of these various motion artifacts relies completely on the subject's breath holding ability and heart beat regularity.

In the 3D segmented turbo-FLASH technique respiratory motion during and between segments dominates all other sources of vessel motion. Prone to ghosting and blurring, this technique must use pseudo-gating and/or retrospective gating to control these image artifacts [33, 46, 86].

The ultrashort scan time of single-shot EPI provides coronary images free of vessel motion blurring. However, the tradeoffs are multiple. Its relatively long signal readout compared to most multi-shot techniques limits the spatial resolution and SNR and increases sensitivity to magnetic susceptibility [10] and in-plane flow artifacts [62].

More detailed imaging of the coronary vessels requires a significantly higher spatial resolution, and hybrid/interleaved sequences have been developed to acquire higher resolution images in the period of a breath-hold. Although much of this work has been carried out using segmented FLASH sequences, there are potential advantages in using EPI. These include a higher SNR and a significantly shorter acquisition time per cardiac cycle, which enable images to be acquired even when the heart is moving most rapidly in systole and early diastole. There are also disadvantages, however, and the implications of these need to be fully understood. These include a sensitivity to both local and general field inhomogeneities, flow-related signal loss, and artifacts due to motion. Meyer and colleagues [55] have demonstrated the possibility of using interleaved spiral EPI by developing a sequence with an acquisition time equivalent to 20 cardiac cycles in which data were acquired for 17 ms of each (Fig. 6). Hu and colleagues [34] from the same group applied the technique by acquiring multiple contiguous slices over the 20 cardiac cycles. Although the different slices were at different times in the cardiac cycle, the set of images could be viewed as a cine loop to help visualize the continuity of the main coronary branches for several centimeters. As yet very little work has been reported on imaging the coronary arteries with the more conventional version of interleaved EPI, although the results might be expected to be similar to those of the spiral version except for a higher sensitivity to flow, a different sensitivity to motion and a different, and probably less debilitating sensitivity to field inhomogeneities and off-resonance errors. (General field inhomogeneities and off-resonance effects result in image distortion on conventional EPI and image blurring on spiral EPI.)

Coronary Flow Measurement

Quantification of Coronary Flow by EPI TOF

Several methods exist to measure flow velocity with MRI, based either on phase contrast or on TOF effects. We chose a TOF-based method because flow velocity can be measured by modeling the effects of blood flow wash-in through a slice [76, 87], probing only the magnitude information integrated over the whole vessel cross-section. This acquisition allows the use of partial k acquisition with much shorter TE and makes the best use of the tradeoff between lower resolution and lower motion artifacts in single-shot EPI.

The coronary vessels are highly mobile as a result of cardiac wall motion. The cyclic shortening of the ventricles (from 13 mm at the base to 2 mm at the apex; [70]) produces significant through-plane motion of these vessels, which complicates the use of MRI techniques for in-flow measurement. To address this we modified the original model presented by Wehrli [88] and adapted it to the coronary configuration by including a presaturation slab larger than the imaging slice [67]. This modification does not suppress per se the translational component of the vessel from an inflow measurement. However, the spatially wider presaturation serves to reduce the effect that "in/out" cardiac wall motion would have on the coronary signal and to maximize the contrast between the coronary vessel and myocardial wall.

The pulse sequence for TOF flow quantification is shown in Fig. 13. By progressive increments of the interval between the saturation and excitation RF pulses for each acquisition we can measure the signal intensity change due to blood wash-in through the slice. The slice excitation pulse timing is fixed to a particular ECG gate delay, and the presaturation interval is lengthened backward in time from the chosen cardiac gate delay. Fixing the gate delay in this fashion

Fig. 13. TOF EPI pulse sequence. Two 90° RF pulses are applied: the first saturates a large slab, and the second excites the imaging slice central to it. Between these pulses is a presaturation delay (T_{sat}). The slice excitation pulse timing is fixed to a particular ECG gate delay, and the presaturation interval is lengthened backward in time from the chosen cardiac gate delay at each cardiac cycle. *Shaded insert* corresponds to the diagram of a single-shot, flow-compensated gradient-echo pulse sequence

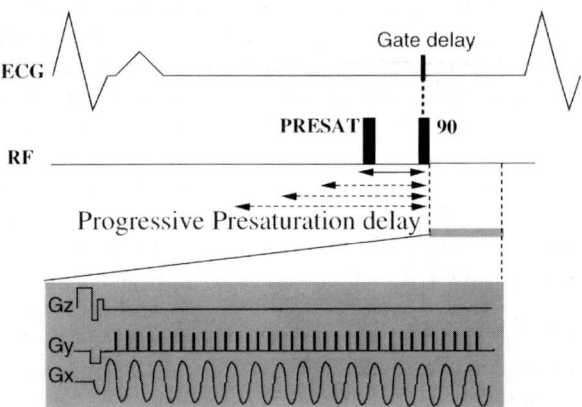

allows us to freeze the position of the heart and measure the wash-in effect at a constant position of the vessel. Any movement of the vessel within the series can be tracked by the operator for subsequent data analysis.

The wash-in function derived in the TOF model describes the signal change of unsaturated spins flowing in a vessel perpendicular to the imaging plane, assuming laminar flow. This flow progressively refreshes the slice that has been saturated by previous excitations. The total signal from the vessel is the sum of two components, $S(t) = F(t)+(1-F(t))\ (1-(1-\cos\ \theta)\ e^{-t/T1})$. The first term corresponds to the fraction $F(t)$ of fresh spins entering the slice, while the second term corresponds to the remaining fraction $(1-F(t))$ of spins presaturated by a RF pulse θ. The function that describes the fraction of fresh spins, $F(t)$, can be derived and split into three parts (see Fig. 14). Maximum flow velocities are determined by fitting the experimental wash-in curves to this model.

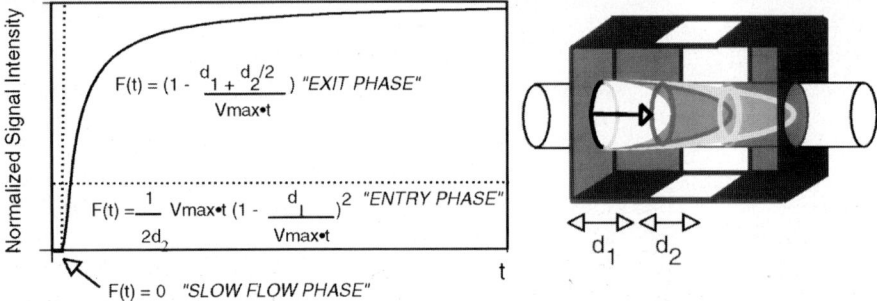

Fig. 14. TOF model describing the fraction of a laminar bolus of fresh spins entering a slice saturated by previous excitations. At first the fraction is zero as long as the fresh bolus traverses only the presaturation slab (d_1). When the laminar bolus of fresh spins reaches the slice, the function starts its "entry phase." Finally, when the laminar bolus has reached the end of the slice (d_2), the function changes and plateaus during its "exit phase"

An important assumption that the TOF model makes is that the blood flow in the vessel is laminar. Such condition is fulfilled in the case of coronary flow, as supported by direct Doppler velocity-profile measurements [28, 37].

Measurement of Coronary Flow in the LAD

To measure flow velocity in the LAD coronary we collected a single-slice series of 20–25 short-axis images of the heart, with each image acquired at the same fixed cardiac gate delay on successive heart beats (see Fig. 15). The first three images of each series were obtained without any presaturation, and were used for reference signal intensity. The next images were collected with a 3-cm presaturation slab overlapping the slice plane and a presaturation interval that was progressively increased by 10-ms increments from 10 ms to 220 ms on successive heart beats. This maximum time window was set in order to avoid excessive velocity averaging over the cardiac cycle. Each series was acquired during a single breath-hold. Note that in this protocol the 3-cm-thick presaturation slab (surrounding the 1-cm-thick slice) allows to fully contain the displacement of the myocardium through the slice that might occur during the presaturation period.

A region-of-interest of 2–4 pixels covering the whole vessel's cross-section was selected, and the change in signal intensity was measured for the complete series collected with the TOF sequence. To avoid errors related to in-plane motion of the vessel through the series the vessel was tracked manually in each image by the operator. Flow velocities were then determined for each series with two iterations of curve fitting to the "exit phase" function of our TOF model:

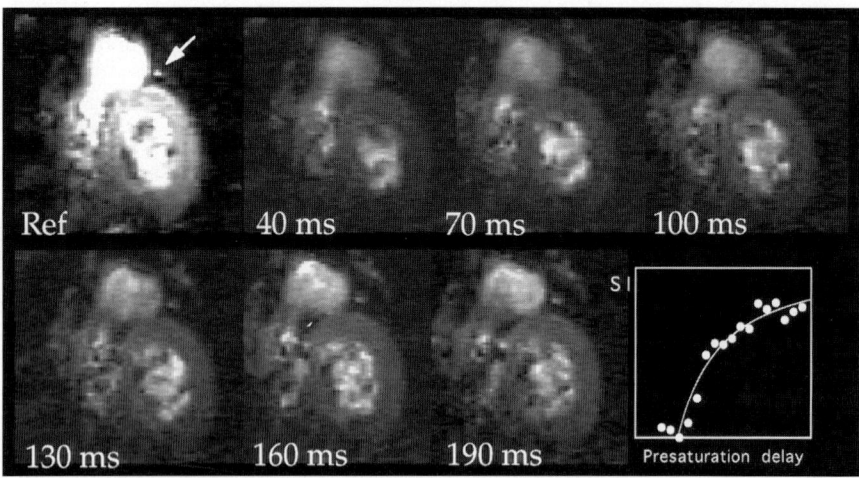

Fig. 15. TOF signal change of the LAD coronary vessel at a fixed delay in diastole. The first image is a reference frame obtained without any presaturation and the next frames were obtained with variable presaturation delays (*lower left*). *Lower right*, the corresponding normalized TOF signal intensity change in the LAD vessel

$$\frac{S_{exit}(t)}{t} = \frac{\alpha(1-1.5cm)}{v_{max}} + m_0$$

where m_0 is the noise or "zero" level determined from the minimum values of the series, α is the asymptote determined from the first iteration of curve fitting, and V_{max} is the maximum flow velocity, derived from the second iteration ($V_{max} = 2\overline{V}$, where $\overline{V}$ is mean flow velocity).

Applications of TOF EPI Coronary Flow Quantification

LAD Coronary Phasic Flow

A first application of the TOF technique is to study coronary flow dynamics across the cardiac cycle. Unlike the cine phase contrast method, the TOF technique can measure flow velocity only at one point in the cardiac cycle per breath-hold. In order to record the full phasic information multiple TOF series were collected at various cardiac delays in systole and diastole (see Fig. 16). We measured velocities in the LAD coronary artery of maximum coronary flow velocity (CFV_{max}) at 10 cm/s or below in systole and peak CFV_{max} of 27 ± 6 cm/s in diastole ($n = 11$). Such pattern with peak velocities during diastole is in good agreement with the phasic behavior of the left coronary flow velocity demonstrated by intracoronary Doppler measurement [37, 52, 97].

Our systolic velocity measurements have remained approximate. This is because the limits of validity of our TOF technique using a long observation period are in conflict with many features of the systolic phase: low flow velocities compared to our level of detection ($V_{max} \geq 8-10$ cm/s), possible periods of flow reversal [97], large translational motion of the heart, and the relatively short duration of this phase.

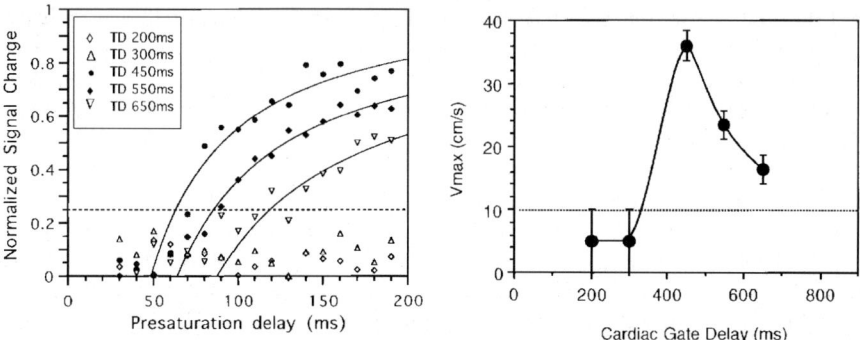

Fig. 16. *Left*, the normalized coronary TOF signal change at different cardiac delays in systole and diastole. Superimposed on the measured points are the fitted curves from our TOF model. *Right*, the derived maximum velocities are represented in function of gate delay from the ECG R wave, along with the extent of a full cardiac cycle

A common source of error to all quantitative methods, the cyclic motion of the heart, with peak velocities in early diastole [39], is likely to affect all MRI studies of phasic coronary flow. With changes in vessel orientation and velocity across the cycle, measurements of instantaneous velocities must be corrected to evaluate ratios such as CFV_{diast}/CFV_{syst} [74].

LAD Coronary Flow Response to Exercise

As a preliminary to our coronary flow reserve study we tested the sensitivity of our TOF technique to changes in coronary flow velocity induced physiologically using for test a continuous isometric hand and lower extremity exercise. Multiple TOF series were obtained at a fixed gate delay in diastole, before, during, and after the exercise. We measured peak diastolic velocity increase of $83\% \pm 43\%$ during the exercise, with a corresponding increase in double product (= heart rate×systolic blood pressure) of $51\% \pm 28\%$ ($n = 8$).

This type of study illustrates well one of the advantages of EPI over conventional MRI in perturbation studies. Within the confined environment of the magnet, sustaining any kind of exercise for the duration of an imaging session results in variable heart rate that produces motion artifacts in conventional imaging. Free of motion artifact, single-shot EPI is, on the other hand, exposed only to the risk of spatial misregistration between images.

Coronary Flow Reserve: LAD Coronary Flow Response to Dipyridamole

The physiological stress from an isometric exercise is insufficient to induce a maximum response. In order to test the capacity of our technique to measure coronary flow reserve we used instead a pharmacological vasodilator stimulus. Focusing, again, our measurements during peak diastolic flow, all TOF series were acquired at a trigger delay set to 100–150 ms after the T wave (the 150 ms offset accounted for the presaturation time window). After several baseline coronary flow measurements 0.56 mg/kg dipyridamole (Persantine) was infused intravenously over 4 min, and the induced changes in coronary flow velocity were measured every 1 or 2 min for 20 min. The dipyridamole effect was then reversed with 50–75 mg aminophylline, and the return to baseline velocities was measured for another 10 min.

We measured in healthy subjects the full time course of diastolic coronary flow velocity changes induced by dipyridamole (see Fig. 17). Diastolic CFV_{max} in the LAD increased from 22 ± 7 cm/s to 90 ± 40 cm/s after dipyridamole and returned to 23 ± 5 cm/s after aminophylline ($n = 10$). The coronary flow velocity reserve (CFVR), defined as the ratio of peak diastolic flow velocity after dipyridamole over baseline velocity, had a mean value of 3.9 ± 1.5.

Our preliminary clinical results show reduced coronary flow reserve in the arteries, with greater than 50% stenoses compared to lesser diseased vessels, with a measured CFVR of 1.9 ± 0.4 vs. 3.3 ± 0.5, respectively ($n = 5$). However,

Fig. 17. Time course of changes in diastolic coronary flow velocity (*CFV*) and heart rate (*HR*) after dipyridamole infusion (0.56 mg/kg) in a normal subject. Coronary flow velocities, derived by curve fitting, are normalized to the average baseline value. The increase in coronary flow velocity is well correlated with the change in heart rate, normal reflex to the induced hyperemia. Both time courses show a peak effect 6 min postinfusion. Full return to baseline velocities is reached after injection of amino-phylline (50 mg)

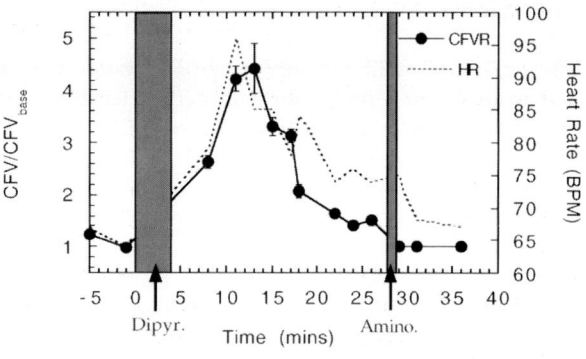

the percentage of lumen narrowing is known to be correlated only modestly with the functional significance of a coronary obstructive lesion [93].

MRI of Coronary Flow and Coronary Flow Reserve

Several methods exist to measure flow velocity with MRI, based on either phase contrast or TOF effects. Except for our work, all studies of coronary blood flow have used cine phase contrast [1, 4, 19, 40, 73, 74, 83].

The TOF technique integrates the information from the full vessel lumen and suffers little effect from the myocardium or pericardial fat because of their respective long T1 or large chemical shift offset. The TOF technique is thus particularly well adapted for low-resolution imaging of the coronary flow. The phase contrast technique, on the other hand, is highly sensitive to the spatial resolution. Prone to partial volume averaging, the phase contrast method can make an error up to 30 % in small vessels no larger than 3 pixels [80].

One method to cope with the small size and difficulty in imaging the coronary arteries by conventional MRI is to measure the distal venous outflow in the coronary sinus (more than twice as wide [83]). Another way is to measure the retrograde blood flow in the ascending aorta (more than 10 times wider [1, 4]). However, these methods provide only an indirect measure of global coronary blood flow.

Since the development of 2D segmented turbo-FLASH techniques, a number of studies of coronary flow velocity have been presented both in the RCA and the LAD [20, 41, 73, 74]. Measurements of phasic flow in the LAD coronary artery have shown similar flow velocities to our results [73]. In a study of coronary flow reserve using adenosine instead of dipyridamole a mean CFVR of 5±2 was measured in normal subjects ($n = 5$ [19]).

Conclusion

The capability of EPI to depict cardiac anatomy, to quantify ejection fractions, and to detect and image the coronary arteries in a real-time fashion has been well demonstrated. In addition, the feasibility has been shown of measuring coronary flow velocity reserve with TOF EPI, both in normal subjects and in patients with coronary disease. Independent validation of the methodology will require correlative intracoronary Doppler flow measurements in patients and correlation with other functional techniques such as PET. In future studies the right and circumflex coronary arteries will be the focus of interest.

Still in its infancy, the study of cardiac and coronary anatomy and blood flow has opened a long-awaited field in cardiovascular MRI – the noninvasive functional assessment of coronary disease. Although not yet capable of replacing current invasive diagnostic techniques, the development of an integrated cardiac MRI examination evaluating function both in the coronary vessels and in the myocardium will play an increasingly important role in clinical screening and therapeutic follow-up of coronary disease. EPI holds great promise to be part of this bright future.

References

1. Bogren HG, Buonocore MH (1992) Coronary artery blood flow measurement by magnetic resonance velocity mapping in the ascending aorta. In: Proceedings of the 11th annual meeting of the Society of Magnetic Resonance in Medicine, Berlin, p 530
2. Brittain JH, Wright GA, Nishimura DG (1994) Coronary angiography with magnetization-prepared T2 contrast. J Magn Reson Imaging 4 (P):80
3. Buckwalter KA, Aisen AM, Dilworth LR, Mancini GBJ, Buda AJ (1986) Gated cardiac MRI: ejection fraction determination using the right anterior oblique view. Am J Roentgenol 147:33–37
4. Buonocore M (1994) Estimation of total coronary artery flow using measurement of flow in the ascending aorta. Magn Reson Med 32:602–611
5. Butts K, Riederer SJ (1992) Analysis of flow effects in echo-planar imaging. JMRI 3:285–293
6. Caputo GR (1991) Coronary arteries: potential for MR imaging. Radiology 181:629–630
7. Cho ZH, Mun CW, Friendenberg RM (1991) NMR Angiography of coronary vessels with 2-D planar images scanning. Magn Reson Med 20:134–143
8. Chrispin A, Small P, Rutter N, Coupland RE, Doyle M, Chapman B, Coxon R, Guilfoyle D, Cawley M, Mansfield P (1986) Echo-planar imaging of normal and abnormal connections of the heart and great arteries. Paediatr Radiol 16:289–292
9. Chrispin A, Small P, Rutter N, Coupland RE, Doyle M, Chapman B, Coxon R, Guilfoyle D, Cawley M, Mansfield P (1986) Transectional echo-planar imaging of the heart in cyanotic congenital heart disease. Paediatr Radiol 16:293–297
10. Cohen MS, Weisskoff RM (1991) Ultra-fast imaging. Magn Reson Imaging 9 (1):1–37
11. Davis CP, McKinnon GC, Debatin JF, Wetter D, Eichenberger AC, Duewell S, Von Schulthess GK (1994) Normal heart: evaluation with echo-planar MR imaging. Radiology 191:691–696
12. Davis CP, McKinnon GC, Debatin JF, Duewell S, Von Schulthess GK (1995) Single-shot versus interleaved echo-planar MR imaging: application to visualization of cardiac valve leaflets. JMRI 5:107–112
13. Doyle M, Mansfield P (1986) Real-time movie image enhancement in NMR. J Phys E (Sci Instr) 19:439–444
14. Doyle M, Scheidegger M, De Graaf R, Vermeulen J, Pohost G (1993) Coronary artery imaging in multiple 1-sec breath holds. Magn Reson Imaging 11:3–6
15. Duerk JL, Simonetti OP (1991) Theoretical aspects of motion sensitivity and compensation in echo-planar imaging. JMRI 1:643–650

16. Dumoulin CL, Souza S (1990) Coronary MR angiography. In: Proceedings of the 9th Annual Meeting of the Society of Magnetic Resonance in Medicine, New York, p 501

17. Edelman RR, Li W (1994) Contrast-enhanced echo-planar MR imaging of myocardial perfusion – preliminary study in humans. Radiology 190:771–777

18. Edelman RR, Manning W, Burstein D, Paulin S (1991) Coronary arteries: breath-hold MR angiography. Radiology 181:641–643

19. Edelman RR, Manning WJ, Gervino E, Li W (1993) Flow velocity quantification in human coronary arteries with fast, breath-hold MR angiography. J Magn Reson Imaging 3:699–703

20. Edelman RR, Gaa J, Li W, Prasad PV, Pearlman JD (1993) Diffusion imaging of the human heart. Proceedings of the SMRM, 12th annual meeting, New York, vol 1, p 286

21. Edelman RR, Wielopolski P, Schmitt F (1994) Echo-planar MR imaging. Radiology 192:600–612

22. Feinberg DA, Crooks LE, Hoenninger J, Arakawa M, Watts J (1984) Pulsatile blood velocity in human arteries displayed by magnetic resonance imaging. Radiology 153:177–180

23. Firmin DN, Nayler GL, Klipstein RH, Underwood SR, Rees RSO, Longmore DB (1987) In vivo validation of MR velocity imaging. J Comput Assist Tomogr 11:751–756

24. Firmin DN, Klipstein RH, Hounsfield GL, Paley MP, Longmore DB (1989) Echo-planar high-resolution flow velocity mapping. Mag Reson in Med 12:316–327

25. Firmin DN, Nayler GL, Kilner PJ, Longmore DB (1990) The application of phase shifts in NMR for flow measurement. Magn Reson Med 14:230–241

26. Firmin DN, Gatehouse PD, Longmore DB (1992) Comparison of snap-shot quantitative flow imaging techniques. Proceedings of the SMRM, 11th annual meeting, Berlin, vol 2, p 2915

27. Gatehouse PD, Firmin DN, Collins S, Longmore DB (1994) Real time blood flow imaging by spiral scan phase velocity mapping. Magn Reson Med 31:504–512

28. Goto M, Flynn AE, Doucette JW, Kimura A, Hiramatsu O, Yamamoto T, Ogasawara Y, Tsujioka K, Hoffman JIE, Kajiya F (1992) Effect of intracoronary nitroglycerin administration on phasic pattern transmural distribution of flow during artery stenosis. Circulation 85:2296–2304

29. Gould KL (1988) Percent coronary stenosis: battered gold standard, pernicious relic or clinical practicality? J Am Coll Cardiol 11:886–888

30. Guilfoyle DN, Gibbs P, Ordidge RJ, Mansfield P (1991) Real-time flow measurements using echo-planar imaging. Magn Reson Med 18:1–8

31. Higgins CB, Wagner S, Kondo C, Suzuki JI, Caputo GR (1991) Evaluation of valvular heart disease with cine gradient echo magnetic resonance imaging. Circulation [Suppl] I:I-198-I-207

32. Hirsch R, Kilner PJ, Connelly M, Redington AN, St John Sutton MG, Somerville J (1994) Diagnosis in adolescents and adults with congenital heart disease. Prospective assessment of the individual and combined roles of magnetic resonance imaging and transesophageal echocardiography. Circulation 90:2937–2951

33. Hofman M, Paschal C, Li D, Haacke E, van Rossum A, Sprenger M (1995) MRI of coronary arteries: 2D breath-hold vs 3D respiratory-gated acquisition. J Comput Assist Tomogr 19 (1):56–62

34. Hu BS, Meyer CH, Macovski A, Nishimura DG (1994) Multi-slice spiral magnetic resonance coronary angiography. Proceedings of the SMR, 2nd meeting, San Francisco, vol 1, p 371

35. Hunter GJ, Hamberg LM, Weisskoff RM, Halpern EF, Brady TJ (1994) Measurement of stroke volume and cardiac output within a single breath hold with echo-planar MR imaging. JMRI 4:51–58

36. Iliceto S, Marangelli V, Memmola C, Rizzon P (1991) Transesophageal Doppler echocardiography evaluation of blood flow velocity in baseline conditions and during dipyridamole-induced coronary vasodilation. Circulation 83:61–69

37. Kajiya F, Ogasawara Y, Tsujioka K, Nakai M, Goto M, Wada Y, Tadaoka S, Matsuoka S, Mito K, Fujiwara T (1986) Evaluation of human coronary blood flow with an 80 channel 20 Mhz pulsed Doppler velocimeter and zero-cross and Fourier transform methods during cardiac surgery. Circulation 74 [Suppl III]:III-53–III-60

38. Kannel W, Abbott R (1984) Incidence and prognosis of unrecognized myocardial infarction. An update of the Framingham Study. N Engl J Med 311:1144–1147

39. Karwatowski SP, Mohiaddin R, Yang GZ, Firmin DN, St. John Sutton M, Underwood DB (1994) Assessment of regional left ventricular long-axis motion with MR velocity mapping in healthy subjects. J Magn Reson Imaging 4:151

40. Keegan J, Firmin D, Gatehouse P, Longmore D (1994a) The application of breath hold phase velocity mapping techniques to the measurement of coronary artery flood flow velocity – phantom data and initial in vivo results. Magn Reson Med 31:526–536

41. Keegan J, Firmin DN, Gatehouse PD, Longmore DB (1994b) Velocity mapping of coronary artery blood flow. Magn Reson Mat Phys Biol Med 2:311–314
42. Kilner PJ, Manzara CC, Mohiaddin RH, Pennell DJ, Sutton MGS, Firmin DN, Underwood SR, Longmore DB (1993) Magnetic resonance jet velocity mapping in mitral and aortic valve stenosis. Circulation 4:1239–1248
43. Langou R, Huang E, Kelley M, Cohen L (1980) Predictive accuracy of coronary artery calcification and abnormal exercise test for coronary artery disease in asymptomatic men. Circulation 62 (6):1196–1203
44. Le Bihan D, Breton E, Lallemand D, Aubin M, Vignaud J, Laval-Jeantet M (1988) Separation of diffusion and perfusion in intravoxel incoherent motion MR imaging. Radiology 168:497–505
45. Lenz GW, Haacke EM, White RD (1989) Retrospective cardiac gating: a review of the technical aspects and future directions. Magn Reson Imaging 7:445–455
46. Li D, Paschal CB, Haacke EM, Adler LP (1993) Three-dimensional magnetic resonance imaging of the coronary arteries with fat saturation and magnetization transfer saturation techniques. Radiology 187:401–407
47. Longmore DB, Klipstein RH, Underwood SR, Firmin DN, Hounsfield GN, Watanabe M, Bland C, Fox KM, Poole-Wilson PA, Rees RSO, Denison DN, McNeilly AM, Burman ED (1985) Dimensional accuracy of magnetic resonance in studies of the heart. Lancet [Suppl] I:1360–1362
48. Lotan CS, Cranney GB, Bouchard A, Bittner V, Pohost GM (1989) The value of cine nuclear magnetic resonance imaging for assessing regional ventricular function. J Am Coll Cardiol 14:1721–1729
49. Lown B (1979) Sudden cardiac death: the major challenge confronting contemporary cardiology. Am J Cardiol 43:313–328
50. Manning WJ, Li W, Boyle NG, Edelman RR (1993) Fat-suppressed breath-hold magnetic resonance coronary angiography. Circulation 1:94–104
51. Mansfield P, Pykett IL (1978) Biological and medical imaging by NMR. J Magn Reson 29:355–373
52. Marcus M, Wright C, Doty D, Eastham C, Laughlin D, Krumm P, Fastenow C, Brody M (1981) Measurements of coronary velocity and reactive hyperemia in the coronary circulation of humans. Circ Res 49:877–891
53. McKinnon GC (1993) Ultrafast interleaved gradient-echo-planar imaging on a standard scanner. Magn Reson Med 30:609–616
54. McKinnon GC, Debatin JF, Wetter DR, von Schulthess GK (1994) Interleaved echo planar flow quantitation. Magn Reson Med 32:263–267
55. Meyer CH, Hu BS, Nishimura DG, Macovski A (1992) Fast spiral coronary artery imaging. Magn Reson Med 28:202–213
56. Mohiaddin RH, Wann SL, Underwood SR, Firmin DN, Rees RSO, Longmore DB (1990) Vena caval flow: assessment with cine MR velocity mapping. Radiology 177:537–541
57. Mohiaddin RH, Kilner PJ, Rees RSO, Longmore DB (1992) Qp/Qs. ratio measured non-invasively by magnetic resonance velocity mapping in patients with intracardiac shunts. Proceedings of the SMRM, 11th annual meeting, Berlin, vol 2, p 2519
58. Mohiaddin RH, Bogren HG, Yang GZ, Kilner PJ, Firmin DN (1994) Magnetic resonance velocity vector mapping in aortic aneurysms. Magn Reson Mat Phys Biol Med 2:335–338
59. Mohiaddin RH, Gatehouse PD, Firmin DN (1995) Exercise related changes in aortic flow measured by spiral echo-planar velocity mapping. JMRI 5:159–163
60. Mostbeck GH, Caputo GR, Higgins CB (1992) MR measurement of blood flow in the cardiovascular system. Am J Roentgenol 3:453–461
61. Nayler GL, Firmin DN, Longmore DB (1986) Blood flow imaging by cine magnetic resonance. J Comput Assist Tomogr 10:715–722
62. Nishimura DG, Irarrazabal P, Meyer CH (1995) A Velocity k-space analysis of flow effects in echo-planar and spiral imaging. Magn Reson Med 33 (4):549–556
63. Ordidge RJ, Mansfield P, Doyle M (1982) Real time movie images by NMR. Br J Radiol 55:729–733
64. Osbakken M, Yuschok T (1986) Evaluation of ventricular function with gated cardiac magnetic resonance imaging. Cath Cardiovasc Diagn 12:156–160
65. Paulin S, von Schulthess GK, Fossel E, Krayenbuehl HP (1987) MR imaging of the aortic root and proximal coronary arteries. Am J Roentgenol 148:665–670
66. Pennell DJ, Keegan J, Firmin DN, Gatehouse PD, Underwood SR, Longmore DB (1993) Magnetic resonance imaging of coronary arteries – technique and preliminary results. Br Heart J 4:315–326

67. Poncelet BP, Kantor H, Weisskoff RM, Holmvang F, Brady TJ, Wedeen VJ (1992) Quantitation of the coronary flow with echo-planar imaging. In: Proceedings of the 11th annual meeting of the Society of Magnetic Resonance in Medicine, Berlin, Germany, p 604
68. Poncelet BP, Weisskoff RM, Wedeen VJ, Brady TJ, Kantor H (1993) Time of flight quantification of coronary flow with echo-planar MRI. Magn Reson Med 30:447–457
69. Poncelet BP, Zervos G, Weisskoff RM, Wedeen VJ, Brady TJ, Kantor H (1994) Measurement of coronary flow reserve with time-of-flight EPI in normal and diseased LAD coronary. In: Proceedings of the 2nd meeting of the Society of Magnetic Resonance, San Francisco, p 374
70. Rogers WJ, Shapiro EP, Weiss JL, Buchalter MB, Rademakers FE, Weisfeldt ML, Zerhouni EA (1991) Quantification of and correction for left ventricular systolic long-axis shortening by magnetic resonance tissue tagging and slice isolation. Circulation 84:721–731
71. Rzedzian RR, Pykett IL (1987) Instant images of the human heart using a new, whole-body MR imaging system. Am J Roentgenol 149:245–250
72. Rzedzian R, Chapman B, Mansfield P, Coupland RE, Doyle M, Chrispin A, Guilfoyle D, Small P (1983) Real-time nuclear magnetic resonance imaging in paediatrics. Lancet [Suppl] II:1281–1282
73. Sakuma H, Globits S, Shimakawa A, Bernstein MA, Higgins CB (1994) Breath-hold coronary flow measurement with a cine phase-contrast technique. In: Proceedings of the 2nd meeting of the Society of Magnetic Resonance, San Francisco, p 375
74. Scheidegger MB, Hess OM, Boesiger P (1994) Assessment of coronary flow over the cardiac cycle and diastolic-to-systolic flow ratio with correction for vessel motion. In: Proceedings of the 2nd meeting of the Society of Magnetic Resonance, San Francisco, p 498
75. Schmitt F, Warach S, Wielopolski P, Edelmann RR (1994) Clinical applications and techniques of echo-planar mapping. Magn Reson Mat Phys Biol Med 2:259–266
76. Singer JR (1959) Blood flow rates by nuclear magnetic resonance measurements. Science 130:1652–1653
77. Steiner RE, Bydder GM, Selwyn A, Deanfield J, Longmore DB, Klipstein RH, Firmin D (1983) Nuclear magnetic resonance imaging of the heart. Current status and future prospects. Br Heart J 50:202–208
78. Stehling M, Chapman B, Glover P, Ordidge RJ, Mansfield P, Dutka D, Howseman A, Coxon R, Turner R, Jaroszkiewicz G, Morris GK, Worthington BS, Coupland RE (1987) Real-time NMR imaging of coronary vessels. Lancet 24:964–965
79. Stehling MJ, Howseman AM, Ordidge RJ, Chapman B, Turner R, Coxon 0R, Glover P, Mansfield P, Coupland RE (1989) Whole-body echo-planar MR imaging at 0.5T. Radiology 170:257–263
80. Tang C, Blatter DD, Parker DL (1993) Accuracy of phase-contrast flow measurements in the presence of partial-volume effects. J Magn Reson Imaging 3:377–385
81. Underwood SR, Firmin DN, Klipstein RH, Rees RSO, Longmore DBL (1987) Magnetic resonance velocity mapping: clinical application of a new technique. Br Heart J 57:404–412
82. Underwood SR, Gill CRW, Firmin DN, Klipstein RH, Mohiaddin RH, Rees RSO, Longmore DB (1988) Left ventricular volume measured rapidly by oblique magnetic resonance imaging. Br Heart J 60:188–195
83. van Rossum AC, Visser FC, Hofman MBM, Galjee MA, Westerhof N, Valk J (1992) Global left ventricular perfusion: noninvasive measurement with cine MR imaging and phase velocity mapping of coronary venous outflow. Radiology 182:685–691
84. Waller B (1989) Anatomy, histology, and pathology of the major epicardial coronary arteries relevant to echocardiographic imaging techniques. J Am Soc Echocardiogr 2:232–252
85. Wang SJ, Hu BS, Macovski A, Nishimura D (1991) Coronary angiography using fast selective inversion recovery. Magn Reson Med 18:417–423
86. Wang Y, Grist TM, Korosec FR, Christy PS, Alley MT, Polzin JA, Mistretta CA (1995) Respiratory blur in 3D coronary MR imaging. Magn Reson Med 33 (4):541–548
87. Wehrli FW, MacFall JR, Axel L, Shutts D, Glover GH, Herfkins RJ (1984) Approaches to in-plane and out-of-plane flow imaging. Noninvasive Med Imaging 1 (2):127–136
88. Wehrli FW, Shimakawa A, Gullberg GT, MacFall JR (1986) Time-of-flight MR flow imaging; selective saturation recovery with gradient refocusing. Radiology 160:781–785
89. Weisskoff RM (1990) Improved hard-pulse sequences or frequency-selective presaturation in magnetic resonance. J Magn Reson 86:170–175
90. Weisskoff RM, Crawley AP, Wedeen V (1990) Flow sensitivity and flow compensation in instant imaging. Proceedings of the SMRM, 9th annual meeting, New York, vol 1, p 398
91. Weisskoff RM, Cohen MS, Rzedzian RR (1993) Nonaxial whole-body instant imaging. Magn Reson Med 29:796–803

92. Wendland MF, Saeed M, Masui T, Derugin N, Moseley ME, Higgins CB (1993) Echo-planar MR Imaging of normal and ischemic myocardium with gadodiamide injection. Radiology 2:535–542

93. White CW, Wright CB, Doty DB, Hiratzaka LF, Eastham CL, Harrison DG, Marcus ML (1984) Does visual interpretation of the coronary angiogram predict the physiologic importance of a coronary stenosis? N Engl J Med 310 (819):819–824

94. Wilke N, Simm C, Zhang J, Ellermann J, Ya X, Merkle H, Path G, Ludemann H, Bache RJ, Ugurbil K (1993) Contrast-enhanced first pass myocardial perfusion imaging – correlation between myocardial blood flow in dogs at rest and during hyperemia. Magn Reson Med 4:485–497

95. Wilke N, Jerosch-Herold M, Stillman AE, Kroll K, Tsekos N, Merkle H, Parrish T, Hu X, Wang Y, Bassingthwaighte J, Bache RJ Ugurbil K (1994) Concepts of myocardial perfusion imaging in magnetic resonance imaging. Magn Reson Q 10:249–286

96. Wright GA, Nishimura DG, Macovski A (1991) Flow independent magnetic resonance projection angiography. Magn Reson Med 17:126–140

97. Yamagishi M, Hotta D, Tamai J, Nakatani S, Miyatake K (1991) Validity of catheter-tip Doppler technique in assessment of coronary flow velocity and application of spectrum analysis method. Am J Cardiol 67:758–762

CHAPTER 13

Perfusion Imaging with Echo-Planar Imaging

M. K. Stehling, R. Brüning, and B. R. Rosen

"Where shall I climb, sound, seek, search, or find that *summum bonum* which may stay my mind? ...
The depth and sea have said 'tis not in me,' With pearl and gold it shall not valued be....
It yieldeth pleasures far beyond conceit, And truly beautifies without deceit.
Nor strength, nor wisdom, nor fresh youth shall fade, Nor death shall see, but are immortal made.
This pearl of price, this tree of life, this spring, Who is possessed of shall reign a king.
Nor change of state nor cares shall ever see, But wear his crown unto eternity.
This satiates the soul, this stays the mind, And all the rest, but vanity we find."
from: *The Vanity of All Worldly Things,*
Anne Bradstreet, ca. 1612–1672

Introduction

The introduction of nuclear magnetic resonance (NMR) into medicine [1] initially created hopes that this totally noninvasive imaging modality would be able to differentiate clearly between healthy and pathological tissue on the basis of T1 and T2 signals [2]. As originally conceived, however, these hopes were overly optimistic as they assumed that parameters characterizing processes on a nuclear or molecular scale could provide a sensitive and specific means of characterizing disease processes which, although ultimately based on molecular derangements, manifest themselves on a micro- and macrostructural and functional level. Thus MRI techniques geared towards elucidating these pathophysiological processes had to be developed.

The development of contrast agents has substantially expanded the capabilities of NMR in this respect. Contrast agents can provide information about the physiology of tissue in several ways. In clinical routine the biodistribution of extracellular agents such as Gd-DTPA^{2-} in the various spaces of the body provides information about their size and about exchange processes between them. This provides an initial, albeit crude, assessment of tissue vascularity. More specific are contrast agents such as mangafodipir trisodium (Mn-DPDP), gadolinium ethoxybenzyl diethylenetriamine pentaacetic acid (Gd-EOB-DTPA) and ultrasmall superparamagnetic iron oxide particles (SPIO, USPIO). These are taken up selectively by specific cells, such as the hepatocytes and phagocytes of the reticuloendothelial system, and therefore allow differentiation between different tissue types [3].

In addition to these "static" uses of contrast agents, dynamic studies carried out during and after the injection of a contrast agent bolus can be used to gather information about hemodynamics and exchange processes between different tissue compartments. The in vivo measurement of regional hemodynamics has wide clinical potential because of the unequivocally established relationship between physiological function, energy metabolism, and localized blood supply [4]. The tracer kinetic approach to measuring perfusion based on indicator dilution theory is not new. It has been used extensively in physiology since the nineteenth century [5], employing various techniques to record the concentration of the employed tracer, such as direct blood sampling with catheters. Functional imaging methods can be used for such measurements, such as positron emission tomography (PET) [6, 7] and contrast-enhanced computed tomography (CT) [8–11], but require exposure to iodine and ionizing radiation and can be imprecise due to poor spatial resolution and low signal to noise ratio (SNR).

Magnetic resonance imaging (MRI) is the latest in this armamentarium of recording devices, with several advantages and disadvantages. One advantage is its high sensitivity to even small amounts of NMR contrast agents, particularly in view of the very slow flow rates in capillaries (about 0.5–1.5 mm/s) and the small volume fractions of the intravascular bed in most tissues (2%–10%) [12]. The other advantage is the fact that NMR is noninvasive and nonhazardous to the human body, which allows extended and repetitive measurements to be performed. On the other hand, NMR also has several disadvantages. The relationship between tracer and signal in general is nonlinear, and to date neither freely diffusible nor intravascular tracers have been available for routine clinical use.

Despite these obstacles MRI techniques to measure blood volume and flow have recently been developed which exploit magnetic susceptibility effects to provide the spatial and temporal resolution needed to determine these parameters on a voxel-by-voxel basis in both normal and neoplastic brain tissue. This development was spurred in the first half of the 1990s by two parallel developments. First, high-speed imaging with gradient-echo (GRE) [13] and echo-planar imaging (EPI) techniques [14, 15], which have been implemented on commercially available equipment, has resulted in greatly increased speed of NMR data collection. Second, a better understanding of the dose-relaxation ratio of exogenous and endogenous NMR contrast agents has been reached.

Most research has focused on measuring tissue blood volume and blood flow. Other investigated parameters include membrane permeabilities, compartmental exchange rates, and blood oxygenation. Hemodynamic parameters are of great clinical significance since they play a key role in the understanding, differential diagnosis, and treatment planning of vascular diseases such as stroke and ischemic heart disease (accounting for over half the deaths in industrialized countries) as well as in cancer, which is characterized by angioneogenesis and consequent changes in blood volume and flow [16, 17].

Because of the extracellular distribution of Gd-DTPA the only tracer available for routine clinical use so far, most medical applications of perfusion and cerebral blood volume (CBV) imaging have focused on the brain. The blood-brain barrier (BBB) renders Gd-DTPA an intravascular contrast agent thus facilitating tracer kinetic modeling.

In the normal brain changes in regional CBV (rCBV) are sensitive reflections of brain function. Although blood volume and flow may be closely related in the normal brain, this is not necessarily the case in pathological states, particularly in the case of brain tumors and other conditions in which the vascular system differs considerably from that in normal brain tissues. Although existing radionuclide data suggest that blood flow measurements alone are not a critical determinant of tumor activity, recent concepts in tumor biology and radiation oncology stress the importance of tumor vascularity (angiogenesis) as critical in the regulation of tumor growth and its malignant potential [18]. It has been previously reported that expression of angiogenic growth factor genes in primary human astrocytomas may contribute to their growth and progression [19]. Measurement of tissue microvascular blood volume appears to be sensitive to the phenotypic expression of angiogenesis, particularly increased microvascular density, providing another important inroad to the understanding and monitoring of this important pathophysiological mechanism.

Three major approaches to hemodynamic imaging have been pursued:

- One, using exogenous tracers, involves the use of rapid ^{1}H MRI techniques to resolve the tissue transit of intravenously administered contrast agents, exploiting either T1 or T2 contrast. These are considered in some detail in this chapter. Exogenous tracers based on nuclei other than ^{1}H, such as D_2O, ^{17}O, and ^{19}F compounds, have also been used and are mentioned only briefly.
- The second approach, relying on endogenous tracers, is based on spin-labeling of water protons without the application of contrast material. These techniques are discussed in detail in Chap. 16 of this volume. Another endogenous tracer, blood hemoglobin, has been exploited in neurofunctional MRI and is treated in Chaps. 15 and 16.
- The third technique exploits signal attenuation in the presence of diffusion gradients interpreting capillary blood flow as a type of "pseudodiffusion." This approach is treated in more detail in Chap. 9.

The Concept of Perfusion

The definition of the term "perfusion" used here is based on the enlightening discussion of the term by Le Bihan and Turner [20]. Heated arguments have erupted about the term "perfusion" because it means different things to different people, and it is thus not always clear whether a particular technique actually measures perfusion or something else. In the broader sense, "perfusion" has been used by pathologists and radiologists to denote the density of microvasculature in a tissue. For the physiologist perfusion refers to the circulation of blood. Blood perfusion assures the delivery of oxygen and nutrient to cells by fresh, oxygenated, arterial blood and the elimination of the waste products of metabolism through the venous drainage. The process of delivery and elimination depends on two major factors: blood microcirculation and the blood-tissue exchange processes. It is the former (i.e., blood flow measured in milliliters of blood per minute per 100 g of tissue) which is determined by conventional perfusion measurement techniques based on the uptake and washout of radionuclide tracers. Blood-tissue exchange is a different, but no less important, process which, however, depends on the molecular species, particles, or cells being investigated.

For freely diffusible tracers blood flow measurements are based on the Fick principle [21] (see also [22]), simply stating mass conservation. The ultimate parameter measured is blood flow and not the exchange of the tracer with the tissue, since most of these tracers are not biological nutrients, so that their diffusion and compartmentalization in the tissue does not reflect physiological blood-tissue exchanges. The diffusion of the tracer is merely a technical artifice to measure blood flow.

For nondiffusible tracers the principle of mass conservation can be reformulated into the central volume theorem [5]:

$$F = V_d/MTT \tag{1}$$

where denotes flow and V_d is the volume of distribution of the tracer. Since the actual mean transit time (MTT) is difficult to determine (see below), intravascular agents are most often used to determine only blood volume, which is not perfusion or blood flow [23].

There is an important difference between freely diffusible and intravascular tracers in respect to the term "perfusion." Measurements using freely diffusible tracers rely on the exchange of the tracer between the capillaries and the tissue and thus measure only the fraction of microscopic blood flow which actively contributes to the process of supply and elimination of metabolites to the tissue. Measurements employing intravascular tracers, on the other hand, measure the total microscopic blood flow, including shunted blood in physiological and pathological arteriovenous connections bypassing the capillaries and thus the physiologically important exchange process.

Perfusion Imaging Using NMR Contrast Agents

Many original and review articles are available on NMR contrast agents in perfusion imaging, to which we refer the interested reader for a comprehensive treatment of this subject. In Particular, the original works by Rosen et al. [24] and Boxerman et al. [25] provide a comprehensive view of the theory and research on susceptibility contrast and have provided the basis for the following paragraphs.

Knowledge of the interaction between NMR contrast agents and tissue is a prerequisite for their use as tracers, and this has been studied extensively [23, 26–31]. Paramagnetic compounds interact with proton nuclear spins through dipolar coupling of their unpaired electrons. This short-reaching effect requires the proton to come into close contact with the paramagnetic compound for its magnetization to be affected. Proton signal thus depends not only on the concentration of the contrast agent but also on the speed of water exchange between different tissue compartments. Paramagnetic compounds predominantly shorten the longitudinal relaxation time T1, thus affecting image contrast mainly on T1-weighted spin-echo (SE) and GRE images. The relaxivity of these compounds has been studied in detail [32].

Rosen et al. [24, 33–35] have demonstrated that the same paramagnetic agents, injected in a compact high-dose bolus, can affect T2 relaxation and thus contrast in T2-weighted SE and GRE images as profoundly as classical dipolar relaxation can effect T1-weighted images. Here the mechanism of proton signal change depends on compartmentalization of the contrast agent rather than direct interaction of tissue water with unpaired spins. Signal attenuation is caused by susceptibility gradients between the intravascular and extravascular space, reaching far beyond the vessels into the surrounding tissue and thus providing a greater effect, particularly in weakly vascularized tissue such as the brain. To apply the pharmaceutical effect to the measurement of tissue blood flow and volume with NMR imaging requires an understanding of the relaxation mechanisms and the relationship between image signal changes and local contrast agent concentration. Particularly important, in addition, is the relationship between compartmentalization of contrast agent delivery and tissue, as well as how these effect NMR image intensity. Analysis of these data, in a properly designed model, allows tissue microcirculation parameters to be determined.

Susceptibility Contrast Imaging

Magnetic susceptibility is the proportionality constant between an applied magnetic field and the resultant magnetization established within material. Unpaired electrons of elements such as iron, gadolinium, and dysprosium have electron magnetic dipoles which respond to an externally applied magnetic field, B_0, in much the same way as the weaker nuclear magnetic dipoles, tending to align themselves with the applied field:

$$M = \chi \, B_0, \quad \chi > 0 \tag{2}$$

As with nuclear spins, only a fraction of the electron spins normally contribute to this induced net magnetization, M. If the unpaired spins are present in sufficient concentration, this effect dominates the weaker diamagnetic properties caused by paired electrons, whose spins align themselves opposite the applied field. Thus in elements with a large number of free electrons the net induced magnetization is aligned with, and not opposed to, the applied field. They have a positive magnetic susceptibility, i.e., $\chi > 0$, and are termed paramagnetic [36, 37]. If a large number of such unpaired spins are contained within crystal structures, the so-called domains, such that their magnetic moments couple synergistically, an even greater number of dipoles align themselves with the applied field. These materials are labeled superparamagnetic or ferromagnetic, depending on the size and precise nature of the crystal domains [38–40].

If homogeneously distributed in aqueous solutions, paramagnetic ions in sufficient concentration display relaxation properties as described by the Solomon [41]-Bloembergen [42] equations. These are discussed below. If heterogeneous in distribution, however, regions of high and low magnetic susceptibility within voxels of an image can cause significant signal losses not predicted by the classical Solomon-Bloembergen theory. These effects can be understood by remembering that magnetic susceptibility differences affect the local resonance frequency by modifying the magnetic field experienced by nearby water protons. This can affect NMR images in three ways:

- By increasing the diversity of magnetic fields within a voxel, variations in magnetic susceptibility lead to an increase in water resonance linewidth. This results in decreased signal from pulse sequences, which do not fully refocus static inhomogeneities, such as gradient echoes or spin echoes with temporal offsets in their 180° pulses [43].
- In these same pulse sequences the variation in magnetic field can lead to a net displacement in the resonance frequency throughout a whole voxel. This in turn results in phase shifts seen with phase-sensitive imaging techniques. In both cases the effect increases with longer TE and with 180° offset times.
- In pulse sequences with complete refocusing of static inhomogeneities, for example, spin echoes, increases in resonance linewidth or shift in resonance frequency do not lead directly to signal loss or phase distortions. If the TE, however, is sufficiently long to allow substantial diffusion of water through areas of different magnetic field during the TE period, the magnetic field variations become essentially a dynamic phenomenon in the reference frame of the spin. This leads to dephasing and hence signal loss. Although this effect is less pronounced than the signal loss on GRE images, with sufficient TE the signal loss can be quite significant. This is often (incorrectly) labeled a T2 effect, although it does not reflect classical T2 relaxation but rather diffusion-related signal attenuation; the signal can indeed be recovered with short TE Carr-Purcell-Meiboom-Gill sequences.

Paramagnetic chelates such as $Gd(DTPA)^{2-}$ or $Dy(DTPA)^{2-}$, because of their large magnetic moments, can transiently alter the magnetic susceptibility of tissues during their passage through the microvascular bed, with resultant changes in T2 and T2*. Figure 1 shows signal-versus-time curves from a susceptibility contrast study performed in a patient with a high-grade (grade 3) right thalamic astrocytoma. Although the vascular space constitutes less than 5 % of the total tissue volume, the compartmentalization of contrast agent within the intravascular space leads to a large, 10 % (white matter) 40 % (tumor) transient drop in signal following the administration of $Gd(DTPA)^{2-}$. This reflects the local field inhomogeneities which extend beyond the vascular space, affecting much of the surrounding brain tissue. Rapid imaging techniques such as EPI are especially suited for studying this phenomenon due to the high temporal resolution

---

Fig. 1. a Series of echo-planar SE images of a patient with a right thalamic tumor. The images were acquired immediately before, during, and after the first pass of a bolus of gadopentetate dimeglumine through the brain. Images were obtained at a rate of one per second; every second image is shown. When the contrast material reaches the brain, it causes signal loss (*middle row*). Regions of greater CBV exhibit greater signal loss, as demonstrated by the greater regional blood volume of gray matter compared to white matter. The tumor has heterogeneous signal loss, greatest in its medial aspect due to focally elevated CBV. Numbers indicate sequence in image acquisition. **b** *Left*, CBV map calculated on a pixel-by-pixel basis from the data set partially presented in **a**. Higher CBV is represented by higher signal intensity (*white area*) on the CBV map. Note the relatively high CBV in the normal cortical gray matter and the deep gray nuclei, as well as within the medial portion of the tumor. *Right*, graph shows normalized signal intensity curves during the transit of the contrast material through the brain for normal gray and white matter regions and for two areas within the tumor. *x-axis*, seconds; *y-axis*, signal intensity values. (With permission of the authors and the publisher, from Aronen et al. [19])

needed to characterize the passage of these agents through the vascular space [44].

Several theoretical models have been proposed to describe this observed behavior [45–48]. These can be divided into three categories.

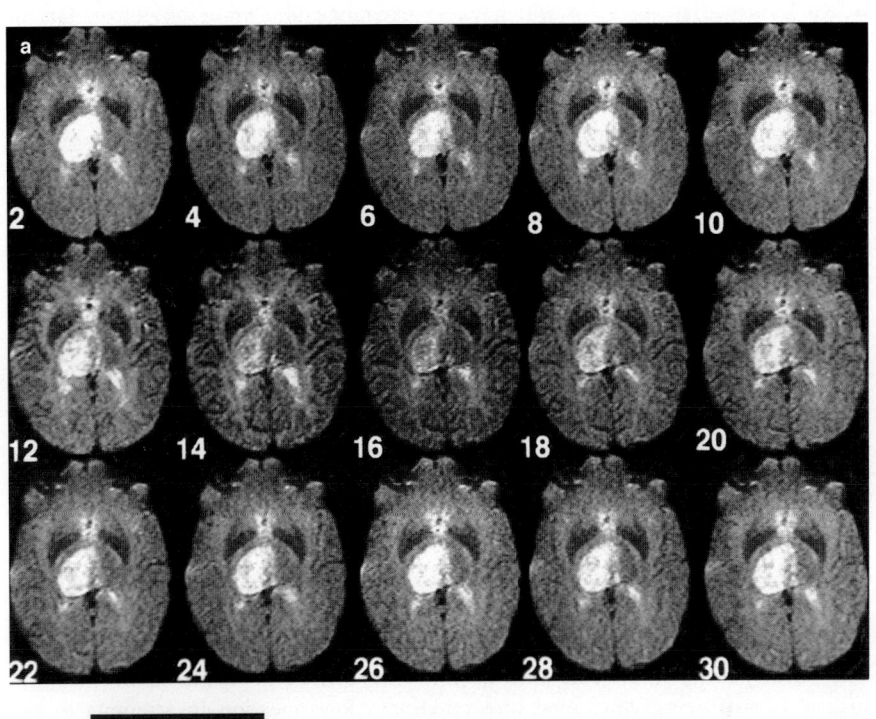

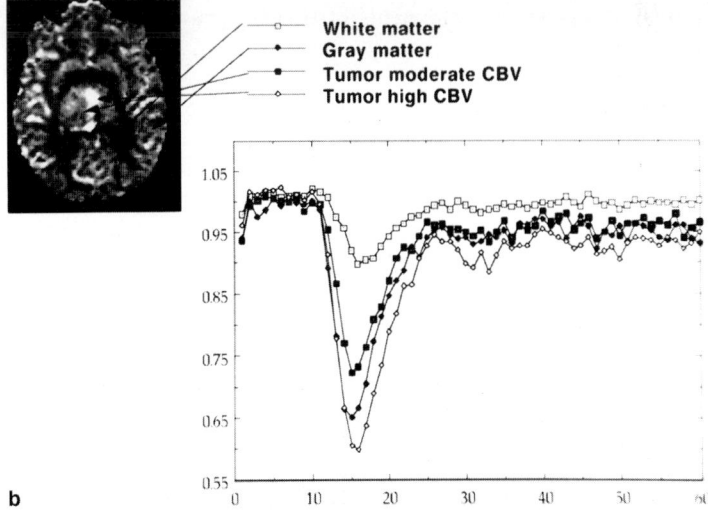

- White matter
- Gray matter
- Tumor moderate CBV
- Tumor high CBV

- A fast exchange model, assuming rapid movement of the water spins across the heterogenous field. This applies best to small, high-susceptibility regions, such as ferritin deposits within hemorrhage.
- A slow exchange model, with the magnetic field experienced by the spins similar to a linear field gradient. This model applies best to large heterogeneous regions or limited water diffusion.
- An intermediate case, in which water exchange is neither obviously fast or slow and analytic expressions are difficult to derive. For this reason, statistical, so-called Monte Carlo techniques have been used to model and predict the distribution of field strength, static lineshapes, and, finally, dynamic, diffusion-related spin dephasing.

Both empirical data and Monte Carlo modeling show a linear relationship between tissue contrast agent concentration and the T2 relaxation rate change:

$$\Delta R_2 = k_2 \, C_{VOI} \tag{3}$$

where k_2 is a field strength and pulse sequence specific constant and C_{VOI} the tracer concentration in tissue. This relationship is analogous to that found with relaxivity agents. Assuming monoexponential behavior, the signal intensity changes following contrast agent injection can be related to the T2 rate change:

$$S(t) = S_0 \exp\{-TE(\Delta R_2(t))\} \tag{4}$$

Combining Eq. 3 and 4, the signal intensity changes can be converted to a tissue concentration-time curve:

$$C_{VOI}(t) = -\ln(S_{VOI}(t)/S_0) \, / \, (k_2 TE) \tag{5}$$

where $C_{VOI}(t)$ is the concentration-time curve, S_0 is the baseline signal intensity before injection, $S_{VOI}(t)$ is the tissue signal with contrast agent present at time t. The validity of the above relationship in normal and pathological states in several organs is still being elucidated and remains a key question in attempts to use NMR contrast agents for measurements of tissue perfusion.

The Blood-Brain Barrier and Susceptibility Contrast

The concept of a BBB was developed by the German cell biologist Ehrlich [49]. He found that the intravenous injection of dyes such as trypan blue was followed by staining of tissues in most organs, but not in the brain and spinal cord. The brain and CSF are selectively protected by this barrier against surging fluctuations of blood constituents. The BBB is not simply composed of a single comprehensive layer but by many different systems [50]. These include tight junctions between capillary endothelial cells, the glial foot processes of astrocytes surrounding the capillaries, and the special functionality of the transport systems of these cells which favor selective transport over general passive diffusion. The rate of exchange across the BBB, however, is also affected by characteristics of the solute. Size is crucial. Small molecules (e.g., 0.5 kDa) cross the BBB much more quickly than larger ones (e.g., 5 kDa). Lipid solubility strongly enhances the exchange. Many pathological processes, such as ischemia-induced energy failure, inflammations, and temporary imbalances in blood constituents can lead to a temporary or lasting failure of the BBB. A defective BBB is also found in brain tumors which stimulate angioneogenesis of structurally and functionally immature vessels.

Gd-DTPA^{2-} and similar compounds available for clinical use cannot cross the intact BBB and thus assume the properties of intravascular contrast agents in the brain. This facilitates susceptibility contrast studies, which make use of long-range magnetic perturbations that are produced by paramagnetic agents when these are compartmentalized in the vascular bed. These perturbations occur even when the "conventional" short-range, T1-enhancing property of such agents as Gd-DTPA^{2-}, which is caused by protons diffusing within the coordination sphere of the gadolinium free electrons, is precluded owing to reduced access of water to the contrast agent (e.g., when the BBB is intact). When compartmentalized, these high magnetic susceptibility materials produce magnetic field distortion susceptibility effects which can act at a distance of many micrometers to relax the transverse magnetization of tissue protons. Thus, sizable signal attenuation effects can be recorded despite the low vascular volume of the brain.

Susceptibility Contrast and Pulse Sequences

The majority of dynamic susceptibility contrast studies have been carried out using either GRE or SE EPI variants. The effect of susceptibility contrast on the two major types of pulse sequences, SE and GRE sequences, has been studied extensively, both theoretically and experimentally, by a number of research groups [51–54]. The excellent article by Boxerman et al. [25] furnishes a comprehensive view of susceptibility contrast mechanisms and provides the basis for the following section. Boxerman et al. have shown that the observed signal attenuation in susceptibility contrast studies depends not only on the concentration of the contrast agent but also on a complex relationship between the type of pulse sequence used and the size of the blood vessels present in the investigated tissue.

Dependence of Relaxivity on Vessel Size

Figure 2 compares plots of $\Delta R2^*(R)$ at TE = 60 ms and $\Delta R2(R)$ at TE = 100 ms for f = 2% (f is the vascular volume fraction) and $\Delta\chi = 1\times10^{-7}$, corresponding to an intravascular Gd-DTPA concentration of approximately 3.6 mM, a typical first-pass concentration for a 0.1 mmol/kg BW injection, at TE values typically used for clinical applications at 1.5 T. This graph also shows the effect of different vascular permeabilities. For this $\Delta\chi$, $\Delta R2$ peaks around R = 5 μm. $\Delta R2^*$ exceeds $\Delta R2$ at all radii, reaches a plateau for large vessels, and is considerably greater for macro- then for microvessels.

Plotting $\Delta R2(R)$ as a function of varying intravascular $\Delta\chi$, it is found that with increasing $\Delta\chi$, i.e., increasing intravascular contrast agent concentration, peak

Fig. 2. Size dependence of
ΔR2* (TE = 60 ms) and ΔR2
(TE = 100 ms) for f = 2 % and
$\Delta\chi = 1\times10^{-7}$ for impermeable
vessels ($p = 0$), freely perme-
able vessels (*dashed line*) and
vessels corresponding to physiological permeability (*solid
line*). At this Δχ, ΔR2(R) peaks
for microvessels. ΔR2* exceeds
ΔR2 at all radii, reaches a
plateau for macrovessels, and
is actually greater for macrovessels than for microvessels.
Permeability marginally

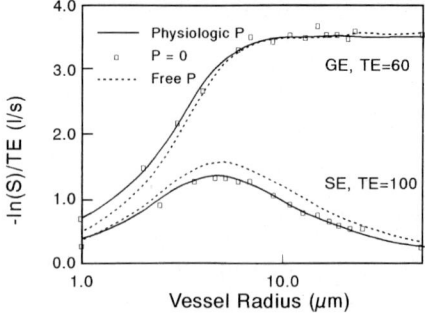

increases ΔR2 for all radii and decreases ΔR2* relaxivity for microvessels only for very large,
unphysiological permeabilities. (Modified from Boxerman et al. [25])

relaxivity shifts toward smaller vessel radii. Figure 3 shows ΔR2 plotted as a
function of vascular radius for $\Delta\chi = 3\times10^{-6}$, corresponding to blood oxygenation
level dependent (BOLD) contrast with 60 % venous oxygenation, and $\Delta\chi = 1\times10^{-7}$,
2×10^{-7}, and 4×10^{-7}, corresponding to vascular Gd-DTPA concentrations of
3.6, 7.1, and 14.3 mM, respectively. While for the two lower Δχ values peak
ΔR2 is obtained for radii between 5 and 8 μm, peak ΔR2 for the two higher
Δχ values is obtained at true capillary radii, i.e., 2–3 μm. With asymmetric spin
echo (ASE) sequences a combination of SE and GRE contrast is obtained. Vascular
selectivity thus becomes a function of the offset τ between spin and gradient echo.
With increasing τ the vessel size dependence of the relaxivity change behaves
more as that for a GRE and less as that for a SE sequence, as is to be expected.

Fig. 3. ΔR2(R) (f = 2 %,
TE = 100 ms) for increasing
Δχ. Over the range of Δχ
applicable to both endogenous
and exogenous contrast-based
fMRI, peak ΔR2 is obtained
for microvessels (R<8 μm).
For Δχ associated with typical
first-pass concentrations of
Gd-DTPA, peak relaxivity is
derived for vessels with true
mean capillary radii. (Modified from Boxerman et al.
[25])

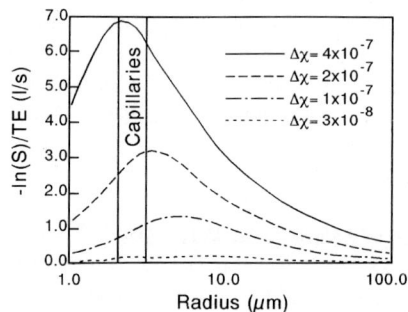

Dependence of Relaxivity on Contrast Agent Concentration

Figure 4 shows plots of ΔR2 (TE = 60 ms) versus vascular contrast agent concentration for a vasculature with total f = 4 %, R_c = 3 μm (weighted by α = 0.25, 0.5
and 1.0) and R_v = 25 μm (weighted by 1–α). Also plotted is ΔR2 (TE = 100 ms)
versus Gd-DTPA concentration for a fixed 2 % capillary volume fraction and various macrovascular compositions [blood volume of 2(1/α–1)%, α = 0.25, 0.5, and

Fig. 4. Dependence of $\Delta R2^*$ (TE = 60 ms) on Gd-DTPA for a vasculature with f = 4% composed of capillaries (R = 3 µm, weighted by α) and venules (R = 25 µm, weighted by 1–α). Also, the dependence of $\Delta R2$ (TE = 100 ms) upon Gd-DTPA for a fixed 2% capillary volume fraction. (Modified from Boxerman et al. [25])

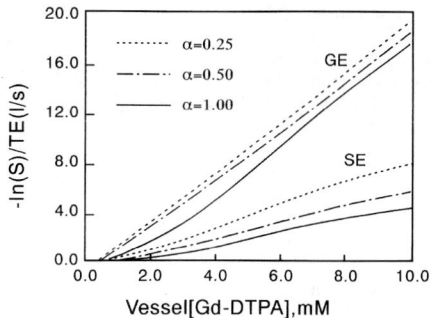

1.0] with R_v = 25 µm. A quadratic increase with Gd-DTPA concentration at low concentrations (<2.0 mM, corresponding to BOLD at 1.5 to 3.0 T) can be observed for both $\Delta R2^*$ and $\Delta R2$ at all vascular weightings. The GRE relationship is generally linear at higher concentrations (>2 mM) with little disparity between vascular weightings. For SE, on the other hand, a more diverse profile is obtained over the range of vascular weightings. With increasing capillary weighting for a fixed capillary volume fraction, both $\Delta R2^*$ and $\Delta R2$ decrease.

Dependence of Relaxivity on Echo Time TE

In Fig. 5 $\Delta R2(R)$ is plotted for TE between 20 and 100 ms, f = 2% and $D_c = 3 \times 10^{-6}$. As TE decreases, $\Delta R2(R)$ shifts downward and slightly to the left; both peak $\Delta R2$ and the radius at which the peak occurs decreases.

Fig. 5. $\Delta R2(R)$ for TE ranging from 20 to 100 ms. f = 2% and $\Delta \chi = 3 \times 10^{-8}$. As TE decreases, the size dependence curve shifts down and to the left; both peak susceptibility change and the radius at which the peak occurs decreases. At lower TE the ratio of relaxivity change for capillary radii (R = 3 µm) to that for venules increases, thereby increasing microvascular selectivity at the cost of overall sensitivity. (Modified from Boxerman et al. [25])

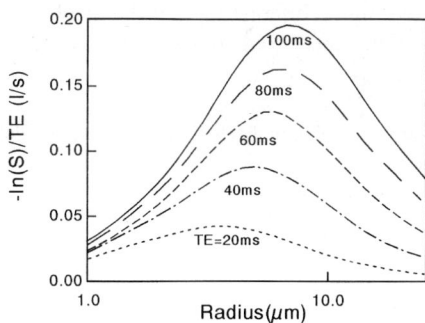

Comparison of Model with In Vivo Data

A mean total blood volume for the whole rat of 5.8 ml/100 g has been measured and agrees well with the 6 ml/100 g reported in the literature. The average measured CBV fraction (whole brain) was 1.5%±0.4%. Figure 6 shows plots of experimental $\Delta R2^*$ and $\Delta R2$ against vascular concentration of AMI-227. Also plotted are the Monte Carlo $\Delta R2^*$ and $\Delta R2$ concentration dependence curves

Fig. 6. Comparison of $\Delta R2^*$ and $\Delta R2$ (TE = 20 ms) for simulation (equidistributed model, f = 1.5% (*solid lines*) and f = 1.5%±0.4% (*dashed lines*), Rv = 25 µm) and experiment as a function of vascular concentration of AMI-227 at 4.7 T. For each cumulative injection, means and standard errors for both intravascular concentration and relaxivity from the data for all three rats were obtained. The experimental data agree with the simulation

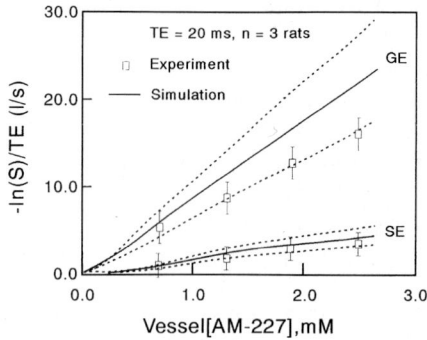

results to within the standard error of the vascular volume fraction. (Modified from Boxerman et al. [25])

for the equidistributed model ($R_v = 25$ µm) with f = 1.5% (solid lines) and f = 1.5%±0.4% (dashed lines). An agreement of the experimental data with the simulation results to within the standard error of the vascular volume fraction was found.

The results of Boxerman and colleagues [25] show that because SE relaxivity peaks for vessels of capillary size or smaller, SE images more heavily weight the contrast distributed within the capillary bed, i.e., microvascular blood volume. In GRE images, however, all vessels are weighted approximately equally. Thus GRE-derived CBV maps more fully represent the total blood volume, including the supplying arteries and draining veins. Because the capillaries deliver substrate to tissue, measurements of capillary blood volume provided by SE imaging may prove more interesting for the study of cerebrovascular disease than total blood volume measured by GRE techniques

Measurement of Tissue Perfusion: The Central Volume Theorem

The guiding principle for the analysis of concentration time data, the central volume theorem, was outlined almost a century ago by Stewart [5] and later reviewed and expanded by Meier and Zierler [55]. Derived simply from mass conservation, this theory states tissue blood flow in tissue, F_t, can be determined by the ratio:

$$F_t = V/MTT \tag{6}$$

where V is the volume of distribution of the agent within the tissue (e.g., the tissue blood volume for an intravascular agent), and MTT is the average time required for any given particle of contrast agent to pass through the tissue. Under these idealized conditions F_t is expressed in units of milliliter of blood per milliliter of tissue. Thus knowledge of V and MTT is required. V can be derived considering mass conservation of the tracer in the volume of interest (VOI). For intracascular tracers this yields:

$$\int C_{VOI}(\tau)d\tau = V \int C_a(\tau)d\tau \qquad (7)$$

where V denotes the volume of distribution, which is equal to the intravascular, extracellular space, i.e., the plasma volume, $C_a(t)$ the concentration of tracer in the arterial input to VOI, and $C_{VOI}(\tau)$ the concentration of contrast in VOI. In the CNS, with an intact BBB, this relationship also applies to extracellular paramagnetic contrast agents. V is thus given by:

$$V = (1 - Hct_m) \, BV \qquad (8)$$

where Hct_m is the microvascular hematocrit and BV the blood volume. Unfortunately, Hct_m is an intricate function of vessel size, flow, and pathophysiological conditions and varies between 40% and 100% of the systemic hematocrit, Hct_S [56]. A working approximation of $Hct_m = 3/2 \, Hct_S$ is reasonable [56].

The MTT for the tracer particles is defined in terms of the density function:

$$MTT \equiv \int \tau h(\tau)d\tau \, / \int h(\tau)d\tau \qquad (9)$$

where h(t) is the probability density function of the transit times of the tracer molecules through the VOI, also termed *transport function*. h(t) reflects the specific properties of the investigated vascular territory and describes the way in which an arterial input $C_a(t)$ is modulated by its passage:

$$C_v(t) = C_a(t) * h(t) = \int C_a(t)h(t - \tau)d\tau \qquad (10)$$

where $C_v(t)$ is the venous output from VOI and "*" denotes convolution. The term h(t) cannot be measured directly but defines the central quantity in bolus-passage experiments, namely the fraction of injected tracer retained in the vasculature at time t, the residue function:

$$R(t) \equiv [1 - \int h(\tau)d\tau] \qquad (11)$$

From this the central equation for the determination of nondiffusible tracers can be derived:

$$C_{VOI}(t) = F_t \int C_a(t)R(t - \tau)d\tau \qquad (12)$$

Considering that the residue function R(t) equals 1 at time 0, R(0) = 1, because all the tracer is still present in the circulation, the initial height of the deconvolved concentration time curve equals the flow, F_t. In practice, however, there are several factors which complicate the issue. The arterial input function $C_a(t)$ may undergo dispersion during its passage from the point of measurement, for example, in the carotid arteries, to more peripheral vessels, for example, the arterioles supplying the tissue of interest. This can be expressed mathematically by convolution of the "true" residue function R(t) with a vascular transport function, h'(t):

$$R'(t) = R(t) * h'(t) \tag{13}$$

The initial height of the deconvolved concentration time curve would thus be underestimated by the dispersion of R'(t) [57]. The arterial input should therefore be measured as closely as possible to the tissue of interest. Solving Eq. 12 for F_t constitutes an inverse problem which involves deconvolution with $C_a(t)$. Two main techniques can be applied, the model-independent and the model-dependent approach. The model-dependent approach assumes a specific analytic expression for R(t), imposing a priori assumptions on the microvasculature. This makes the deconvolution process more stable. Usually a single [58, 59] or multiple exponential function [60] is assumed:

$$R(t,MTT) = e^{-t/MTT} \tag{14}$$

This approach can, however, introduce large systematic errors when flows in two regions with different residue functions are compared [23, 57, 61].

Model-independent approaches, on the other hand, make no assumptions for R(t) but try to solve Eq. 12 for F_t. They require high SNR data to avoid instabilities of the deconvolution process. The transform approach invokes the convolution theorem of the Fourier transform:

$$R(t) = 1/F_t \; FT^{-1}\{FT \; [C_{VOI}(t)]/FT \; [C_a(t)]\} \tag{15}$$

where FT and FT^{-1} denote the forward and reverse Fourier transform. This approach tends severely to underestimate flow, even in the absence of noise, particularly when the MTT is short compared to the sampling rate, and when filters are used as a means to suppress noise [61]. The underestimation of flow for short MTT also means that in regions with high blood volume and thus long MTT flow appears high, rendering the estimated blood volume weighted.

In the algebraic approach [62–64] the convolution integrals of Eqs. 10 and 12 are expressed as discrete matrix equations:

$$A \times B = C \tag{16}$$

where A is a matrix containing $C_a(t_i)$ at different points in time, B and C vectors containing the elements of $R(t_i)$ and $C_{VOI}(t_i)$, respectively, with $i = 1, 2, ..., N$. This can be solved iteratively for B. This approach, employing regularization and, in particular, single value decomposition (SVD) provides the best estimation of flow. While regularization is still somewhat blood volume dependent, SVD is most independent from the underlying vascular structure and volume.

Figure 7 provides an in vivo comparison of these different approaches in a case of a right temporal tumor. For a systematic comparison of these different techniques in theory and experiment we refer the interested reader to the excellent works by Østergaard and coworkers [64, 65].

In practice, $C_a(t)$ can be measured directly with arterial blood sampling, as is conventionally carried out with PET imaging, or directly from NMR images if sufficient temporal and contrast resolution is present. The function $C_{VOI}(t)$ could, subject to the limitations discussed, be determined regionally or on a voxel-by-voxel basis from the imaging study. The measured $C_{VOI}(t)$ curves can, however, include contributions due to tracer recirculation which must be elimi-

Fig. 7. A Calculated CBV map displaying tumor localized to the right temporal lobe. **B** Also shown is a CBF-weighted image acquired with a noncontrast T1 flow-sensitive technique. **C,D** Calculated CBF map using model-dependent (exponential residue model) (C) and SVD (D) deconvolution, both display areas of high flow shown by the T1 technique (*arrows*). This regional heterogeneity was not clearly demonstrated by the accompanying CBV map (A). **E** A flow map was also generated by using a gaussian residue model. Note that the area with high flow is not qualitatively displayed.

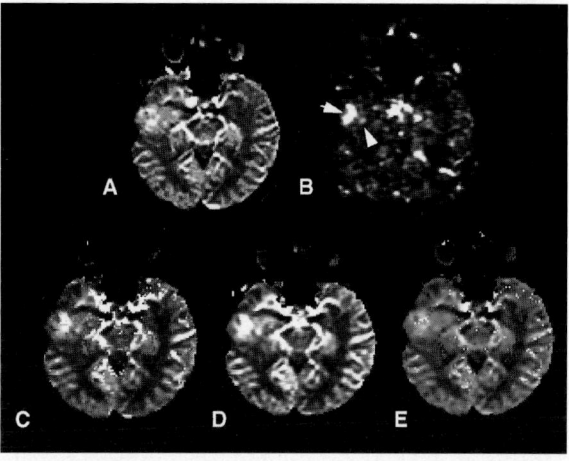

The χ^2 of the fit to the concentration time curve was increased in the same area. Also, note that gray–white matter flow ratio is noticeably lower in the gaussian fit, as was found in the normal volunteers. Symmetric areas of high flow around the brainstem and corresponding to the course of the MCA are artifacts due to susceptibility effects around large vessels. (With permission of the authors and the publisher, from Østergaard et al. [65])

nated prior to deconvolution in order to extract volume and flow information. This can be accomplished by exponential extrapolation, numerical integration, or fitting to a γ-variate function with a recirculation cutoff [66–68]:

$$C_{VOI}(t) = Q \ t^r \ e^{-(t/b)} \tag{17}$$

where Q, r, and b are constants. A variety of functional parameters can be analytically calculated, including the area under the concentration-time curve, which is proportional to the local blood volume [23, 69, 70].

The accuracy with which the MTT can be determined depends on the quality of both the $C_a(t)$ and the $C_{VOI}(t)$ data. In the case of freely diffusible tracers this is facilitated by the slower transit times through the tissues; thus the measurement of MTT is less dependent on the arterial input curve. For purely intravascular tracers the transit is so rapid that a well-characterized bolus is needed to obtain accurate measurements of the MTT [71].

Determination of blood flow, in addition to measuring the MTT, requires knowledge of the volume of distribution of the contrast agent. For intravascular agents this is the tissue blood volume, V, an important physiological parameter itself. V can be determined by integrating the tissue concentration-time curve and normalizing to the integrated arterial (input) data [31, 32, 35, 72]:

$$V = \int Tissue(t) \ / \int Art(t) \tag{18}$$

This has several important consequences.

- Because the blood volume determination is reflected in the time-integrated tissue and blood concentration data, measurement of blood volume alone has somewhat diminished the need for very high temporal resolution measurements. In the measurement of arterial blood data this can mean that samples collected over time do not need to be fractionally measured and can simply be pooled from an average determination.

● Because the arterial input to an organ is ultimately derived from a common source, measurement of *relative* blood volume can be made without any knowledge of the arterial concentration-time data.

For these reasons attempts to quantify microcirculatory parameters from NMR data have so far focused on the somewhat simpler measurement of blood volume, as a necessary and important first step towards complete characterization of tissue perfusion.

Rempp et al. [73, 72], however, have reported cerebral blood flow (CBF) measurements in a group of 12 subjects without intracranial pathology. They used a simultaneous dual fast low-angle shot (FLASH) sequence as first proposed by Perman et al. [74] to acquire two different parallel images with different TE values, which allowed them to measure simultaneously the concentration time curves from brain tissue (single slice) and the arterial input in the carotids or vertebral arteries. They used a combination of model-dependent and model-independent approaches, fitting a γ-variate function to the concentration-time data and using deconvolution analysis to determine regional CBF. To control instabilities with the algorithm, a Wiener filter was applied to the frequency domain data [75]. They obtained rCBV values of 8.0 ± 3.1 ml/100 g tissue for gray matter and 4.2 ± 1.0 ml/100 g tissue for white matter, corresponding to an average of 6.5 ± 2.0 ml/100 g tissue assuming a 60:40 ratio of gray to white matter. Within the SDs these values agree with PET [76, 77] data, although they were slightly too high.

Clinical Applications

A variety of different noninvasive techniques to measure CBF have been developed over the past 25 years, including SPECT, PET and CT, employing a variety of diffusible and intravascular tracers [78–80]. Radionuclide tracer methods are hampered by two major disadvantages: their limited resolution and the fact that the recorded signal originates to a large extent from the macrovasculature. As outlined above, susceptibility-contrast MRI methods provide better spatial resolution and are more sensitive to the microvasculature than radionuclide methods and thus come closer to the goal of revealing the microvascular architecture and the mechanisms by which the brain regulates its needs for metabolic substrates.

Because of the difficulties experienced in determining true blood flow, as outlined above, the determination of blood volume is the most frequently used method. This method has so far been evaluated in more than 1000 brain tumor studies worldwide [81]. The studies reported show that CBV mapping can easily be added to a conventional NMR imaging study simply by collecting functional data during the contrast injection, without compromising the routine postcontrast studies.

Brain Tumors

CBV mapping using susceptibility contrast has become an established method in the evaluation of patients with malignant brain tumors and is now used routinely in the work-up and follow-up of these patients in many centers worldwide.

Because of the induction of capillary proliferation by humoral factors released by the neoplasm, malignant tumors typically have regions of elevated CBV. This is in accordance with PET data which also show hypermetabolism in these vital areas of the tumor. High-grade tumors typically are characterized by regions of higher CBV than normal brain. This is illustrated in Fig. 8 by comparison of conventional MRI, CBV, and PET studies in the case of a high-grade oligoastrocytoma. On the CBV maps, however, the tumor appears heterogeneous with areas of increased and decreased blood volume, revealing the typical biological characteristics of high-grade tumors. Another high-grade tumor, an oligoastrocytoma, with histopathological correlation, is shown in Fig. 9.

Low-grade lesions typically display lower CBV than corresponding normal brain and are more homogeneous, as illustrated by the CBV map of a benign, low-grade glioma in Fig. 10. Remarkable heterogeneity, however, has been observed in tumors originally classified as low grade that later revealed features consistent with a greater degree of malignancy. Central necrosis has low or missing rCBV values, and the surrounding edema also shows decreased values.

Just as PET studies with fluorodeoxy glucose (FDG) are powerful predictors of prognosis, results from ongoing studies indicate that CBV mapping by MRI may be of great use in assessing the prognosis of glioma patients [82–86]. Data show that the results of MRI blood volume mapping is well correlated with PET-FDG findings in most gliomas studied. Studies of patients with primary brain tumor have shown that MRI CBV maps can characterize these lesions based on their microvasculature structure and may provide information on new tissue characteristics based on the pathophysiological properties of the tumor itself. Theses results also indicate that MRI CBV mapping may be of use in the grading of primary gliomas.

The largest study on the value of CBV mapping for the diagnostic assessment of cerebral gliomas was conducted by Aronen et al. [81] who evaluated 19 patients. They obtained CBV maps from SE EPI studies performed in either a single or multiple (eight) axial planes with the following parameters: TE = 100 ms, TR = 1000 ms (single-) to 1500 ms (multislice), thickness = 7 mm, 128×256 matrix with 20×40 cm field-of-view ($1.5 \times 1.5 \times 7$ mm^3 voxel size). They used various gadolinium chelates (Magnevist, Schering; Omniscan, Nycomed; and Prohance, Squibb Diagnostics) in concentrations of 0.1 or 0.2 mmol/kg BW, injected at a rate of 5 ml/s with a Medrad Spectris powerinjector. Three patients with suspected interruption of the BBB received two consecutive injections of Gd-chelate to saturate the interstitial space before the second measurement from which the CBV map calculated. Because the method yields relative rather than absolute CBV values, white matter was used as an internal standard. All results were compared with findings on conventional MRI and tumor specimens obtained at biopsy or surgery and graded according to the World Health Organization [87] and Daumas-Duport [88] grading systems.

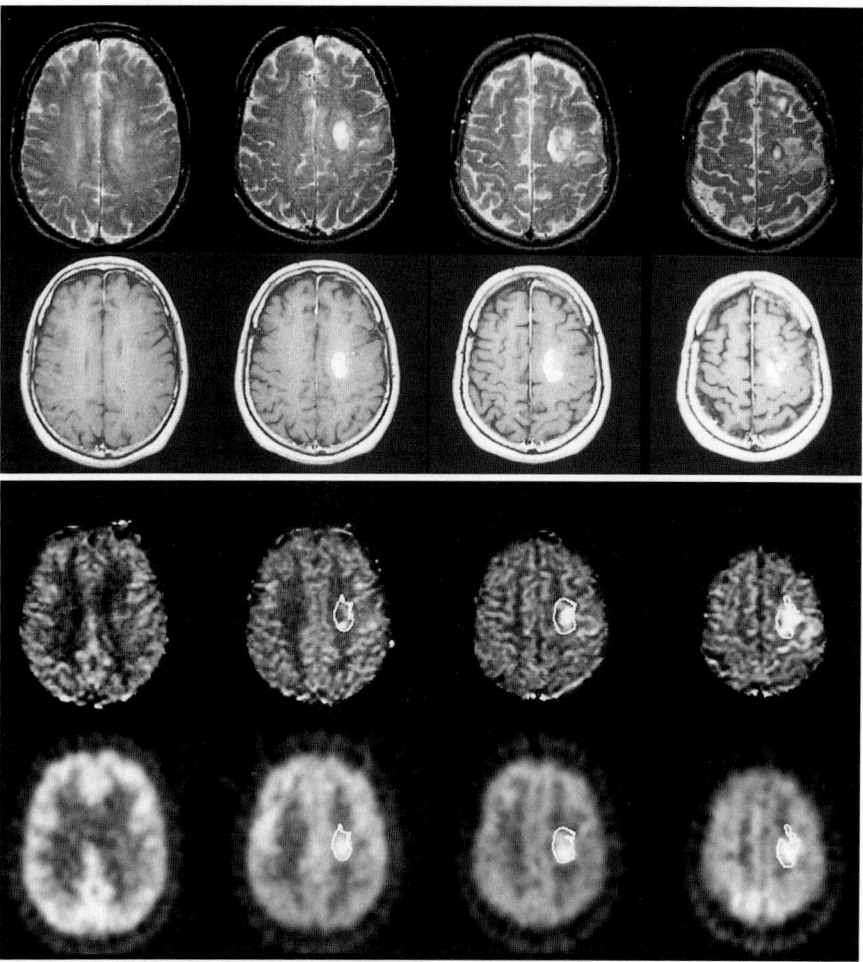

Fig. 8. T2-weighted NMR images (2000/80) (*top row*), contrast enhanced T1-weighted images (700/20; *second row*), multisection CBV maps (*third row*), and PET-FDG scans (*lower row*) from a patient with a grade III oligoastrocytoma. Four of the eight sections obtained are shown. The areas of high CBV identified on the CBV maps show substantial overlap with areas of increased signal intensity on the T2-weighted images but are partially distinct from enhancing regions on the T1-weighted images. They are well correlated with the areas of high activity on the PET-FDG scans. The diagnosis was confirmed at biopsy. Focal regions of high CBV are present in regions of high signal intensity on T2-weighted images (*arrow*), with and without associated edema; this could indicate tumor, edema, or both. High CBV suggests the presence of active tumor. (Modified, with permission of the authors and the publisher, from Aronen et al. [19])

Fig. 9a–c. A Precontrast (*top left*) and postcontrast (*top right*) T1-weighted NMR images (700/20), T2-weighted NMR image (2000/80) (*bottom left*), and CBV map (*bottom right*) of two enhancing foci in the right temporal lobe. The CBV map, obtained after injection of 0.2 mmol/kg BW gadodiamide, shows elevated CBV in both foci, suggesting a high-grade glioma. The diagnosis was confirmed at surgery. B,C Corresponding histological specimens show increased capillary density in the high-grade oligoastrocytoma. B,C Densely cellular areas (cellularity = 3) with numerous branching vessels (vascularity = 3; B) and many wider vessels and conspicuous endothelial cells (vascularity = 3; C) are seen. Thus the tumor demonstrated both heterogeneity of vessel diameter and high vascularity at histopathological examination and heterogeneously increased CBV. (With permission of the authors and the publisher from Aronen et al. [19])

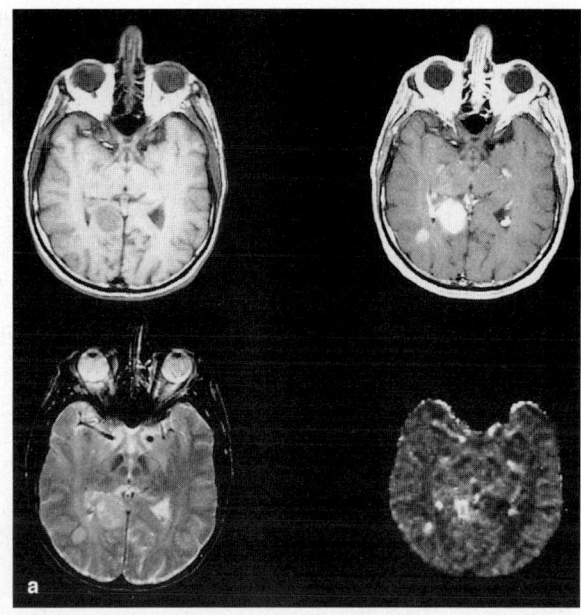

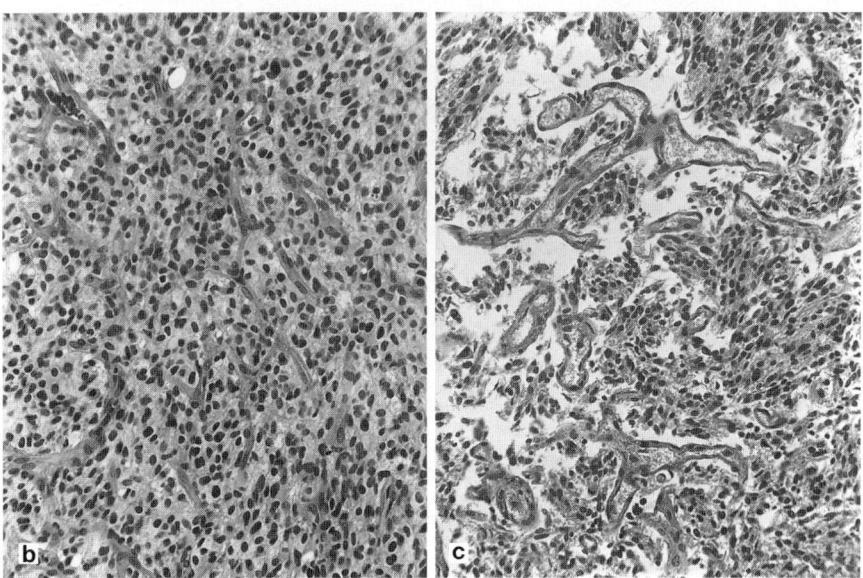

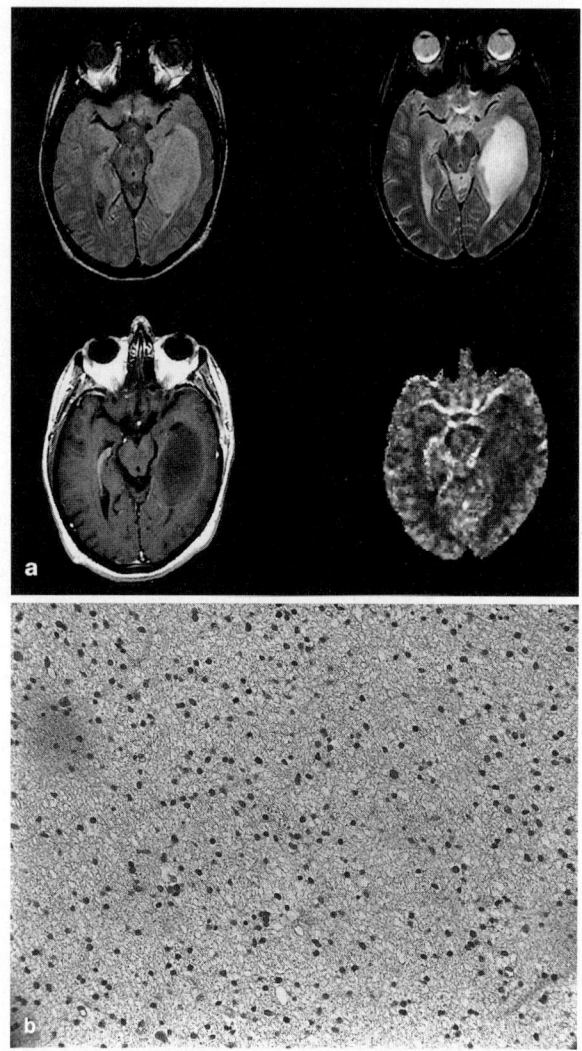

Fig. 10. a Proton density weighted (2000/30; *top left*), T2-weighted (2000/80; *top right*), and contrast-enhanced T1-weighted (700/20) (*bottom left*) NMR images; *bottom right*, the CBV map of a
left temporal lobe tumor. The appearance of the tumor on all studies was consistent with that of
a low-grade glioma, which was verified at biopsy. The tumor is nonenhancing and shows a relatively low blood volume on the CBV map. Note the relatively high CBV content in the normal
choroid plexus and larger vessels. **b** Histological specimen. A grade 2 astrocytoma was diag-
nosed. The tumor was mildly hypercellular (cellularity = 1) with rare, thin-walled capillaries
(vascularity = 1). (With permission of the authors and the publisher, from Aronen et al. [19])

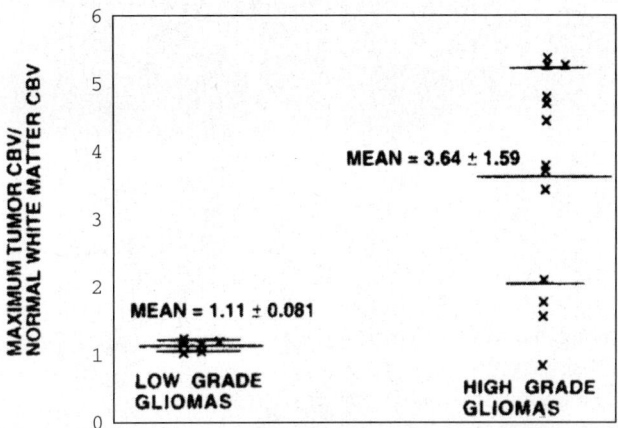

Fig. 11. Maximal tumor/normal white matter CBV ratio. The ratio is higher in the high-grade gliomas than in the low grade gliomas. The highest CBV value (mean±standard deviation) in the low-grade ($n = 6$, 1.11 ± 0.081) and in the high-grade ($n = 13$, 3.64 ± 1.59) glioma groups were compared to that of the normal white matter. The difference in means is statistically significant ($p = 0.0001$, Student's t test for unequal variances). Mean and 1 SD lines are shown for each group. (With permission of the authors and the publisher, from Aronen et al. [19])

They found a ratio of gray matter/white matter CBV in normal areas of 2.32 ± 0.27, in accordance with physiological values. The relationship of maximal tumor CBV and tumor grade is shown in Fig. 11. Only one high-grade glioma had low CBV values overlapping with the values in the low-grade group. As was to be expected, the range of CBV values was larger in the high-grade group (2.94 ± 1.5) than in the low-grade group (0.22 ± 0.22; $p = 0.0001$). Tumor vascularity was correlated with CBV ($p = 0.09$) but not with tumor cellularity ($p = 0.1$). A positive correlation of CBV with mitotic activity ($p = 0.006$) was also found. Interestingly, of the findings at conventional MRI only enhancement was associated with tumor grade ($p = 0.001$), but edema ($p = 0.011$), heterogeneity ($p = 0.046$), necrosis ($p = 0.11$), cyst formation ($p = 1.0$), delineation ($p = 0.62$), hemorrhage ($p = 0.26$), and mass effect ($p = 0.079$) were not. The comparison between CBV and conventional MRI showed a positive correlation only for tumor heterogeneity and CBV ($p = 0.023$) but not for enhancement ($p = 0.12$).

Experience with blood volume mapping of extra-axial lesions has been limited. In meningiomas the benefits of preoperative embolization with the goal of decreasing intraoperative blood loss has been evaluated. Bruening et al. [89] have shown that Gd-enhanced T1-weighted imaging underestimates the response to embolization therapy. CBV mapping, on the other hand, proved to be a more exact measure of the extent of successful embolization than the intraoperative findings. Figure 12 shows an example. Embolization was taken to be successful when the ratio of tumor to gray matter CBV decreased to 20 % or less of the pre-embolization value of the tumor. In six of the examined nine meningiomas T1 enhancement suggested residual perfusion in the embolized areas on conventional MRI, but the dynamic susceptibility studies showed no signal decline dur-

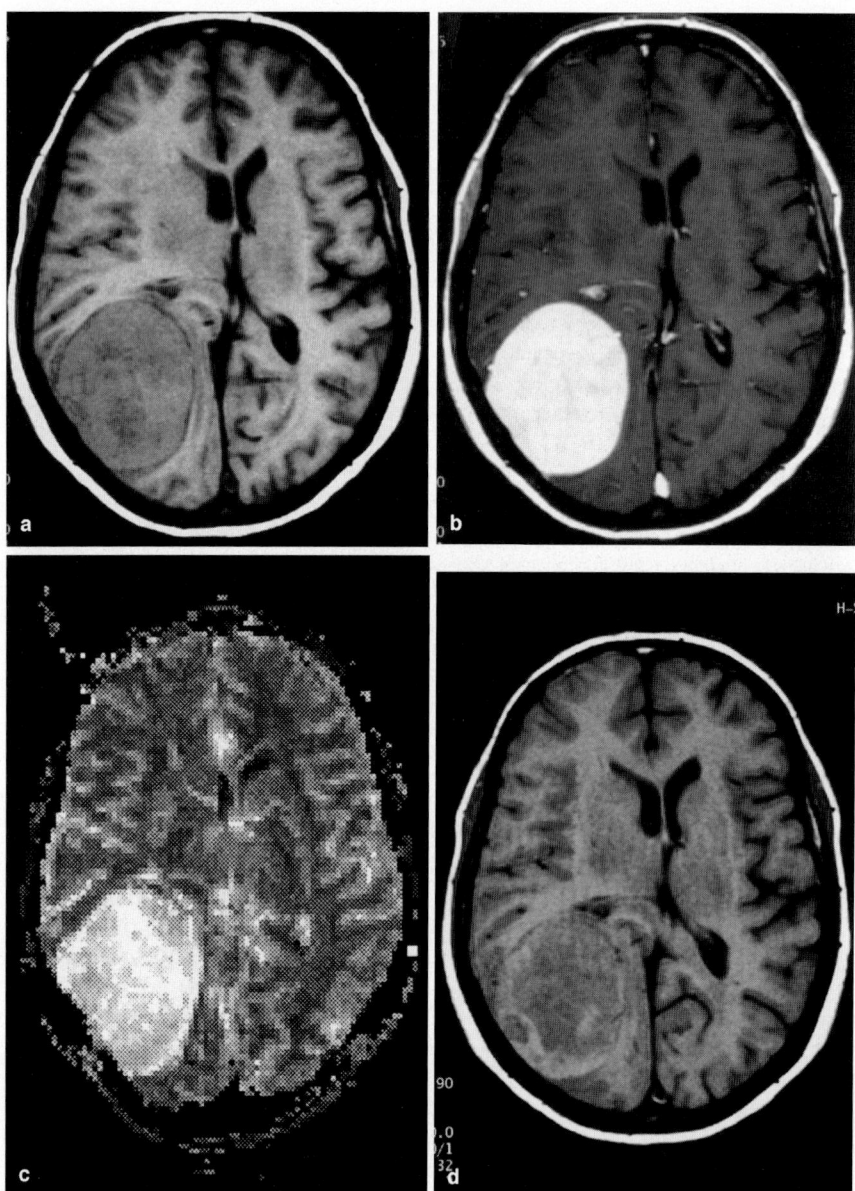

Fig. 12a–f. Right temporoparietal convexity meningioma in a 61-year-old woman. Preemboliza-
tion. **a** T1-weighted unenhanced SE-image. **b** T1-weighted Gd-enhanced (0.2 mmol/kg BW)
image. **c** Regional blood volume map. Postembolization. **d** T1-weighted unenhanced SE image.
e T1-weighted Gd-enhanced (0.2 mmol/kg BW) SE image. **f** Regional blood volume map.
Good correlation between the T1-weighted Gd-enhanced image and the regional blood volume
map is observed in this patient both before and after embolization. After embolization, the
Gd-enhanced T1 w-image underestimates the embolized area, which is more realistically represented on the BV-map

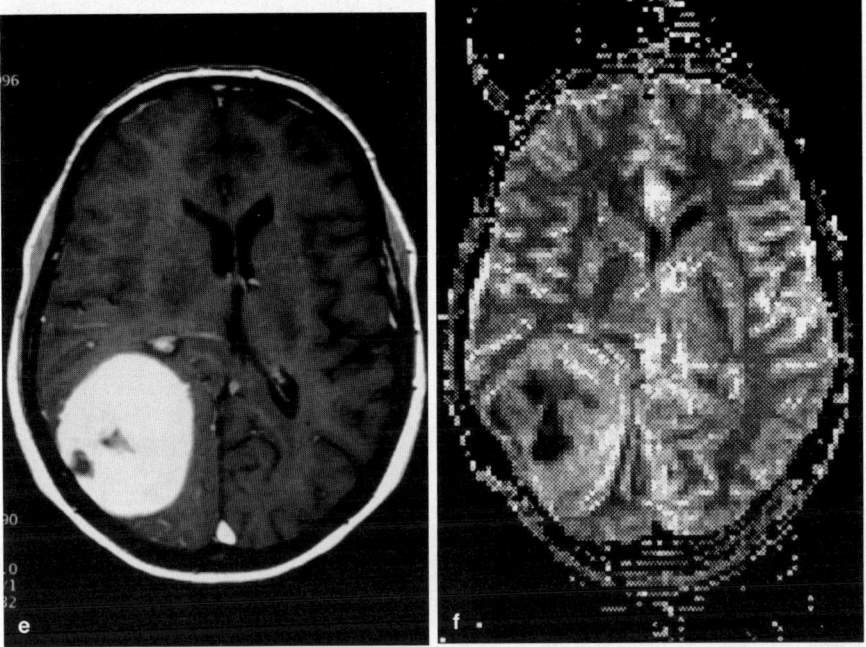

ing the bolus passage. These data suggest that even in the absence of measurable perfusion Gd-DTPA leaks into the interstitium by plasma circulation, diffusion, or slow collateral flow.

Radiation Treatment: Follow-Up and Necrosis

A particularly challenging problem in neuro-oncological imaging is the monitoring of radiation therapy and in particular the diagnosis of radiation necrosis and its distinction from tumor recurrence since they require different therapeutic approaches. Because both radiation damage and tumor regrowth may show enhancement on CT and conventional MRI studies, conventional imaging modalities cannot reliably distinguish these pathological entities. PET-FDG studies have been shown to be useful in this regard and can differentiate suspected radiation necrosis from tumor regrowth. Results from preliminary studies using MRI blood volume mapping techniques suggest, however, that MRI can provide similar information less invasively, at lower cost and with higher spatial resolution. Areas of radiation necrosis are characterized by lower blood volume and perfusion than recurrent gliomas [18, 89]. Figure 13 illustrates this differential diagnostic dilemma in a patient with recurrent glioma of the brain.

Wenz at al. [18] have shown that the reduction in blood volume in astrocytomas and normal brain after radiation therapy can be quantified using dynamic susceptibility contrast NMR imaging, making functional monitoring of tumor

Fig. 13a–c. Patient with high grade (IV) astrocytoma in surgically nonaccessible location 6 months after fractionated radiation therapy. **a** T1-weighted Gd-enhanced SE-image. **b** Regional blood volume obtained with T1-weighted dynamic EPI study. **c** Regional blood volume map obtained with dynamic susceptibility weighted EPI study. Since both radiation necrosis and recurrent gliomas show enhancement on conventional Gd-enhanced T1-weighted studies, clear differentiation between these twentities is often impossible. The high blood volume values on the regional blood volume maps, however, clearly indicate recurrent tumor

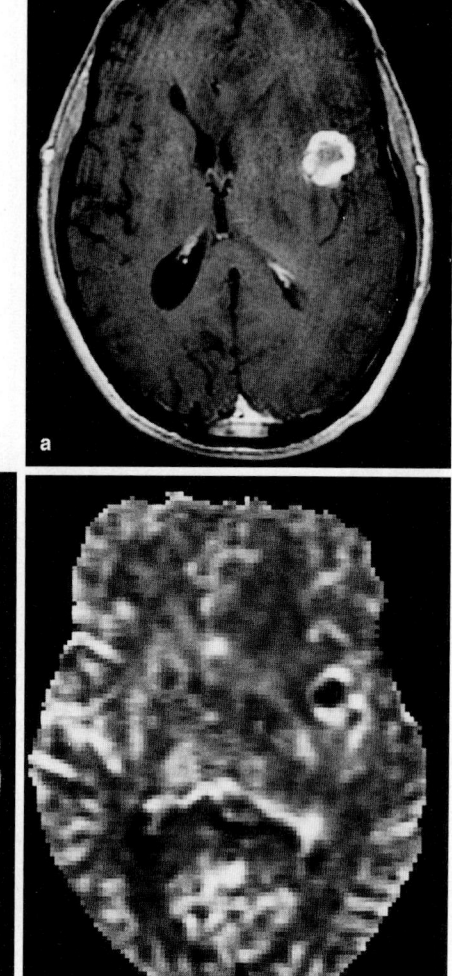

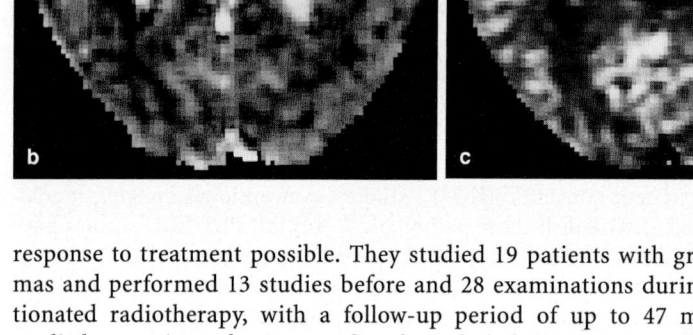

response to treatment possible. They studied 19 patients with grade II astrocytomas and performed 13 studies before and 28 examinations during and after fractionated radiotherapy, with a follow-up period of up to 47 month. They also studied 13 patients for 79 months after whole-brain irradiation. They calculated quantitative CBV maps using their two-slice GRE technique, which allows monitoring of the arterial input function at the level of the carotid arteries while the second slice located at the level of the tumor to record records the tissue signal-time-curve. The results of their study are summarized in Table 1.

Their blood volume values for gray and white matter were in good agreement with data from PET [91]. Patients with whole-brain irradiation had significantly decreased blood volume in normal brain tissue than in nonirradiated brain, which may at least in part have been due to concomitant chemotherapy and higher age in this group. Patients undergoing conformation therapy, because of the steep dose gradient outside the target volume, showed only a very moderate

Table 1. Blood volumes for normal gray and white matter and grade II astrocytomas before and after conformation radiotherapy (modified from [18])

Time of study	No. of exams	Blood volume (ml/100 g)		
		Gray matter	White matter	Astrocytomas
Before radiation therapy	13	9.2±2.8	4.4±1.9	12.2±8.7
After conformation radiotherapy (8.0±9.5 months; median 5.5)	28	7.4±3.2	4.1±2.3	6.5±5.3
After whole-brain radiotherapy (15±26 months; median 3)	13	6.3±1.2	3.1±1.0	n/a

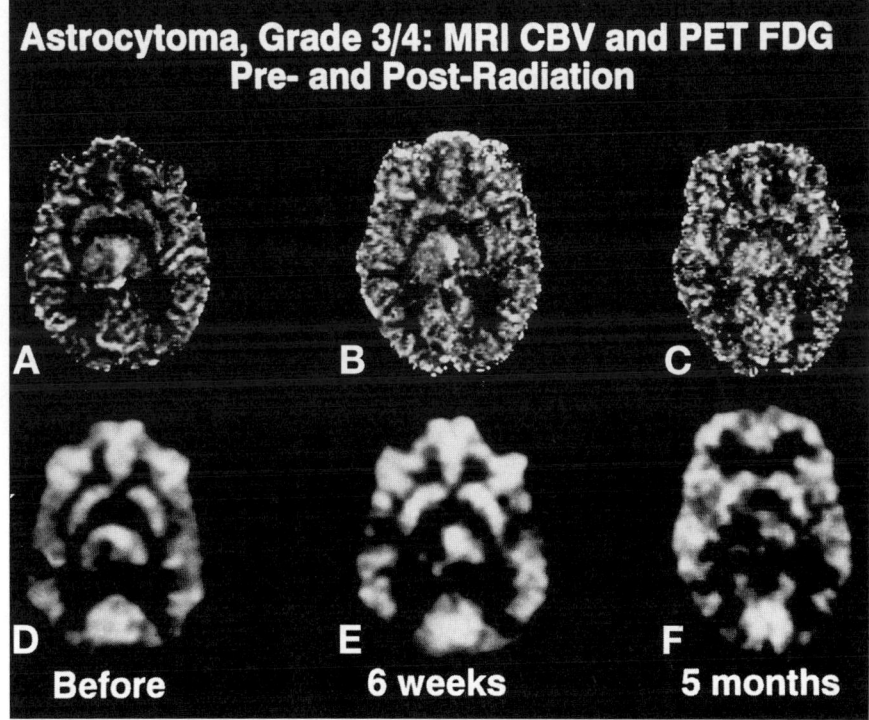

Fig. 14A–F. Inoperable grade III/IV astrocytoma involving the basal ganglia. *Upper row,* EPI blood volume maps (**A–C**); *lower row,* PET-FDG study (**D–F**), before (**A,D**), during (**B,E**) and after fractionated radiation therapy. Both PET metabolic activity and blood volume of the tumor decrease in parallel during treatment and indicate tumor necrosis. Note better resolution of NMR study. (Courtesy of B.R. Rosen et al., Massachusetts General Hospital, Boston)

decrease in normal tissue blood volume after therapy. Of the 13 grade II astro-cytomas, 10 had higher, but none lower, blood volumes than normal gray matter. These findings were in contradiction to the reports from Maeda et al. [84] and Aronen et al. [19] who, using EPI and different postprocessing, obtained rela-tively reduced blood volumes in the tumors. After radiation therapy most of the tumors in their study in agreement with cases from other groups [84, 92] showed decreased vascularity after radiation therapy. Figure 14 shows a time-course study of a grade III/IV astrocytoma under radiation therapy in correlation with the PET-FDG study. They conclude that dynamic susceptibility contrast MRI allows the quantification of radiation effects in low-grade astrocytomas and nor-mal brain tissue. The generally low blood volumes of radiation necrosis may not, however, be sufficient evidence to exclude tumor recurrence.

Biopsy Guidance

CT-guided, stereotactic needle biopsy has become a commonly used procedure in the diagnostic work-up of intracranial tumors. Because of the pronounced het-erogeneity of primary gliomas successful diagnosis and grading based on stereo-tactic biopsies depends to a large extent on the sampling site. Although contrast enhancement on T1w images is useful for the characterization of these tumors, it does not provide sufficient guidance to the optimal biopsy site, because areas of enhancement are not necessarily correlated to the areas of most active tumor metabolism and tumor growth.

Only PET-FDG studies can so far locate the optimal biopsy site by identifying most active part of the tumor. Because of the correlation between PET-FDG activity and blood volume maps, dynamic susceptibility enhanced MRI may in future be used to locate optimal biopsy sites in gliomas. This would obviate the need for matching the coordinates of the PET study with those of CT or MRI since both functional and imaging study and possibly even the biopsy pro-cedure can be carried out in one scanner, with the added benefit of higher reso-lution and lower cost.

Figure 15 illustrates the way in which CBV maps can facilitate the localization of the optimal biopsy site in a case of a high-grade astrocytoma.

Ischemia

MRI is known to be highly sensitive for changes associated with ischemic stroke; however, acute cerebral infarction in humans with a time interval less than 12 h usually is not reliable on conventional imaging. Since this time interval is too long to influence acute stroke therapy, there is a strong demand for an imaging technique providing information of the location, size, and nature of the lesion. Also, therapy is influenced by the degree of perfusion deficit and by the collat-eral blood supply. Despite the successful demonstration of protection in a variety of animal models of cerebral infarction the transfer of such results to human stroke has been largely unsuccessful. As a result, no current therapy concept is

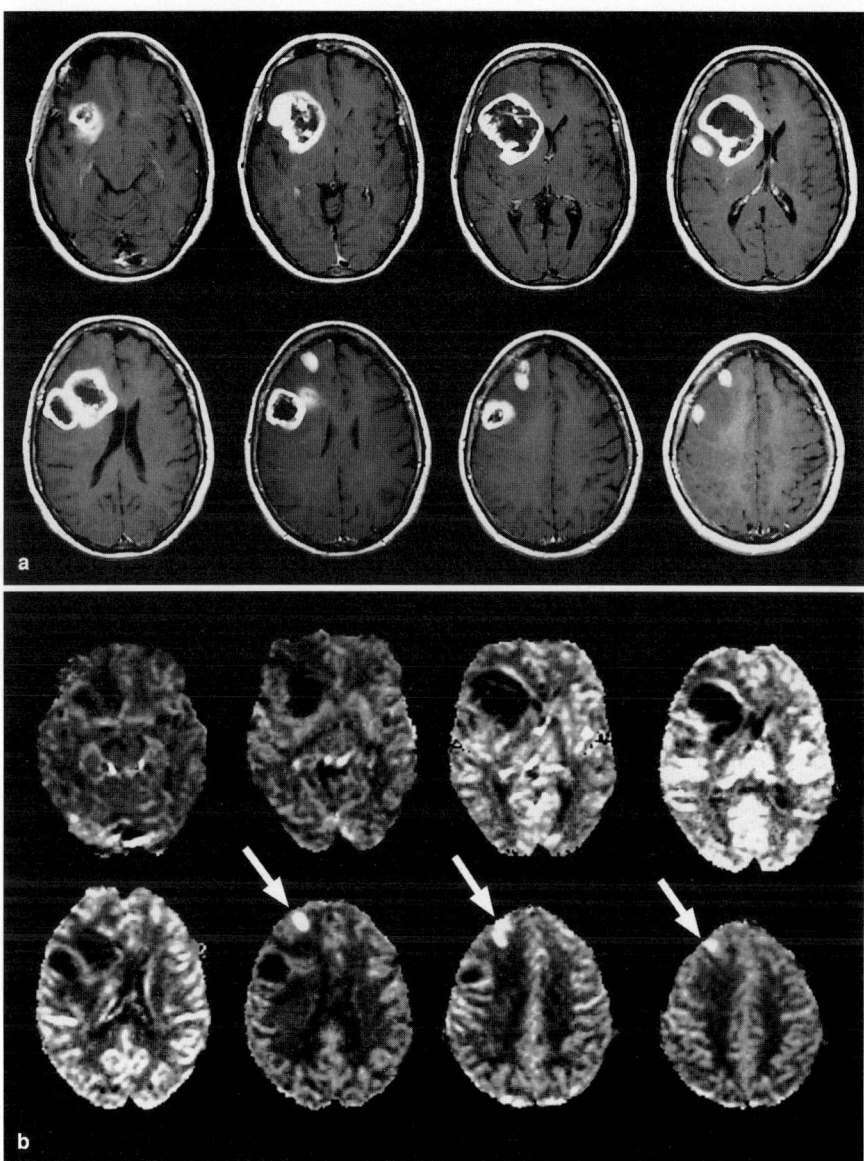

Fig. 15. Contrast-enhanced T1-weighted NMR images (700/20; **a**) and multisection CBV maps (**b**) obtained before surgical resection of a high-grade astrocytoma with multifocal enhancement. Regions of varying CBV were noted within the enhancing area. Biopsy material obtained from the region of the highest CBV (*arrows* in **b**) exhibited high capillary density and a high tumor grade. (With permission of the authors and the publisher, from Aronen et al. [19])

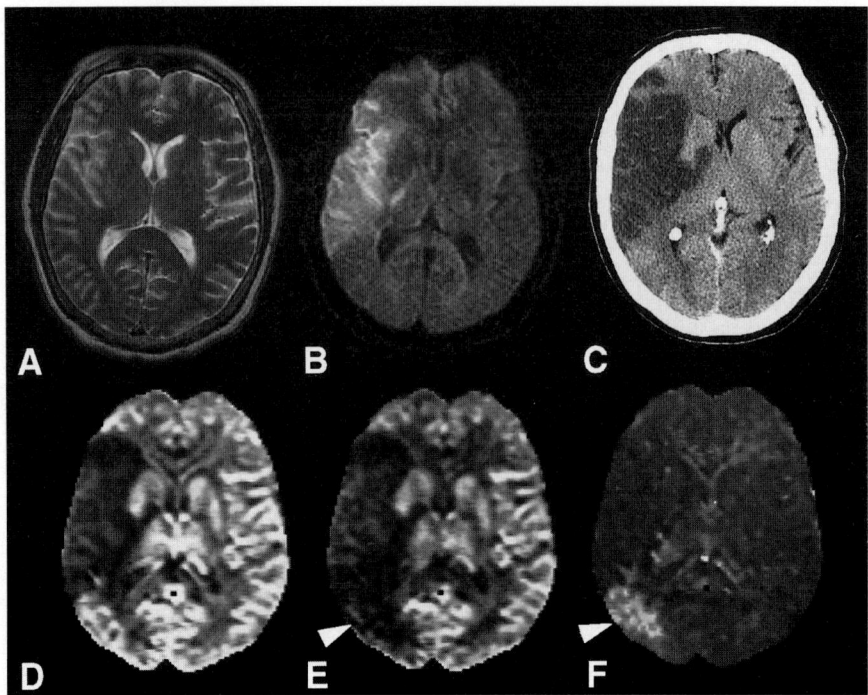

Fig. 16A–F. Images of a 53-year-old man 3 h after acute onset of left hemiparesis. T2-weighted FSE (**A**) shows minimal sulcal effacement in the right hemisphere. The isotropic diffusion weighted image (**B**) is well correlated with the size of the infarcted area and the follow-up CT scan 3 days later (**C**). The CBV (**D**) and SVD CBF (**E**) maps show a small region with low flow and high volume that survived the stroke (*arrow*). The region of flow-volume mismatch is clearly visible in the MTT map (**F**). (With permission of the authors and the publisher, from Østergaard at al. [65].)

universally accepted for acute ischemia. Recent NMR imaging studies demonstrate that discrimination between partial and total ischemic lesions is possible by the use of rCBV mapping [93, 94]. In these cases susceptibility sequences and diffusion-weighted sequences were used as an adjunct to the routine protocol on an emergency basis (Fig. 16).

The efficacy of thrombolytic therapy in reducing ischemic cell injury is greatest in the first hours after stroke onset, as shown in animal models [95–98]. The safe and efficient use of thrombolytic agents, however, is limited as standard neuroimaging procedures such as CT and MRI fail to detect salvagable brain tissue within this time range. It has been shown, however, that a combination of blood flow and diffusion imaging can be used to identify salvagable brain tissue at the periphery of an ischemic area, the so-called "ischemic penumbra." In the latter the water diffusion is decreased due to partial (functional) energy failure, but blood flow is preserved at a level sufficient to prevent structural breakdown of the cells. As has been shown in rodent studies (Fig. 17), the ischemic pen-

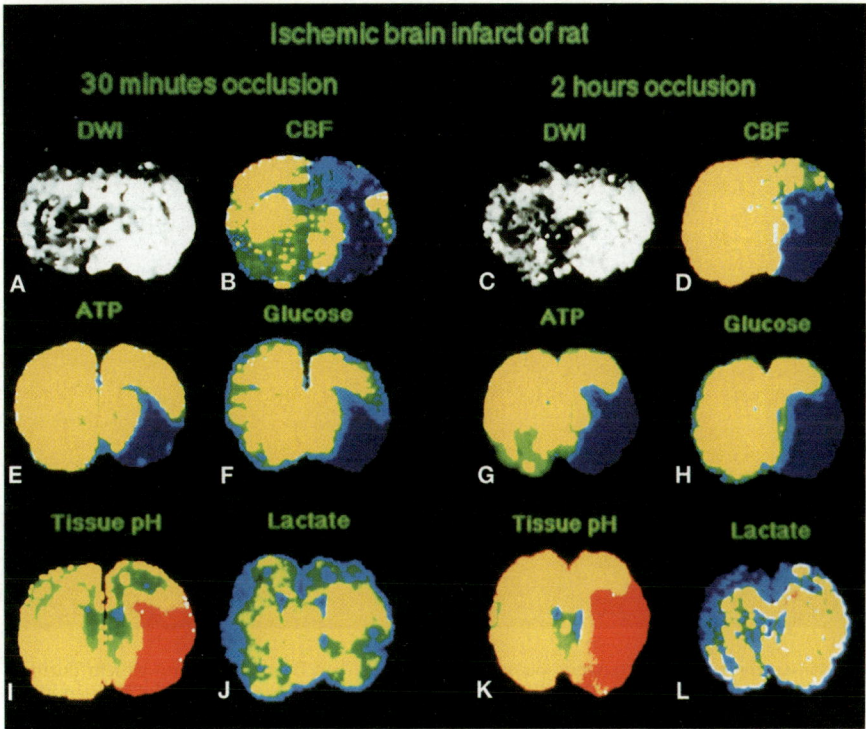

Fig. 17A–L. Evolution of stroke induced by left middle cerebral artery (*MCA*) occlusion in a rat. *Left block* (**A–F**), 30 min after MCA occlusion. **A** High signal intensity on diffusion-weighted EPI image (*DWI*) delineates area of ischemia-induced cytotoxic edema (high signal area = D1). **B** Blood flow map shows central area of severe flow deficit (dark blue area = F1) compared to normal contralateral MCA territory. Note that area F1 is smaller than area D1. **C** Map of ATP concentration. Note that area correlates well with the area of severe ATP depletion (dark blue area = A1). In the borderline area (B1 = F1–D1) flow and ATP concentration are maintained at a sufficient level to prevent tissue necrosis. This is the so called "ischemic penumbra," i.e., salvagable brain tissue. **D** Map of glucose concentration. **E** Map of tissue pH. **F** Map of lactate concentration. *Right block* (**G–L**), 2 h after MCA occlusion. **G** DW image has not changed significantly. Note that both areas F1 and A1 have increased (**H**), now equaling roughly area D1, indicating complete energy failure in the previously preserved ischemic borderzone. (Courtesy of Back T and Höhn-Berlage M, Max Planck Institut Köln, Germany)

umbra as defined by MRI is well correlated with metabolic indicators of energy failure and gradually disappears with increasing time from the onset of stroke. If an ischemic penumbra cannot be identified, tissue necrosis is irreversible at the current level of understanding. Thrombolytic therapy at this stage is probably contraindicated since it exposes the patient to the risk of hemorrhage without having any beneficial effect.

Only sporadic studies of the hemodynamic effects of patients with migraine can be found. An interesting case was reported by Østergaard at al. [65] and is shown in Fig. 18.

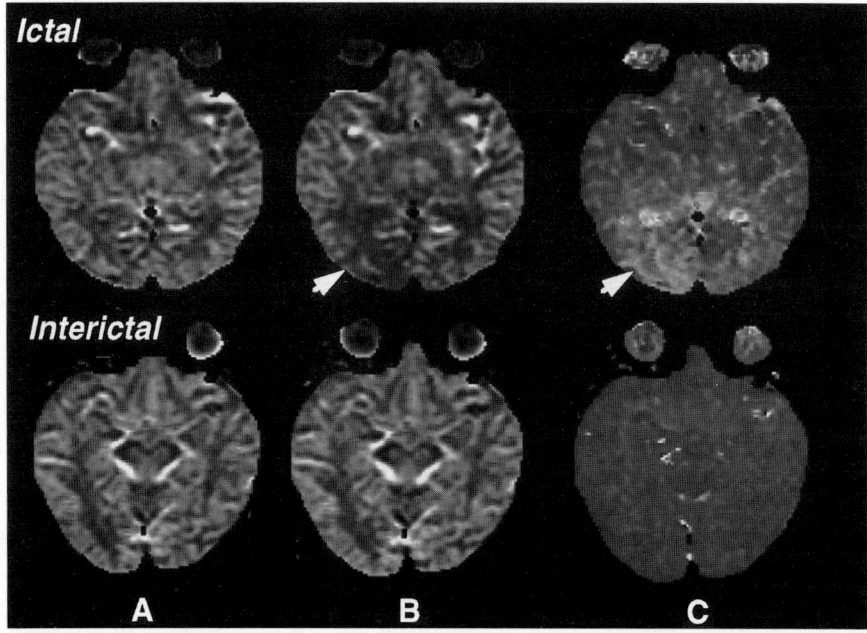

Fig. 18A–C. *Top row,* hemodynamic parameter maps obtained from a migraine patient during a left visual hemifield aura. **A** The CBV map shows only subtle changes. **B** The CBF map shows an area with decreased flow localized to the right occipital lobe. **C** The mismatch between volume and flow, indicating altered vascular tone, is clearly demonstrated by the MTT map and is correlated with the patient's symptoms. The maps clearly demonstrate the congruence between left hemifield aura and right occipital hypoperfusion. *Bottom row,* interictal control study. Perfusion and MTT maps display no changes in the occipital cortex. (With permission of the authors and the publisher, from Østergaard et al. [65])

Epilepsy

Few reports exist in the current literature on the use of hemodynamic MRI in patients with epilepsy. Localization of the seizure focus is crucial prior to performing surgical resection, which can cure epilepsy in up to 90%. Although electroencephalography (EEG), SPECT (Vattino), and PET (Spencer) can be used for this purpose, they lack spatial precision. Conventional MRI, particularly using the inversion recovery (IR) technique, can be used to localize epileptic foci based on its high resolution and contrast (Jackson) but does not provide sufficient sensitivity and specificity in all cases.

Warach et al. [998] reported a patient with focal status epilepticus who presented with left visual field hemianopsia and visual hallucinations with left body convulsions. He was investigated with a dynamic susceptibility contrast technique employing a T2*-weighted FLASH sequence (35/25/10) and bolus injection of 20 cc Gd-DTPA. Relative rCBV values were calculated from DR2*. They found markedly increased rCBV (+91%) in the right temporoparietal region during seizure activity, corresponding to marked hyperperfusion (+50 %) on SPECT. After the seizure activity had stopped, both MRI rCBV and SPECT perfusion measurements became symmetric. They also found that the estimated time to maximal signal decrease was the same for both ictal and control regions and used these values as substitutes for MTT, which could not be determined in this study. Flow being the ratio of CBV and MTT, the increased rCBV in the seizure focus also suggested increased flow, in accordance with the SPECT study.

Wu et al. [100] in a CBV study of interictal epileptic patients found lower relative CBV values in the left hippocampus than the right in eight of the ten investigated patients. The mean CBV ratio (hippocampus/white matter) was 1.80 (mean, SD not provided) on the left to 2.21 on the right ($p<0.01$). The CBV findings agreed with the EEG and PET results.

In one 32-year-old female patient with mitochondrial myopathy, encephalopathy, lactic acidosis, and strokelike episodes (MELAS) investigated during the seizure, they found elevated CBV values in the epileptogenic lesions, with CBV ratios of 2.82 (mean, SD not provided) versus 1.94 in the presumably normal contralateral brain area.

These intial data fuel hope that blood volume mapping may become a useful adjunct to conventional NMR in the preoperative workup of epileptic patients.

Neurodegenerative Disorders

Only a single report on the application of blood volume mapping for the diagnosis of Alzheimer's disease was available at the time of writing. Harris et al. [101] compared the temporoparietal and sensorimotor rCBV of 13 patients with Alzheimer's disease (Mini-Mental State, MMS, examination [102] score 19.6±4.1) with the rCBV of an age- and size-matched control group (MMS score 28.7±1.0). Ratios of rCBV to cerebellar CBV were analyzed since the cerebellum is less affected than the cortex in Alzheimer's disease. They used a multislice EPI protocol with TE = 100 ms, TR = 2 s, 50 sets of ten image planes over 100 s, 128×256 matrix, 1.5×1.5 mm in-plane resolution, 7-mm slice thickness, and 3-mm gap with a 6-s 0.2 mmol/kg BW Gd-DTPA bolus. A comparison of rCBV maps from a patient with Alzheimer's disease and a normal control subject is shown in Fig. 19.

Harris and colleagues found an average 17 % rCBV reduction in the temporoparietal regions in Alzheimer patients, with only 8 %–9 % rCBV reduction in the sensorimotor areas. These results were consistent with those of prior SPECT [103] and PET [104] data which yielded 18 % temporoparietal and 8.5 % sensorimotor rCBV reduction in Alzheimer patients. The results are summarized in Table 2.

The effect of cocaine on CBV and MTT has been investigated by Li et al. [105]. Using fast- imaging with steady precession (FISP) sequence with 1.12-s time resolution on a 4.7-T Bruker Biopsec system. Four groups of rats were investigated: group I, control; group II, no prior drug exposure; group III, 8–11 day withdrawal; group IV, 18–24 days withdrawal. They found a 32.5 %±20.3 % increase ($p<0.05$) in MTT and a trend to increased rCBV in group III versus a

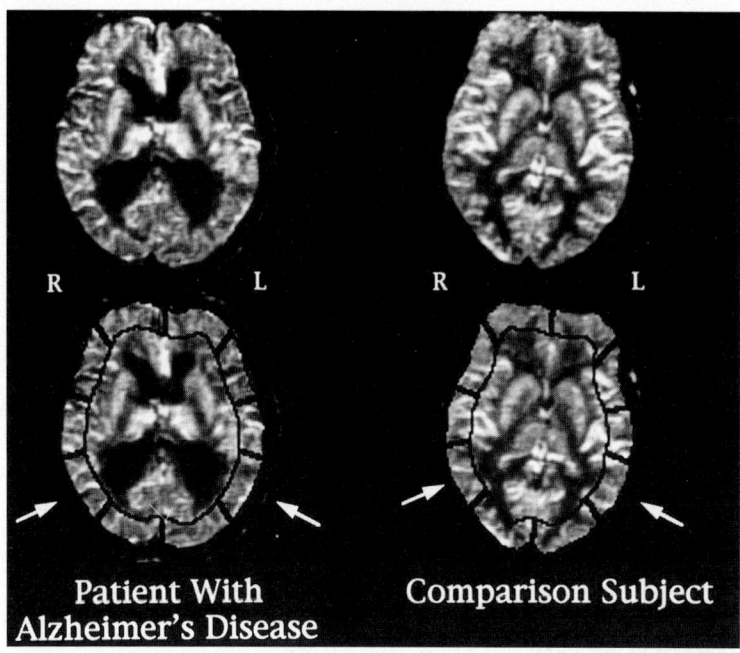

Fig. 19. Dynamic susceptibility contrast EPI of rCBV in an 86-year-old male patient with Alzheimer's disease (MMS score = 25) and an 83-year-old male comparison subject (MMS score = 29). The left temporoparietal cortex-cerebellum blood volume ratio was 93 % in the Alzheimer patient versus 115 % in the normal control. The cortical rings an regional divisions used for quantitative analysis are displayed on the lower pair of images. The arrow points to the temporoparietal cortex. (Modified, with permission of the author and the publishers, from Harris et al. [101])

Table 2. rCBV as a percentage of regional cerebellar blood volume in elderly patients with Alzheimer's disease and normal matched comparison subjects (data obtained with dynamic susceptibility contrast EPI study)

Region	Alzheimer patients	Control group	Difference (%)	p
Temporoparietal				
Right	94±17	113±7	17	0.002
Left	93±11	112±7	17	<0.0001
Sensorimotor				
Right	98±18	108±14	9	0.12
Left	98±13	106±11	8	0.07

decrease of both MTT ($-28.5 \% \pm 10.5 \%$, $p<0.05$) and rCBV ($-21.2 \% \pm 8.1 \%$, $p<0.05$) in group IV (all measurements versus control animals). Group II showed variable increases and decreases. Their results suggest that previous discrepancies between human [106] and animal [107] studies are in part due to the human subjects' previous drug exposure. Since PET studies have shown that the ratio of rCBV/rCBF, i.e., MTT, is well correlated with the regional oxygen extraction fraction of the brain, which in turn is an index of cerebral circulatory reserve [108], some investigators have suggested that the rCBV/rCBF ratio is the most sensitive indicator of hemodynamic risk to the brain [109]. Since dopamine-rich areas are primarily affected, cocaine-related cerebral ischemia could be ameliorated by dopamine antagonist therapy. Functional MRI may help to shed light on these questions.

T1 Contrast Techniques

Although the majority of NMR perfusion studies have made use of susceptibility contrast, there are a number problems with this technique, such as the need for large doses [33], short injection times requiring power injectors [19], and the need for high-flow intravascular access. Moreover, when the BBB is defective or not present, such as in tissues outside the CNS, competing T1 effects from the extracellular distribution of the paramagnetic contrast agents can lead to an underestimation of blood volume and flow values calculated from T2-weighted images [19].

The relationship between paramagnetic lanthanides, such as gadolinium, in aqueous solution and proton relaxation has been described by Solomon [41] and Bloembergen [42]. The dominant relaxation mechanism is the dipole-dipole interaction between the large free electron spin of the paramagnetic ion and the proton spin. In most tissues examined so far under equilibrium condition, i.e., with an equal intravascular and extracellular contrast agent concentration, an essentially linear relationship between contrast agent concentration and relaxation change has been found [110, 111]:

$$\Delta(1/\text{T1}_{\text{bulk}}) = \Delta \text{R1}_{\text{bulk}} = k_1 \, C_{\text{VOI}} \tag{19}$$

where k_1 is a tissue and field strength specific constant and C_{VOI} the concentration of the contrast agent in the tissue VOI. This monoexponential relaxation rate enhancement requires fast and free access of the water molecules to the relaxation center, the so-called "fast exchange" situation. Unfortunately, these assumptions have yet to be confirmed for dynamic studies, where most of the contrast agent is intravascular and the fast exchange conditions may not apply [112]. In the brain the BBB hinders this exchange sufficiently (intermediate or slow exchange) such that only small T1 effects are observed.

Blood Volume Mapping Using T1 Contrast

Several investigators have shown that changes in T1 relaxivity from the intravenous injection of a contrast material can also be used to calculate cerebral hemodynamics [28, 113, 114]. There are two major differences between T1- and T2*-based blood volume maps. First, in the presence of tissues without an intact BBB the T1 method tends to overestimate blood volume while the T2* method tends to underestimate it. The apparent regions of high blood volume evident on the map obtained by the T1 method may reflect leakage of the contrast agent into the extracellular space during the first pass rather than truly increased blood volume. The T1-based blood volume values are at least partially weighted by the permeability surface area (PS) product [8, 91, 115–117], in contrast to the negative weighting in T2 rCBV maps [15] in the case of BBB destruction [118]. Although this PS weighting may limit the possibility to define the T1 maps as rCBV weighted maps under all circumstances, PS itself may have an important physiological importance in the evaluation of brain tumors.

Second, due to the physics of susceptibility-based contrast on SE images, SE T2 rCBV maps show significant microvascular weighting [24]. T1-weighted rCBV maps exhibit sensitivity to the total vascular space, including small and large vessels. This is apparent in the visual appearance on the maps. In this respect one may anticipate that T1-based rCBV maps will prove more closely correlated with blood volume maps obtained with nuclear medicine studies (such as with [11]Co-PET imaging). However, whether sensitivity to the total vascular or microvascular space confers a specific advantage in evaluating cerebral diseases has not yet been definitely determined. Initial studies evaluating brain tumors demonstrated no substantial differences in the two methods in low-grade tumors but significant differences in high-grade tumors [119]. Further studies comparing T1 and T2 rCBV maps are required to answer the specific clinical questions, for example, tumor recurrence versus necrosis.

Several other points distinguish the T1- and T2-based methods. From an economic standpoint, the most important is the large difference in the amount of contrast dose required, with T1 rCBV maps using about one-tenth as much as T2-based methods. However, this comes at the loss of about one-half of the contrast to noise ration in the raw data [119], a difference which cannot be compensated by use of an additional contrast agent, due to T1 saturation effects [113]. The use of a narrow, better defined bolus with the T1 rCBV method provides the additional advantage of being able to extract relative CBF information from first-pass data. Finally, the use of short repetition times in T1-w techniques limits the number of slices that can be acquired, in contrary to T2-weighted sequences. The use of IR sequences may improve this in the future.

Assessment of Tumor Angiogenesis and Microcirculation

In addition to the measurement of hemodynamic parameters, dynamic contrast-enhanced MRI has been shown to provide information about tumor angiogenesis and microcirculation. These factors are critical elements in the growth, spread (formation of metastases), characterization, and response to treatment of neoplasms.

Without angiogenesis tumors are restricted to sizes of only 1–2 mm, relying on nutrient supply by diffusion rather then perfusion. Being derived from a single cell line, tumors cannot form vessels themselves. They stimulate the growth of host vessels through humoral factors. The hyperpermeability of tumor vessels facilitates the entry of tumor cells into the circulation and is one of the prerequisites for metastatic deposits. The inhibition of angiogenesis prevents the growth of tumor cells both at the primary and secondary sites [120].

Being a prerequisite for tumor growth and spread, it has been shown by histological assays that microvascular density is correlated with and is a useful predictor of local aggressiveness and metastatic rate, and in turn of adverse prognosis in a variety of human malignancies [121]. Microvascular density, however, is not an ideal clinical tool because it requires invasive tissue sampling with the risk of sampling errors in the notoriously heterogenous tumors.

The macromolecular contrast media (MMCM) currently being developed for both MRI and CT have molecular sizes approximating those of serum proteins and are well suited to defining the hypervascularity and hyperpermeability inherent to tumor microvasculature [122–124]. MMCM diffuse very slowly, if at all, through normal endothelial walls.

Van Dijke et al. [123] have obtained measurements of blood volumes and permeability surface area products (PS) in rodent mammary adenocarcinomas using MRI with enhancement by albumin Gd-DTPA$_{35}$ (MW = 92 kDa, plasma half-life approx. 3.5 h). Their measurements are closely correlated ($r^2 = 0.8$) with histological measurements of microvascular density. Based on the noninvasive MRI data two tumor types, one slowly growing, the other rapidly growing and aggressive, can be differentiated and graded with respect to their angiogenesis profiles.

Brasch et al. have show the ability of MMCM-enhanced MRI to monitor the acute (≤ 24 h) effects of antiangiogenesis treatment with anti-vascular endothelial growth factor of human breast cancer carrying nude rats. They used a spoiled grass sequence to obtain pre- and postcontrast R1 measurements and assumed a linear relationship between the concentration of Gd-DTPA$_{35}$ and ΔR1 in tumor tissue. Dynamic measurements were obtained every few minutes, sufficient to characterize the relatively slow leakage of Gd macromolecules into the tumor. Fitted to a two-compartment model [125], estimates of the fractional leak rate (FLR; h-1), fractional reflux rate (FRR; h^{-1}), plasma volume (PV: ml cm^{-3}) and permeability surface area product (PS; ml h^{-1} cm^{-3}) were obtained before and after treatment. After 24 h of anti-vascular endothelial growth factor treatment, they found an obvious decrease in the tumor accumulation of albumin Gd-DTPA$_{35}$. Although there was no significant change in fractional tumor blood volume (0.0475 pre- vs. 0.0541 posttreatment, $p > 0.05$), a 98 % decrease in FLR (from 0.056 to 0.001 min^{-1}, $p < 0.005$) and FRR (from 0.089 to 0.001 min^{-1}, $p < 0.005$) and a 97 % decrease in PS (from 0.084 to 0.002 ml h^{-1} cm^{-3}, $p < 0.001$) was observed, confirming the expected reduction in vascular permeability during treatment. Their study also confirmed the utility of MMCM-enhanced MRI for the detection and quantitation of changes in tumor microvascular permeability in response to antiangiogenesis intervention.

Because smaller macromolecules, such as Gd-DTPA, leak much more rapidly into the interstitium (10 %–70 % during the first passage, depending on tissue type capillary structure), they have inherent limitations for measuring blood volume and capillary permeability outside the CNS. Faster data acquisition with EPI, however, can compensate at least partially for this disadvantage, as has been shown by Gowland et al. [82].

Another important application of perfusion imaging lies in the assessment of the responsiveness of tumors to cytotoxic treatment. In chemotherapy and immunotherapy, tumor perfusion, capillary permeability, and interstitial pressure are crucial factors in the delivery of therapeutic agents [126]. In hyperthermia temperature distribution [127] and in radiation therapy local oxygen concentration [128] are both crucial factors affecting the efficacy of treatment. Monitoring of microcirculatory parameters with MRI may thus guide the choice of the optimal therapy regime and help to predict which patients are likely to fail therapy. Unfortunately, small molecular weight gadolinium compounds such as Gd-DTPA behave intermediately between intravascular and freely diffusible tracers. Thus neither tracer-kinetic methods such as that proposed by Meier and Zierler [55] nor Kety's model [129] for freely diffusible tracers describe the circumstances accurately. Modifications of Kety's model [130, 131] have been proposed but require both the first-pass extravasation of the tracer and tissue perfusion to be determined, which is problematic in vivo. Griebel et al. [17] have introduced a tracer-kinetic modeling based on Fick's conservation principle, which extends the approach used by Meier and Zierler to extravascular tracers:

$$C_{VOI}(t) = P_t[\int C_a(\tau)d\tau - (\int C_a(\tau)d\tau) * h(t)] \tag{20}$$

where $C_a(t)$ and $C_{VOI}(t)$ are the concentration-time curves as measured in arterial blood and tumor and P_t tissue perfusion and RF(t) the residue function, i.e., the distribution of the transit times of the tracer molecules through the tissue following an instantaneous bolus. For an extracellular tracer such as Gd-DTPA the capillary permeability is such that a fraction, α, enters the interstitial space, while the remainder $(1-\alpha)$ behaves as an intravascular tracer. RF(t) thus breaks down into two components:

$$RF(t) = (1 - \alpha)RF_{iv}(t) + \alpha Rf_{ec}(t) \tag{21}$$

where iv and ec denote the intravascular and extracellular components, respectively. Introducing the interstitial residue function $RF_{is}(t)$ which describes the transit from capillary through interstitium back to capillary, $Rf_{ec}(t)$ can be written as:

$$Rf_{ec}(t) = Rf_{iv}(t) * Rf_{is}(t) \tag{22}$$

If the intravascular and interstitial residue functions of transit are $Rf_{iv}(t) = I_b\exp\{-I_bt\}$ and $Rf_{is}(t) = I_d\exp\{-I_dt\}$, C_{VOI} can be expressed analytically and P_t and α estimated by least squares fit. Thus the problem of simultaneous estimation of perfusion and extraction fraction is possible.

Spin Labeling Techniques

Saturation Technique

The simplest spin labeling technique, described by Detre et al. [132], employs a steady-state imaging sequence downstream from a saturation band used to label the spins of flowing blood, producing an endogenous, freely diffusible tracer. Subtraction of an image without saturation band from one with saturation band results in a flow-weighted image. The following expression for flow can be derived for this technique:

$$f = \lambda/T1_{app} \{1 - S_{sat}(TR)/S_{control}(TR)\} \tag{23}$$

where $T1_{app}$ is the apparent T1 of tissue, f flow (in milliliters per gram per second) and λ the blood-tissue water partition coefficient, defined as (quantity of tracer/gram of tissue)/(quantity of tracer/milliliter of blood) [133]. Detre at al. [134] and other researchers have obtained very precise quantitative perfusion measurements using this technique in animals and humans.

Inversion Recovery Techniques

Two spin labeling techniques based on an angiography technique proposed by Nishiimura et al. [135] have been developed to measure perfusion without extrinsic contrast agents. In the technique proposed by Kwong et al. [136] subtraction of a flow-insensitive IR-EPI image obtained with a nonselective 180° pulse from a flow-sensitive IR-EPI image obtained with a selective 180° pulse provides flow-weighted EPI images. These flow images can be used to study steady-state blood flow and have been shown to provide good gray-white matter flow contrast in the cortex (3.2 % ± 0.5 %), white matter (1.0 % ± 0.2 %), and deep structures such as the thalamus and the basal ganglia (2.3 % ± 0.3 %). In contrast to the technique of signal targeting with alternating radiofrequency (EPISTAR) as suggested by Edelman et al. [137], which labels blood upstream from the read-out slice with a single inversion pulse, the double-inversion technique developed by Kwong tags and reads in the same slice and does not suffer from T1 relaxation during the inflow of blood from the tagging location to the read-out slice. It also avoids magnetization transfer artifacts [132], which can dominate the perfusion effects. The signal of the flow sensitive subtraction image S_{flow} is given by:

$$S_{flow} = S_{sel} - S_{non-sel} \approx 2 \, S_0 \, TI \, f/\lambda \, e^{-TI/T1} \, [e^{-Tx/T1}] \tag{24}$$

where S_{sel} and $S_{non-sel}$ denotes the signal of the selective and nonselective IR-EPI image and TI the inversion time. For EPISTAR the time taken by the blood traveling from the inversion plane to the read out slice, Tx, causes an additional attenuation of the signal:

$$S_{flow} \approx 2 \, S_0 \, (TI - Tx) \, f/\lambda \, e^{-(TI - Tx)/T1} \, e^{-Tx/T1} \tag{25}$$

These expressions demonstrate a disadvantage of both techniques: Flow contrast is "amplified" by proton density and long T1, thus distorting comparisons of flow between different tissues. Quantitative steady- state flow maps can be generated by varying TI to quantify T1. An example of a flow map obtained with the double-inversion technique in the case of a brain tumor is shown in Fig. 7 in comparison with flow maps obtained with susceptibility contrast agents. A more detailed description of this technique can be found in Chap. 16 of this volume.

Perfusion maps obtained in this previously described way give reasonable blood flow values for gray matter, but the maps usually show poor gray-white matter flow contrast. This may be associated with two problems. First, the partial volume effects of CSF and gray matter flow value. Second, a blood T1 time which is much longer than white matter T1 leads to an overestimation of white matter blood flow value. Blood T1, being slightly longer than gray matter T1, has little impact on gray matter blood flow value. Using this technique, a typical volunteer demonstrates in gray matter a single increase of 3.2 %, while a white matter region show a difference of 1.0 %.

Blood Oxygenation Level Dependent Techniques

Instead of using water as a freely diffusible tracer, hemoglobin can utilized as an intravascular tracer. First reported by Ogawa et al. [138], it has been shown that the susceptibility of blood changes dramatically when oxyhemoglobin is converted into deoxyhemoglobin, the transverse relaxation T2 changing by a factor of 3 at 65 MHz and 6 at 270 MHz. This effect has been used extensively for neuroactivation studies, and this application is described in detail in Chaps. 15 and 16 of this volume. Blood oxygenation changes, however, can also be used to evaluate perfusion changes and oxygen extraction in tissue by tracer-kinetic methods pertaining to intravascular tracers. In contrast to exogenous tracers and labeled water, the arterial blood oxygen saturation and, knowing the hematocrit, concentration, are easily measured using a pulse oxymeter. Several authors have also shown that blood oxygen changes can be introduced externally by ventilation with various gases such as carbogen, nitrogen, and pure oxygen or simply by breathholding.

Intravoxel Incoherent Motion

Le Bihan was the first to suggest that intervoxel incoherent motion [139], basically the application of the Stejskal-Tanner NMR method [140] to MRI, can be used to measure not only water diffusion in tissue but also perfusion [141]. This is based on the assumption that capillary microcirculation can be modeled as a pseudodiffusive process. This method is described in detail in Chap. 9 of this volume, and only a brief overview is provided here.

The effect of a dipolar gradient pulse, G(t,), on nonstationary spins is given by:

$$S(b) = S_0 \ e^{-bD} \tag{26}$$

with:

$$b = \gamma^2 \int \left| \int G(t'')dt'' \right|^2 dt' \tag{27}$$

where D is the diffusion coefficient. In perfused tissue blood microcirculation also contributes to the attenuation of S_0. Assuming a quasirandom geometric disposition of the capillary network, an assumption which is correct at least in the brain, blood microcirculation can be treated as a pseudo-diffusion process characterized by a pseudodiffusion coefficient D^*:

$$D^* = \langle l \rangle \langle v \rangle / 6 \tag{28}$$

where $\langle l \rangle$ is the mean capillary segment length and $\langle v \rangle$ the average blood velocity [141]. Under the assumption that D^* is about ten times larger than D the attenuation of S_0 becomes a biexponential process:

$$S(b) = S_0 \left[(1 - f)\ e^{-bD} + f\ e^{-bD^*} \right] \tag{29}$$

where f is the ratio of the volume of NMR-visible water flowing in the capillary compartment, V_d, to the total voxel volume of NMR-visible water, V_{H2O}:

$$f = V_d / V_{H2O} \tag{30}$$

or, knowing the NMR-visible water fraction $fw = V_{H2O}/V$:

$$f = V_d / f_w V = CBV / f_w \tag{31}$$

If L is the total capillary length, Eq. 28 provides an expression for the MTT:

$$MTT = L / \langle v \rangle = L \langle l \rangle / 6D^* \tag{32}$$

Combining Eqs. 28 and 31 according to the central volume therorem and expression for blood flow can be derived:

$$CBF = CBV/MTT = f_w f\ /\ MTT = (6f_w\ /\ L\langle v \rangle)\ fD^* \tag{33}$$

The expression in brackets is tissue specific, and relative perfusion or blood flow can be estimated from the product fD^*. Absolute measurements require a comprehensive knowledge of the microvascular anatomy [12, 141, 143] but, where available, have provided very encouraging results [77]. Problematic remains the separation of the massive contribution of bulk tissue water from perfusion, which is easier in highly perfused organs such as the kidneys [145] but has proven extremely difficult in the brain [145, 146].

The advantage of this method, on the other hand, is its complete noninvasiveness using blood as a physiological, internal tracer. Assuming that water exchange between blood and capillaries is negligible during the few tens of milliseconds of the measurement, which at least in the brain is a reasonable assumption [148, 149], IVIM is similar to methods using intravascular tracers. There are, however, no contributions from large vessels because the signal from higher velocity blood becomes spoiled in the presence of the bipolar diffusion gradients.

Other Nuclei

It may suffice here to note that other nuclear species which provide an NMR signal at various other Lamor frequencies than protons can also be used as tracer for NMR perfusion measurements. This has the advantage that the tracer signal can be easily discriminated from the ^1H proton signal of biological specimens. Among those that have been used in animal experiments are D_2O, ^{19}F, and ^{17}O, in various chemical compounds. D_2O behaves as the more abundant water molecule H_2O and thus constitutes an ideal (freely diffusible) tracer. ^{19}F has been used in macromolecules to provide intravascular tracers. ^{17}O can be used either as a gas or in various chemical compounds. Since these tracers have been used neither in humans nor with high-speed imaging we refer the interested reader to the original articles for more detail on these techniques [149, 150].

Conclusion

During the past decade the MRI measurement of hemodynamic parameters has matured into a tool suitable for application in both basic research and clinical diagnostics. Several factors underlie this development, particularly the availability of fast imaging techniques such as EPI and the development and better understanding of the mechanism of action of contrast agents and the "translation" of tracer-kinetic theory to MRI. Although a number of NMR-visible tracers have been evaluated in vitro and in animal studies, only few have yet been approved for clinical use. Gd-DTPA and its analogue, low molecular weight chelates, have the disadvantage of being neither freely diffusible not truly intravascular, with the exception of the brain's circulation when the BBB is intact. Even there the measurement of microcirculatory blood flow is difficult because of the difficulties involved in determining the "true" MTT.

Thus most applications have focused on CBV mapping. With the soon to be expected availability for clinical use of a number of truly intravascular contrast agents, these problems may be overcome, and the clinical applications can be expected to expand rapidly. In addition to flow and blood volume, the structure of the capillary wall, its permeability, and the size of the various tissue compartments are of great interest to the physiologist and clinician because they are sensitive parameters in characterizing the biological behavior of malignant tumors. It has already been shown that this type of functional MRI may be used to grade the aggressiveness of tumors and predict their response to cytotoxic treatment. The use of hemodynamic imaging in the diagnosis and treatment planning of ischemic diseases such as stroke has been amply illustrated.

In comparison with other functional imaging modalities such as PET and SPECT, MRI has several advantages: It is noninvasive, it does not require the generation, storage, and handling of nuclear isotopes, it provides higher resolution, it allows structural and functional studies to be performed in one session, obviating the need for complicated image fusion, it is cheaper than nuclear medicine studies, and it is more widely available. Thus a large percentage of the population could profit from this technology once it has developed to the point that it becomes commercially available for routine use.

References

1. Lauerbur PC (1973) Image formation by induced local interactions: examples employing nuclear magnetic resonance. Nature 242:190
2. Damadian R, Zaner K, Hor D et al (1973) Human tumors by NMR. Physiol Chem Phys 5:381–402
3. Low RN (1997) Contrast agents for MR imaging of the liver. J Magn Reson Imaging 7:56–67
4. Leenders KL, Perani D et al (1990) Cerebral blood flow, blood volume and oxygen utilization. Normal values and effect of age. Brain 113:27–47
5. Steward GN (1894) Researches on the circulation time and on influences which affect it. J Physiol (London) 15:1
6. Pappata S, Fiorelli M et al (1993) PET study of changes in local brain hemodynamics and oxygen metabolism after unilateral middle cerebral artery occlusion in baboons. J Cereb Blood Flow Metab 13(3):416–24
7. Heiss WD, Graf R et al (1994) Dynamic penumbra demonstrated by sequential multitracer PET after middle cerebral artery occlusion in cats. J Cereb Blood Flow Metab 14(6):892–902
8. Bartolini A, Gasparetto B et al (1993) Functional vascular volume and blood-brain barrier permeability images by angio-CT in the diagnosis of cerebral lesions. Comput Med Imaging Graph 17(1):35–44
9. Feldmann HJ, Sievers K et al (1993) Evaluation of tumor blood perfusion by dynamic MRI and CT in patients undergoing thermoradiotherapy. Eur J Radiol 16(3):224–229
10. Grosset, DG, McDonald I et al (1994) Prediction of delayed neurological deficit after subarachnoid haemorrhage: a CT blood load and Doppler velocity approach. Neuroradiology 36(6):418–21
11. Nambu K, Suzuki R et al (1995) Cerebral blood flow: measurement with xenon-enhanced dynamic helical CT. Radiology 195(1):53–57
12. Pawlik G, Rackl A, Bing RJ (1981) Quantitative capillary topography and blood flow in the cerebral cortex of cats: an in vivo microscopic study. Brain Res 208:35–58
13. Frahm J, Merbold KO et al (1992) Functional MRI of human brain activation at high spatial resolution. Magn Reson Med 29:139–144
14. Stehling MK, Turner R, Mansfield P (1991) Echo-planar imaging: magnetic resonance imaging in a fraction of a second. Science 254(5028):43–50
15. Cohen MS, Weisskoff RM (1991) Ultrafast imaging. Magn Reson Imaging 9:1–37
16. Brasch R, Pham C, Shames D et al (1997) Assessing tumor angiogenesis using macromolecular MR imaging contrast media. J Magn Reson Imaging 7:68–74
17. Griebel J, Mayr NA, de Vries A et al (1997) Assessment of tumor microcirculation: a new role of dynamic contrast mr imaging. J Magn Reson Imaging 7:111–119
18. Wenz F, Rempp K et al (1996) Effect of radiation on blood volume in low-grade astrocytomas and normal brain tissue: quantification with dynamic susceptibility contrast MR imaging. Am J Roentgenol 166(1):187–193
19. Aronen HJ, Gazit IE et al (1994) Cerebral blood volume maps of gliomas: comparison with tumor grade and histologic findings. Radiology 191(1):41–51
20. Le Bihan D, Turner R (1992) The capillary network: a link between IVIM and clssical perfusion. Magn Reson Med 27:171–178
21. Fick A (1948) Verhandl dtsch physmed Gesellschaft zu Würzburg 1870, p 36
22. Hoff HE, Scott HJ (1948) N Engl J Med 239:122
23. Lassen NA (1984) Cerebral transit of an intravascular tracer may allow measurement of regional blood volume but not regional blood flow. J Cereb Blood Flow Metab 4:633–634
24. Rosen BR, Belliveau JW et al (1990) Perfusion imaging with NMR contrast agents. Magn Reson Med 14(2):249–265
25. Boxerman JL, Hamberg LM, Rosen BR, Weisskoff RM (1995) MR contrast due to intravascular magnetic susceptibility pertubations. Magn Reson Med 34:555–566
26. Rosen BR, Belliveau JW et al (1991) Contrast agents and cerebral hemodynamics. Magn Reson Med 19(2):285–292
27. Canty JM, Judd RM et al (1991) First-pass entry of nonionic contrast agent into the myocardial extravascular space. Circulation 84:2071–2078
28. Dean BL, Lee C et al (1992) Cerebral hemodynamics and cerebral blood volume: MR assessment using gadolinium contrast agents and T1-weighted Turbo-FLASH imaging. Am J Neuroradiol 13(1):39–48
29. Judd RM, Atalay MK et al (1995) Effects of myocardial water exchange on T1 enhancement during bolus administration of MR contrast agents. Magn Reson Med 33(2):215–223

30. Mathur-De Vre R, Lemort M (1995) Invited review: biophysical properties and clinical applications of magnetic resonance imaging contrast agents. Br J Radiol 68(807):225–247
31. Reith W, Forsting M et al (1995) Early MR detection of experimentally induced cerebral ischemia using magnetic susceptibility contrast agents: comparison between gadopentetate dimeglumine and iron oxide particles. Am J Neuroradiol 16(1):53–60
32. Dwek RA (1973) Nuclear magnetic resonance in biochemistry: applications to enzyme systems. Clarendon, Oxford
33. Villringer A, Rosen BR (1988) et al Dynamic imaging with lanthanide chelates in normal brain: contrast due to magnetic susceptibility effects. Magn Reson Med 6(2):164–174
34. Fisel CR, Ackerman JL et al (1991) MR contrast due to microscopically heterogeneous magnetic susceptibility: numerical simulations and applications to cerebral physiology. Magn Reson Med 17(2):336–347
35. Rosen BR, Belliveau JW et al (1991) Susceptibility contrast imaging of cerebral blood volume: human experience. Magn Reson Med 22(2):293–299
36. Goodstein DL (1975) States of matter. Prentice-Hall, Englewood Cliffs
37. Chu SCK, Xu Y, Balschi JA, Springer CS (1990) Magn Reson Med 13:239
38. Boudreaux EA, Mulay LN (1976) Theory and application of molecular paramagnetism. Wiley, New York
39. Burke HE (1986) Handbook of magnetic phenomena. Van Nostrad-Reinhold, New York
40. Bean CP, Livingston JD (1959) J Appl Phys 30:1205
41. Solomon I (1955) Relaxation processes in a system of two spins. Phys Rev 99:559–565
42. Bloembergen N (1957) J Chem Phys 27:572
43. Wismer GL, Buxton RB, Rosen BR et al (1988) Susceptibility induced MR line broadening: applications to brain iron mapping. J Comput Assist Tomogr 12:259
44. Belliveau JW, Rosen BR, Kantor HL et al (1990) Functional cerebral imaging by susceptibility contrast NMR. Magn Reson Med 14(3):538–546
45. Gillis P, Koenig SH (1987) Transverse relaxation of solvent protons induced by magnetized spheres: application to ferritin, erythrocytes and magnetite. Magn Reson Med 5:323–345
46. Majumdar S, Gore JC (1989) Regional differences in rat brain displayed by fast MRI with superparamagnetic contrast agents. Magn Reson, C Med 6(6):611-5
47. Case TA, Durney CH, Ailion DC et al (1987) J Magn Reson 73:304
48. Fisel CR, Ackerman JL, Buxton RB et al (1991) MR contrast due to microscopically heterogenous magnetic susceptibility: numerical simulations and applications to cerebral physiology. Magn Reson Med 17(2):336–347
49. Ehrlich P (1913) Chemotherapeutics: Scientific principles, methods, and results. Lancet 2:445–451
50. Kndel ER, Schwartz JH (eds) (1981) Principles of neural science. Edward Arnold, London
51. Weisskoff RM, Zuo CS, Boxerman JL, Rosen BR (1994) Microscopic susceptibility variation and transverse relaxation: theory and experiment. Magn Reson Med 31:601–610
52. Yablonskiy DA, Haacke EM (1994) Theory of NMR signal behaviour in magnetically inhomogenous tissues: the static dephasing regime. Magn Reson Med 32:749–763
53. Kennan RP, Zhong J, Gore JC (1994) Intravascular susceptibility contrast mechanisms in tissues. Magn Reson Med 31:9–21
54. Gillis P, Petö S, Moiny F, Mispelter J, Cuenod C-A (1995) Proton transverse nuclear magnetic relaxation in oxidized blood: a numerical approach. Magn Reson Med 33:93–100
55. Meier P, Zierler K (1954) On the theory of the indicator-dilution method for assessment of blood flow and volume. J Appl Physiol 6:731–744
56. Larsen OA, Lassen NA (1964) Cerebral hematocrit in normal man. J Appl Physiol 19(4):571–574
57. Weisskoff RM, Chesler D, Boxerman JL, Rosen BR (1993) Pitfalls in MR measurements of tissue blood flow with intravascular tracers: which mean transit time? Magn Reson Med 29:553–559
58. Bassingthwaithe JB, Goresky CA (1984) In: Renkin EM, Michel CG (eds) Handbook of physiology, sect 2. American Physiology Society, Bethesda, pp 549–626
59. Lassen NA, Henriksen O, Sejrsen P (1984) In: Shepherd JT, Abboud FM Handbook of physiology, sect 2. American Physiology Society, Bethesda, pp 21–64
60. Jacquez JA (1972) In: Compartmental analysis in biology an medicine. Kinetics and distribution of tracer labeled materials. Elsevier, Amsterdam, pp 84–101
61. Østergaard L, Weisskoff RM, Chesler DA, Gyldensted C, Rosen BR (1996) High resolution measurement of cerebral blood flow using intravascular tracer bolus passages. I. Mathematical approach and statistical analysis. Magn Reson Med 36:715–725
62. Valentinuzzi ME, Volachec MM (1975) Discrete deconvolution. Med Biol Eng 13:123–125

63. Todd-Pokropek A (1988) In: Rescigno A, Boicelli A (eds) Cerebral blood flow. Mathematical models, instrumentation, and imaging techniques. Plenum, New York, pp 107–119
64. Bronikowski TA, Dawson CA, Linehan JH (1983) Model-free deconvolution techniques for estimating vascular transport functions. Int J Biomed Comput 14:411–429
65. Østergaard L, Sorensen AG, Kwong KK et al (1996) High resolution measurement of cerebral blood flow using intravascular tracer bolus passages. II. Experimental comparison and preliminary results. Magn Reson Med 36:726–736
66. Thompson HK, Starmer CF, Whalen RE, McIntosh HD (1964) Indicator transit time considered as a gamma variate. Circ Res 14:502–515
67. Starmer CF, Clark DO (1970) Computer computations of cardiac output using the gamma function. J Appl Physiol 28:219–20
68. Berninger WH, Axel L, Norman D, Napel S, Redington RW (1981) Functional imaging of the brain using computed tomography [published erratum appears in Radiology 1989 Jun; 171(3):878. Radiology 138(3):711–6
69. Axel L (1980) Cerebral blood flow determination by rapid sequence computed tomography. Radiology 137:679–686
70. Zierler KL (1965) Theoretical basis of indicator-dilution methods for measuring flow and volume. Circ Res 16:393–407
71. Axel L (1983) Tissue mean transit time from dynamic computer tomography by a simple deconvolution technique. Invest Radiol 18:94–9
72. Lassen NA, Perl W (1979) Tracer kinetic methods in medical physiology. Raven, New York
73. Rempp KA, Brix G, Wenz F et al (1994) Quantification of regional cerebral blood flow and volume with dynamic susceptibility contrast-enhanced MR imaging. Radiology 193:637–641
74. Perman WH, Gado MH, Larson KB, Perlmutter JS (1992) Simultaneous MR acquisition of arterial and brain signal-time curves. Magn Reson Med 28:74–83
75. Press WH, Flannary BR, Teukolsky SA, Vetterling WT (1986) Numerical recipes: the art of scientific computing. Cambridge University Press, Cambridge, pp 417–420
76. Phelps ME, Hawkins RA (1988), PET in clinical oncology. Cancer metastasis Rev 7(2):119–42
77. Grubb RL, Raichle ME, Eichling JO, Ter-Pogossian MM (1974) The effects of changes in PaCO2 on cerebral blood volume "blood flow" and vascular mean transit time. Stroke 5:630–9
78. Raichle ME (1987) In: Plum F (eds) Handbook of physiology: the nervous system, vol V. American Physiological Society, Bethesda, p 643
79. Phelps ME, Mazziotta JC (1985) Positron emission tomography: human brain function and biochemistry. Science 28:799–809
80. Archer DP, Labrecque P et al (1990) Measurement of cerebral blood flow and volume with positron emission tomography during isoflurane administration in the hypocapnic baboon. Anesthesiology 72(6):1031–1037 [published erratum appears in 73(4):798]
81. Aronen HJ, Glass J et al (1995) Echo-planar MR cerebral blood volume mapping of gliomas. Clinical utility. Acta Radiol 36(5):520–528
82. Gowland P, Mansfield P et al (1992/93) Dynamic studies of gadolinium uptake in brain tumors using inversion-recovery echo planar imaging. Magn Reson Med 192(26):241–258
83. Groshar D, McEwan AJ et al (1993) Imaging tumor hypoxia and tumor perfusion. J Nucl Med 34(6):885–888
84. Maeda M, Itoh S et al (1993) Tumor vascularity in the brain: evaluation with dynamic susceptibility-contrast MR imaging. Radiology 189(1):233–238
85. Wenz F, Lohr F et al (1994) Flow cytometric measurement of proliferating cell nuclear antigen (PCNA) in solid tumors. Strahlenther Onkol 170(4):235–242
86. Boeck J, Wlodarczyk W et al (1995) Regional cerebral blood volume of intracranial tumors determined by MRI. Eur Radiol 5:528–533
87. Kleihues P, Burger PC, Scheithauer BW (1993) Histological typing of tumors of the central nervous system, 2nd edn. Springer, Berlin Heidelberg New York
88. Daumas-Duport C, Scheithauer B, O'Fallon J, Kelly P (1988) Grading of astrocytomas: a simple and reproducible method. Cancer 62:2152–2165
89. Bruening R, Wu RH, Yousry TA et al (1998) Regional relative blood volume (rBV) MR maps of meningiomas before and after partial embolization. J Comput Assist Tomogr (accepted)
90. Krueck WG, Schmiedl UD et al (1994) MR Assessment of radiation-induced blood-brain barrier permeability changes in a rat glioma model. Am J Neuroradiol 15:625–632
91. Frackowiak RSJ, Lenzi GL, Jones T, Heather JD (1980) Quantitative assessment of regional cerebral blood flow and oxygen metabolism in man using 15O and positron emission tomography: theory, procedure and normal values. J Comput Assist Tomogr 4:727–736

92. Gückel F, Brix G, Rempp K et al (1994) Assessment of cerebral blood volume with dynamic susceptibility contrast-enhanced gradient echo imaging. J Comput Assist Tomogr 18:344–351

93. Rother J, Guckel F et al (1996) Assessment of regional cerebral blood volume in acute human stroke by use of single-slice dynamic susceptibility contrast-enhanced magnetic resonance imaging. Stroke 27(6):1088–1093

94. Sorensen A, Buonanno F et al (1996) Hyperacute stroke: evaluation with combined multisection diffusion-weighted and hemodynamically weighted echo-planar MR imaging. Radiology 199:391–401

95. Moseley ME, Kucharczyk J et al (1990) Diffusion-weighted MR imaging of acute stroke: correlation with T2-weighted and magnetic susceptibility-enhanced MR imaging in cats. Am J Neuroradiol 11:423–429

96. Moseley ME, Mintorovitch J et al (1990) Early detection of ischemic injury: comparison of spectroscopy, diffusion-, T2-, and magnetic susceptibility-weighted MRI in cats. Acta Neurochirurgica 51 [Suppl]:207–209

97. De Crespigny AJ, Wendland MF et al (1992) Real-time observation of transient focal ischemia and hyperthermia in cat brain. Magn Reson Med 27:391–397

98. De Crespigny AJ, Tsuura M et al (1993) Perfusion and diffusion MR imaging of thromboembolic stroke. J Magn Reson Imaging 3(5):746–754

99. Warach S, Levin JM, Schomer DL, Holman BL, Edelman RR (1994) Hyperperfusion of ictal seizure focus demonstrated by MR perfusion imaging. AJNR Am J Neuroradiol 15:965–968

100. Wu RH, Bruening R, Noachter S et al (1998) MR measurement of regional relative cerebral blood volume in epilepsy. AJNR Am J Neuroradiol (submitted)

101. Harris GJ, Lewis RF, Satlin A et al (1996) Dynamic susceptibility contrast MRI of regional cerebral blood volume in Alzheimer's disease. Am J Psychiatry 153(5):721–724

102. Folstein MF, Folstein SE, McHugh PR (1975) "Mini-mental state": a practical method for grading the cognitive state of patients for the clinician. J Psychiatr Res 12:189 198

103. Pearlson GD, Harris GJ, Powers RE et al (1992) Quantitative changes in mesial temporal volume, regional cerebral blood flow, and cognition in Alzheimer's disease. Arch Gen Psychiatry 49:402–408

104. Fazekas F, Alavi A, Chawluk JB et al (1989) Comparison of CT, MR, and PET in Alzheimer's dementia and normal aging. J Nucl Med 30:1607–1615

105. Li K-L (1987) Protective effects of captopril and enalapril on myocardial ischemia and reperfusion damage of rat. J Mol Cell Cardiol

106. Volkow ND, Mullani N, Gould KL, Adler S, Drajewski K (1988) Cerebral blood flow in chronic cocaine users: A study with positron emission tomography. Br J Psychiatry 152:641–648

107. Stein EA, Fuller SA (1993) Cocaine's time action profile on regional cerebral blood flow in the rat. Brain Res 626:117–126

108. Toyama H, Takeshita G, Tekeuchi A et al (1990) Cerebral hemodynamics in patients with chronic obstructive carotid disease by rCBF, rCBV, and rCBV/rCBF ratio using SPECT. J Nucl Med 31:55–60

109. Knapp WH, Kummer RV, Kybler W (1986) Imaging of cerebral blood flow-to-volume distribution using SPECT. J Nucl Med 27:465–470

110. Alsaadi BM, Rossotti FJC, Williams RJP (1980) A pmr study of the effects of pH and anion and metal ion binding of the histidyl residues of ovotransferrin. J Inorg Biochem

111. Strich G, Hagan PL, Gerber KH, Slutsky RA (1985) Radiology 154:723

112. Donahue KM, Burtsein D, Manning WJ, Gray ML (1994) Studies of Gd-DTPA relaxivity and proton exchange rates in tissue. Magn Reson Med 32:66–76

113. Hacklaender T (1995) Parametric images of cerebral blood volume with T1 FLASH sequences. Roentgenpraxis 48:146–152

114. Hacklaender T, Hofer M et al (1995) Kernspintomographische Blutvolumenmessungen in der Diagnostik des Schlaganfalls: Ergebnisse einer klinischen Pilotstudie. ROFO Fortschr Geb Röntgenstr Neuen Bildgeb Verfahr 164:206–211

115. Bartolini A, Gasparetto B et al (1994) Functional circulation and blood-brain permeability images by angio CT in the assessment of cerebral ischemia. Comput Med Imaging Graph 18(3):151–161

116. Bartolini A, Gasparetto B et al (1994) Functional perfusion and blood-brain barrier permeability images in the diagnosis of cerebral tumors by Angio CT. Comput Med Imaging Graph 18(3):145–150

117. Di Rocco RJ, Silva DA et al (1993) The single-pass cerebral extraction and capillary permeability-surface area product of several putative cerebral blood flow imaging agents. J Nucl Med 34:641–648

118. Sage MR, Wilson AJ (1994) The blood-brain barrier: An important concept in neuroimaging. AJNR Am J Neuroradiol 15(4):601–622
119. Bruening R, Kwong KK, Vevea MJ et al (1996) Echo-planar MR determination of regional cerebral blood volume in human brain tumors: T1 versus T2 weighting. AJNR Am J Neuroradiol 17:831–840
120. Fidler I, Ellis L (1994) The implication of angiogenesis for the biology and therapy of cancer metastases. Cell 79:185–188
121. Weidner N (1995) Intratumoral microvascular density as a prognostic factor in cancer. Am J Pathol 147:9–19
122. Aicher KP, Dupon JW, White DL et al (1990) Contrast-enhanced magnetic resonance imaging of tumor-bearing mice treated with human recombinant tumor necrosis factor alpha. Cancer Res 50:7376–7381
123. van Dijke C, Brasch R, Roberts T et al (1996) Mammary carcinoma model: correlation of macromolecular contrast enhanced MR imaging characterizations of tumor microvasculature and histologic capillary density. Radiology 198:813–818
124. Schwickert H, Stiskal M, Roberts T et al (1996) Contrast-enhanced MRI assessment of tumor capillary permeability: the effect of pre-irradiation on the tumor delivery of chemotherapy. Radiology 198:893–898
125. Shames D, Kuwatsuru R, Vexler V, Muehler A, Brasch R (1993) Measurement of capillary permeability to macromolecules by dyamic magnetic resonance imaging: a quantitative non-invasive technique. Magn Reson Med 29:616–622
126. Jain R (1994) Barriers to drug delivery in solid tumors. Sci Am 58–65
127. Song C (1984) Effect of local hyperthermia in blood flow and microenvironment: a review. Cancer Res 44:4721S–4730S
128. Gray LH, Conger AD, Ebert M (1953) The concentration of oxygen dissolved in tissues at the time of irradiation as a factor in radiotherapy. Br J Radiol 26:638–648
129. Kety S (1949) Measurement of regional circulation by the local clearance of radioactive sodium. Am Heart J 38:321–328
130. Kety S (1951) The theory and application of the exchange of inert gas at the lungs and tissues. Pharmacol Rev 3:1–41
131. Larsson H, Fritz-Hansen T, Rostrup E, Sondergaard L (1996) Myocardial perfusion modeling using MRI. Magn Reson Med 35:716–726
132. Detre J, Leigh J, Williams D, Koretzsky A (1992) Perfusion imaging. Magn Reson Med 23:37–45
133. Raichle ME, Eichling JO, Straatmann MG et al (1976) Blood-brain barrier permeability of 11C-labeled alcohols and 15O-labeled water. Amer J Physiol 230:543–552
134. Detre JA, Zhang W, Roberts DA, Silva DS, Grandis DJ, Koretsky AP, Leigh JS (1994) Tissue specific perfusion imaging using arterial spin labeling. NMR Biomed 7(1–2):75–82
135. Nishiimura DG, Macovski A, Pauly JM, Conolly AM (1987) MR angiography by selective inversion recovery. Magn Reson Med 4:193–202
136. Kwong KK, Chesler DA, Weisskoff RM et al (1995) MR perfusion studies with T1 weighted echo planar imaging. Magn Reson Med 34:878–87
137. Edelman RR, Siewert B, Darby DG et al (1994) Qualitative mapping of cerebral blood flow and functional localization with echo-planar MR imaging and signal targeting with alternating radio frequency. Radiology 192:513–520
138. Ogawa S, Lee TM, Kay AR, Tank DW (1990) Brain magnetic resonance imaging with contrast dependent on blood oxygenation. Proc Natl Acad Sci USA 87(24):9868–72
139. Le Bihan D, Breton E, Lallemand D et al (1986) MR imaging of intravoxel incoherent motions: application to diffusion and perfusion in neurologic disorders. Radiology 161:401–407
140. Stejskal EO, Tanner JE (1965) Use of spin echo in a pulsed magnetic field gradient to study anisotropic restricted diffusion and flow. J Chem Phys 43:3579
141. Le Bihan D, Breton E, Lallemand D et al (1988) Separation of diffusion and perfusion in intravoxel incoherent motion (IVIM) MR imaging. Radiology 168:497–505
142. Le Bihan D, Moonen CTW, Van Zijl PCM, Pekar J, DesPres D (1991) Measuring random microscopic motion of water in tissues with MR imaging: a cat brain study. J Comput Assist Tomogr 15:19–25
143. Fatouros PP, Marmarou A (1991) In vivo brain water determination by T1 measurements: effect of total water content' hydration fraction' and field strength Mag Reson Med 17(2):402–13
144. Powers TA, Lorentz CH, Holburn GE, Prince RR (1991) Renal artery stenosis: in vivo perfusion MR imaging. Radiology 178:543–8

145. McKinstry RC, Belliveau JW, Moore JB et al (1992) Ultrafast MR imaging of water mobility, animal models of altered cerebral perfusion. J Magn Reson Imaging 2:377–84
146. Kwong KK, Reimer P, Weisskoff R, Cohen MS, Brady TJ, Weissleder R (1992) Dynamic signal intensity changes in liver with superparamagnetic MR contrast agents 2(2):177–81
147. Eichling JO, Raichle ME, Grubb RL, Ter-Pogossian MM (1974) Evidence of the limitations of water as freely diffusible tracer in brain of the rhesus monkey. Circ Res 35(3):358–64
148. Frase PA, Dallas AD (1990) Measurement of filtration coefficient in single cerebral microvessets of the frog. J Physiol 423:343–61
149. Kim S-G, Ackerman JH (1988) Multicompartment analysis of blood flow and tissue perfusion employing D2O as a freely diffusible tracer: a novel deuterium NMR technique demonstrated with murine RIF-1 tumors. Magn Reson Med 8:410–426
150. Kim S-G, Ackerman JH (1988) Quantitative determination of tumor blood flow and perfusion via deuterium nuclear magnetic resonance spectroscopy in mice. Cancer Res 48(12):3449–53

CHAPTER 14

Clinical Applications of Neuroimaging Using Echo-Planar Imaging

B. Siewert and S. Warach

Introduction

Diagnostic Imaging

With echo-planar imaging (EPI) images may be acquired in less than 1 s [98], providing many advantages relevant to clinical diagnosis. In addition to the practical virtues of faster image acquisition and reduced sensitivity to motion artifact, the technique allows investigation of physiological processes such as diffusion and perfusion.

Diffusion Imaging

With conventional magnetic resonance imaging (MRI) diffusion imaging can be performed using spin-echo techniques (SE [54]) or turboSTEAM sequences [62]. However, since diffusion-weighted imaging (DWI) is extremely sensitive to any net translational movement of water molecules, even slight movement of the head and brain during image acquisition severely impairs the quality of the images and invalidates diffusion measurements. Asking patients, particularly those with acute stroke, to maintain the head in a completely immobile position for the 10 min or more required for DWI with conventional MRI is not feasible. Navigated SE sequences [25, 81] can be applied to correct for patient motions, but this does not satisfactorily overcome the imaging time for eight slices in the order of 15 min or more or the problem of substantial motion. EPI can provide multi-slice DWI of higher spatial and temporal resolution [106] in as little as 48 s for multiple b values [114].

Perfusion Imaging

Perfusion imaging can be performed with various techniques, including single photon emission computed tomography, sequential computed tomography, and positron emission tomography. Perfusion imaging with MRI is performed without radiation, provides better spatial resolution, and may not require intravenous contrast media.

Techniques employing an intravenous contrast agent measure either the relaxivity or susceptibility effect of the passage of the contrast media through the capillary bed. The injection of the contrast media leads to T1 shortening and results either in increased signal intensity on T1-weighted images [7, 58, 84, 96] or in T2* shortening because of differences in susceptibility and therefore T2 or T2* signal loss [109]. For susceptibility-based techniques tissues with higher perfusion experience higher signal loss due to phase incoherences from inhomogeneity of the magnetic field [85]. Using these techniques, cerebral blood volume (CBV) has been calculated in healthy volunteers [5] and in patients with ischemia, tumors, and arteriovenous malformations [28].

Techniques not requiring administration of contrast media rely either on changes that are blood oxygenation level dependent (BOLD [4, 51, 79]) or on applied inversion pulses to tag blood flowing into the slice [29, 83, 122]. Signal changes in BOLD are due to the fact that deoxyhemoglobin is paramagnetic while oxygenated blood and surrounding tissue are diamagnetic [51, 78, 107]. These differences in magnetic susceptibility generate local magnetic field gradients and lead to signal attenuation [35, 78, 102]. With task activation, for example, an increase in perfusion results in an increase in oxygenated blood and a decrease in the amount of deoxygenated blood. Since oxygenated blood has a longer T2* than deoxygenated blood, the signal intensity of the activated area increases. The advantage of these techniques is that they can be repeated multiple times since no injection of contrast media is necessary.

Diffusion Imaging of Normal Brain Tissue

DWI has recently been applied in healthy volunteers for the diagnosis of ischemia and in tumor imaging [15, 16, 20, 53, 54, 103, 111].

The DWI pulse sequences apply diffusion-sensitizing gradients before and after the 180° pulse of a SE sequence to dephase and rephase spins (Fig. 1). In the absence of diffusion, spins are completely refocused at the time of the echo, and the gradients have no effect on signal amplitude. If diffusion is present, spins precess with different frequencies when moving along the gradients and are not completely refocused at the time of the echo. This results in signal loss due to phase dispersion, with the amount of signal loss dependent on the amount of

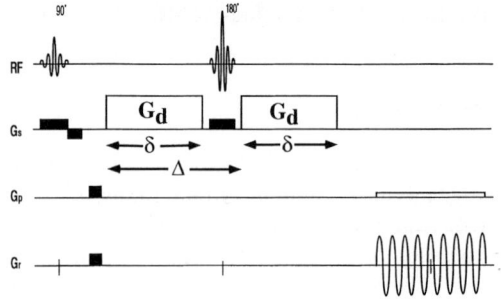

Fig. 1. Pulse sequence diagram of a diffusion-weighted sequence. Relative timings of radiofrequency (RF) pulses and gradients are illustrated (not to scale). Between the 90° and 180° pulses a dephasing gradient (Gd) is applied with duration δ, and an equivalent rephasing gradient is applied after the 180° RF pulse. The time between the leading edge of the two diffusion gradients is the diffusion time. A continuous echo planar readout follows

diffusion [101]. The less the net diffusion, the less is the signal loss, and the brighter the region appears in contrast to areas with greater diffusion.

Using the equation of Stejskal and Tanner [101], the diffusion coefficient can be calculated when a minimum of two images with different diffusion sensitivity are acquired. This factor is called the apparent diffusion coefficient (ADC) since in biological tissues barriers exist to unrestricted diffusion, and motion due to processes other than diffusion may contribute to its value. An ADC map, which shows the ADC at each pixel, can then be generated based on the signal change between images acquired with different diffusion gradient strengths. This value is derived as the negative slope of the regression line fitting the diffusion sensitivity (b value) to the natural log of the signal intensity. The ADC map represents water diffusion at each pixel, independently of T1 and T2 relaxation times, such that areas of low diffusion (e.g., acute cerebral infarcts) are depicted as low signal intensity lesions on ADC maps.

It is noteworthy that ADC measurements are affected by a number of parameters such as TE, diffusion time, diffusion encoding direction, cardiac gating, and cerebrospinal fluid (CSF) flow which affect the accuracy and the value of the diffusion coefficient measured [15]. There is an optimal TE for quantitative diffusion imaging at which diffusion effects are maximized while signal loss due to T2 relaxation is minimized. The accuracy of the measurement is greater for spins having more significant diffusion-related signal change than signal loss due to T2 relaxation. Pulsation of CSF can increase the measured ADC as much as 200 % in the periventricular region; via extension into the surrounding tissues. Cardiac gating should be performed in diastole to minimize pulsation effects and motion in the brain itself which might artificially increase the ADC. Because of these variables the direct comparison of ADC measurements from different institutions may not be feasible. With single-shot EPI gating may not be necessary, but variability in ADC calculation could occur because of variations in brain or CSF motion during different phases of the cardiac cycle. Single-shot EPI acquired at different diffusion sensitivities may therefore show different effects of motion without cardiac gating.

Several authors have measured ADC in brain tissue (Table 1.). The ADC for CSF has been reported to vary with location due to differences in CSF flow. It was found to be the same as pure water in the horns of the lateral ventricles but was significantly higher in the third and fourth ventricles [54].

Table 1. ADC in normal brain tissue reported in the literature (from Le Bihan et al. 1986; Chien et al. 1988; Le Bihan et Turner 1990)

Tissue	Gradients	ADC ($\times 10^{-3}$ mm^{-2}/s^{-1})	
		Minimum	Maximum
Gray matter	All	0.66 ± 0.06	2.0 ± 0.1
White matter	All	0.73 ± 0.19	1.7 ± 0.1
	Parallel	1.00 ± 0.05	1.07 ± 0.06
	Perpendicular	0.43 ± 0.03	0.64 ± 0.05
Cerebrospinal fluid	All	2.5 ± 0.2	3.44

Ischemia

The early diagnosis of acute stroke has been a dilemma in diagnostic imaging since, on computed tomography or conventional MRI, changes in damaged brain tissue cannot reliably be seen until 8 h after clinical onset [13, 124]. Furthermore, the initial clinical diagnosis is incorrect in up to 30 % of patients in predicting location, size, and mechanism of pathological changes [17, 75, 77, 110]. Early establishment of the diagnosis is all the more critical with the advent of pharmacological agents which promise to improve clinical outcome of stroke patients, if treated early.

A means of diagnosing ischemia is required as soon as possible after the onset of symptoms and distinguishing acute from chronic ischemic changes. Information about tissue viability and consequently the utility of pharmacotherapy would be helpful. As transient ischemia requires different therapeutic response, it would be helpful to be able to differentiate with the onset of symptoms whether ischemia is transient or fixed.

Diagnosis of Acute Ischemia

Animal experiments have investigated changes in diffusion and perfusion after controlled occlusion of a cerebral artery [14, 23, 50, 121] in order to determine the time interval between occlusion of an artery and earliest detectable changes on MRI.

Moseley et al. [70, 71] demonstrated DWI to be more sensitive in detection of ischemic changes than is T2-weighted SE. Within minutes after the unilateral occlusion of the MCA they reported foci of hyperintense signal on diffusion-weighted images [21, 71], correlated with a lower ADC for water in these areas. The decrease in ADC is thought to be due to cytotoxic edema from water uptake of the ischemic cells [3, 68, 70, 91]. A modern theory of cytotoxic edema, still debated, is that cellular calcium channels open due to the excitation of N-methyl-D-aspartate receptors by the release and accumulation of neurotoxic dicarboxylic amino acids, such as glutamate, in the extracellular spaces [37]. This results in the cell release of potassium ions and the massive entry of sodium ions (and subsequently water), which quickly overtake the capacity of the ionic trans-membrane pumps. Alternative explanations include local drop in temperature and brain pulsation due to decrease in local cerebral blood flow [3]. In the Moseley et al. study the areas of high signal intensity on DWI matched the areas of hypoperfusion on the perfusion images. These results have been confirmed by others in a variety of different animal experiments [64, 68, 69].

First clinical experience with 32 patients demonstrated hyperacute infarcts in four patients, initially seen only on DWI (Fig. 2). The time interval between imaging and clinical onset of symptoms varied between 105 min and 4 h for these patients. On follow-up computed tomography and MRI examinations these abnormalities were seen in the same distribution [111]. Patients imaged 24 h after the onset of symptoms showed lesions of the same extent on diffusion and T2-weighted SE images.

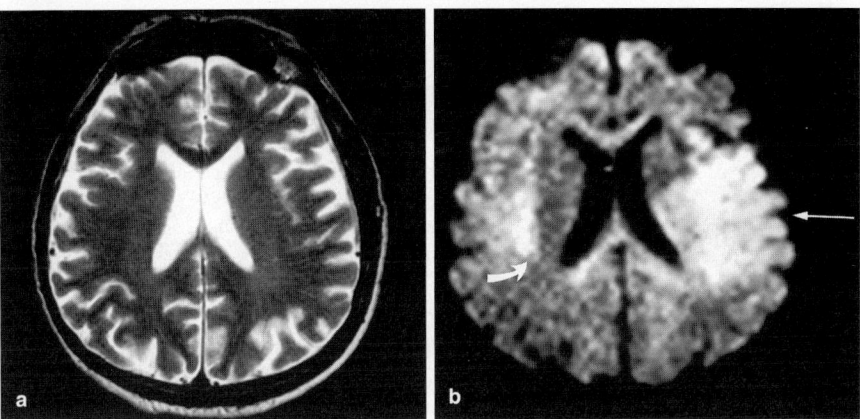

Fig. 2a,b. Four-hour infarct shown by diffusion-weighted EPI. **a** T2-weighted SE image 4 h after the onset of stroke shows no abnormal signal intensity. **b** Diffusion-weighted EPI 2 h after stroke onset shows increased signal in the vascular distribution of the left middle cerebral artery (*arrow*), indicative of acute injury, and reduced ADC. Area of increased signal intensity on the right (*curved arrow*) is due to anisotropic diffusion within normal white matter tracts

The study mentioned above used a turboSTEAM sequence on a conventional MRI scanner, which is not ideal for DWI. The use of EPI for DWI has several advantages over conventional DWI:

● The whole brain can be imaged in seconds, and degradation of image quality from motion artifacts is less of a problem. Motion artifacts can arise from gross patient motion and/or from physiological brain motion due to cardiac or respiratory pulsations [32]. The increased sensitivity to patient motion is accentuated by the long imaging times for conventional DWI.

● Unlike conventional DWI, EPI can be performed for multiple slices. Therefore the full extent of lesions can be determined, and errors in clinical localization may not result in false-negative results. In addition, the evolution of an ischemic lesion can be demonstrated in full extent. Small lesions can be depicted in adjacent slice positions, thus improving sensitivity to detect diffusion abnormalities. This is particularly useful for infarcts in the brainstem (Fig. 3). Using this technique lesions as small as 4 mm have been demonstrated [114].

● With diffusion-weighted EPI multiple diffusion sensitivities can be applied, giving more accurate calculation of the ADC, in contrast to conventional DWI in which fewer diffusion sensitivities can be obtained in a time period practical for clinical use.

Other conditions have been demonstrated to cause decrease in ADC. These include experimental status epilepticus [125], decreased temperature [55], hyponatremia [91], and, possibly, spreading depression [39, 43].

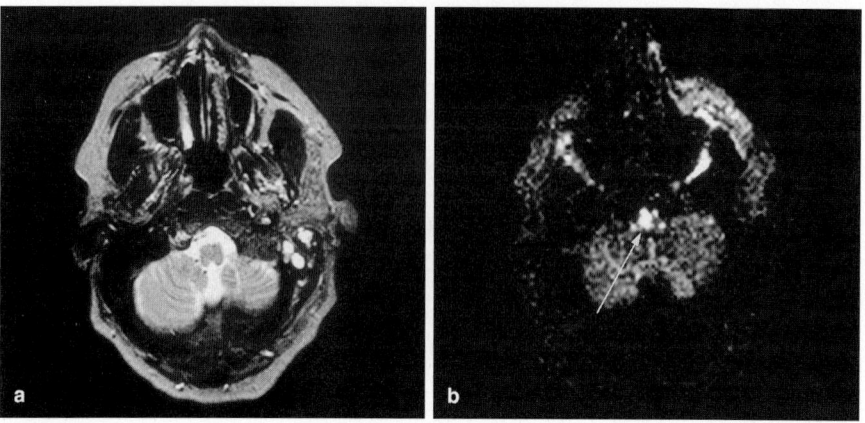

Fig. 3a,b. Two-hour infarct shown by diffusion-weighted EPI. **a** T2-weighted SE image 2 h after the onset of stroke shows no abnormal signal intensity. **b** Diffusion-weighted EPI 2 h after stroke onset shows increased signal in the medulla (*arrow*) indicative of acute injury and reduced ADC. (Reprinted with permission from [93])

Differentiating Acute from Chronic Ischemic Changes

Chronic infarcts (older than 8–10 weeks) can be distinguished from acute infarcts since mass effect and contrast enhancement on T1-weighted images are absent, and calcifications or signs of old hemorrhage may be found. However, difficulties may arise in differentiating acute from chronic ischemic changes older than 2 weeks on standard SE sequences since T1 and T2 relaxation times can be prolonged in both [59] or in new white matter lesions occurring in a field of extensive white matter changes.

On DWI old infarcts may demonstrate a characteristic appearance after 11 days. They appear relatively isointense with the surrounding tissue whereas acute infarcts demonstrate high signal intensity. Thus, old infarcts may be indistinguishable from normal tissue on DWI. Acute and chronic infarcts may be distinguishable on qualitative criteria alone in combination with T2-weighted SE with acute infarcts demonstrating hyperintense signal on both sequences and old infarcts demonstrating hyperintensity on the T2-weighted SE sequence and being isointense or hypointense on diffusion-weighted EPI.

With turboSTEAM ADC measurements of these two conditions vary from $1.41-1.21\times10^{-3}$ mm^{-2} s^{-1} for acute changes (<12–48 h) to 2.68×10^{-3} mm^{-2} s^{-1} for chronic changes (ADC for normal brain tissue varies between 1.95 and 2.32×10^{-3} mm^{-2} s^{-1} [112]). On ADC maps chronic infarcts therefore appear as high signal intensity regions and are distinguishable form normal brain tissue. The increase in ADC in chronic infarcts may initially be due to vasogenic edema with bulk water motion in the extracellular space and later be due to tissue necrosis with concomitantly increased extracellular spaces and CSF in the area of the chronic infarct. Using all three methods a differentiation of acute and chronic infarct can be made (Fig. 4; Table 2).

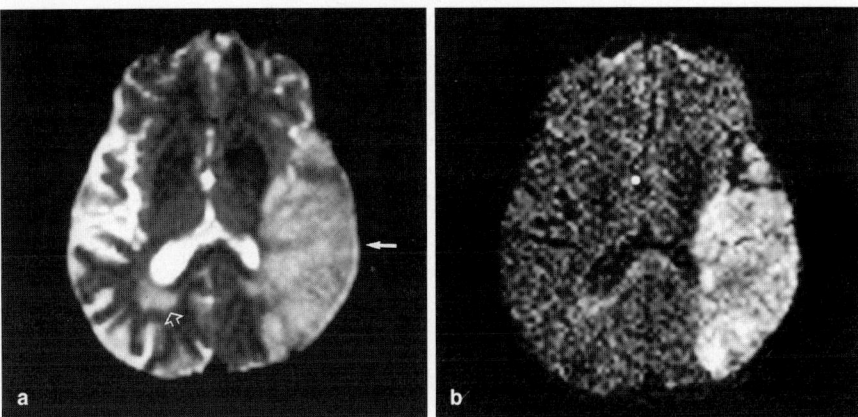

Fig. 4a,b. Diffusion-weighted EPI distinguishes acute from chronic lesions. **a** T2-weighted SE image demonstrates increased signal in the left middle cerebral artery territory with sulcal effacement (*arrow*). In addition, a moderate sized hyperintense area is seen contralaterally (*open arrow*). Acute and chronic changes cannot be distinguished on signal characteristics alone. **b** Diffusion-weighted EPI shows acute infarct as hyperintense lesion whereas chronic right parietal infarct is indistinguishable from normal brain tissue. (Reprinted with permission from [93])

Table 2. Signal characteristics and ADC typical at each stroke stage (from Warach et al. 1995)

Stage	Time after clinical onset	T2 SE	DWI	ADC
Hyperacute	0–6 hours	Normal	Increased	Decreased
Acute	6–48 hours	Normal-increased	Increased	Decreased
Subacute	3–10 days	Increased	Increased	Decreased-normal
Chronic	>10 days	Increased	Decreased-increased	Increased

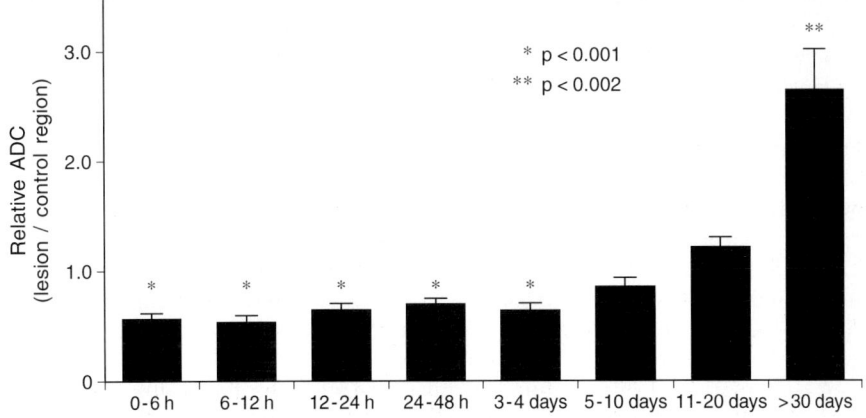

Fig. 5. Mean ADC ratio at time from onset after stroke

Changes on diffusion-weighted images evolve over time (Fig. 5), appearing less intense and relatively more restricted to cerebrocortical gray matter in the first 12 h, with ADC values around $1.41 \times 10{-3}$ mm^{-2}. Over the subsequent 12 h signal intensity on DWI increases, and ADC drops to 1.15×10^{-3} mm^{-2}. ADC values then increase again, and ADC becomes pseudonormalized at 5–10 days. Thereafter ADC increases while signal intensity decreases; after weeks to months the infarcted area is isointense to the surrounding tissue [16, 112, 114].

Assessment of Tissue Viability

Animal experiments have demonstrated that substances which suppress the transmission of glutamate, an important neurotoxic substance in ischemia, reduce the area of decreased diffusion [48, 49, 64, 67, 92]. The efficacy of such agents in the treatment of stroke patients is now being studied in many centers. In the future the assessment of tissue viability and the evaluation of the usefulness of therapies will therefore be of major importance, particularly since the reperfusion of irreversibly ischemic tissue may be hazardous, possibly exacerbating brain edema or promoting hemorrhagic transformation. Of crucial importance is therefore the definition of the penumbra, an area of reduced perfusion sufficient to cause potentially reversible clinical deficits but insufficient to cause energy failure [2, 42].

Others have asked whether the ADC measured initially can be predictive of the severity of the ischemia and risk of infarction and have demonstrated that hyperintense lesions with less ADC decline are more likely to improve than those with a greater fall in ADC [50]. Dardzinski et al. [20] found that the threshold for a lesion becoming an infarct is an ADC of lower than 0.55×10^{-3} mm^{-2} $^{s-1}$. This value was determined in an animal model following a 2-h occlusion of the MCA and subsequent reperfusion with the diffusion-sensitizing gradient applied along the z-axis.

Several investigators have demonstrated that hyperintense areas on DWI in animal models of focal cerebral ischemia are in part reversible [50, 65, 67, 68]. The time window for significant reversal of ischemic lesions in animals is between 1 and 2 h of ischemia. When reflow is begun within 33 min of arterial occlusion scans normalize completely after 4 h of reperfusion [22, 68]. Within 60 min luxury perfusion is generally observed initially, and minimal brain damage results [50]. However, postreperfusion injury is observed on MR perfusion-sensitive images, and this is correlated with mild to moderate neuronal cell damage. Attempted reflow after 60 min of occlusion demonstrates delayed contrast agent transit, suggesting some element of ischemic tissue injury [50]. Producing reflow after 2 h of occlusion does not restore brain perfusion and results in histopathological brain damage and persistent hyperintensity on the DWI [66]. A 6-h occlusion is associated with pronounced perfusion deficits.

A combination of diffusion and perfusion imaging can be used in the evaluation of stroke to identify the area of penumbra. This region is identified as an area of decreased perfusion with no abnormality on DWI ([113]; Fig. 6).

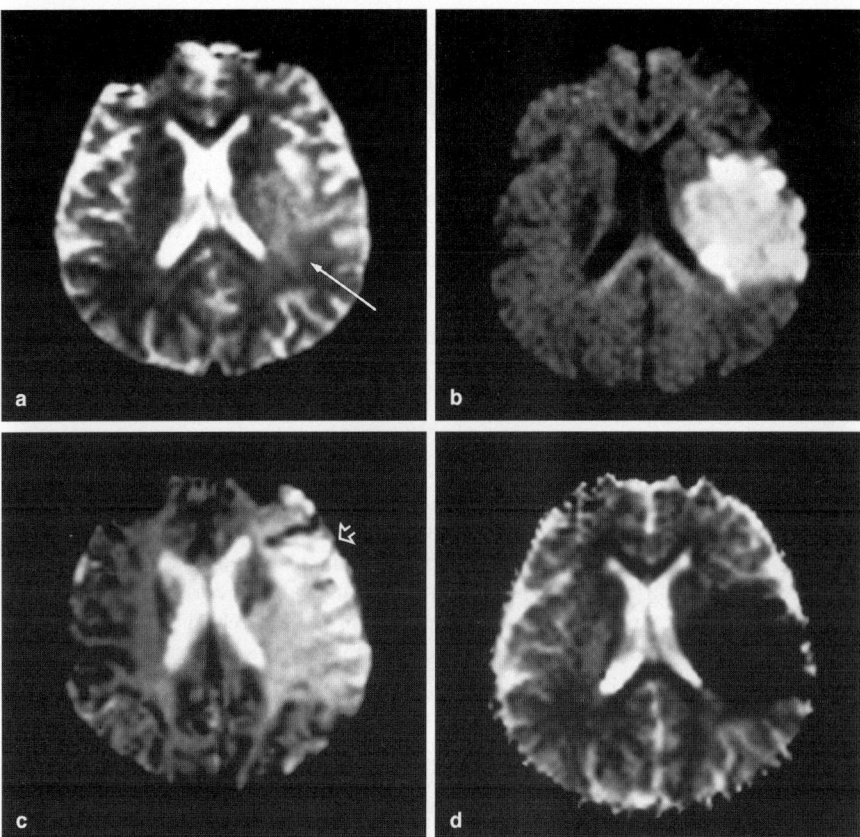

Fig. 6a–d. Demonstration of the penumbra phenomena. **a** T2-weighted EPI 24 h after the onset of stroke demonstrates slight hyperintensity in the vascular distribution of the left middle cerebral artery (*arrow*). **b** Diffusion-weighted image readily demonstrates acute infarct. **c** Perfusion-image (8 s after first pass of contrast media) demonstrates perfusion defect to be larger than diffusion abnormality (*open arrow*). This difference is felt to represent the penumbra. **d** ADC map shows reduced ADC in acute infarct as dark area. (Reprinted with permission from [93])

Differentiation of Acute Infarction and Transient Ischemia

Along similar lines, the differentiation of acute infarction and transient ischemia may be possible. If symptoms are caused by transient ischemia, no abnormalities are found on either diffusion or perfusion imaging [113]. If abnormalities are present on DWI, perfusion imaging is normal. These patients' symptoms have been shown to resolve without therapy. These and other preliminary data suggest that DWI is more accurate than the clinical examination not only in localizing early lesions, but that in combination with perfusion it might be possible to distinguish progression to infarction from potential resolution of deficits at a time when the patient is still symptomatic.

In animal experiments De Crespigny et al. [22] could not demonstrate changes on DWI up to 2.5 min of occlusion, while changes consistent with hyperemia were seen on BOLD images. BOLD imaging initially demonstrates signal loss reflecting the deoxygenation of static blood which is no longer being replaced. Time-resolved observations of ADC changes after occlusion show that the ADC decreases much more slowly, over the course of 10 or 20 min [73]. With reperfusion, signal increase results from hyperoxia due to reactive hyperemic response of tissues on resumption of blood supply. The duration of the overshoot is strongly related to the length of occlusion. Transient ischemic changes during apnea have also been demonstrated using the BOLD technique [24, 100] in animal experiments and healthy volunteers.

Complete Evaluation of Ischemia

The complete MR workup of a possible acute infarct includes T2-weighted dual SE sequences, diffusion-weighted sequences with multiple b values, perfusion images, and, in cases of questionable areas of high signal intensity on DWI images, anisotropic diffusion images. The assessment of a stroke patient is not complete without an angiographic study to evaluate the underlying disease process. This can be carried out in the same setting using cerebral MR angiography ([112]; Fig. 7). In the future even faster EPI angiographic sequences may be available.

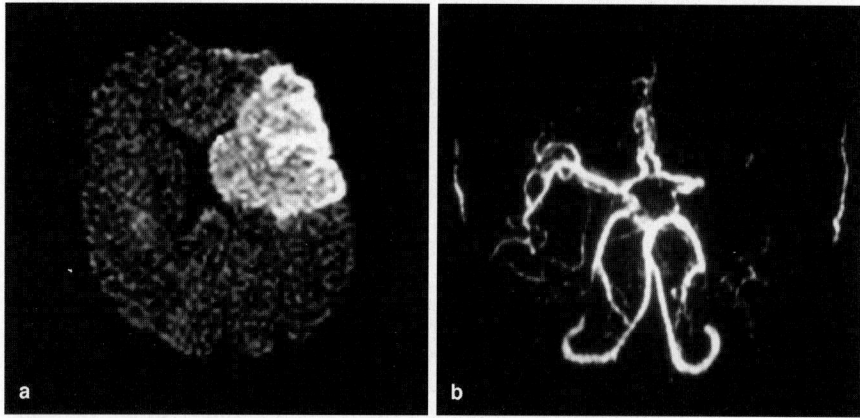

Fig. 7a,b. Acute embolic infarct in the vascular distribution of the middle cerebral artery. **a** Diffusion-weighted EPI demonstrates acute infarct as hyperintensity. **b** MR angiography demonstrates occlusion of the middle cerebral artery consistent with embolus. (Reprinted with permission from [93])

Problems in Study Interpretation

It should be noted that ADC may vary both within and between lesions, particularly in older infarcts, and that measurements may be heterogeneous in the same lesion. In an acute lesion the ADC is typically lower in the core of the lesion, with a rim of less severe ADC decrease. Over time the core of the lesion pseudonormalizes, and a rim of expanding infarction may demonstrate a lower ADC.

Susceptibility artifacts in the anterior frontal and temporal lobes, adjacent to the paranasal sinuses, can mimic acute infarcts. On higher diffusion sensitivities they appear as small hyperintense distortions of the images. However, since these are rare locations for strokes to occur in isolation, this should generally not constitute a problem.

Diffusion measurements are affected by directional barriers. The diffusion of water molecules occurs with relative ease along the long axis of fiber pathways but is relatively restricted when perpendicular to this axis. This is termed anisotropy and has been demonstrated as a normal phenomenon in cortical and deep

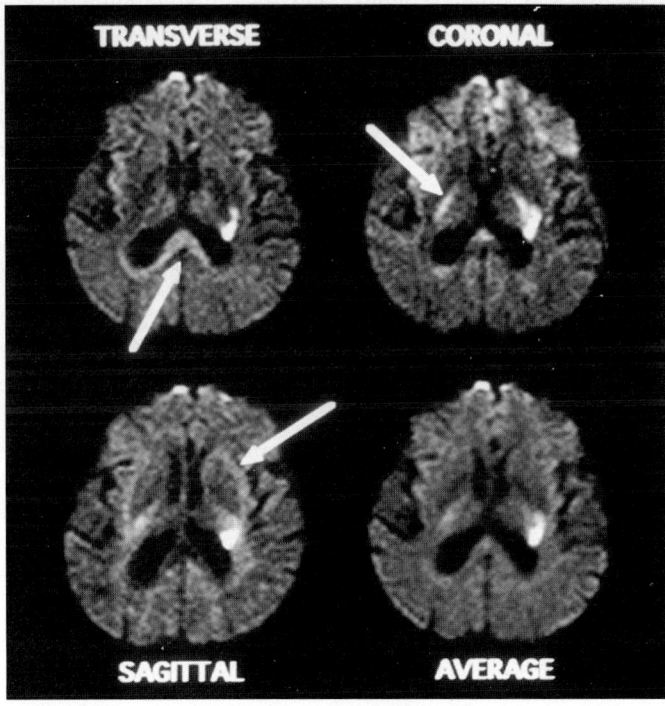

Fig. 8. Seven-hour lesion in the left internal capsule with diffusion gradients applied in transverse, coronal, and sagittal directions. White matter tracts oriented perpendicularly to the orientation of the diffusion gradient appear relatively hyperintense (*arrows*) whereas those parallel to the diffusion gradient appear isointense or hypointense. The infarct is present regardless of direction of diffusion. The average of the three diffusion directions produces an image relatively free from anisotropy. Hyperintensity at the inferior frontal poles at the top of this image is caused by susceptibility artifact. (Reprinted with permission from [114])

white matter in healthy volunteers [105]. Gray matter, although it restricts movement of water molecules, does not show this net directional restriction of diffusion and is therefore isotropic [27, 56, 74]. Thus, faster diffusion occurs when the diffusion-sensitizing gradient is applied parallel to the long axes of white matter tracts, whereas decreased water diffusion is observed with the diffusion-gradient applied perpendicular to the long axis [72]. These areas may be confused with the decreased diffusion that is measured in acute ischemic injury. Differentiation is possible when the diffusion gradient is applied in a different direction with the area demonstrating normal diffusion (Fig. 8).

Tumors

Several shortcomings still apply when conventional MRI is used in the preoperative evaluation of brain tumors. Among those problems are the differentiation of nonenhancing tumor and peritumoral vasogenic edema [97], occasionally the distinction between solid and cystic tumor components, difficulties in assessing tumor vascularity and tumor grading, and the differentiation of postsurgical changes from nonenhancing tumor recurrence. The administration of intravenous contrast media has increased the sensitivity and specificity of MRI of the brain, and at present contrast media are used whenever tumor is suspected [33, 90]. However, important limitations exist when conventional imaging techniques are used in the diagnosis of primary brain tumors. Measurements of T1, T2, and proton-density, and combinations thereof, are not sufficiently specific to help distinguish between low-grade and high-grade tumor [46]. Moreover, contrast enhancement or lack thereof is not specific for tumor grading, even though greater likelihood for contrast enhancement exists in low-grade tumors [8, 9].

Tissue Characterization

DWI has been performed to differentiate various tumor histologies. ADC measurements vary from less than 1.5×10^{-3} mm^{-2} s^{-1} for low-grade astrocytomas to more than 3.5×10^{-3} mm^{-2} s^{-1} for metastases (Table 3). The low ADC for astrocytomas (being lower than for normal brain tissue) has been explained by the restriction of diffusion due to the small cell size and the low volume of perfusion.

Table 3. ADC for various brain tumors and edema (from Le Bihan et al. 1986; Harada et al. 1990; Tien et al. 1994)

	Tissue	ADC ($\times 10^{-3}$ mm^{-2}/s^{-1})
Primary Tissue	Astrocytoma	<1.5
	Glioma	1.1±0.2
	Metastases	>3.5
	Cyst	2.65
Tumor components	Tumor necrosis	2.38
	cystic	2.5±0.2
	Edema	2.49

The high ADC for metastases being higher than the ADC of water (ADC of water $= 2.5 \times 10^{-3}$ mm^{-2} s^{-1}) could be due to the enhanced perfusion in this tissue [54].

Differentiation of Tumor Components and Peritumoral Edema

The differentiation of nonenhancing tumor and peritumoral vasogenic edema is important for determining sites for biopsy, radiation, and surgical therapy and for evaluating response to therapy. Accurate definition of tumor boundaries may allow restricted resection and radiation. DWI may be used to distinguish various tumor components and might be helpful in differentiating nonenhancing tumor from peritumoral edema (Table 4 [41, 103]).

Cystic or necrotic areas demonstrate the greatest signal suppression on DWI along with the highest ADC values. These findings represent a lack of significant restriction of diffusion of water molecules within the cystic or necrotic area, similar to results for CSF in the ventricles [27, 54]. Diffusion within necrotic areas has been found to be greater than within living tissue [44, 57]. This feature becomes clinically useful in some complicated cystic lesions with high paramagnetic protein content, with T1 and T2 times similar to a solid tumor [40]. In these cases DWI clearly shows the liquid nature of the lesion [54, 56]. Similar findings have been reported for arachnoid cysts, which demonstrate diffusion similar to that of stationary water [104], unlike more solid lesions, such as epidermoids with signal intensities closer to that of brain parenchyma (Fig. 9).

Solid tumors demonstrate less signal suppression on DWI than cystic or necrotic tumors ([27, 54]; Fig. 10). Similarly, enhancing tumors on T1-weighted SE images are hyperintense on DWI, with lower ADCs than nonenhancing or peritumoral edema [103]. This is thought to be due to the underlying histological pattern of densely packed, randomly organized tumor cells, which would inhibit effective motion of water molecules and restrict diffusion [54].

Table 4. Signal characteristics and ADC for various tumor components (from Tsuruda et al. 1990; Tien et al. 1994)

Tumor component	T2 SE	T1 SE, postcontrast	DWI	ADC
Cystic	Increased	Decreased	Markedly decreased	Markedly increased
Necrotic	Increased	Decreased	Markedly decreased	Markedly increased
Solid (nonenhancing)	Increased	Decreased	Moderately decreased	Intermediate
Solid (enhancing)	Increased	Increased	Increased	Decreased
Edema	Increased	Decreased	Markedly decreased	Moderately increased
Postsurgical	Increased	Decreased	Intermediate	Intermediate

Fig. 9a–c. Differentiation of
arachnoid cyst and epidermoid using DWI. **a** T2-
weighted SE. **b** Single-shot T2-
weighted EPI. **c** Diffusion-
weighted EPI. T2-weighted SE
demonstrates a hyperintense
prepontine lesion (isointense
to CSF) with widening of the
prepontine cistern. The lesion
compresses the right cerebral
peduncle and encases the
basilar artery. Differential
diagnosis includes epidermoid
and arachnoid cyst. Note signal loss of CSF on DWI (**c**)
due to a high ADC. The lesion
remains hyperintense con-
firming diagnosis of epidermoid

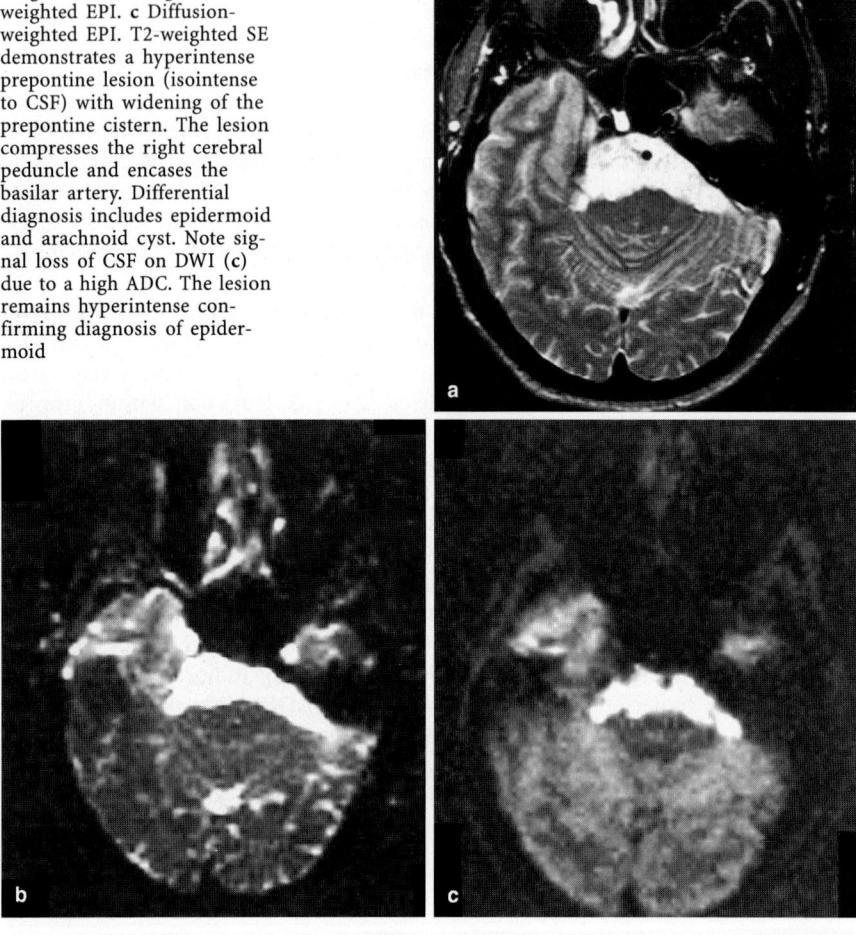

Nonenhancing tumor has signal intensities on DWI and ADCs between those
of enhancing tumors and cystic/necrotic lesions. These differences in diffusion
between nonenhancing and enhancing tumor components can be due to differences in tumor differentiation, tumor cytoarchitecture, or the degree of tumor
infiltration.

When nonenhancing tumors infiltrate white matter tracts oriented parallel to
the diffusion gradient, their ADCs are dependent on the direction of the diffusion
gradient, with resulting differences in anisotropic diffusion. This result can be
used to distinguish nonenhancing tumor from peritumoral edema. Since the
two entities can have similar ADCs, such distinction might be problematic.
With the application of anisotropic diffusion, a marked difference can be found
[12, 41]. This is due to the fact that tumor-invading corticospinal tracts causes

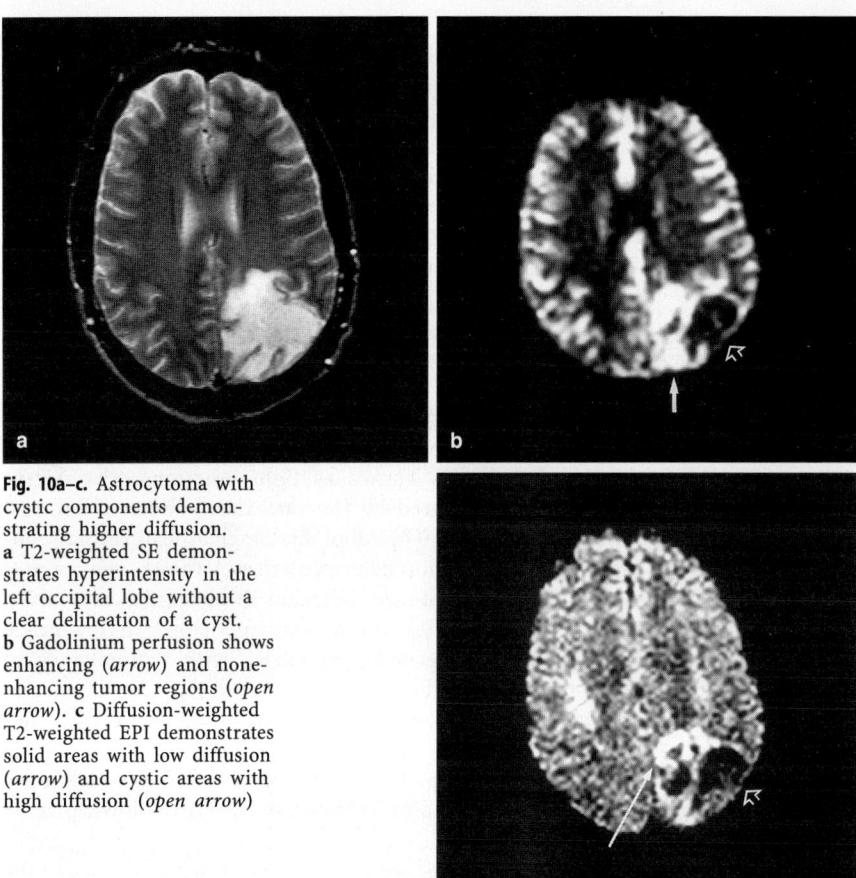

Fig. 10a-c. Astrocytoma with cystic components demonstrating higher diffusion.
a T2-weighted SE demonstrates hyperintensity in the left occipital lobe without a clear delineation of a cyst.
b Gadolinium perfusion shows enhancing (*arrow*) and nonenhancing tumor regions (*open arrow*). c Diffusion-weighted T2-weighted EPI demonstrates solid areas with low diffusion (*arrow*) and cystic areas with high diffusion (*open arrow*)

greater restriction to water molecules traveling in the direction of the white matter than does vasogenic edema. The latter can increase diffusion by virtue of increasing free water in the white matter tracts and, possibly, by increasing the distance between areas of relative diffusion restriction. This results in peritumoral edema demonstrating marked signal suppression with higher ADC and nonenhancing tumor showing less signal suppression with lower ADCs than those of edema.

When comparing anisotropic diffusion, it is important to take into account the amount of mass effect which by reorienting the white matter tracts may change the rate of diffusion. This phenomenon may affect both the ADC measurements and the images, and the problem is compounded by the finding that tumor cells can coexist with areas of edema [115].

Separating postsurgical changes from recurrent tumor is problematic since recent postsurgical changes may enhance and, depending on the tumor histology, recurrent tumor may enhance as well. DWI may permit such distinctions, as shown by Tsuruda et al. [104] reporting a recurrent epidermoid and postsurgical changes with differing ADCs (the ADC of the tumor was decreased, while the ADC of the surgical lesion was intermediate compared to CSF which demonstrated a high ADC). Another possibility in differentiating tumor recurrence from radiation necrosis is the analysis of CBV maps [86]. Radiation necrosis demonstrates significant T2 elevation and enhancement on postcontrast T1-weighted images because of blood-brain barrier (BBB) breakdown. These changes can also be due to tumor recurrence, and the two entities thus cannot be distinguished. The finding of diminished blood volume within this lesion on CBV maps is likely to exclude tumor recurrence.

Assessment of Tumor Vascularity and Tumor Grading

The BBB comprises the following histological characteristics of cerebral capillaries: continuous basement membrane, narrow intercellular gaps, paucity of pinocytosis, and fused endothelial cells known as tight junctions. The degree of breakdown of the BBB can be measured by the rate and amount of contrast accumulating in the extracellular space. The other histological feature that contributes to contrast enhancement is tumor neovascularity. A tumor may release an angiogenic factor which stimulates the proliferation of abnormal capillaries, most prominently at its peripheral boundary or growing edge. In low-grade tumors the vessels resemble normal cerebral capillaries with maintenance of the BBB so that no enhancement occurs. In malignant tumors the capillaries are fenestrated, and pinocytosis is present. They have a deficient BBB and show enhancement [38].

Evaluation of tumor vascularity is important in planning of stereotactic biopsy or surgical resection; for the former the area of maximal BBB breakdown is most suitable.

The breakdown of BBB in tumors has been investigated with EPI using the dynamics of Gd-DTPA uptake [38, 123]. The diffusion of Gd-DTPA across the BBB causes enhancement, and the time for transfer across the BBB varies between 20 and 1050 ms [38]. Analyzing the temporal profile of enhancement may allow discrimination of different histologies and provide information on tumor grade.

MRI techniques employing contrast enhancement to measure tumor vascularity are limited to pathological vessels with defects in the BBB. On the other hand, CBV maps calculated from MR images can depict the microvasculature [34, 119]. This allows the detection of neovascularity at the capillary level, as well as its quantification in relative terms [5, 86] even when the BBB is still intact.

CBV mapping can be obtained from either T1- or T2-weighted (susceptibility contrast) images since Gd produces both T2 and T1 relaxation. Since signal drop on T2 is masked by signal increase in regions where T1 effects are significant, such as areas with disruption of the BBB in high-grade gliomas, T2 CBV maps underestimate the real microvascular blood volume in such cases. This effect can be corrected for when disruption of the BBB is moderate [120]. Other advantages of T1 CBV maps are the low amount of contrast agent necessary and the conspicuity of pathological tissue in the T1 maps.

CBV maps calculated from dynamic EPI SE during intravenous injection of contrast media have been found to be correlated with histopathological tumor vascularity [1]. In addition, functional parameters for assessing glioma grade and regions of focal activity are now available [1]. An association between high CBV and pathological grade of gliomas has been demonstrated: high CBV has been found to be associated with mitotic activity and vascularity and may signify dedifferentiation or high-grade tumor. Low CBV is found in low-grade tumors and patients without tumor recurrence [10]. The appearance of a tumor on a CBV map can be heterogeneous with such variations, particularly common within a high grade tumor. An area of high CBV within an otherwise homogeneous tumor with low CBV is believed to be a specific marker for the existence of a high-grade glioma. No relationship has been shown between CBV and cellular atypia, endothelial proliferation, necrosis, or cellularity.

White Matter Disease

Early studies have used DWI to elucidate white matter diseases such as multiple sclerosis, wallerian degeneration, and delayed myelination in neonates [87, 88].

Diffusional anisotropy is closely related to brain maturation and is not found in neonates without myelination [88]. Since the ADC depends strongly on barrier permeability, the addition of even one layer of myelin would be expected to significantly reduce the ADC of unmyelinated axons. In contrast, the reduction in T1 associated with myelination of white matter requires many layers of myelin [47]. This is supported by the finding that diffusion anisotropy is observed earlier than changes on T1-weighted images starting at 38 weeks of gestational age [87], raising the possibility of earlier detection of abnormal neonatal brain development with diffusion-weighted MRI.

In chronic plaques of multiple sclerosis the ADC is increased, consistently with less effective myelin barrier [52, 63].

Fast Imaging

EPI acquisition times on the order of milliseconds may be particularly useful in patients with claustrophobia and in unstable patients who are unable to cooperate for imaging. Good results have been obtained for brain imaging with EPI at various field strengths [60, 89]. With EPI at 3.0 T spatial resolution can be improved tremendously up to 0.75×0.75 mm for a 2.5-mm slice thickness; thus susceptibility artifacts at the bone-air interface do not constitute a problem [60].

EPI suffers from lower contrast-to-noise ratios than conventional SE sequences. Therefore detailed information may be lost on EPI images. Similar problems have been reported for fast SE sequences [76]. In a study comparing single-shot and segmented EPI sequences to conventional MRI for lesion detection in multiple sclerosis, segmented EPI offered greater lesion detection than single-shot EPI such that lesions larger than 10 mm could be depicted with confidence ([94]; Figs. 11, 12). Other investigators have compared EPI to conventional MRI using larger lesions. EPI was found to be slightly inferior in tumor visualization, border definition, and detail information, whereas the extent of edema was equally well depicted with the two techniques [11].

Lesion conspicuity on EPI images can be improved with the use of an EPI fluid-attenuated inversion recovery (FLAIR) technique. With this technique signal from CSF is suppressed [95], and lesions, particularly those near CSF boundaries become more evident.

With very short acquisition times EPI images are less degraded by motion or pulsation artifacts [11] but may suffer from susceptibility artifacts. However, segmented EPI sequences, acquired in one-eight of the acquisition time of conventional SE sequences, suffer less from susceptibility artifacts and combine the advantages of EPI and those of conventional SE techniques.

Although they may interfere with image quality, susceptibility artifacts can be used for diagnostic imaging. Thus, lesions containing blood products, as with contusions and arachnoid cysts, have been demonstrated more clearly with EPI than with conventional T2-weighted SE [95].

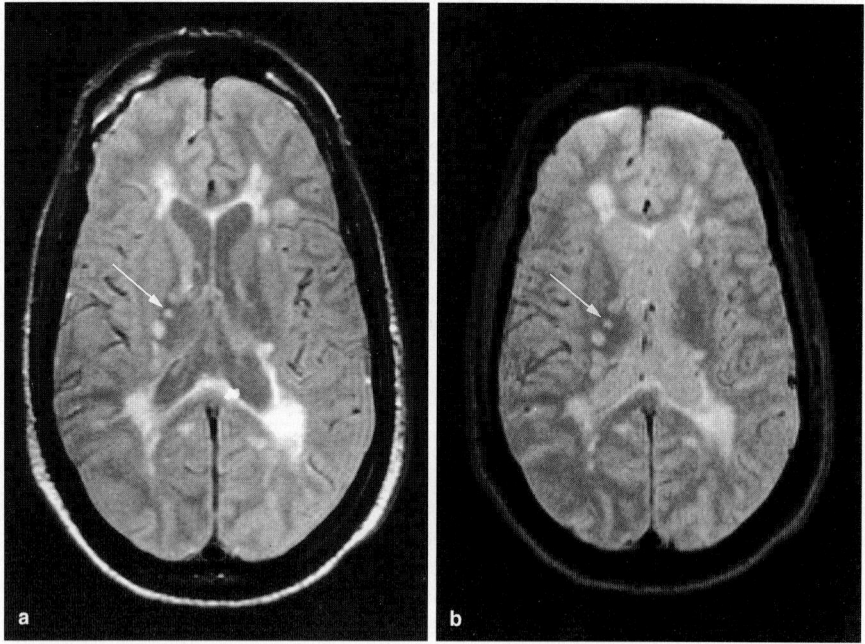

Fig. 11a–g. Sequence comparison in a patient with multiple sclerosis. **a** Proton density weighted SE. **b** Segmented proton density weighted EPI.

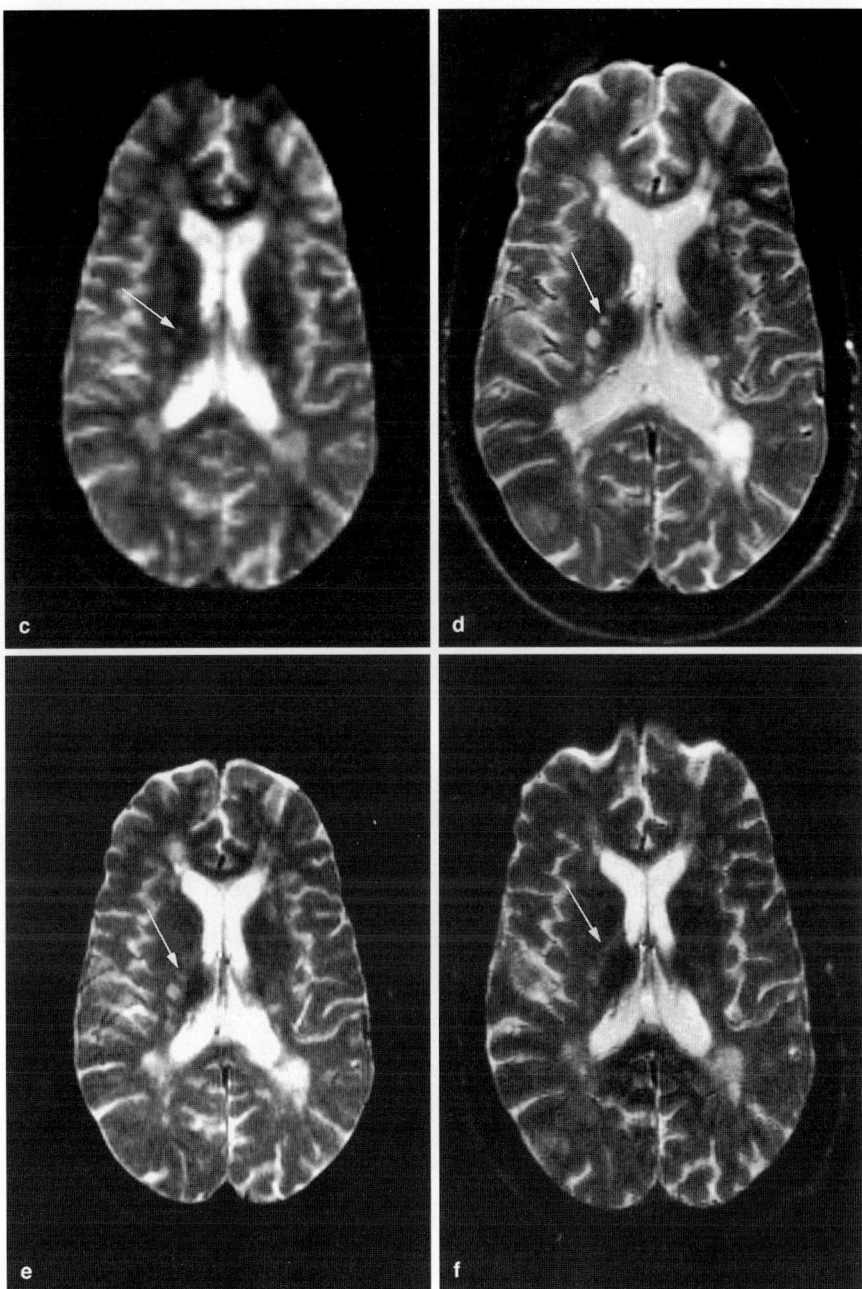

Fig. 11a–g. c Single-shot proton density weighted EPI. **d** T2-weighted SE. **e** Segmented EPI T2. **f** Single-shot high-resolution EPI.

Fig. 11a–g. (continued) **g** Single-shot EPI T2. Larger lesions are well seen with the segmented sequences and less conspicuously with single-shot EPI. Smaller lesions (*arrow*) are well depicted with segmented sequences but may be missed with single-shot EPI

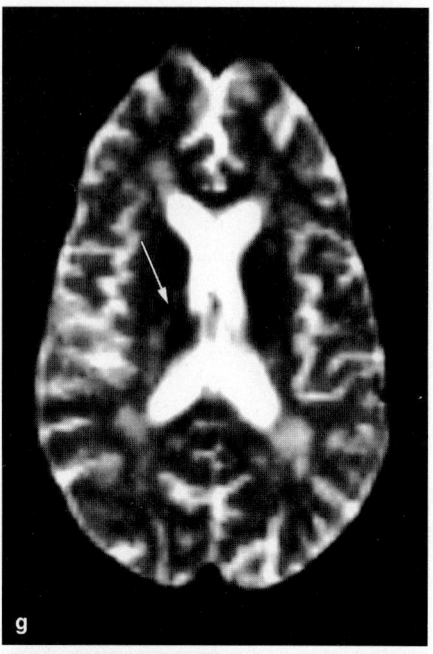

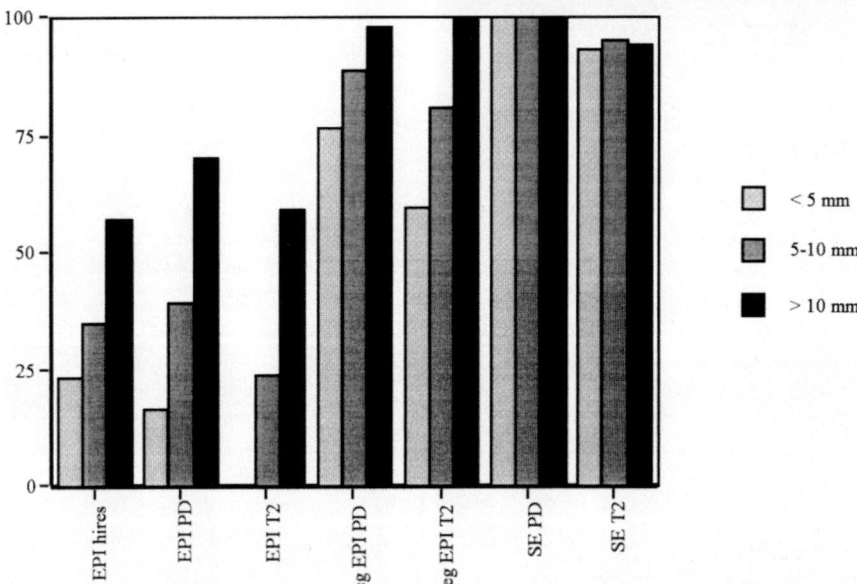

Fig. 12. Sequence comparison for lesion detection. *X-axis*, sequences. *EPI hires*, High-resolution T2-weighted EPI; *EPI PD*, single-shot proton density weighted EPI; *EPI T2*, single-shot T2-weighted EPI; *seg EPI PD*, segmented proton density weighted EPI; *seg EPI T2*, segmented T2-weighted EPI; *SE PD*, proton density weighted spin echo; *SE T2*, T2-weighted spin-echo. *Y-axis*, Percentage of lesions detected with each sequence

CSF Flow

CSF flow is influenced by respiratory and cardiac pulsatile flows. The mechanisms of CSF propulsion is still incompletely understood. Cardiac-dependent CSF motion occurs secondary to cerebral perfusion. Thus far flow data have been best explained by postulating synchronous pulsatile flow of CSF at the foramen of Monro and at the aqueduct, with antegrade flow during systole and retrograde but smaller flow during diastole, resulting in net antegrade flow of CSF into the basal cisterns [61]. Pulsatile flow has been observed at the foramen of Monro, suggesting that the lateral ventricles do play a part in generating CSF flow, perhaps via expansion of the choroid plexus.

CSF flow patterns have been studied using EPI, and transient intraventricular flow has been observed [99]. With T2-weighted sequences rapid flow is seen as a signal void due to dephasing. In healthy volunteers rapid CSF flow between intracranial and intraspinal compartments has been demonstrated. A patent aqueduct is seen as a systolic signal void originating from the aqueduct and extending to the fourth ventricle. The flow plume decays away in diastole. This has been found in patients with communicating hydrocephalus. In the syringohydromyelia complex CSF flow patterns can be seen within syrinx cavities as areas of signal loss which travel caudally during systole.

CSF dynamics can be quantitatively measured when a flow sensitive sequence is used [80]. Signal intensity is proportional to flow and flow maps can be generated.

Systematic analysis of large patient series has not yet been performed, and the role of EPI in the diagnosis of the conditions mentioned above is unclear.

Clinical Functional Imaging

Functional EPI has been performed using both the BOLD technique [108] and the EPI signal targeting with alternating radiofrequency technique [29]. The physiological phenomena involved with cognitive tasks may be studied in order to perform brain mapping [19, 51], and information from functional imaging can be valuable in patients when investigating brain plasticity. For clinical purposes, topics of interest include the assessment of functional reorganization in patients following brain injury (ischemia) and preoperative delineation of primary cortical areas.

Positron emission tomography studies have demonstrated functional reorganization of intact cortex following recovery from stroke [18, 36, 116–118], including lateral extension of the sensorimotor cortex and bilateral activation of the motor system and/or recruitment of additional motor areas with use of ipsilateral pathways [6]. Initial studies using conventional MRI have shown that functional imaging can assess the recovery of brain function in stroke patients [30], demonstrate brain function in patients with congenital hemiplegia [82], and show sparing or recovery of function in cases of infantile hemiplegia [31].

Functional EPI would be extremely valuable in the evaluation of patients with brain tumors prior to neurosurgery. The significant morbidity associated with surgical procedures involving the cerebral cortex results from disruption of primary sensory (visual, auditory, and somatosensory) and motor cortical areas. Neurosurgeons attempt to preserve these areas during therapeutic interventions but are handicapped by the normal variation in organization of these areas as well as by the reorganization that may follow neurological disease [118], particularly in children and in patients with slowly growing tumors. To overcome this difficulty intraoperative cortical mapping in the awake patient has been used in an attempt to define the extent of a primary area in an individual patient and to allow a decision that balances therapeutic need against potential functional impairment [19]. EPI as a noninvasive means of identifying the primary areas and their relationship to tumor tissue preoperatively would clearly be of value in clinical management.

Interventional EPI

In the future EPI may prove useful in interventional radiology because of its ability to measure temperature with diffusion techniques. Temperature changes induced within the magnet bore when a dedicated hyperthermia device or laser beam is used have been demonstrated and measured with diffusion-weighted MRI. Temperature-diffusion imaging, combined with fast imaging, may play a role in the real-time monitoring of interventional or neurosurgical procedures performed within the magnet bore [26, 45, 55].

Prospects

In conclusion, given further refinements in EPI and the development of effective therapy for acute stroke, whole-brain EPI DWI may well become the essential emergency diagnostic test to guide patient management. Additional sophistication is expected in the diagnosis of patients with brain tumors. Beyond the role of EPI as a very fast imaging tool that allows the imaging of unstable, uncooperative, and claustrophobic patients in a few minutes, major improvements in diagnosis should follow the integration of functional imaging into patient evaluation.

References

1. Aronen HJ, Gazit IE, Louis DN et al (1994) Cerebral blood volume maps of gliomas: comparison with tumor grade and histologic findings. Radiology 191:41–51
2 Astrup J, Siesjo BK, Symon L (1981) Thresholds in cerebral ischemia- the ischemic penumbra. Stroke 12:723–725
3. Baker LL, Kucharczyk J, Sevick RJ, Minotorovitch J, Moseley M (1991) Recent advances of MR imaging/spectroscopy of cerebral ischemia. AJR 156:1133–1143
4. Bandettini PA, Wong EC, Hinks RS et al (1992) Time course EPI of human brain function during task activation. Magn Reson Med 25:390–397
5. Belliveau JW, Rosen BR, Kantor HL et al (1990) Functional cerebral imaging by susceptibility-contrast NMR. Magn Reson Med 14:538–546

6. Benecke R, Meyer B, Freund H-J (1991) Reorganisation of descending motor pathways in patients after hemispherectomy and severe hemispheric lesions demonstrated by magnetic brain stimulation. Exp Brain Res 83:419–426
7. Bloembergen N (1957) Proton relaxation times in paramagnetic solutions. J Chem Phys 27:527
8. Brant-Zawadzki M (1991) Pitfalls of contrast-enhanced imaging in the nervous system. Magn Reson Med 22:243–248
9. Brant-Zawadzki M, Berry I, Osaki L et al (1986) Gd-DTPA in clinical MR of the brain. I. Intraaxial lesions. AJNR 8:781–788
10. Bruening R, Kwong K, Vevea M et al (1994a) Cerebral blood volume (CBV) maps in primary brain tumors – implementation of T1-effects using echo planar imaging (EPI). In: Proceedings of the Society for Magnetic Resonance, p 196
11. Bruening R, Campbell T, Niemi P, Rosen BR (1994b) T2-weighted imaging of human brain tumors using 512" Echo planar imaging (EPI) In: Proceedings of the Society for Magnetic Resonance, p 521
12. Brunberg JA, Chenevert TL, Ross DA et al (1993) In vivo MR determination of water diffusion coefficients and diffusion anisotropy: correlation with structural alteration in astrocytes of the cerebral hemispheres (abstract). In: Book of abstracts. American Society of Neuroradiology, Chicago, p 71
13. Bryan RN, Levy LM, Whitlow WD et al (1991) Diagnosis of acute cerebral infarction: comparison of CT and MR imaging. AJNR 12:611–620
14. Busza AL, Allen KL, King MD et al (1992) Diffusion-weighted imaging studies of cerebral ischemia in gerbils. Potential relevance to energy failure. Stroke 23:1602–1612
15. Chien D, Buxton RB, Kwong KK et al (1990) MR diffusion imaging of the human brain. J Comput Assist Tomogr 14:514–520
16. Chien D, Kwong KK, Gress DR et al (1992) MR diffusion imaging of cerebral infarction in humans. AJNR 13:1097–1102
17. Chimowitz MI, Logogian EL, Caplan LR (1990) The accuracy of bedside neurological diagnosis. Ann Neurol 28:78–85
18. Chollet F, DiPiero V, Wise RJS et al (1991) The functional anatomy of motor cortex recovery after stroke in humans: a study with positron emission tomography. Ann Neurol 29:63–71
19. Connelly A, Jackson GD, Frackowiak RSJ et al (1993) Functional mapping of activated human primary cortex with a clinical MR imaging system. Radiology 188:125–130
20. Dardzinski BJ, Sotak CH, Fisher M et al (1993) Apparent diffusion coefficient mapping of experimental focal cerebral ischemia using diffusion-weighted echo-planar imaging. Magn Reson Med 30:318–25
21. Davis D, Ulatowski J, Eleff S et al (1994) Rapid monitoring of changes in water diffusion coefficients during reversible ischemia in cat and rat brain. Magn Reson Med 31:454–460
22. de Crespigny AJ, Wendland MF, Derugin N, Koznieska E, Moseley ME (1992) Real-time observation of transient focal ischemia and hyperemia in cat brain. Magn Reson Med 27:391–397
23. de Crespigny AJ, Wendland MF, Derugin N et al (1993a) Rapid MR imaging of a vascular challenge to focal ischemia in cat brain. J Magn Reson Imaging 4:475–481
24. de Crespigny AJ, Tsuura M, Mosely ME, Kucharczyk J (1993b) Perfusion and diffusion MR imaging of thromboembolic stroke. J Magn Reson Imaging 3:746–54
25. de Crespigny A, Yenari M, Enzmann D et al (1994) Navigated spin-echo diffusion imaging of human stroke. In: Proceedings of the Society for Magnetic Resonance, p 137
26. Delannoy J, Le Bihan D, Hoult D, Levin R (1990) Hyperthermia system combined with an MRI unit. Med Phys 17:855–860
27. Douek P, Turner R, Pekar J et al (1991) MR color mapping of myelin fiber orientation. J Comput Assist Tomogr 15:923–929
28. Edelman RR, Mattle HP, Atkinson DJ et al (1990) Cerebral blood flow: assessment with dynamic contrast-enhanced T2*-weighted MR imaging at 1.5 T. Radiology 176:211–220
29. Edelman RR, Siewert B, Darby DG, Thangaraj V, Nobre AC, Mesulam MM, Warach S (1994) Qualitative mapping of cerebral blood flow and functional localization with echo-planar MR imaging and signal targeting with alternating radio frequency. Radiology 192:513–520
30. Faiss JH, Rijntjes M, Weiller CS et al (1994) Motor recovery following cerebral infarction visualized by functional MRI. In: Proceedings of the Society for Magnetic Resonance, p 333
31. Farmer SF, Harrison LM, Ingram DA, Stephens JA (1991) Plasticity of central motor pathways in children with hemiplegic cerebral palsy. Neurology 41:1505–1510
32. Feinberg D, Mark A (1987) Human brain motion and cerebrospinal fluid circulation demonstrated with MR velocity imaging. Radiology 163:793–799

33. Felix R, Schoerner W, Lanaido M et al (1985) Brain tumors: MR imaging with Gadolinium-DTPA. Radiology 156:681–688
34. Fisel CR, Moore Jr, Garrido L et al (1989) A general model for susceptibility-based MR contrast (abstract). In: Book of abstracts. Society of Magnetic Resonance in Medicine, Berkeley, p 324
35. Frahm J, Bruhn H, Merbolt KD, Hänicke W (1992) Dynamic MR imaging of human brain oxygenation and photic stimulation. JMRI 2:501–505
36. Fries W, Danek A, Scheidtmann K, Hamburger C (1993) Motor recovery following capsular stroke. Brain 116:369–382
37. Garcia JH, Anderson ML (1989) Physiopathology of cerebral ischemia. Crit Rev Neurobiol 4:303–324
38. Gowland P, Mansfield P, Bullock P et al (1992) Dynamic studies of gadolinium uptake in brain tumors using inversion recovery echo-planar imaging. Magn Reson Imaging 26:241–58
39. Gyngell ML, Back T, Hoehn-Berlage M et al (1994) Transient cell depolarization after permanent middle cerebral artery occlusion: an observation between diffusion-weighted MRI and localized 1H-MRS. Magn Reson Med 31:337–341
40. Haimes AB, Zimmerman RD, Morgello S et al (1989) MR imaging of brain abscesses. AJR 152:1073–1085
41. Hajnal JV, Doran M, Hall AS et al (1991) MR imaging of anisotropically restricted diffusion of water in the nervous system: technical, anatomic, and pathologic considerations. J Comput Assist Tomogr 15:1–18
42. Hakim AM (1987) The cerebral ischemic penumbra. Can J Neurol Sci 14:557–559
43. Hasegawa Y, Latour LL, Sotak CH et al (1994) Spreading waves of reduced diffusion coefficient of water in the rat brain. Neurology 44 [Suppl 2]:A341
44. Henkelman RM (1990) Diffusion-weighted MR imaging: a useful adjunct to clinical diagnosis or a scientific curiosity? AJNR 11:932–934
45. Jolescz FA, Higuchi N, Bleier AR, Jakab P (1990) MRI of laser effects on tissue. Magn Reson Imaging 8(P):156
46. Just M, Thelen M (1988) Tissue characterization with T1, T2, and proton density values: results in 160 patients with brain tumors. Radiology 169:779–785
47. Koenig SH, Brown RD III, Spiller M, Lundbom N (1990) Relaxometry of the brain: why white matter appears bright in MRI. Magn Reson Med 14:482–495
48. Kucharczyk J, Chew W, Derugin N et al (1989) Nicardipine reduces ischemic brain injury: magnetic resonance imaging/spectroscopy study in cats. Stroke 20:268–274
49. Kucharczyk J, Mintorovitch J, Mosely ME et al (1991) Ischemic brain damage: reduction by sodium channel ion channel modulator RS-87476. Radiology 179:221–227
50. Kucharczyk J, Vexler ZS, Roberts TP et al (1993) Echo-planar perfusion-sensitive MR imaging of acute cerebral ischemia. Radiology 188:711–717
51. Kwong K, Belliveau JW, Chesler DA et al (1992) Dynamic magnetic resonance imaging of human brain activity during primary sensory stimulation. Proc Natl Acad Sci USA 89:5675–5679
52. Larsson HBW, Christiansen P, Thomsen C et al (1990) In vivo measurement of water self diffusion in patients with chronic multiple sclerosis. Book of abstracts. Society of Magnetic Resonance in Medicine, 9th annual meeting, New York, p 150
53. Le Bihan D (1991) Molecular diffusion nuclear magnetic resonance imaging. Magn Reson Q 7:1–30
54. Le Bihan D, Breton E, Lallemand D et al (1986) MR imaging of intravoxel incoherent motion: applications to diffusion and perfusion in neurologic disorders. Radiology 161:401–407
55. Le Bihan D, Delannoy J, Levin RL (1989) Temperature mapping with MR imaging of molecular diffusion: application to hyperthermia. Radiology 171:853–857
56. Le Bihan D, Turner R, Moonen CTW, Pekar J (1991) Imaging of diffusion and microcirculation with gradient sensitization: design, strategy and significance. J Magn Reson Imaging 1:7–28
57. Le Bihan D, Douek P, Argyropoulou M et al (1993) Diffusion and perfusion magnetic resonance imaging in brain tumors. Top Magn Reson Imaging 5:25–31
58. Lee C, Dean BL, Kirsch JE et al (1992) Cerebral infarction: assessment of patterns using ultra-fast MR contrast imaging. AJNR 13:277–279
59. Lundblom N, Katevuo K, Kuomo M et al (1992) T1 in subacute and chronic brain infarctions: time-dependent development. Invest Radiol 27:673–680
60. Mansfield P, Coxon R, Glover P (1994) Echo-planar imaging of the brain at 3.0 T: first normal volunteer results. J Comput Assist Tomogr 18:339–343

61. Mark AS, Feinberg DA, Brant-Zawasski MN (1987) Changes in size and magnetic resonance signal intensity of the cerebral CSF spaces during the cardiac cycle, as studied by gated, high resolution MRI. Invest Radiol 22:290–297

62. Merboldt KD, Hanicke W, Bruhn H, Gynell ML, Frahm J (1992) Diffusion imaging of the human brain in vivo using high speed STEAM MRI. Magn Reson Med 23:179–192

63. Mikulis D, Chien D, Kwong K et al (1988) Diffusion magnetic resonance imaging in multiple sclerosis. Book of abstracts. Society of Magnetic Resonance in Medicine, 7th annual meeting, New York, p 762

64. Minematsu K, Fischer M, Li L et al (1992a) A non-competitive NMDA antagonist, CNS-1102, reduces ischemic injury in vivo and postmortem infarction area (abstract). Neurology 42 [Suppl 3]:292

65. Minematsu K, Li L, Sotak M et al (1992b) Reversible focal ischemic injury demonstrated by diffusion-weighted magnetic resonance imaging in rats. Stroke 23:1304–1311

66. Minematsu K, Li L, Fischer M et al (1992c) Diffusion-weighted magnetic resonance imaging: rapid and quantitative detection of focal brain ischemia. Neurology 42:235–240

67. Minematsu K, Fisher M, Li L et al (1993) Effects of a novel NMDA antagonist on experimental stroke rapidly and quantitatively assessed by diffusion-weighted MRI. Neurology 43:397–406

68. Mintorovitch J, Mosely ME, Chileuitt L et al (1991) Comparison of diffusion- and T2-weighted MRI for the early detection of cerebral ischemia and reperfusion in rats. Magn Reson Med 18:39–50

69. Moonen CTW, Pekar J, de Vleeschouwer MHM et al (1991) Restricted and anisotropic displacement of water in healthy cat brain and in stroke studied by NMR diffusion imaging. Magn Reson Med 19:317–322

70. Moseley ME, Cohen Y, Mintorovitch J et al (1990a) Early detection of regional cerebral ischemia in cats: comparison of diffusion- and T2-weighted MRI and spectroscopy. Magn Reson Med 14:330–346

71. Moseley ME, KucharczykJ, Mintorovitch J et al (1990b) Diffusion-weighted MR imaging of acute stroke: correlation with T2-weighted and magnetic susceptibility-enhanced MR imaging in cats. AJNR 11:423–42

72. Moseley ME, Cohen Y, Kucharczyk J et al (1990c) Diffusion-weighted MR imaging of anisotropic water diffusion in cat central nervous system. Radiology 176:439–445

73. Moseley ME, Wendland MF, Kucharzyk J (1991a) Magnetic resonance imaging of diffusion and perfusion. Top Magn Reson Imaging 3:50–67

74. Moseley M, Kucharczyk J, Asgari HS, Norman D (1991b) Anisotropy in diffusion-weighted MRI. Magn Reson Med 19:321–326

75. National Institute of Neurological Disorders and Stroke (NINDS) (1990) Special report: classification of cerebrovascular diseases. III. Stroke 21:637–676

76. Norbash AM, Glover GH, Enzmann DR (1992) Intracerebral lesion contrast with spin-echo and fast spin-echo pulse sequences. Radiology 185:661–665

77. Norris JW, Hachinski VC (1982) Misdiagnosis of stroke. Lancet 1:328–331

78. Ogawa S, Lee TM, Kay AR, Tank DW (1990) Brain magnetic resonance imaging with contrast dependent on blood oxygenation. Proc Natl Acad Sci USA 87:9868–9872

79. Ogawa S, Tank DW Menon R et al (1992) Intrinsic signal changes accompanying sensory stimulation: functional brain mapping with magnetic resonance imaging. Proc Natl Acad Sci USA 89:5951–5955

80. Ordidge RJ, Guilfoyle DN, Gibbs P, Mansfield P (1989) Real-time flow measurements using echo-planar imaging. Proceedings of the 8th annual meeting of the Society of Magnetic Resonance in Medicine (SMRM), Amsterdam, vol 2, p 889

81. Ordidge RJ, Helpern JA, Qing ZX, Knight RA, Nagesh V (1994) Correction of motional artifacts in diffusion-weighted MR images using navigator echoes. Magn Reson Imaging 12:455–460

82. Rimmington JE, Lin J.-P., Santosh C, Best JJK (1994) Functional MRI at 1 tesla: activation of primary motor cortex and supplementary motor area during complex finger tasks in control and hemiplegic subjects. In: Proceedings of the Society for Magnetic Resonance, p 671

83. Roberts DA, Detre JA, Insko EK et al (1992) Cerebral perfusion imaging in human brain at 1.5T using adiabatic inversion of the arterial input (abstract). 11th annual meeting of the Society of Magnetic Resonance in Medicine, book of abstracts. Society of Magnetic Resonance in Medicine, Berkley, vol 1, p 305

84. Rosen BR, Belliveau JW, Chien D (1989) Perfusion imaging by nuclear magnetic resonance. Magn Reson Q 5:263–281

85. Rosen BR, Belliveau JW, Verea JM, Brady TJ (1990) Perfusion imaging with NMR contrast agents. Magn Reson Med 14:249–265
86. Rosen BR, Belliveau JW, Aronen HJ et al (1991) Susceptibility contrast imaging of cerebral blood volume: human experience. Magn Reson Med 22:293–299
87. Rutherford MA, Cowan FM, Manzur AY et al (1991) MR imaging of anisotropically restricted diffusion in the brain of neonates and infants. J Comput Assist Tomogr 15:188–198
88. Sakuma H, Nomura Y, Takeda K et al (1991) Adult and neonatal human brain: diffusional anisotropy and myelination with diffusion-weighted MR imaging. Radiology 180:229–233
89. Schmitt F, Stehling MK, Ladebeck R, Fang M, Quaiyumi A, Barschneider E, Huk WJ (1992) Echo-Planar imaging of the central nervous system at 1.0 T. J Magn Reson Imaging 2:473–478
90. Schwaighofer BW, Klein MV, Wesbey G et al (1990) Clinical experience with routine Gd-DTPA administration for MR imaging of the brain. J Comput Assist Tomogr 14:11–17
91. Sevick RJ, Kanda F, Mintorovich J et al (1992) Cytotoxic brain edema: assessment with diffusion-weighted MR imaging. Radiology 185:687–690
92. Sibson NR, Gill R, Maskell L et al (1994) The neuroprotective effect of MK-801 in a permanent model of focal cerebral ischemia in the rat assessed using diffusion weighted magnetic resonance imaging. In: Proceedings of the Society for Magnetic Resonance, p 1376
93. Siewert B et al (1995) Stroke and ischemia. MRI Clin North Am 3:529–540
94. Siewert B, Patel MR, Mueller MF, Gaa J, Darby DG, Poser CM, Wielopolski PA, Edelman RR, Warach S (1995) Detection of brain lesions using echo-planar imaging: multiple sclerosis. Radiology 162:765–771
95. Simonson TM, Crosby DL, Fisher DJ et al (1994) Echo-planar FLAIR in the evaluation of intracranial lesions. In: Proceedings of the Society for Magnetic Resonance, p 522
96. Solomon I (1955) Relaxation processes in a system of two spins. Phys Rev 99:559
97. Steen RG (1992) Edema and tumor perfusion: characterization by quantitative 1H MR imaging. AJR 158:259–264
98. Stehling MK, Turner R, Mansfield P (1991a) Echo-planar imaging: magnetic resonance imaging in a fraction of a second. Science 254:43–50
99. Stehling MK, Firth JL, Worthington BS et al (1991b) Observation of cerebrospinal fluid flow with echo-planar magnetic resonance imaging. BR J Radiol 64:89–97
100. Stehling MK, Schmitt F, Ladebeck R (1993) Echo-planar MR imaging of human brain oxygenation changes. J Magn Reson Imaging 4:471–474
101. Stejskal EO, Tanner JE (1965) Spin diffusion measurements: spin echoes in the presence of a time-dependent field gradient. J Chem Phys 42:288–292
102. Thulborn KR, Waterton JC, Matthews PM, Radda GK (1982) Oxygenation dependence of the transverse relaxation time of water protons in whole blood at high field. Biochem Biophys Acta 714:265–270
103. Tien RD, Felsberg GJ, Friedman H et al (1994) MR imaging of high grade cerebral gliomas: value of diffusion-weighted echoplanar pulse sequences. AJR 162:671–677
104. Tsuruda JS, Chew WM, Mosely ME, Norman D (1990) Diffusion-weighted MR imaging of the brain: value of differentiating between extraaxial cysts and epidermoid tumors. AJNR 11:925–931
105. Turner R, Le Bihan D, Maier J et al (1990) Echo-planar imaging of intravoxel incoherent motion. Radiology 177:407–414
106. Turner R, LeBihan D, Chesnick AS (1991a) Echo-planar imaging of diffusion and perfusion. Magn Reson Med 19:247–253
107. Turner R, Le Bihan D, Moonen CTW et al (1991b) Echo planar time course MRI of cat brain oxygenation changes. Magn Reson Med 22:159–166
108. Turner R, Jezzard P, Wen H et al (1993) Functional mapping of the human visual cortex at 4 and 1.5 tesla using deoxygenation contrast EPI. Magn Reson Med 29:227–229
109. Villringer A, Rosen RB, Belliveau JW et al (1988) Dynamic imaging with lanthanide chelates in normal brain: contrast due to magnetic susceptibility effects. Magn Reson Med 6:164–174
110. von Arbin M, Britton M, de Faire U et al (1981) Accuracy of bedside diagnosis in stroke. Stroke 12:288–293
111. Warach S, Chien D, Li W et al (1992a) Fast magnetic resonance diffusion-weighted imaging of acute human stroke. Neurology 42:1717–1723
112. Warach S, Li W, Ronthal M, Edelman RR (1992b) Acute cerebral ischemia: evaluation with dynamic contrast-enhanced MR and MR angiography. Radiology 182:41–47

113. Warach S, Wielopolski P, Edelman RR (1993) Identification of the ischemic penumbra of acute human stroke using echo planar diffusion and perfusion imaging. Proceedings of the 12th annual scientific meeting of the Society of Magnetic Resonance in Medicine, p 263
114. Warach S, Gaa J, Siewert B, Wielopolski PA, Edelman RR (1995) Acute human stroke studied by whole brain echo planar diffusion weighted MRI. Ann Neurol 161:233–236
115. Watanabe M, Tanaka R, Takeda N (1992) Magnetic resonance imaging and histopathology of cerebral gliomas. Neuroradiology 34:463–469
116. Weder B, Knorr U, Herzog H et al (1994) Tactile exploration of shape after subcortical ischemic infarction studied with PET. Brain 117:593–605
117. Weiller CS, Chollet F, Friston KJ et al (1992) Functional reorganization of the brain in recovery from striatocapsular infarction in man. Ann Neurol 31:463–472
118. Weiller C, Ramsay SC, Wise RJS, Friston KJ, Frackowiak RSJ (1993) Individual patterns of functional reorganization in the human cerebral cortex after capsular infarction. Ann Neurol 33:181–189
119. Weisskopf R, Belliveau J, Kwong K, Rosen B (1992) Functional MR imaging of capillary hemodynamics. In: Potchen E (ed) Magnetic resonance angiography: concepts and applications. St Louis, Mosby, pp 473–484
120. Weisskopf RM, Boxerman JL, Sorensen AG et al (1994) Simultaneous blood volume and permeability mapping using a single Gd-based contrast injection. In: Proceedings of the Society for Magnetic Resonance, p 279
121. Wendland MF, White DL, Aicher KP et al (1991) Detection of echo-planar MR imaging of transit susceptibility contrast medium in a rat model of regional brain ischemia. J Magn Reson Imaging 1:285–292
122. Williams DS, Detre JA, Leigh JS, Koretsky AP (1992) Magnetic resonance imaging of perfusion using spin echo inversion of arterial water. Proc Natl Acad Sci USA 82:212–216
123. Worthington BS, Bullock P, Stehling M et al (1991) Clinical experience with contrast enhanced echo-planar imaging of the brain. Magn Reson Med 22:255–258
124. Yuh WTC, Crain MR, Loes DJ et al (1991) MR imaging of cerebral ischemia: findings in the first 24 hours. AJNR 12:621–629
125. Zhong J, Petroff OA, Prichard JW, Gore JC (1993) Changes in water diffusion and relaxation properties of rat cerebrum during status epilepticus. Magn Reson Med 30:241–246

CHAPTER 15

Echo-Planar Magnetic Resonance Imaging of Human Brain Activation

P. A. Bandettini and E. C. Wong

Introduction

Development of new methods to image the thinking human brain is fundamental to unraveling the principles of its workings. The latest and most promising functional brain activation imaging techniques to emerge have been those which use magnetic resonance imaging (MRI). The array of MRI-based techniques used for the study of brain activation has been termed functional MRI (fMRI). Echo-planar imaging (EPI), an ultrafast MRI technique [1–5], has been and continues to be ubiquitous in the ongoing development and application of fMRI in general. In the growing number of centers that have EPI capability, it is the fMRI method of choice. An overview of EPI in the study of human brain function is given in this chapter. A brief overview of fMRI is first given. Second, details regarding the implementation of EPI for fMRI, as of May, 1995, are described. Lastly, EPI is discussed in the context of four developing areas in fMRI: imaging platform or methodology development, contrast mechanism research, postprocessing development, and applications. In the areas of imaging platform development and contrast mechanism research, several examples demonstrating the utility of EPI are given.

fMRI Overview

Brain Activation

When a population of neurons experiences membrane polarity changes during activation, measurable electrical and magnetic changes in the brain are created [6–12]. Because of the energy requirements of membrane repolarization and neurotransmitter synthesis, brain activation also causes a measurable increase in neuronal metabolism [6–8, 13–18]. Through incompletely understood mechanisms [6, 19–30] these changes are accompanied by changes in blood flow [6–8, 19–36], volume [37–40], and oxygenation [39–43]. All techniques for assessing human brain function are based on the detection and measurement of these electrical, magnetic, metabolic, and hemodynamic changes that are spatially and temporally associated with neuronal activation.

MRI of Cerebrovascular Physiology

Pioneering work has shown that MRI can be used to map several types of cerebrovascular information. With MRI, one can create (a) maps of cerebral blood volume [38, 44–50] and flow [3, 51–53] and (b) maps of *changes* in cerebral blood volume [38], flow [3, 53, 54], and oxygenation [54–65].

Blood Volume

A technique developed by Belliveau and Rosen et al. [44–46] utilizes the susceptibility contrast produced by intravascular paramagnetic contrast agents and the high-speed imaging capabilities of EPI to create maps of human cerebral blood volume. A bolus of paramagnetic contrast agent is injected and T2- or T2*-weighted images are obtained at the rate of about one image per second. As the contrast agent passes through the microvasculature, susceptibility gradients (magnetic field distortions) are produced. These gradients cause an intravoxel dephasing of extravascular proton spins, resulting in a transient signal attenuation. The signal attenuation is linearly proportional to the concentration of contrast agent [44, 45, 66], which in turn is a function of blood volume.

Changes in blood volume that occur during hemodynamic stresses or during brain activation may then created by subtraction of two maps: one during a "resting" state and one during the hemodynamic stress or during activation [38]. The use of this method marked the first time that hemodynamic changes accompanying human brain activation were mapped with MRI.

Blood Flow

Blood flow spans several size and velocity scales. Imaging of large cerebral vessels having rapid flow rates by MR cerebral angiography [50, 67, 68] has been a clinical technique since the middle 1980s.

Imaging and quantification of microvascular flow in the brain has been not yet been fully realized. Two techniques for MRI of cerebral microvasculature have been proposed. LeBihan et al. proposed a technique in which capillary flow is modeled as a fast diffusive process [69–72]. With this intravoxel incoherent motion (IVIM) model, it has been suggested that techniques used to measure diffusion can be used to measure microvascular flow. This technique, while theoretically feasible, has practical limitations which include contamination from cerebral spinal fluid and other tissue motion on the same velocity scales [73] and the requirement of a signal-to-noise ratio (SNR) that is not practically achieved in most imaging studies [74].

A second technique for quantifying microvascular blood flow entails MR detection of inflowing labeled arterial water spins, and was first demonstrated in animals [51, 52]. With this technique blood water flowing to the brain is radiofrequency (RF) saturated outside the imaging plane (usually in the neck region). Because of the relatively long blood T1 times, saturated spins are able to maintain much of their magnetization state as they travel into the plane of interest and exchange, at the capillary level, longitudinal magnetization with bulk water in the brain. The resulting regional concentration of labeled spins in tissue is a function of regional tissue blood flow.

A recently developed extension of this flow imaging technique, named echo-planar imaging with signal targeting and alternating RF (EPISTAR), has been used to map both macrovascular and microvascular flow [3, 75] in humans. This technique is based on the idea of subtracting two image data sets that are identical except for differences in longitudinal magnetization arising from inflowing spins. One data set is acquired after a remote 180° pulse is applied to invert the inflowing arterial spins. The first set is subtracted from a second data set, acquired without the inversion pulse, thus giving a difference map which is a function of flow.

This technique can be made sensitive to different levels of flow velocity by varying the delay time between the inversion pulse and the image acquisition. Maps of arterial flow are created using a relatively short inversion pulse-acquisition delay time of 400 ms. Maps of microvascular flow and exchange processes are created using an inversion pulse-acquisition delay time of 1000 ms or more. After the 1000-ms waiting period tagged magnetization is either within the capillary bed or in the extravascular space in the immediate vicinity of capillaries.

With the use of flow map subtraction changes in blood flow corresponding to hemodynamic stress or brain activation can be mapped as well. The two maps can then be subtracted to reveal regions where changes in flow have occurred [3, 75].

An alternative flow sensitive method is performed by application of the inversion pulse in the same plane. In this case the image intensity is weighted not only by modulation of longitudinal magnetization by flowing spins but also by other MR parameters that normally contribute to image intensity and contrast (proton density, T1, T2). Therefore the application of an inversion pulse in the same plane only allows for observation of changes in flow that occur with hemodynamic stress or brain activation. This technique was first implemented by Kwong et al. [54] to observe activation-induced flow changes in the human brain. In this seminal study activation-induced signal changes associated with local changes in blood oxygenation were also observed.

Blood Oxygenation

In 1932 Pauling et al. [76] discovered that the magnetic susceptibility of hemoglobin is sensitive to its oxygen saturation. The susceptibility of red blood cells decreases linearly from a fully oxygenated value of $-0.26\pm0.07\times10^{-6}$ (CGS units) to a fully deoxygenated value of $0.157\pm0.07\times10^{-6}$, giving a difference in susceptibility of 0.18×10^{-6} between 100% blood oxygenation and 0% blood oxygenation states [77]. This susceptibility difference results from the fact that oxyhemoglobin contains diamagnetic oxygen-bound iron and deoxyhemoglobin contains paramagnetic iron [76, 78, 79].

In 1982 Thulborn et al. [79] demonstrated that the transverse relaxation rate, R2 (or 1/T2), of blood decreases with an increase in blood oxygenation. Because minimal changes in T1 of whole blood were observed upon the oxygenation changes, it was suggested that the primary mechanism of relaxation change is related to diffusion of spins through susceptibility-induced gradients (which affects T2 relaxation) and not due to dipolar interactions (which affects T1 and T2 relaxation). The R2 dependence of blood on its oxygen saturation has been confirmed by several other studies [77, 80–90].

In 1990 pioneering work of Ogawa et al. [59–61] and Turner et al. [63] demonstrated that MR signal in the vicinity of vessels and in perfused brain tissue decreases with a decrease in blood oxygenation. This type of physiological contrast was coined blood oxygenation level dependent (BOLD) contrast by Ogawa et al. [61].

The use of BOLD contrast for the observation of brain activation was first demonstrated in August of 1991 at the 10th Annual Meeting of the Society of Magnetic Resonance in Medicine [91]. The first papers demonstrating the technique, published in July 1992, reported human brain activation in the primary visual cortex [54, 62] and motor cortex [54, 56]. Two [54, 56] of the first three reports of this technique involved the use of EPI. In these experiments a small but significant local signal increase in activated cortical regions was observed using susceptibility-weighted, gradient-echo pulse sequences.

The working model constructed to explain these observations was that an increase in neuronal activity causes local vasodilatation which, in turn, causes an increase in blood flow. This results in an excess of oxygenated hemoglobin beyond the metabolic need, thus *reducing* the proportion of paramagnetic deoxyhemoglobin in the vasculature. This hemodynamic phenomenon had previously been suggested using other techniques [40–42], and later came to the attention of MR investigators attempting to explain these localized activation-induced MR signal increases. A reduction in deoxyhemoglobin in the vasculature causes a reduction in susceptibility differences in the vicinity of venules, veins, and red blood cells within veins, thereby causing an increase in spin coherence (increase in T2 and T2*) and therefore an increase in signal in T2*- and/or T2-weighted sequences.

Presently the most widely used fMRI technique for the noninvasive mapping of human brain activity is high-speed gradient-echo imaging using BOLD contrast. The reasons for this are that (a) gradient-echo T2*-sensitive techniques have demonstrated higher activation-induced signal change contrast than techniques having T2-weighed, flow-sensitive, and blood volume-sensitive techniques, and (b) BOLD contrast can be obtained using more widely available high-speed multi-shot non-EPI techniques.

Several ongoing issues regarding interpretation, postprocessing, and the limits of applicability of fMRI remain. As is shown below, EPI is a technique that because of its speed, efficiency, and robustness lends itself well to the understanding and resolution of these issues.

Implementation of EPI for fMRI

Several issues regarding the implementation of EPI are briefly addressed here in the context of fMRI. These include issues of spatial resolution, hardware, biological limitations, artifacts, software, and data handling.

Spatial resolution in single-shot EPI is limited either by the area of k space that can be critically sampled in approximately one T2* period or by the system bandwidth [92]. The area of k space that can be covered can be limited by the velocity in k space (gradient amplitude) or the acceleration in k space (gradient slew rate) and is typically limited by both. The tradeoff between gradient amplitude and gradient slew rate in the design of the gradient system is one that has application-specific optima; systems that are designed specifically for single-shot EPI therefore generally perform this function most efficiently.

The requirement for strong and rapidly switching gradients can be satisfied by increasing the gradient amplifier power, implementing resonant gradient technology, or by reducing the inductance of the gradient coils such that they can be driven by conventional gradient amplifiers. The latter strategy may be implemented by using a gradient coil that is localized only to the head. Figure 1 illustrates an example of a local gradient coil used for EPI on an otherwise conventional system. The three-axis balanced torque gradient coil (ID = 30 cm, length = 37 cm) was designed and constructed by Wong [93]. The method of design was gradient descent [94]. The gradient fields were optimized for a region that covers the human brain (cylinder of diameter 18.75 cm and length 16.5 cm.) The maximum gradient strengths (G/cm 100 A) are 2.272 G/cm for X, 2.336 G/cm for Y, and 2.487 G/cm for Z. As a result of the low coil inductance (0.149 mH for X, 0.174 mH for Y, and 0.076 mH for Z), the minimum rise time from zero amplitude to full scale is approximately 50 µs. For a comprehensive review on techniques for designing gradient coils, please refer to Turner [95]. While the use of local gradient coils makes single-shot EPI possible on standard clinical systems, the system bandwidth may limit its implementation. Inadequate bandwidths may limit the useful gradient amplitude, thereby reducing spatial resolution. Lastly, single-shot EPI can be carried out on a conventional imaging system

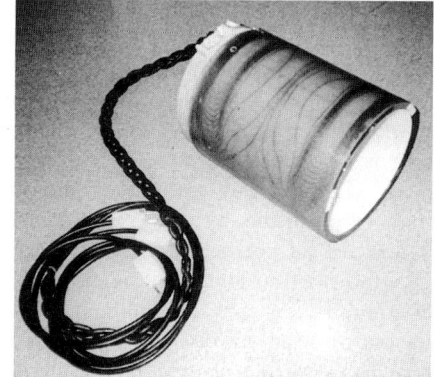

Fig. 1. The three-axis balanced torque head gradient coil used for EPI on conventional clinical MRI scanners. ID = 30 cm; length = 37 cm. The maximum gradient strengths (G/cm at 100 A) are 2.272 G/cm for X, 2.336 G/cm for Y, and 2.487 G/cm for Z. Inductances are 0.149 mH for X, 0.174 mH for Y, and 0.076 mH for Z. Minimum rise time from zero amplitude to full scale is approximately 50 µs

without the use of local gradient coils by simply using a large field of view and/ or a small image matrix size [96].

A major non-hardware-related limitation on gradient slew rate is the biological threshold for neuronal stimulation due to time-varying magnetic fields. At present high-performance gradient systems (either local gradient coils or high-powered whole body systems) are capable of exceeding the guidelines of the United States Food and Drug Administration on field slew rate (dB/dt), and the optimization of EPI pulse sequences is strongly affected by dB/dt considerations. Taking all these considerations into account, optimal spatial resolution in the human head for single-shot EPI is achieved at these approximate values: matrix of 128×128, bandwidth of 250 kHz, gradient strength of 4 G/cm, and data acquisition window of 80 ms.

The requirements for successful implementation of EPI for fMRI are not limited to hardware. In most cases phase correction algorithms are a necessity to compensate for timing errors related to imperfections in the gradients, gradient-induced eddy currents, and static field inhomogeneities. The timing errors generally manifest themselves as Nyquist ghosts. Even if the ghosts are not completely eliminated from each image, they usually remain stable in intensity and location from image to image over time. Also, since the location of the ghosts is usually outside of the head, they usually do not cause significant problems in the interpretation of the functional images.

Because of the long-sampling time and artifactual phase modulation, two other types of off-resonance related artifacts exist in EPI: signal dropout, and image distortion.

Signal dropout is primarily due to intravoxel phase dispersion resulting from through plane variation of magnetic field. This effect is common to all gradient-recalled imaging techniques, and is dependent primarily on the TE and slice thickness and the local shim in specific regions of the brain. The problem of signal dropout in gradient-echo sequences can be reduced by reduction of the voxel volume. Therefore gradient-echo image quality, if acquired at the base of the brain where large susceptibility gradients exits, is improved by reduction of voxel volume. Also, this effect is greatly reduced in spin-echo EPI as well as other spin-echo techniques because the macroscopic off-resonance effects are refocused at the echo time.

Image distortion is caused by the phase modulation that occurs during data acquisition. Because the artifactual phase modulation is linear in time, it is directly proportional to the data acquisition time. In EPI this linear phase modulation creates primarily a linear distortion of the image in the phase encode direction whose magnitude is given by the Fourier shift theorem. If the phase modulation is 2π across the data acquisition window, the shift in image space is one pixel. Thus for a 40-ms data acquisition window a signal that is 25 Hz off resonance is shifted by one pixel. Several postprocessing methods have been put forward for correcting image distortion in EPI [97–99].

The image distortion effect is present in conventional imaging techniques as well. For example, if a conventional spin-warp technique is used with the same resolution and the same data acquisition time as used with EPI, the distortion is the same. However, the distortion in spin-warp imaging techniques is typically smaller because the data acquisition times are shorter and the resolution is higher, both of which decrease the magnitude of the distortion. It should be noted, however, that it is exactly these two parameters, higher resolution and shorter data acquisition times, that decreases the SNR per unit time of spin-warp techniques relative to EPI.

The artifacts caused by macroscopic off-resonance effects are also dependent on k space traversal path. In the case of spiral imaging off-resonance effects are not manifested as Nyquist ghosts or image distortion but as blurring [4, 100]. Figure 2 shows a comparison of single-shot blipped EPI (40 ms acquisition window) and single-shot spiral EPI (28 ms acquisition window). The anatomical images differ in that the blipped image is sharper but more distorted. The spiral image shows apparently less distortion but much more blurring in the radial direction. A time course of blipped and spiral images were collected during which the subject performed periodic bilateral finger tapping. Functional correlation images, shown below the anatomical images, were created by calculation of the vector product of a reference waveform with the time course of each voxel [101]. Note that both sequences reveal signal enhancement in the supplementary and primary motor cortex and possibly the somatosensory cortex. The locations and extents of the activated regions appear different due to the different sensitivity to gross off-resonance effects. It should also be noted that because the central part of k space is usually covered very early in the spiral path, the sequence is less sensitive to flow than blipped sequences are [100, 102].

Another practical but significant factor to be considered when performing fMRI with EPI is the rapidity with which large amounts of data are collected. This data may then go through several additional transformations (adding to the total required data storage capacity) before a functional image is created. If ten slices having 64×64 resolution are acquired every 2 s (typical for multislice fMRI), the data acquisition rate is approximately 2 MB per minute.

Fig. 2. Demonstration of the relative sensitivity of single-shot blipped and spiral EPI to off-resonance effects. *Left,* single-shot blipped EPI is sharper but distorted; *right,* single-shot circular spiral EPI is not distorted but is more blurred. Functional correlation images demonstrate similar functional contrast but slightly different locations

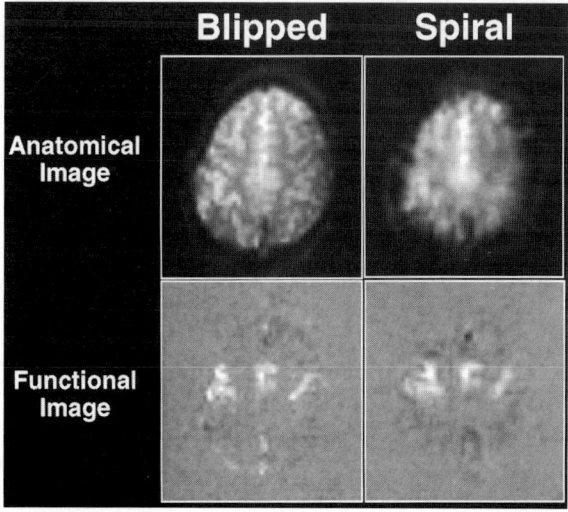

Research in fMRI

Research in fMRI can be divided into four overlapping and interdependent categories: functional imaging hardware and pulse sequence development, contrast mechanism research, postprocessing development, and applications. In all of these categories the use of EPI has been extensive, primarily because for most applications its robustness outweighs its limitations. In the remainder of the chapter the role of EPI in each of these research categories is discussed.

fMRI Hardware and Pulse Sequence Development

The first fMRI experiments were carried out using EPI at 1.0 [103], 1.5 [54, 56, 64, 91, 104, 105], 2.1 [57], 3.0 [106], and 4 T [64], and fast multi-shot gradient-recalled imaging techniques at 1.5 [64], 2 [58, 107], and 4 T [62]. Platforms for fMRI vary considerably in terms of pulse sequence, field strength, gradient hardware, and RF coil hardware. Generally, fMRI platform evolution has been in the direction of increased functional contrast-to-noise ratio (CNR), temporal resolution, spatial resolution, and hemodynamic specificity.

Functional Contrast-to-Noise Ratio

Functional contrast relates to the detection of activation-induced signal changes in space (as opposed to nonactivated regions) and time (as opposed resting state signal). The most fundamental of needs in fMRI is a high functional CNR to detect small signal changes. When using gradient-echo sequences, maximal susceptibility contrast is achieved by using TE approximately equal to $T2^*$ [57, 108, 109]. In addition, studies have shown, largely in agreement with predictions of several susceptibility contrast models [66, 110–114], that BOLD contrast increases with field strength [62, 64, 106, 108, 115, 116]. However, because of its sensitivity to off-resonance effects, performance of EPI is more difficult, but still possible, at higher field strengths [64, 106, 116–118].

An alternative to increasing contrast is reduction in the noise relative to the image signal intensity. Several simple strategies are commonly used in fMRI to increase SNR – most of which EPI is well suited for. The use of a relatively long TR, 90° flip angle, and temporal averaging of several hundred images can be performed in an experimentally feasible amount of time using EPI. Also, with EPI the long data acquisition times that are typically used in order to achieve acceptable spatial resolution are approximately equal to the $T2^*$ of gray matter – optimal from the point of view of maximizing the SNR.

Many of the sources of signal contamination are not from system or thermal noise but rather from cardiac and respiration-related pulsatile motion [100, 102, 119–123] or subject movement [124] or possibly from susceptibility gradient variations related to spontaneous changes in flow [125, 126] or respiration-related changes in chest cavity size, which has been suggested to cause changes in B_0 as far away as the head region (Ugurbil, personal communication). Therefore the CNR can also be increased by reduction of signal fluctuations that contribute to the noise.

In conventional multi-shot techniques pulsatile motion during data acquisition has been shown to cause variation in k space registration which primarily causes nonrepeatable ghosting variations across each image, adding significantly to the noise [100, 102]. With EPI physiological motion is "frozen" by the short 40-ms acquisition time of all k space, enabling stable line-to-line registration across each image during acquisition – thus reducing this source of noise significantly.

In EPI gross displacement generally manifests itself as misregistration at edges and as some isolated signal propagation in the phase encode direction from rapidly flowing or moving spins [127]. Asymmetric spin-echo EPI, with similar contrast weighting as gradient-echo EPI, has demonstrated a reduction in artifacts caused by rapidly flowing and pulsatile spins because the 180° pulse does not refocus rapidly flowing spins [128].

Among non-EPI techniques multi-shot spiral-scan sequences [100, 102], sequences employing oblique motion compensation [129], and sequences employing navigator pulses [130] have all demonstrated more signal stability over time and less artifactual signal changes than standard two- or three-dimensional Fourier transform multi-shot techniques.

The SNR can also be increased by the use of region-selective RF coils. Optimally, the RF coil should couple only to the regions that are being studied, such as surface coils over the occipital pole in visual stimulation studies. However, it is becoming increasingly desirable for most functional imaging studies to observe the entire brain. For whole-brain studies whole-head quadrature coils commonly used clinically for head and neck imaging are suboptimal because they couple to other tissue that is not of interest, causing an unnecessary increase in noise. Recently quadrature whole-brain transmit-receive coils that couple predominantly to the brain have been implemented for fMRI [131, 132].

Temporal Resolution

Because the fMRI signal change is based on hemodynamic changes, the practical upper limit on functional temporal resolution is determined by MRI SNR and by the variation of the hemodynamic response latency in space and in time [133–139]. These variations may be due to differences in neuronal activation characteristics across tasks [137, 138], to differences in vessel size [133, 134], or to other physiological or anatomical differences. In primary visual and motor cortex the latency of the hemodynamic response is approximately 5–8 s from stimulus onset to 90 % maximum, and 5–9 s from stimulus cessation to 10 % above baseline [54, 57, 101, 138–141]. This latency has been described as a shifting and smoothing transformation of the neuronal input [142]. Given the variations of the hemodynamic response, the upper limit of temporal resolution discrimination has been empirically determined to be on the order of 1 s [136] or less [143]. With greater specificity for hemodynamic scale, higher SNR, and innovative experimental design this upper limit on temporal resolution may be increased even further.

For many types of investigations it may be desirable to use experimental paradigms similar to those used in event-related potential recordings or magnetoencephalography [144], in which multiple runs of transient stimuli are averaged together. For this type of paradigm, requiring rapid sampling and high SNR for a very brief duration, EPI is optimal. As a side note, because of the brief collection time of EPI relative to typical TR values the between-image waiting time allows performance of EEG in the scanner during the imaging session [145].

The type of neuronal and/or hemodynamic information that may be obtained from signals elicited from brief stimuli paradigms may be different from the information elicited by longer duration activation times. Transient activation durations (<1 s) are detectable as MR signal changes which begin to increase 2 s after the activation onset and plateau at 3–4 s after activation [135, 139, 140, 143, 146]. Figure 3 shows signal intensity vs. time from a region in motor cortex in which the subject performed a finger tapping task for 0.5 s.

Unique information may also be obtained from rapidly sampled and highly averaged time course data. As an example of unique hemodynamic information obtained in this manner, a small decrease in signal before the subsequent signal increase with photic stimulation has been observed by Menon et al. [117, 118] using EPI at 4 T.

The study of the underlying noise from which activation-induced signal changes must be separated is also highly important for both detailed physiological studies and postprocessing development. Frequency components contained in signal fluctuations have been characterized using EPI [120, 121, 147]. An example is given of how the use of EPI allows for characterization of signal fluctuations. In this study the a time course of images were rapidly collected during rest. After reaching steady state magnetization 125 images were collected in 25 s (voxel volume = 3.75×3.75×10 mm^3, flip angle = 60°. TR = 200 ms). Signal intensity was measured from a voxel in the sagittal sinus. Figure 4 shows a plot of signal vs. time from a region containing the sagittal sinus and the Fourier transform of that signal. The peak at about 45 beats per minute corresponds to the volunteer's heart rate (a marathon runner). An anatomical image of the axial slice observed

Fig. 3. Signal intensity (from a single run) vs. time from a region in motor cortex. TR/TE = 1000 ms/40 ms. Two 0.5-s episodes of finger movement were performed. Signal intensity begins to increase 2 s after activation, peaks 4–5 s after activation, then returns to baseline 8–9 s after activation

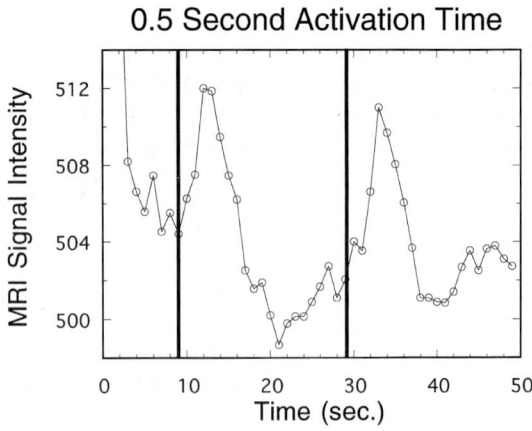

Fig. 4. Signal intensity vs. time from a voxel in the sagittal sinus. TE/TR = 40 ms/200 ms. *Below*, Fourier transform of the signal vs. time plot, revealing a peak at the heart-rate

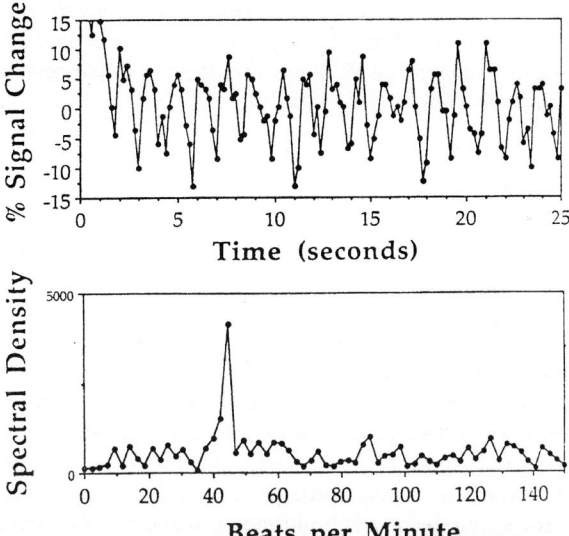

and the spectral density image at that frequency is shown in Fig. 5. High signal intensity regions in this spectral density image correspond to voxels containing cerebral spinal fluid and large vessels. The source of these signal changes is likely periodic time-of-flight inflow effects of unsaturated magnetization.

With the use of EPI approximately ten images may be obtained per second – giving the option to image the entire brain in under 2 s or to sample a smaller number of imaging planes to allow a more dense sampling of the time course. Another possibility in EPI is to sample less densely in space but to cover a large volume in a single shot. This technique is known as echo-volume imaging [1, 5, 148].

The more rapid the feedback of fMRI data, the more easily experiments can be fine-tuned or appropriately adjusted. If EPI is used in conjunction with real-time functional image formation [149], the quality of functional images can be monitored during time course scanning until the desired functional image quality is

Fig. 5. Anatomical image and spectral density image at the above heart rate frequency peak, revealing regions of periodic signal changes in the brain

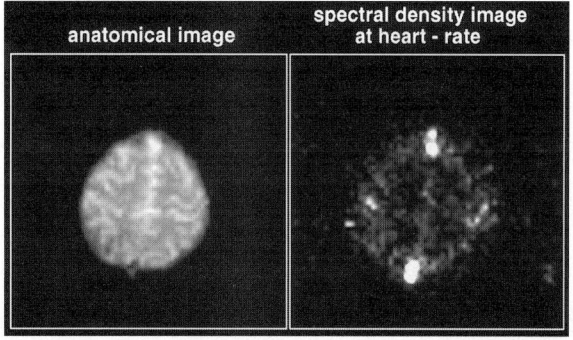

obtained. Also, if single slice studies are desired, the use of EPI can allow for an iterative search until the appropriate region is located – similar to a clinical scout scan. In general, EPI allows this type of iterative approach to be performed in a reasonable amount of time.

Spatial Resolution

The upper limit on functional spatial resolution, similarly to the limit of temporal resolution, is likely determined not by MRI resolution limits but by the hemodynamics through which neuronal activation is transduced. Evidence from in vivo high-resolution optical imaging of the activation of ocular dominance columns [41–43] suggests that neuronal control of blood oxygenation occurs on a spatial scale of less than 0.5 mm. On the other hand, MR evidence exists which suggests that the blood oxygenation increases that occur upon brain activation may be more extensive than the actual activated regions [133, 134, 150–153]. In other words, it is possible that, while the local oxygenation may be regulated on a submillimeter scale, the subsequent changes in oxygenation may occur on a larger scale due to a "spill-over" effect.

To achieve the goal of high spatial resolution fMRI a high functional CNR and reduced signal contribution from draining veins is necessary. Greater hemodynamic specificity, accomplished by proper pulse sequence choice, innovative activation protocol design, or proper interpretation of signal change latency, may allow greater functional spatial resolution. If the contribution to activation-induced signal changes from larger collecting veins or arteries can be easily identified and/or eliminated, not only is confidence in the brain activation localization increased, but also the upper limits of spatial resolution are determined by scanner resolution and BOLD CNR rather than variations in vessel architecture.

Currently voxel volumes as low as 1.2 µl have been obtained by functional fast low-angle shot techniques at 4 T [115], and experiments specifically devoted to probing the upper limits of functional spatial resolution, using spiral scan techniques, have shown that fMRI can reveal activity localized to patches of cortex having a size of about 1.35 mm [154]. These studies and others carried out using EPI [155] and multi-shot spiral scanning [154, 156] have observed a close tracking of MR signal change along the calcarine fissure as the location of visual stimuli was varied.

The voxel dimensions typically used in single-shot EPI studies are in the range of 3–4 mm, in plane, and have 4- to 10-mm slice thicknesses. As mentioned, these dimensions are determined by practical limitations such as readout window length, sampling bandwidth, limits of dB/dt, SNR, and data storage capacity. In spite of these limitations higher resolution single-shot EPI can be performed in some situations. Figure 6 presents an example of four functional studies using progressively higher resolution single-shot gradient-echo EPI. The imaging plane contains the motor cortex. The subject was instructed to perform periodic bilateral finger tapping. Anatomical and functional correlation images and corresponding voxel dimensions are shown. The size of the activated region appears

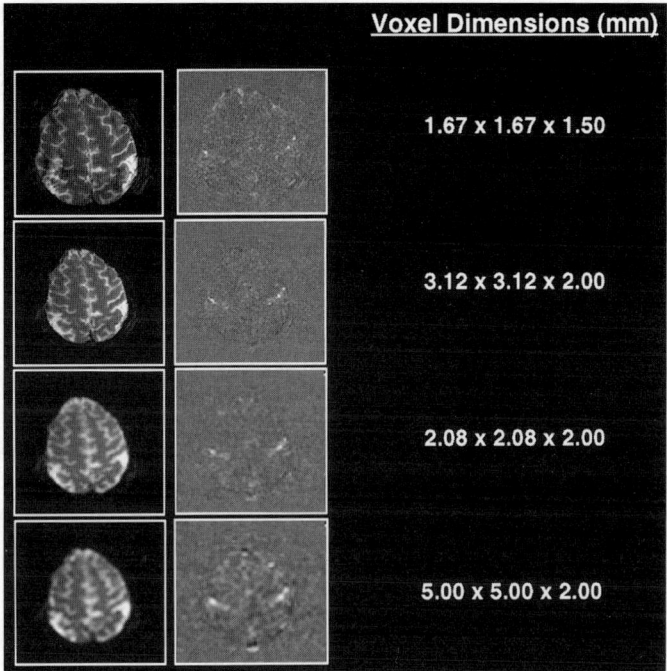

Fig. 6. Demonstration of progressively higher resolution single-shot gradient-echo EPI. Anatomical and functional correlation images from a single subject performing bilateral finger movement

to decrease as the spatial resolution is increased. At low resolution either more subtle capillary-related signal changes are being observed (due to the higher SNR) along with large vessel effects, or large vessel effects are simply being partial volumed with inactive areas in the same large voxels.

Other ways to bypass the practical scanner limits in spatial resolution include partial k space acquisition [4] and multi-shot mosaic or interleaved EPI [4, 157, 158]. An example of multi-shot interleaved EPI in the context of fMRI is given in Fig. 7 (images provided by S. Tan). Axial anatomical and corresponding functional correlation images containing motor cortex are shown. The subject performed cyclic bilateral finger tapping. The highest resolution image was obtained in 4 s. The voxel dimensions for this image are $0.937 \times 0.937 \times 5$ mm. The activated regions, while reduced in size, are clearly visible. In many fMRI situations multi-shot EPI may be the optimum compromise between spatial resolution, SNR, and temporal resolution for fMRI.

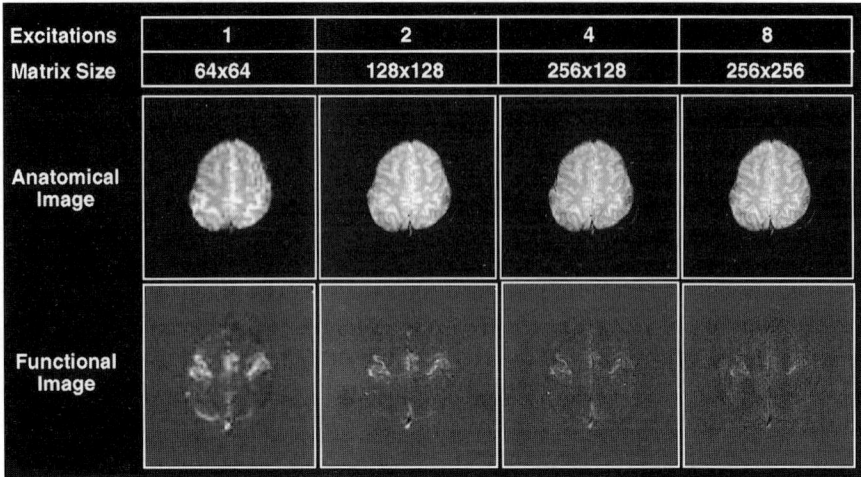

Excitations	1	2	4	8
Matrix Size	64x64	128x128	256x128	256x256
Anatomical Image				
Functional Image				

Fig. 7. Demonstration of progressively higher resolution multi-shot interleaved EPI. Anatomical and functional correlation images from a single subject performing bilateral finger movement. (Images were provided by S. Tan)

Hemodynamic Specificity

The interpretability of fMRI depends to a large degree on the specific hemodynamic sensitization that is possible. Changes in flow, volume, and oxygenation can be selectively observed with fMRI: volume changes – using rapidly obtained T2*- or T2-weighted sequences in combination with bolus administration of a paramagnetic contrast agent [38], flow changes – using inversion recovery [53, 54] or short TR/short TE sequences [151, 159], and oxygenation changes – using T2*- or T2-weighted sequences [54, 56–65, 109]. Also, intravascular vs. extravascular effects may be discerned by appropriate choice of velocity-dephasing gradients [160–163]. Large vessel vs. small vessel effects may be selectively observed by careful interpretation of relative activation -induced R2 and R2* changes [109, 113, 164, 165] as well as by inspection of high resolution T2*-weighted images at high field strength [108]. Veins in the latter case show up as dark spots in the high resolution T2*-weighted images. Because the typical implementation of single-shot EPI involves the acquisition of one image every RF excitation followed by a waiting period of about 1 s, many of the above-mentioned hemodynamic-specific pulse-sequence manipulations can be applied without any sacrifice in imaging time and without additional contamination from motion artifacts which is especially important in the case of diffusion weighting. Figure 8 illustrates schematically, the types of manipulations that can be easily implemented for hemodynamic specificity using EPI.

A comparison of activation-induced signal change locations across several pulse sequence weightings, keeping all else constant, is given below. Each time course series consisted of 240 sequential images. (TR = 2 s, voxel

Fig. 8. Schematic illustration of the types of contrast manipulations that can be implemented for achieving hemodynamic specificity with EPI

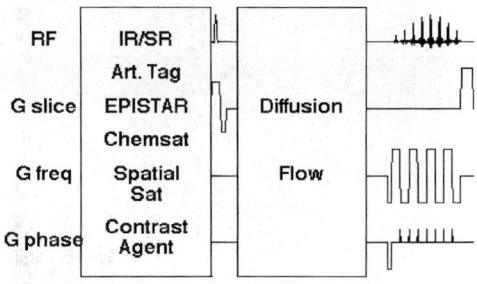

volume = 3.75×3.75×5 mm.) Total time course length was 480 s. Table 1 displays the EPI pulse sequence parameters used and their respective contrast weightings, based on what has been hypothesized in the literature [3, 51, 52, 54, 113]. During each time course series, sequential, bilateral finger tapping was performed in alternating 20-s rest and 20-s activation cycles. Functional correlation images were then created. Figure 9 displays the first image in each of the six time course series. Figure 10 displays the corresponding functional correlation images showing activation in primary motor cortex regions. In spite of the different hemodynamic specificity of each sequence, the activated regions are similar in location, extent, and shape. However, on closer inspection of a magnification of the images, shown in Fig. 11, a systematic shift in activation foci is apparent. In the T2*-weighted images the focal points of activation appear more lateral on

Table 1. Pulse sequences and the corresponding image contrast and functional contrast weightings

Sequence	Parameters	Contrast weighting	Flow	Oxygenation	
				BOLD (>20 μm)	BOLD (<20 μm)
Inversion recovery	TI = 1200 TR = 2000 TE = 60	High T1 Slight T2	y		x
Asymmetric spin-echo inversion recovery	TI = 1200 TR = 2000 TE = 60 τ = 40	High T1 High T2* Slight T2	y	y	x
Asymmetric spin-echo	TR = 2000 TE = 60 τ = 40	High T2* Slight T2		y	x
Spin-echo	TR = 2000 TE = 60, 100	Slight T2 High T2			x,y
Gradient-echo	TR = 2000 TE = 40	High T2*		y	y

y = high sensitivity, x = low sensitivity, according to the current models, to flow or to changes in blood oxygenation in large (greater than 20 μm) compartments and small (less than 20 μm) compartments.

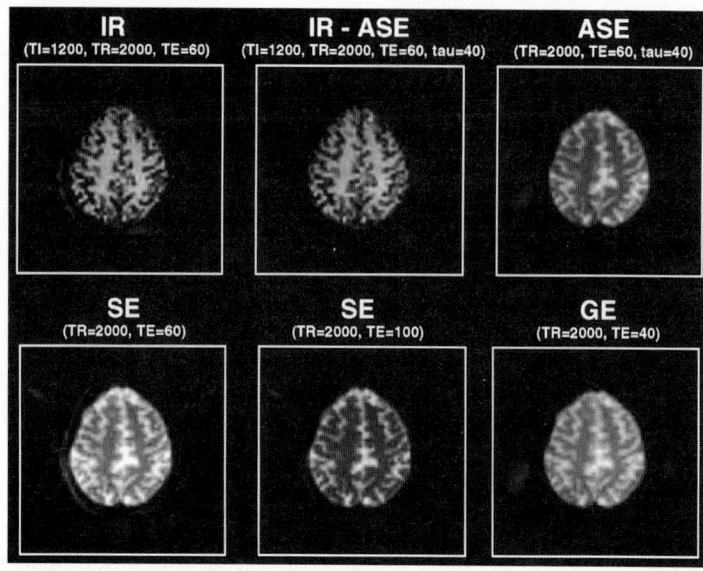

Fig. 9. First image in each of the EPI time course series having different contrast weightings. *IR*, inversion recovery; *ASE*, asymmetric spin echo; *SE*, spin echo; *GE*, gradient echo

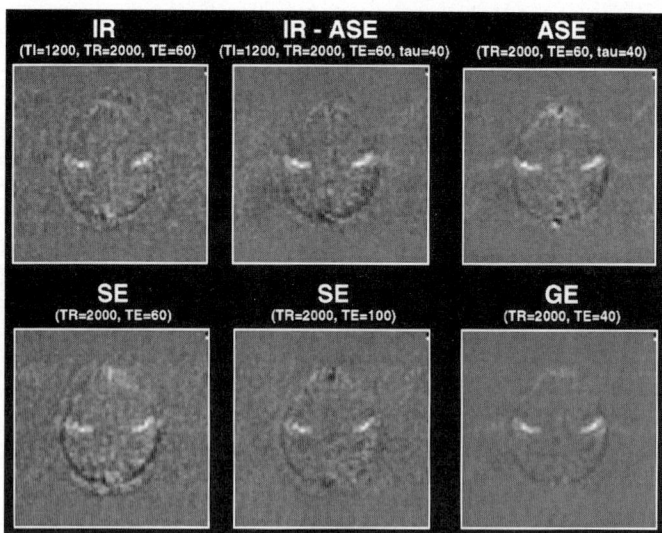

Fig. 10. Functional correlation images created from time course series of corresponding images (Fig. 9). Differences can be seen in functional contrast to noise and actifactual contamination. Overall similarity of activated region locations and extents is apparent. For abbreviations, see Table 1

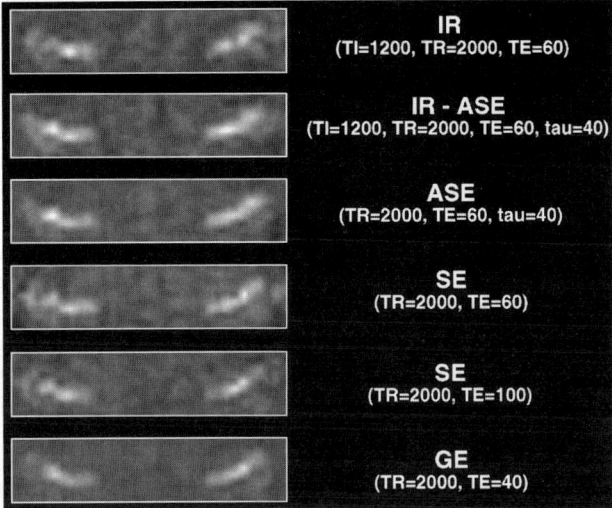

Fig. 11. Magnification of functional correlation images given in Fig. 10. Comparison of the different pulse sequences demonstrates subtle and systematic shifts in activation locations. For abbreviations, see Fig. 9

both sides. In the T1- and the T2-weighted images the focal points are located several millimeters more centrally. In the correlation image that was obtained using the asymmetric spin-echo inversion-recovery sequence, which is both T2*- and T1-weighted, two foci appear on the left side of the image that correspond to the individual foci obtained separately using the other sequences.

While not giving any definitive conclusion about underlying hemodynamic processes, these studies illustrate the flexibility that EPI offers in the time-efficient collection of images having several different contrast weightings. Regardless of the hemodynamic weighting of the pulse sequence it is heartening to note that the regions showing activation in this study predominantly overlap.

Contrast Mechanism Research

Research performed to characterize the details of the fMRI contrast mechanisms has been motivated by the desire to determine a correlation of the magnitude, spatial extent, and timing of the observed MR signal changes with underlying neuronal activation magnitude, extent, and timing. While it is generally accepted that MR signal changes are transduced through neuronally induced hemodynamic changes, the following two relationships are not clear: (a) the relationship between the magnitude, timing, and spatial extent of neuronal activation and the magnitude, timing, and spatial extent of the hemodynamic changes, and (b) the relationship between the degree, timing, and spatial extent of induced hemodynamic changes and the degree, timing, and spatial extent of the MR signal changes.

The difficulty in activation-induced signal change contrast mechanism research is that the *actual* location, magnitude, and timing of neuronal activation is imprecisely known. In general, contrast mechanism studies have involved well-controlled modulation of many potentially significant parameters. By parameter modulation and subsequent comparison with an ever-growing model which includes MR physics, cerebral physiology, and neurology a large amount of convergent information about the relative contributions to MR signal changes has been and continues to be obtained.

Strategies for a more complete understanding of fMRI contrast mechanisms have involved: (a) observation of the dependence of the magnitude, timing, and spatial extent of activation-induced signal changes upon MR parameters such as TE [62, 108, 109, 116, 164–167], TI [3], flip angle [151], B_0 [62, 64, 106, 108, 116], slice thickness and resolution [107, 152, 153, 166], outer volume saturation [159], and diffusion weighting [160–163], (b) observation of the resting signal, and activation-induced signal changes, during different degrees of hemodynamic stress [59–61, 63, 168–173] or during different degrees of neuronal activity (visual flicker rate, finger tapping rate, syllable presentation rate) [54, 135, 139, 140, 174, 175], (c) comparison of signal locations with macroscopic vessel maps [108, 133, 134, 152, 153] or neuronal activation maps [176–178], and (d) modeling of activation-induced MR signal changes based upon knowledge of MR physics and human cerebral physiology [66, 111–114, 179–181].

EPI lends itself well to many of these contrast mechanism studies since its pulse sequence parameters are easily modulated, and many images can be obtained rapidly with minimal systematic artifacts which can become more problematic with longer image time course acquisition times. Presented below is an example of how EPI can be utilized in the study of fMRI contrast mechanisms.

Relaxation Rate Comparison

As mentioned above, many variables can contribute to the a change in MR signal intensity during brain activation. Among the possible sources of activation-induced MR signal changes are a decrease in R2* and R2, movement near a high signal intensity gradient, a net frequency shift causing a subvoxel spatial shift, an increase in apparent T1 relaxation rate caused by perfusion changes, and a possible change in proton density. The extent to which these parameters contribute depends on the pulse sequence parameters and conditions of the experiment.

The degree to which each parameter contributes to the signal intensity change under specific pulse-sequence conditions is a question that is central to a large proportion of contrast mechanism studies. For example, the issue of flow vs. oxygenation contrast entails understanding how much of the signal change (or what areas) are related primarily to oxygenation changes and how much is due to non-susceptibility related flow changes. It is essentially a question of localization, interpretation, and ultimately quantification. The proportion and location of large draining veins vs. capillary contributions affects BOLD contrast. Large draining veins may cause oxygenation-related signal changes far removed from regions of activation due to the fact that the blood volume in each voxel heavily weights the magnitude of susceptibility-related signal change. Also, large vessels may give artificial "hot spots" that may be misinterpreted as the location of highest neuronal activation. These issues are not yet been fully understood. The study described below demonstrates the manner in which EPI can be used to address such issues.

The study below demonstrates (a) that the predominant mechanism of signal changes with susceptibility-weighted sequences having TR of 1 s or greater is from alterations in transverse relaxation rate due to changes in the susceptibility of hemoglobin during activation and has minimal non-susceptibility-related contributions [108, 109, 116, 164, 165], and (b) the predominant vascular scale contributing to BOLD contrast during brain activation varies significantly over space.

In this study, the assumption was made that the resting and activated MRI signal intensity, Sr and Sa respectively, may be approximated by:

$$Sr = Sr_o \ e^{-(R2r \ TE)} \quad and \quad Sa = Sa_o \ e^{-(R2a \ TE)}$$

Resting and activated signal at TE = 0, Sr_o and Sa_o can be altered by changes in proton density and/or T1. Resting and activated transverse relaxation rates, R2r (1/T2r), and R2a (1/T2a), can be altered in this context by changes in the magnetic susceptibility of blood, which causes changes in R2' (R2* = R2+R2'). Temporally and spatially registered time course measurements of R2, R2*, and S_o during rest and activation enables accurate separation of these flow (non-susceptibility-related) and oxygenation (susceptibility-related) effects.

Using a combined spin-echo and gradient-echo EPI sequence (SEGE EPI) [165] (Fig. 12), a pair of spin-echo and gradient-echo single-shot echo-planar time course series were collected simultaneously and processed in an identical manner. In Fig. 12 the missing phase-encode blips are incorporated to allow for two line phase correction for each image [182, 183]. SEGE EPI has proven

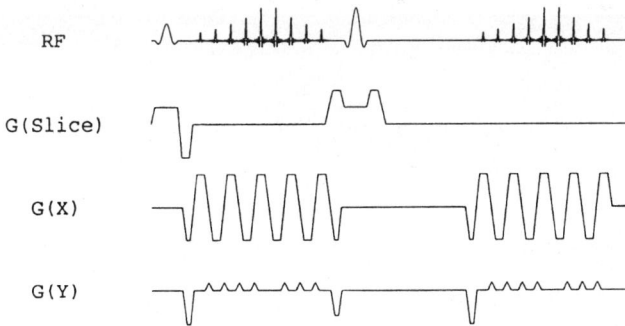

Fig. 12. SEGE-EPI. This sequence allows for the collection of spin-echo (T2-weighted) and gradient-echo (T2*-weighted) echo planar image pairs within about 50 ms of each other. This sequence is used to obtain spatially and temporally registered gradient-echo and spin-echo time course series for voxelwise comparison of activation-induced signal change dynamics and locations with different contrast weightings. Systematic incrementation of the two TE values in each sequential time course image also enables the simultaneous mapping of relative transverse relaxation rates (R2*, R2, and R2') and steady-state magnetizations

Fig. 13. The first pair of anatomical images and the corresponding functional correlation images obtained simultaneously from a SEGE EPI time course series. The gradient-echo functional image (*GE*) appears to have a higher functional CNR than the spin-echo image (*SE*). The signal change locations also show differences

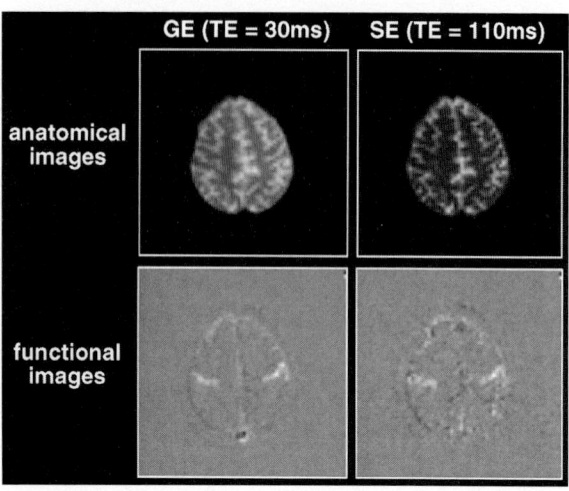

useful for voxel-wise comparisons of relative R2* and R2 contrast [165, 184]. Imaging was performed on a 1.5-T GE Signa scanner using a local three-axis gradient coil and a quadrature transmit/receive birdcage RF coil. Voxel volume was 3.75×3.75×5 mm^3.

The first part of the experiment entailed obtaining SEGE EPI time course series (TR = 1 s) during cyclic on/off finger movement using single TE values of 30 ms (gradient-echo) and 110 ms (spin-echo). With this protocol the relative signal change latencies can be compared and the relative relaxation rates (R2*/R2) mapped. Figure 13 shows the first pair of anatomical images and the corresponding functional correlation images obtained. The gradient-echo functional image more clearly shows activation-induced signal changes. Also, the signal change locations differ. Figure 14 shows a magnification of motor cortex and

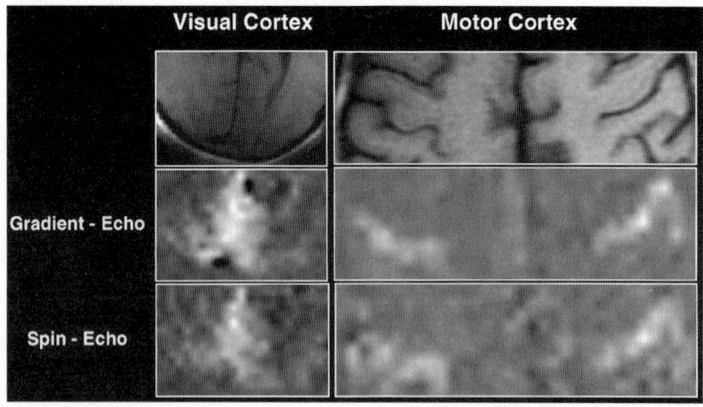

Fig. 14. Magnification of simultaneously obtained and identically processed gradient-echo (TE = 30 ms) and spin-echo (TE = 110 ms) functional correlation images of visual and motor cortex activation

visual cortex functional correlation images. Corresponding high-resolution anatomical images are shown for reference. In spin-echo sequences pulsatile and/or large vessel artifacts are significantly reduced at some expense in functional CNR.

Figure 15 shows gradient-echo and spin-echo time course signals from the same motor cortex region of interest obtained simultaneously using the SEGE sequence. The vertical scales are the same to illustrate the relative contrasts typically obtained. To compare the relative latencies of the signal changes each activation/rest cycle was averaged over time and then normalized. This comparison is shown in Fig. 16. A monoexponential model of the signal change onset is an oversimplification of the behavior of the MR signal change on activation, but for the purpose of comparison with the literature values [54], similar monoexponential fits to the initial rise in signal were performed. The fitted onset time constants were 3.67 ± 0.30 s for the gradient-echo sequence and 4.19 ± 0.46 for the spin-echo sequence. Within the certainty of experimental noise the two onset latencies are the same.

As discussed above, mathematical models of the BOLD effect have suggested that the $\Delta R2^*/\Delta R2$ ratio is highly dependent on compartment (red blood cell and vessel) size, activation-induced susceptibility change, and the diffusion coef-

Fig. 15. Simultaneously obtained gradient-echo (*GE*; TE = 30 ms) and spin-echo (*SE*; TE = 110 ms) time-course signal from the same region of interest in motor cortex. *Vertical scales* have the same range to illustrate the relative contrasts. *Horizontal bars* indicate when bilateral finger tapping was performed

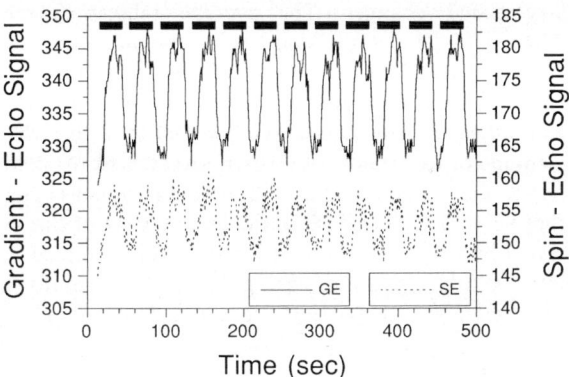

Fig. 16. Normalized gradient-echo and spin-echo time course created by averaging all of the 12 on-off cycles in Fig. 15. The signal change shapes do not show significant differences

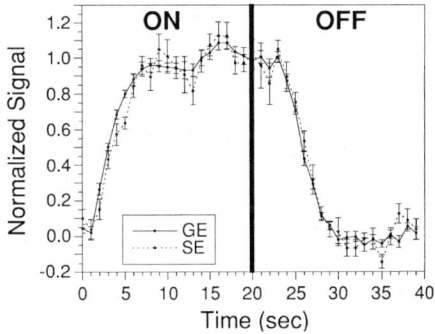

Fig. 17. Relative activation-induced $\Delta R2^*/\Delta R2$ map created from voxels showing activation with both the gradient-echo and spin-echo contrast weightings. The ratio varies considerably in space and has an average value of 3.52 ± 0.48

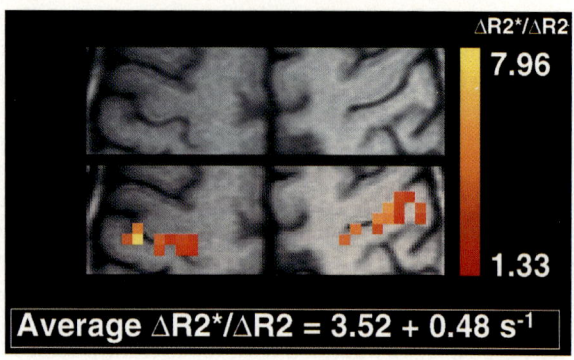

ficient. The relative change in relaxation rates, [determined by $\Delta R2(*) = -\mathrm{Ln}(Sa/Sr)$], were compared on a voxelwise basis, in regions showing common activation, directly from the signal changes in the SEGE-EPI time course series. Figure 17 shows the map of $\Delta R2^*/\Delta R2$ values. The variation in $\Delta R2^*/\Delta R2$ values suggests a heterogeneous distribution of predominant vascular scales. The highest ratio is observed directly within a sulcus where a large vessel appears to be. Lower ratios appear to be predominantly within gray matter regions, indicating capillary-related changes. The average relaxation rate ratio was found to be 3.52 ± 48 s. This ratio suggests an average compartment size of approximately 10 μm [113]. One caveat in the interpretation of these maps is that the ratios reflect *compartment* size and not *vessel* size. Within vessels there are many smaller compartments (red blood cells) which tend to reduce this ratio in large vessels.

Maps of $\Delta R2^*$ and $\Delta R2$ which are created using single TE values may be inaccurate due to non-susceptibility-related signal changes. The assumption is made that $So_a = So_r$. Therefore in the second part of the experiment this assumption is tested by time course collection of highly sampled R2 and R2* decay curves during rest and activation. Extrapolating these curves to TE = 0, the nonsusceptibility component of the signal, So, was determined.

Figure 18 shows a plot from the same voxels in the motor cortex of the Ln(S) vs. TE, collected during rest and activation. Each curve has 100 points (gradient-echo TE = 25–74.5 ms, spin-echo TE = 100–199 ms). All data for this plot were obtained in under 17 min using SEGE EPI. Activation-induced changes in the relaxation rates, $\Delta R2^*$ and $\Delta R2$, were measured to be -0.81 ± 0.02 s^{-1} and -0.19 ± 0.02 s^{-1}, respectively. The interpolated change in So using the $\Delta R2^*$ curves was significant.

Using this same data set, the percentage of signal change vs. TE was computed (Fig. 19). The percentage change shows a linear TE dependence. The ΔSo at TE = 0 corresponds closely to the apparent T1-related signal changes predicted at TR = 1 s ($\approx0.6\%$) using the perfusion model of Kwong et al. [54].

A plot of Sa–Sr vs. TE is shown in Fig. 20. Bold lines indicate Sa–Sr values calculated using the measured $\Delta R2^*$, $\Delta R2$ as well as extrapolated ΔS_o values. Lighter lines are calculated using the measured $\Delta R2^*$, $\Delta R2$ values and assuming $So_r = So_a$. Once again, the more precise fit to the ΔS curve was that which used

Fig. 18. Resting and active R2, R2* curves obtained simultaneously during rest and activation from identical regions in motor cortex. Each curve has 100 points. Gradient-echo (*GE*) TE = 25 to 74.5 ms; spin-echo (*SE*) TE = 100–199 ms). All data for this plot were obtained in under 17 min using SEGE EPI. The observed change in So, when using the ΔR2* curves, was significant

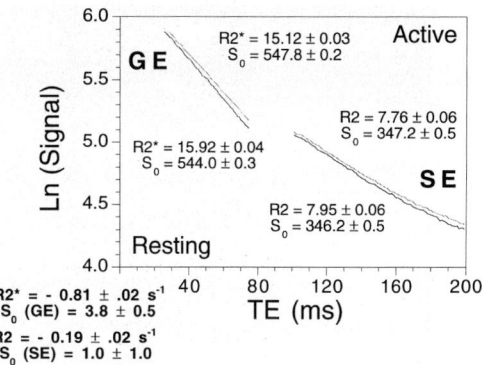

Fig. 19. Percentage of gradient-echo (*GE*) and spin-echo (*SE*) signal change vs. TE from the same data set as in Fig. 18. The TE dependence of the fractional signal change appears linear, and the zero intercept shows a positive change with activation

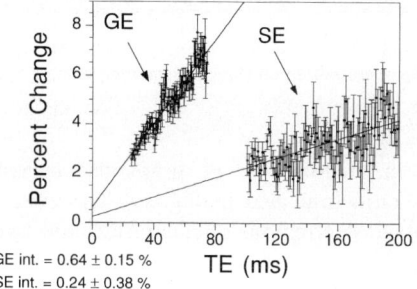

Fig. 20. Signal difference vs. TE from the same data set as in Figs. 18 and 19. *Bold lines* were calculated using the measured resting and active R2, R2*, and So values; *lighter lines* were calculated using the measured R2 and R2* values and assuming that $S_a o = S_r o$. The more precise fit to the Δ S curve was that which used the So$_r$ and So$_a$ values obtained by interpolation of the decay curves to TE = 0

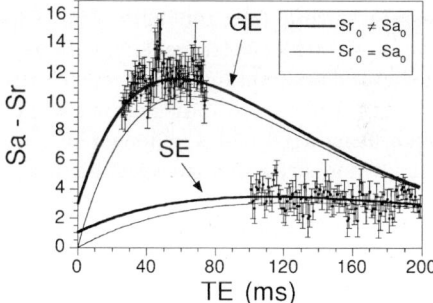

the So$_r$ and So$_a$ values obtained by interpolation of the decay curves to TE = 0. The ratio in contrast at TE$\approx$T2* between gradient-echo and spin-echo sequences is about 3.5–1.

Lastly, using similarly acquired data, maps of So, R2, R2', and R2* as well as maps of activation-induced changes in So, R2, R2', and R2* may be created (Fig. 21). The R2' maps (direct measure of proton resonance linewidth) were calculated from R2*–R2. Decreases in R2* and R2' are observed most easily. Using this method of analysis, a decrease in R2 is minimally perceptible, and S$_o$ changes are relatively imperceptible. The "hot spot" in the ΔR2' map (indicating

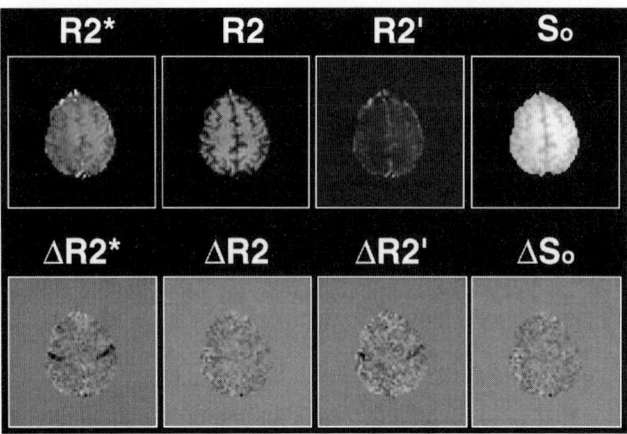

Fig. 21. Maps of resting state and changes in R2*, R2, and So, created using SEGE EPI, in which the TE values were systematically incremented during the time-course collection of images

a change in macroscopic B_o gradients) corresponds closely with the largest $\Delta R2*/\Delta R2$ ratio indicated in Fig. 17. The evidence indicates that this region is likely a vessel. The regions of small $\Delta R2'$ and larger $\Delta R2$ are likely smaller vessels or capillaries.

The use of SEGE EPI enables acquisition of spatially and temporally registered, high-SNR measurements of R2* and R2 in a reasonable amount of time. In this study R2*, R2, and interpolated TE = 0 signal were measured over time in the brain during rest and activation. These studies typically demonstrate large spatial $\Delta R2*/\Delta R2$ heterogeneity, with an average ratio of about 3.5, indicating, with several assumptions, an "average" susceptibility compartment size of 8–10 μm. These studies also indicate that, while susceptibility effects clearly dominate when using a TR of 1 s or longer in gradient-echo or spin-echo sequences, a very small non-susceptibility-related component contributes.

Postprocessing Development

The challenge of accurately determining regions of significant activation from fMRI data is nontrivial and has yet to be solved. Some of the developments addressing this issue include: (a) the development of accurate and robust motion correction [186, 187] and/or suppression methods, (b) the determination of the noise distribution [120, 121, 155], (c) the determination of the temporal [142] and spatial [187] correlation of activation-induced MR signal changes and of baseline MR signal, (d) the characterization or assessment of the temporal behavior or shape of activation-induced signal changes [136–138, 155, 174], and e) the characterization of how the above-mentioned factors vary in time, space [133, 134], across tasks [137, 138, 155], and with different pulse sequence parameters [54].

Several of the postprocessing issues may be bypassed or addressed more effectively using the flexibility and rapid image sampling capabilities of EPI. Examples are given of how EPI can aid in the reduction of various manifestations of motion artifacts, including pulsatile, sudden, gradual, and stimulus-correlated motion. First, because the rapid image sampling rate of EPI allows for critical sampling of many problematic noise frequencies, these frequencies can be rejected using simple band stop filters [121]. With single-shot EPI motion effects above the time scale of 40–100 ms are virtually eliminated. Slower motion that occurs between each shot (100 ms, 6 s) cause primarily misregistration. These effects can be reduced by the use of currently available image registration algorithms [185, 186]. In two-dimensional Fourier transform techniques motion on this time scale is manifested not only as misregistration but also as ghosting that is propagated throughout the image [100, 102]. With EPI very slow motion, manifested as a drift in the time course, is reduced simply by the ability to collect a larger number of on/off activation cycles (40 s per cycle) in a single time course whose duration is less than the time during which signal drift manifests itself (five on/off cycles in under 4 min). Lastly, stimulus correlated motion generally has a different signal change latency than activation-induced signal changes. This fact allows differentiation, using a sampling rate of at least one image every 2 s, of stimulus-correlated signal changes from activation-induced signal changes, based simply on the different temporal "shapes."

Recently a real-time updatable cross-correlation algorithm has been successfully implemented in conjunction with EPI [149]. This algorithm allows images to be continually obtained until the quality of the functional correlation images (updated at a rate of one per second) is suitable. Rapid acquisition of echo-planar images can allow rapid feedback in functional image quality and subsequently a high degree of experimental tuning and an increase in the rate of successful fMRI experiments per imaging session. Consider an investigation (clinical or research) in which different stimuli are to be applied in ten runs. If there is only a 5% chance that one run will be bad, there is a $0.95^{10} = 60\%$ chance that all ten will be good. If all ten are required to be good, the experiment results must be rejected 40% of the time. Immediate feedback can alleviate this problem.

One can also imagine performing experiments whose procedure depends on knowing results from just completed runs. For clinical use one can be sure, if using the real-time fMRI technique, that good results are present before the patient leaves the scanner.

In general, an array of statistical and prestatistical postprocessing methods have been put forward. The statistical methods include the use of Z scores [188], analysis of variance [189], split-half t test [100, 190], the Kolmogrov-Smirnov test [191], and other nonparametric tests [192]. Prestatistical methods include cross-correlation analysis [101], auto-correlation analysis [167], phase tagging [133, 134, 154, 155], principle-components analysis [193], time-frequency analysis [147], and power-spectrum analysis [101, 120, 121, 194]. Currently no one best postprocessing technique exists, or may ever exist, because of the large number of changing variables which contribute to the activation-induced signal change and underlying noise. The best types of postprocessing methods are likely to be those that are adaptable to variations (across scans, regions, tasks, and pulse-sequences) in signal and noise characteristics.

Applications

Most studies involving the development of fMRI from a contrast mechanism, pulse-sequence, and postprocessing standpoint have used primary motor and visual cortex activation due to the easily elicited signal changes. Listed below are some of the applications of fMRI that have gone beyond simple finger tapping or visual stimulation. Most of the studies were performed using EPI. The primary auditory cortex [195–201] and the cerebellum [202–204] have been studied using fMRI. Detailed mapping of regions activated in the primary motor cortex [205–208] and visual cortex [154–156, 209, 210] has been performed as well. Subcortical activity has been observed during visual stimulation [167] and finger movement [211]. Activity elicited in the gustatory cortex has also been mapped [212]. Other studies using fMRI have observed organizational differences related to handedness [213]. Activation changes during motor task learning have been observed in the primary motor cortex [214] and cerebellum [215, 216].

Cognitive studies in normal subjects have included word generation [217–219], mental imagery [220, 221], mental rehearsal of motor tasks and complex motor control [211, 222, 223], speech perception [195, 197, 198, 224, 225], single-word semantic processing [197, 198, 224, 225], working memory [226, 227], spatial memory [228], and visual recall [229]. Studies have observed modulation of activity by attention modulation [155].

fMRI has been extremely useful in mapping visual cortex in humans [155, 190, 209, 230–234]. In particular, because of its high image acquisition rate EPI lends itself to the mapping specific types of neuronal activation. The illusion of motion is transiently perceived following particular stimuli. Recently Tootell et al. [233], using EPI with BOLD contrast at 1.5 T, have been able to observe transient activation in MT/V5 elicited by the illusion of motion following stimulation by radially moving concentric rings.

Studies have also been performed involving specific pathologies. Abnormal connectivity of the visual pathways in human albinos has been demonstrated [235]. Changes in organization in the sensorimotor area after brain injury has been observed [236]. One study has demonstrated larger fMRI signal changes, on the average, in schizophrenic patients [237]. The ability to localize seizure activity has also been demonstrated by fMRI [238]. In addition, preliminary data demonstrating the effects of drugs on brain activation have been presented [239]. Activity associated with obsessive-compulsive behavior has also been observed [240, 241]

The immediate potential for clinical application is currently being explored. "Essential" areas of the sensory and motor cortex as well as language centers have been mapped using both fMRI and electrical stimulation techniques [178, 242]. Activity foci observed across the two methods have shown a high spatial correlation, demonstrating the potential for fMRI to compliment or replace the invasive technique in the identification of cortical regions which should be avoided during surgery. Along this avenue of research fMRI has developed the ability to reliably identify the hemisphere where language functions reside, potentially complimenting or replacing the Wada test (hemisphere specific application of an anesthetic amobarbital) for language localization that is also currently used clinically prior to surgery [243].

Several review articles and chapters on fMRI techniques and applications are currently available [135, 144, 187, 196, 244-248]. In general, the several fMRI research avenues – functional imaging platform development, contrast mechanism research, postprocessing development, and applications – are progressing in a manner that is both complimentary and synergistic. Because of the rigor and creativity of the investigators in this newly created and interdisciplinary field and, in part, because of the robustness of EPI as a functional imaging tool, fMRI is progressing at an accelerating pace.

Acknowledgements. The writing of this chapter benefited from enlightening discussions with Jeffrey Binder, Bharat Biswal, Robert Cox, Ted DeYoe, Victor Haughton, James Hyde, Andrej Jesmanowicz, Stephen Rao, Allen Song, Elliot Stein, and Steven Tan from the Medical College of Wisconsin; and John Baker, Jack Belliveau, Jerry Boxerman, Timothy Davis, Kathleen Donahue, Ken Kwong, Bruce Rosen, Robert Savoy, Roger Tootell, and Robert Weisskoff from the Massachusetts General Hospital. Thanks also to Steven Tan for providing the interleaved echo-planar images.

References

1. Mansfield P (1977) Multi-planar image formation using NMR spin echoes. J Phys C10:L55–L58
2. Stehling MK, Turner R, Mansfield P (1991) Echo-planar imaging: magnetic resonance imaging in a fraction of a second. Science 254:43–50
3. Edelman R, Wielopolski P, Schmitt F (1994) Echo-planar MR imaging. Radiology 192:600–612
4. Cohen MS, Weisskoff RM (1991) Ultra-fast imaging. Magn Reson Imaging 9:1–37
5. Mansfield P, Morris PG (1982) NMR imaging in biomedicine. Academic, New York
6. Roland PE (1993) Brain activation. Wiley-Liss, New York
7. Churchland PS, Sejnowski TJ (1992) The computational brain. MIT Press, Cambridge
8. Kuffler SW, Nicholls JG, Martin AR (1984) From neuron to brain. Sinauer Associates, Sunderland
9. Krnjevic K (1975) Coupling of neuronal metabolism and electrical activity. In: Ingvar DH, Lassen NA (eds) Brain work. Munksgaard, Copenhagen, p 65
10. Hillyard SG, Picton TW (1987) In: Handbook of physiology, section 1: neurophysiology. American Physiological Society, New York, p 519
11. Hari R (1991) On brain's magnetic responses to sensory stimuli. J Clin Neurophysiol 8:157–169
12. Kaufman L, Williamson SJ (1982) Magnetic location of cortical activity. Ann N Y Acad Sci 388:197–213
13. Prichard J, Rothman D, Novotny E, Petroff O, Kuwabara T, Avison M, Howsman A, Hanstock C, Shulman R (1991) Lactate rise detected by 1H NMR in human visual cortex during physiologic stimulation. Proc Natl Acad Sci USA 88:5829–5831
14. Merboldt K-D, Bruhn H, Hanicke W, Michaelis T, Frahm J, (1992) Decrease of glucose in the human visual cortex during photic stimulation. Magn Reson Med 25:187–194
15. Fox PT, Raichle ME, Mintun MA, Dence C (1988) Nonoxidative glucose consumption during focal physiologic neural activity. Science 241:462
16. Phelps ME, Kuhl DE, Mazziotta JC (1981) Metabolic mapping of the brain's response to visual stimulation: studies in humans. Science 211:1445–1448
17. Mazziotta JC, Phelps ME (1985) Human neuropsychological imaging studies of local brain metabolism: strategies and results. In: Sokoloff L (ed) Brain imaging and brain function. Raven, New York, p 121

18. Haxby JL, Grady CL, Ungerleider LG, Horowitz B (1991) Mapping the functional neuroanatomy of the intact human brain with brain work imaging. Neuropsychologia 29:539–555
19. Roy CS, Sherrington CS (1890) On the regulation of the blood-supply of the brain. J Physiol 11:85–108
20. Gotoh F, Tanaka K (1987) In: Vinkin PJ, Bruyn GW, Klawans HL (eds) Handbook of clinical neurology. Elsevier Science, New York, p 47
21. Kushinsky W (1982/1983) Coupling between functional activity, metabolism, and blood flow in the brain: state of the art. Microcirculation 2:357–378
22. Busija DW, Heistad DD (1984) Factors involved in the physiological regulation of the cerebral circulation. Springer, Berlin Heidelberg New York
23. Ursino M (1991) Mechanisms of cerebral blood flow regulation. Crit Rev Biomed Eng 18:255–288
24. Lou HC, Edvinsson L, MacKenzie ET (1987) The concept of coupling blood flow to brain function: revision required? Ann Neurol 22:289–297
25. Kuschinsky W (1991) Physiology of cerebral blood flow and metabolism. Arzneimittelforschung 41:284–288
26. Moskalenko YE, Weinstein GB, Demchenko IT, Kislyakov YY, Krivchenko AI (1980) Biophysical aspects of cerebral circulation. Pergamon, Oxford
27. Estrada C, Mengual E, Gonzalez C (1993) Local NADPH-diaphorase neurons innervate pial arteries and lie close or project to intracerebral blood vessels: a possible role for nitric oxide in the regulation of cerebral blood flow. J Cereb Blood Flow Metab 13:978–984
28. Dirnagl U, Lindauer U, Villringer A (1993) Role of nitric oxide in the coupling of cerebral blood flow to neuronal activation in rats. Neuroscience Lett 149:43–46
29. Iadecola C (1993) Regulation of cerebral microcirculaton during neural activity: is nitric oxide the missing link? Trends Neurosci 16:206–214
30. Mchedlishvili G (1986) Arterial behavior and blood circulation in the brain. Plenum, New York
31. Ingvar DH (1975) In: Ingvar DH, Lassen NA (eds) Brain work. Munksgaard, Copenhagen, p 397
32. Grafton ST, Woods RP, Mazziotta JC, Phelps ME (1991) Somatotopic mapping of the primary motor cortex in humans: activation studies with cerebral blood flow and positron emission tomography. J Neurophysiol 66:735–743
33. Colebatch JG, Deiber M-P, Passingham RE, Friston KJ, Frackowiack RSJ (1991) Regional cerebral blood flow during voluntary arm and hand movements in human subjects. J Neurophysiol 65:1392–1401
34. Fox PT, Raichle ME (1985) Stimulus rate determines regional brain blood flow in striate cortex. Ann Neurol 17:303–305
35. Fox PT, Raichl ME (1991) Stimulus rate dependence of regional cerebral blood flow in human striate cortex, demonstrated by positron emission tomography. J Neurophysiol 51:1109–1120
36. Cameron OG, Modell JG, Hichwa RD, Agranoff BW, Koeppe RA (1990) Changes in sensory-cognitive input: effects on cerebral blood flow. J Cereb Blood Flow Metab 10:38–42
37. Sandman CA, O'Halloran JP, Isenhart R (1984) Is there an evoked vascular response? Science 224:1355–1356
38. Belliveau JW, Kennedy DN, McKinstry RC, Buchbinder BR, Weisskoff RM, Cohen MS, Vevea JM, Brady TJ, Rosen BR (1991) Functional mapping of the human visual cortex by magnetic resonance imaging. Science 254:716–719
39. Villringer A, Planck J, Hock C, Scheinkofer L, Dirnagl U (1993) Near infrared spectroscopy (NIRS): a new tool to study hemodynamic changes during activation of brain function in human adults. Neurosci Lett 154:101–104
40. Fox PT, Raichle ME (1986) Focal physiological uncoupling of cerebral blood flow and oxidative metabolism during somatosensory stimulation in human subjects. Proc Natl Acad Sci USA 83:1140–1144
41. Frostig RD, Lieke EE, Ts'o DY, Grinvald A (1990) Cortical functional architecture and local coupling between neuronal activity and the microcirculation revealed by in vivo high-resolution optical imaging of intrinsic signals. Proc Natl Acad Sci USA 87:6082–6086
42. Grinvald A, Frostig RD, Siegel RM, Bratfeld E (1991) High-resolution optical imaging of functional brain architecture in the awake monkey. Proc Natl Acad Sci USA 88:11559–11563
43. Frostig RD (1994) What does in vivo optical imaging tell us about the primary visual cortex in primates? In: Peters A, Rockland KS (eds) Cerebral cortex, vol 10. Plenum, New York, p 331

44. Rosen BR, Belliveau JW, Chien D (1989) Perfusion imaging by nuclear magnetic resonance. Magn Reson Q 5:263–281
45. Rosen BR, Belliveau JW, Vevea JM, Brady TJ (1990) Perfusion imaging with NMR contrast agents. Magn Reson Med 14:249–265
46. Belliveau JW, Rosen BR, Kantor HL, Rzedzian RR, Kennedy DN, McKinstry RC, Vevea JM, Cohen MS, Pykett IL, Brady TJ (1990) Functional cerebral imaging by susceptibility-contrast NMR. Magn Reson Med 14:538–546
47. Rosen BR, Belliveau JW, Aronen HJ, Kennedy D, Buchbinder BR, Fischman A, Gruber M, Glas J, Weisskoff RM, Cohen MS, Hochberg FH, Brady TJ (1991) Susceptibility contrast imaging of cerebral blood volume: human experience. Magn Reson Med 22:293–299
48. Villringer A, Rosen BR, Belliveau JW, Ackerman JL, Lauffer RB, Buxton RB, Chao Y-S, Wedeen VJ, Brady TJ (1988) Dynamic imaging with lanthanide chelates in normal brain: contrast due to magnetic susceptibility effects. Magn Reson Med 6:164–174
49. Moonen CT, Liu G, van Gelderen P, Sobering G (1992) A fast gradient-recalled MRI technique with increased sensitivity to dynamic susceptibility effects. Magn Reson Med 26:184–189
50. Moonen CTW, van Zijl PCM, Frank JA, LeBihan D, Becker ED (1990) Functional magnetic resonance imaging in medicine and physiology. Science 250:53–61
51. Williams DS, Detre JA, Leigh JS, Koretsky AS (1992) Magnetic resonance imaging of perfusion using spin-inversion of arterial water. Proc Natl Acad Sci USA 89:212–216
52. Detre JA, Leigh JS, Williams DS, Koretsky AP (1992) Perfusion imaging. Magn Reson Med 23:37–45
53. Edelman RR, Sievert B, Wielopolski P, Pearlman J, Warach S (1994) Noninvasive mapping of cerebral perfusion by using EPISTAR MR angiography. JMRI 4(P):68 (abstract)
54. Kwong KK, Belliveau JW, Chesler DA, Goldberg IE, Weisskoff RM, Poncelet BP, Kennedy DN, Hoppel BE, Cohen MS, Turner R, Cheng HM, Brady TJ, Rosen BR (1992) Dynamic magnetic resonance imaging of human brain activity during primary sensory stimulation. Proc Natl Acad Sci USA 89:5675–5679
55. Stehling MK, Schmitt F, Ladebeck R (1993) Echo-planar MR imaging of human brain oxygenation changes. JMRI 3:471–474
56. Bandettini PA, Wong EC, Hinks RS, Tikofsky RS, Hyde JS (1992) Time course EPI of human brain function during task activation. Magn Reson Med 25:390–397
57. Blamire AM, Ogawa S, Ugurbil K, Rothman D, McCarthy G, Ellermann JM, Hyder F, Rattner Z, Shulman RG (1992) Dynamic mapping of the human visual cortex by high-speed magnetic resonance imaging. Proc Natl Acad Sci USA 89:11069–11073
58. Frahm J, Bruhn H, Merboldt K-D, Hanicke W, Math D (1992) Dynamic MR imaging of human brain oxygenation during rest and photic stimulation. JMRI 2:501–505
59. Ogawa S, Lee T-M, Nayak AS, Glynn P (1990) Oxygenation-sensitive contrast in magnetic resonance image of rodent brain at high magnetic fields. Magn Reson Med 14:68–78
60. Ogawa S, Lee T-M (1990) Magnetic resonance imaging of blood vessels at high fields: in vivo and in vitro measurements and image simulation. Magn Reson Med 16:9–18
61. Ogawa S, Lee TM, Kay AR, Tank DW (1990) Brain magnetic resonance imaging with contrast dependent on blood oxygenation. Proc Natl Acad Sci USA 87:9868–9872
62. Ogawa S, Tank DW, Menon R, Ellermann JM, Kim S-G, Merkle H, Ugurbil K (1992) Intrinsic signal changes accompanying sensory stimulation: functional brain mapping with magnetic resonance imaging. Proc Natl Acad Sci USA 89:5951–5955
63. Turner R, LeBihan D, Moonen CTW, Despres D, Frank J (1991) Echo-planar time course MRI of cat brain oxygenation changes. Magn Reson Med 27:159–166
64. Turner R, Jezzard P, Wen H, Kwong KK, Bihan DL, Zeffiro T, Balaban RS (1993) Functional mapping of the human visual cortex at 4 and 1.5 tesla using deoxygenation contrast EPI. Magn Reson Med 29:277–279
65. Jezzard P, Heinmann F, Taylor J, Despres D, Wen H, Balaban RS, Turner R (1994) Comparison of EPI gradient-echo contrast changes in cat brain caused by respiratory challenges with direct simultaneous evaluation of cerebral oxygenation via a cranial window. NMR Biomed 7:35–44
66. Weisskoff RM, Zuo CS, Boxerman JL, Rosen BR (1994) Microscopic susceptibility variation and transverse relaxation: theory and experiment. Magn Reson Med 31:601–610
67. Edelman RR, Mattle HP, Atkinson DJ, Hoogewood HM, (1990) MR angiography. AJR 154:937–946
68. Listerud J (1991) First principles of magnetic resonance angiography. Magn Reson Q 7:136–170

69. LeBihan D, Breton E, Lallemand D, Aubin M-L, Vignaud J, Laval-Jeantet M (1988) Separation of diffusion and perfusion in intravoxel incoherent motion MR imaging. Radiology 168:497–505
70. LeBihan D (1990) Magnetic resonance imaging of perfusion. Magn Reson Med 14:283–292
71. LeBihan D, Turner R, Moonen CT, Pekar J (1991) Imaging of diffusion and microcirculation with gradient sensitization: design, strategy, and significance. JMRI 1:7–28
72. LeBihan D (1992) Theoretical principles of perfusion imaging: applications to magnetic resonance imaging. Invest Radiol 27:S6–S11
73. Kwong KK, McKinstry RC, Chien D, Crawley AB, Pearlman JD, Rosen BR (1991) CSF-suppressed quantitative single-shot diffusion imaging. Magn Reson Med 21:157–163
74. J Pekar, C. T. Moonen, P. C. van Zijl, On the precision of diffusion/perfusion imaging by gradient sensitization. Magn Reson Med 23:122–129 (1992)
75. Edelman RR, Siewert B, Adamis M, Gaa J, Laub GP, Wielopolski P (1994) Signal targeting with alternating radiofrequency (STAR) sequences: application to MR angiography. Magn Reson Med 31:233–238
76. Pauling L, Coryell CD (1936) The magnetic properties and structure of hemoglobin, oxyhemoglobin, and carbonmonoxyhemoglobin. Proc Natl Acad Sci USA 22:210–216
77. Weisskoff RW, Kiihne S (1992) MRI susceptometry: image-based measurement of absolute susceptibility of MR contrast agents and human blood. Magn Reson Med 24:375–383
78. Schenck JF (1992) Health and physiological effects of human exposure to whole-body four-tesla magnetic fields during MRI. Ann N Y Acad Sci 649:285–301
79. Thulborn KR, Waterton JC, Matthews PM, Radda GK (1982) Oxygenation dependence of the transverse relaxation time of water protons in whole blood at high field. Biochim Biophys Acta 714:265–270
80. Brindle KM, Brown FF, Campbell ID, Grathwohl C, Kuchell PW (1979) Application of spin-echo nuclear magnetic resonance to whole-cell systems. Biochem J 180:37–44
81. Brooks RA, Chiro GD (1987) Magnetic resonance imaging of stationary blood: a review. Med Phys 14:903–913
82. Gomori JM, Grossman RJ, Yu-Ip C, Asakura T (1987) NMR relaxation times of blood: dependence on field strength, oxidation state, and cell integrity. J Comput Assist Tomogr 11:684–690
83. Matwiyoff NA, Gasparovic C, Mazurchuk R, Matwiyoff G (1990) The line shapes of the water proton resonances of red blood cells containing carbonyl hemoglobin, deoxyhemoglobin, and methemoglobin: implications for the interpretation of proton MRI at 1.5 T and below. Magn Reson Imag 8:295–301
84. Hayman LA, Ford JJ, Taber KH, Saleem A, Round ME, Bryan RN (1988) T2 effects of hemoglobin concentration: assessment with in vitro MR spectroscopy. Magn Reson Imag 168:489–491
85. Janick PA, Hackney DB, Grossman RI, Asakura T (1991) MR imaging of various oxidation states of intracellular and extracellular hemoglobin. AJNR 12:891–897
86. Wright GA, Nishimura DG, Macovski A (1991) Flow-independent magnetic resonance projection angiography. Magn Reson Med 17:126–140
87. Wright GA, Hu BS, Macovski A (1991) Estimating oxygen saturation of blood in vivo with MR imaging at 1.5 T. JMRI 1:275–283
88. Thulborn KR, Brady TJ (1989) Iron in magnetic resonance imaging of cerebral hemorrhage. Magn Reson Q 5:23–38
89. Hoppel BE, Weisskoff RM, Thulborn KR, Moore JB, Kwong KK, Rosen BR (1993) Measurement of regional blood oxygenation and cerebral hemodynamics. Magn Reson Med 30:715–723
90. Gilles P, Peto S, Moiny F, Mispelter J, Cuenod C-A (1995) Proton transverse nuclear magnetic relation in oxidized blood: a numerical approach. Magn Reson Med 33:93–100
91. Brady TJ (1991) Future prospects for MR imaging. In: Proceedings of the SMRM, 10th annual meeting, San Francisco, p 2
92. Farzaneh F, Riederer SJ, Pelc NJ (1990) Analysis of T2 limitations and off-resonance effects in spatial resolution and artifacts in echo-planar imaging. Magn Reson Med 14:123–139
93. Wong EC, Bandettini PA, Hyde JS (1992) Echo-planar imaging of the human brain using a three axis local gradient coil. In: Proceedings of the SMRM, 11th annual meeting, Berlin, p 105
94. Wong EC, Jesmanowicz A, Hyde JS (1991) Coil optimization for MRI by conjugate gradient descent. Magn Reson Med 21:39–48
95. Turner R (1993) Gradient coil design: a review of methods. Magn Reson Imag 11:903–920

96. Blamire AM, Shulman RG (1994) Implementation of echo-planar imaging on an unmodified spectrometer at 2.1 tesla for functional imaging. Magn Reson Imag 12:669–671
97. Jesmanowicz A, Wong EC, DeYoe EA, Hyde J S (1992) Method to correct anatomic distortion in echo-planar images. In: Proceedings of the SMRM, 11th annual meeting, Berlin, p 4260
98. Jezzard P, Balaban R (1995) Correction for geometric distortion in echo planar images from B_o field distortions. Magn Reson Med 34:65–73
99. Weisskoff RM, Davis TL (1992) Correcting gross distortion on echo planar images. In: Proceedings of the SMRM, 11th annual meeting, Berlin, p 4515
100. Noll DC, Cohen JD, Meyer CH, Schneider W (1995) Spiral k-space MR imaging of cortical activation. JMRI 5:49–56
101. Bandettini PA, Jesmanowicz A, Wong EC, Hyde JS (1993) Processing strategies for time-course data sets in functional MRI of the human brain. Magn Reson Med 30:161–173
102. Glover GH, Lee AT, Meyers CH (1993) Motion artifacts in fMRI: comparison of 2DFT with PR and spiral scan methods. In: Proceedings of the SMRM, 12th annual meeting, New York, p 197
103. Stehling M, Fang M, Ladebeck R, Schmitt F (1992) Functional echo-planar MR imaging at 1 T. JMRI 2(P):76 (abstract)
104. Kwong KK, Belliveau JW, Stern CE, Chesler DA, Goldberg IE, Poncelet BP, Kennedy DN, Weisskoff RM, Cohen MS, Turner R, Cheng H-M, Brady TJ, Rosen BR (1992) Functional MR imaging of primary visual and motor cortex. JMRI 2(P):76 (abstract)
105. Bandettini PA, Wong EC, Tikofsky RS, Hinks RS, Hyde JS (1992) Echo-planar imaging of cerebral capillary percent deoxyhemoglobin change on task activation. JMRI 2(P):76 (abstract)
106. Jesmanowicz A, Bandettini PA, Wong EC, Tan G, Hyde JS (1993) Spin-echo and gradient-echo EPI of human brain function at 3 tesla. In: Proceedings of the SMRM, 12th annual meeting, New York, p 1390
107. Frahm J, Merboldt K-D, Hanicke W (1993) Functional MRI of human brain activation at high spatial resolution. Magn Reson Med 29:139–144
108. Menon RS, Ogawa S, Tank DW, Ugurbil K (1993) 4 tesla gradient recalled echo characteristics of photic stimulation-induced signal changes in the human primary visual cortex. Magn Reson Med 30:380–386
109. Bandettini PA, Wong EC, Jesmanowicz A, Hinks RS, Hyde JS (1994) Spin-echo and gradient-echo EPI of human brain activation using BOLD contrast: a comparative study at 1.5 tesla. NMR Biomed 7:12–19
110. Weisskoff RM, Boxerman JL, Zuo CS, Rosen BR (1993) Functional MRI of the brain. Society of Magnetic Resonance in Medicine, Berkeley, p 103
111. Kennan RP, Zhong J, Gore JC (1994) Intravascular susceptibility contrast mechanisms in tissues. Magn Reson Med 31:9–21
112. Fisel CR, Ackerman JL, Buxton RB, Garrido L, Belliveau JW, Rosen BR, Brady TJ (1991) MR contrast due to microscopically heterogeneous magnetic susceptibility: numerical simulations and applications to cerebral physiology. Magn Reson Med 17:336–347
113. Ogawa S, Menon RS, Tank DW, Kim S-G, Merkle H, Ellerman JM, Ugurbil K (1993) Functional brain mapping by blood oxygenation level-dependent contrast magnetic resonance imaging: a comparison of signal characteristics with a biophysical model. Biophys J 64:803–812
114. Boxerman JL, Weisskoff RM, Hoppel BE, Rosen BR (1993) MR contrast due to microscopically heterogeneous magnetic susceptibility: cylindrical geometry. In: Proceedings of the SMRM, 12th annual meeting, New York, p 389
115. Ugurbil K, Garwood M, Ellermann J, Hendrich K, Hinke R, Hu X, Kim S-G, Menon R, Merkle H, Ogawa S, Salmi R (1993) Imaging at high magnetic fields: initial experiences at 4 T. Magn Reson Q 9:259–277
116. Bandettini PA, Wong EC, Jesmanowicz A, Prost R, Cox RW, Hinks RS, Hyde JS (1994) MRI of human brain activation at 0.5 T, 1.5 T, and 3 T: comparisons of $\Delta R2^*$ and functional contrast to noise ratio. In: Proceedings of the SMR, 2nd annual meeting, San Francisco, p 434
117. Menon RS, Ogawa S, Strupp JP, Anderson P, Ugurbil K (1995) BOLD based functional MRI at 4 tesla includes a capillary bed contribution: echo-planar imaging mirrors previous optical imaging using intrinsic signals. Magn Reson Med 33:453–459
118. Menon RS, Hu X, Anderson P, Ugurbil K, Ogawa S (1994) Cerebral oxy/deoxy hemoglobin changes during neural activation: MRI timecourse correlates to optical reflectance measurements. In: Proceedings of the SMR, 2nd annual meeting, San Francisco, p 68

119. Poncelet B, Wedeen VJ, Weisskoff RM, Cohen MS (1992) Measurement of brain parenchyma motion with cine echo-planar MRI. In: Proceedings of the SMRM, 11th annual meeting, Berlin, p 809

120. Weisskoff RM, Baker J, Belliveau J, Davis TL, Kwong KK, Cohen MS, Rosen BR (1993) Power spectrum analysis of functionally-weighted MR data: what's in the noise? In: Proceedings of the SMRM, 12th annual meeting, New York, p 7

121. Jezzard P, LeBihan D, Cuenod C, Pannier L, Prinster A, Turner R (1993) An investigation of the contributions of physiological noise in human functional MRI studies at 1.5 tesla and 4 tesla. In: Proceedings of the SMRM, 12th annual meeting, New York, p 1392

122. Biswal B, DeYoe EA, Jesmanowicz A, Hyde JS (1994) Removal of physiological fluctuations from functional MRI signals. In: Proceedings of the SMR, 2nd annual meeting, San Francisco, p 653

123. Feinberg DA, Mark AS (1987) Human brain motion and cerebrospinal fluid circulation demonstrated with MR velocity imaging. Radiology 163:793-799

124. Hajnal JV, Myers R, Oatridge A, Schwieso JE, Young IR, Bydder GM (1994) Artifacts due to stimulus correlated motion in functional imaging of the brain. Magn Reson Med 31:283-291

125. Golanov EV, Yamamoto S, Reis DJ (1994) Spontaneous waves of cerebral blood flow associated with a pattern of electrocortical activity. Am J Physiol 266:R204-R214

126. Hudetz AG, Roman RJ, Harder DR (1992) Spontaneous flow oscillations in the cerebral cortex during acute changes in mean arterial pressure. J Cereb Blood Flow Metab 12:491-499

127. Butts K, Riederer SJ (1992) Analysis of flow effects in echo-planar imaging. JMRI 2:285-293

128. Baker JR, Hoppel BE, Stern CE, Kwong KK, Weisskoff RM, Rosen BR (1993) Dynamic functional imaging of the complete human cortex using gradient-echo and asymmetric spin-echo echo-planar magnetic resonance imaging. In: Proceedings of the SMRM, 12th annual meeting, New York, p 1400

129. Frank LR, Stout JC, Archibald S, Buxton RB (1993) Oblique flow compensation for improved functional imaging. In: Proceedings of the SMRM, 12th annual meeting, New York, p 1375

130. Hu X, Kim S-G (1994) Reduction of signal fluctuations in functional MRI using navigator echoes. Magn Reson Med 31:495-503

131. Wong EC, Boskamp E, Hyde JS (1992) A volume optimized quadrature elliptical endcap birdcage brain coil. In: Proceedings of the SMRM, 11th annual meeting, Berlin, p 4015

132. Wong EC, Tan G, Hyde JS (1993) A quadrature transmit-receive endcapped birdcage coil for imaging of the human head at 125 MHz. In: Proceedings of the SMRM, 12th annual meeting, New York, p 1344

133. Lee AT, Glover GH, Meyer CH (1995) Discrimination of large venous vessels in time-course spiral blood-oxygen-level-dependent magnetic-resonance functional neuroimaging. Magn Reson Med 33:745-754

134. Lee AT, Meyer CH, Glover GH (1993) Discrimination of large veins in time-course functional neuroimaging with spiral k-space trajectories. JMRI 3(P):59-60 (abstract)

135. Bandettini PA, Wong EC, Binder JR, Rao SM, Jesmanowicz A, Aaron EA, Lowry TF, Forster HV, Hinks RS, Hyde JS (1995) Functional MRI using the BOLD approach: dynamic characteristics and data analysis methods. In: LeBihan D (ed) Perfusion and diffusion imaging: MRI. Raven, New York, pp 335-349

136. Binder JR, Jesmanowicz A, Rao SM, Bandettini PA, Hammeke TA, Hyde JS (1993) Analysis of phase differences in periodic functional MRI activation data. In: Proceedings of the SMRM, 12th annual meeting, New York, p 1383

137. Binder JR, Rao SM, Hammeke TA, Bandettini PA, Jesmanowicz A, Frost JA, Wong EC, Haughton VM, Hyde JS (1993) Temporal characteristics of functional magnetic resonance signal changes in lateral frontal and auditory cortex. In: Proceedings of the SMRM, 12th annual meeting, New York, p 5

138. DeYoe EA, Neitz J, Bandettini PA, Wong EC, Hyde JS (1992) Time course of event-related MR signal enhancement in visual and motor cortex. In: Proceedings of the SMRM, 11th annual meeting, Berlin, p 1824

139. Bandettini PA, Wong EC, Yoe EAD, Binder JR, Rao SM, Birzer D, Estkowski LD, Jesmaniowicz A, Hinks RS, Hyde JS (1993) The functional dynamics of blood oxygen level dependent contrast in the motor cortex. In: Proceedings of the SMRM, 12th annual meeting, New York, p 1382

140. Bandettini PA (1993) Functional MRI of the brain. Society of Magnetic Resonance in Medicine, Berkeley, p 143

141. Belliveau JW, Kwong KK, Kennedy DN, Baker JR, Benson R, Chesler DA, Weisskoff RM, Cohen MS, Tootell RBH, Fox PT, Brady TJ, Rosen BR (1992) Magnetic resonance imaging mapping of brain function: human visual cortex. Invest Radiol 27:S59–S65
142. Friston KJ, Jezzard P, Turner R (1994) Analysis of functional MRI time-series. Human Brain Mapping 1:153–171
144. Savoy RL, O'Craven KM, Weisskoff RM, Davis TL, Baker J, Rosen B (1994) Exploring the temporal boundaries of fMRI: measuring responses to very brief visual stimuli. In: Book of abstracts, Society for Neuroscience, 24th annual meeting, Miami, p 1264
144. Orrison WW, Lewine JD, Sanders JA, Hartshorne MF (1995) Functional brain imaging. Mosby Year Book, St Louis
145. Ives JR, Warach S, Schmitt F, Edelman RR, Schomer DL (1993) Monitoring the patient's EEG during echo planar MRI. EEG Clin Neurophys 87:417–420
146. Ernst T, Hennig J (1994) Observation of a fast response in functional MR. Magn Reson Med 32:146–149
147. Biswal B, Bandettini PA, Jesmanowicz A, Hyde JS (1993) Time-frequency analysis of functional EPI time-course series. In: Proceedings of the SMRM, 12th annual meeting, New York, p 722
148. Song AW, Wong EC, Hyde JS (1994) Echo-volume imaging. Magn Reson Med 32:668–671
149. Cox RW, Jesmanowicz A, Hyde JS (1995) Real-time functional magnetic resonance imaging. Magn Reson Med 33:230–236
150. Turner R, Jezzard P, Bihan DL, Prinster A (1993) Contrast mechanisms and vessel size effects in BOLD contrast functional neuroimaging. In: Proceedings of the SMRM, 12th annual meeting, New York, p 173
151. Frahm J, Merboldt K-D, Hanicke W, Kleinschmidt A, Boecker H (1994) Brain or vein-oxygenation or flow? On signal physiology in functional MRI of human brain activation. NMR Biomed 7:45–53
152. Haacke EM, Hopkins A, Lai S, Buckley P, Friedman L, Meltzer H, Hedera P, Friedland R, Thompson L, Detterman D, Tkach J, Lewin JS (1994) 2D and 3D high resolution gradient-echo functional imaging of the brain: venous contributions to signal in motor cortex studies. NMR Biomed 7:54–62
153. Lai S, Hopkins AL, Haacke EM, Li D, Wasserman BA, Buckley P, Friedman L, Meltzer H, Hedera P, Friedland R (1993) Identification of vascular structures as a major source of signal contrast in high resolution 2D and 3D functional activation imaging of the motor cortex at 1.5T: preliminary results. Magn Reson Med 30:387–392
154. Engel SA, Rumelhart DE, Wandell BA, Lee AT, Glover GH, Chichilnisky EJ, Shadlen MN (1994) fMRI of human visual cortex. Nature 369:370 [erratum], 525:106 [erratum]
155. DeYoe EA, Bandettini P, Neitz J, Miller D, Winans P (1994) Methods for functional magnetic resonance imaging (FMRI) of the human brain. J Neurosci Methods 54:171–187
156. Schneider W, Noll DC, Cohen JD (1993) Functional topographic mapping of the cortical ribbon in human vision with conventional MRI scanners. Nature 365:150–153
157. Butts K, Riederer SJ, Ehman RL, Thompson RM, Jack CR (1994) Interleaved echo planar imaging on a standard MRI system. Magn Reson Med 31:67–72
158. McKinnon GC (1993) Ultrafast interleaved gradient-echo-planar imaging on a standard scanner. Magn Reson Med 30:609–616
159. Duyn JH, Moonen CTW, vanYperen GH, de Boer RW, Luyten PR (1994) Inflow versus deoxyhemoglobin effects in BOLD functional MRI using gradient-echoes at 1.5 T. NMR Biomed 7:83–88
160. Boxerman JL, Bandettini PA, Kwong KK, Baker JR, Davis TL, Rosen BR, Weisskoff RM (1995) The intravascular contribution to fMRI signal change: Monte Carlo modeling and diffusion-weighted studies in vivo Magn Reson Med 34:4–10
161. Song AW, Wong EC, Bandettini PA, Hyde JS (1994) The effect of diffusion weighting on task-induced functional MRI. In: Proceedings of the SMR, 2nd annual meeting, San Francisco, p 643
162. Boxerman JL, Weisskoff RM, Kwong KK, Davis TL, Rosen BR (1994) The intravascular contribution to fMRI signal change. Modeling and diffusion-weighted in vivo studies. In: Proceedings of the SMR, 2nd annual meeting, San Francisco, p 619
163. Menon RS, Hu X, Adriany G, Anderson P, Ogawa S, Ugurbil K (1994) Comparison of spin-echo EPI, asymmetric spin-echo EPI and conventional EPI applied to functional neuroimaging. The effect of flow crushing gradients on the BOLD signal. In: Proceedings of the SMR, 2nd annual meeting, San Francisco, p 622

164. Bandettini PA, Wong EC, Hinks RS, Estkowski L, Hyde JS (1992) Quantification of changes in relaxation rates R2* and R2 in activated brain tissue. In: Proceedings of the SMRM, 11th annual meeting, Berlin, p 719

165. Bandettini PA, Wong EC, Jesmanowicz A, Hinks RS, Hyde JS (1993) Simultaneous mapping of activation-induced ΔR2* and ΔR2 in the human brain using a combined gradient-echo and spin-echo EPI pulse sequence. In: Proceedings of the SMRM, 12th annual meeting, New York, p 169

166. Baker JR, Cohen MS, Stern CE, Kwong KK, Belliveau JW, Rosen BR (1992) The effect of slice thickness and echo time on the detection of signal changes during echo-planar functional neruroimaging. In: Proceedings of the SMRM, 11th annual meeting, Berlin, p 1822

167. Frahm J, Merboldt KD, Hanicke W, Kleinschmidt A, Steinmetz H (1993) High-resolution functional MRI of focal subcortical activity in the human brain. Long-echo time FLASH of the lateral geniculate nucleus during visual stimulation. In: Proceedings of the SMRM, 12th annual meeting, New York, p 57

168. Bruhn H, Kleinschmidt A, Boecker H, Merboldt K-D, Hanicke W, Frahm J (1994) The effect of acetazolamide on regional cerebral blood oxygenation at rest and under stimulation as assessed by MRI. J Cereb Blood Flow Metab 14:742–748

169. Ogawa S, Lee TM, Barrere B (1993) The sensitivity of magnetic resonance image signals of a rat brain to changes in the cerebral venous blood oxygenation. Magn Reson Med 29:205–210

170. deCrespigny AJ, Wendland MF, Derugin N, Kozniewska E, Moseley ME (1992) Real-time observation of transient focal ischemia and hyperemia in cat brain. Magn Reson Med 27:391–397

171. deCrespigny AJ, Wendland MF, Derugin N, Vexler ZS, Moseley ME (1993) Rapid MR imaging of a vascular challenge to focal ischemia in cat brain. JMRI 3:475–481

172. Bandettini PA, Aaron EA, Wong EC, Lowry TF, Hinks RS, Hyde JS, Forster HV (1994) Hypercapnia and hypoxia in the human brain: effects on resting and activation-induced MRI signal. In: Proceedings of the SMR, 2nd annual meeting, San Francisco, p 700

173. Prielmeier F, Nagatomo Y, Frahm J (1994) Cerebral blood oxygenation in rat brain during hypoxic hypoxia. Quantitative MRI of effective transverse relaxation rates. Magn Reson Med 31:678–681

174. Binder JR, Rao SM, Hammeke TA, Frost JA, Bandettini PA, Hyde JS (1994) Effects of stimulus rate on signal response during functional magnetic resonance imaging of auditory cortex. Cogn Brain Res 2:31–38

175. Rao SM, Bandettini PA, Bobholz J, Binder J, Hammeke TA, Frost JA, Hyde JS (1996) Relationship between movement rate and functional magnetic resonance signal change in primary motor cortex. J Cereb Blood Flow Metab 16:1250–1254

176. Sanders JA, Lewine JD, George JS, Caprihan A, Orrison WS (1993) Correlation of FMRI with MEG. In: Proceedings of the SMRM, 12th annual meeting, New York, p 1418

177. Connelly A, Jackson GD, Frackowiak RSJ, Belliveau JW, Vargha-Khadem F, Gadian DS (1993) Functional mapping of activated human primary cortex with a clinical MR imaging system. Radiology 188:125–130

178. Jack CR, Thompson RM, Butts RK, Sharbrough FW, Kelly PJ, Hanson DP, Riederer SJ, Ehman RL, Hangiandreou NJ, Cascino GD (1994) Sensory motor cortex: correlation of presurgical mapping with functional MR imaging and invasive cortical mapping. Radiology 190:85–92

179. Yablonsky DA, Haacke EM (1994) Theory of NMR signal formation in magnetically inhomogeneous tissue. Fast dephasing regime. Magn Reson Med 32:749–763

180. Wong EC, Bandettini PA (1993) A deterministic method for computer modelling of diffusion effects in MRI with application to BOLD contrast imaging. In: Proceedings of the SMRM, 12th annual meeting, New York, p 10

181. Boxerman JL, Hamberg LM, Rosen BR, Weisskoff RM (1995) MR contrast due to intravascular magnetic susceptibility perturbations. Magn Reson Med 34:555–566

182. Jesmanowicz A, Wong EC, Hyde JS (1993) Phase correction for EPI using internal reference lines. In: Proceedings of the SMRM, 12th annual meeting, New York, p 1239

183. Wong EC (1992) Shim insensitive phase correction for EPI using a two echo reference scan. In: Proceedings of the SMRM, 11th annual meeting, Berlin, p 4514

184. Prinster A, Pierpaoli C, Jezzard P, Turner R (1994) Simultaneous measurement of ΔR2 and ΔR2* in cat brain during hypoxia and hypercapnia. In: Proceedings of the SMR, 2nd annual meeting, San Francisco, p 439

185. Woods RP, Cherry SR, Mazziotta JC (1992) Rapid automated algorithm for aligning and reslicing PET images. J Comput Assist Tomogr 115:565–587

186. Friston KJ, Ashburner J, Frith CD, Poline J-B, Heather JD, Frackowiak R (1996) Spatial registration and normalization of images. Human Brain Mapping (in press)
187. Cohen JD, Noll DC, Schneider W (1993) Functional magnetic resonance imaging: overview and methods for psychological research. Behav Res Methods Instr Comput 25:101–113
188. LeBihan D, Jezzard P, Turner R, Cuenod CA, Pannier L, Prinster A (1993) Practical problems and limitations in using Z-maps for processing of brain function MR images. In: Proceedings of the SMRM, 12th annual meeting, New York, p 11
189. Sanders JA, Orrison WW (1993) ANOVA tests for identification of FMRI activation. In: Proceedings of the SMRM, 12th annual meeting, New York, p 1376
190. Schneider W, Casey BJ, Noll D (1994) Functional MRI mapping of stimulus rate effects across visual processing stages. Human Brain Mapping 1:117–133
191. Baker JR, Weisskoff RM, Stern CE, Kennedy DN, Jiand A, Kwong KK, Kolodny LB, Davis TL, Boxerman JL, Buchbinder BR, Wedeen VJ, Belliveau JW, Rosen BR (1994) Statistical assessment of functional MRI signal change. In: Proceedings of the SMRM, 2nd annual meeting, San Francisco, p 626
192. Biswal B, DeYoe EA, Cox RW, Hyde JS (1994) FMRI analysis for aperiodic task activation using nonparametric statistics. In: Proceedings of the SMR, 2nd annual meeting, San Francisco, p 624
193. Sychra JJ, Bandettini PA, Bhatttacharya N, Lin Q (1994) Synthetic images by subspace transforms. I. Principal components images and related filters. Med Phys 21:193–201
194. Bandettini PA, Wong EC, DeYoe EA, Binder JR, Hinks RS, Hyde JS (1993) Fourier analysis of functional EPI time-course series. JMRI 3(P):89 (abstract)
195. Binder JR, Rao SM, Hammeke TA, Yetkin FZ, Jesmanowicz A, Bandettini PA, Wong EC, Estkowski LD, Goldstein MD, Haughton VM, Hyde JS (1994) Functional magnetic resonance imaging of human auditory cortex. Ann Neurol 35:662–672
196. Binder JR, Rao SM (1994) Human brain mapping with functional magnetic resonance imaging. In: Kertesz A (ed) Localization and neuroimaging in neuropsychology. Academic, San Diego, p 185
197. Binder JR, Rao SM, Hammeke TA, Frost JA, Cox RW, Wong EC, Bandettini PA, Jesmanowicz A, Hyde JS (1994) A lateralized, distributed network for semantic processing demonstrated with whole brain functional MRI. In: Proceedings of the SMR, 2nd annual meeting, San Francisco, p 694
198. Binder JR, Rao SM, Hammeke TA, Frost JA, Cox RW, Bandettini PA, Hyde JS (1994) Identification of auditory, linguistic, and attention systems with task subtraction functional MRI. In: Proceedings of the SMR, 2nd annual meeting, San Francisco, p 681
199. Singh M, Kim H, Kim T, Khosla D, Colletti P (1993) Functional MRI at 1.5 T during auditory stimulation. In: Proceedings of the SMRM, 12th annual meeting, New York, p 1431
200. Turner R, Jezzard P, LeBihan D, Prinster A, Pannier L, Zeffiro T (1993) BOLD contrast imaging of cortical regions used in processing auditory stimuli. In: Proceedings of the SMRM, 12th annual meeting, New York, p 1411
201. Rao SM, Bandettini PA, Wong EC, Yetkin FZ, Hammeke TA, Mueller WM, Goldman S, Morris GL, Antuono PG, Estkowski LD, Haughton VM, Hyde JS (1992) Gradient-echo EPI demonstrates bilateral superior temporal gyrus activation during passive word presentation. In: Proceedings of the SMRM, 11th annual meeting, Berlin, p 1827
202. Bates SR, Yetkin FZ, Bandettini PA, Jesmanowicz A, Estkowski L, Haughton VM (1993) Activation of the human cerebellum demonstrated by functional magnetic resonance imaging. In: Proceedings of the SMRM, 12th annual meeting, New York, p 1420
203. Cuenod CA, Zeffiro T, Pannier L, Posse S, Bonnerot V, Jezzard P, Turner R, Frank JA, LeBihan D (1993) Functional imaging of the human cerebellum during finger movement with a conventional 1.5 T MRI scanner. In: Proceedings of the SMRM, 12th annual meeting, New York, p 1421
204. Ellerman JM, Flament D, Kim S-G, Fu Q-G, Merkle H, Ebner TJ, Ugurbil K (1994) Spatial patterns of functional activation of the cerebellum investigated using high field (4 T) MRI. NMR Biomed 7:63–68
205. Kim S-G, Hendrich K, Hu X, Merkle H, Ugurbil K (1994) Potential pitfalls of functional MRI using conventional gradient-recalled echo techniques. NMR Biomed 7:69–74
206. Kim S-G, Ashe J, Georgopoulos AP, Merkle H, Ellermann JM, Menon RS, Ogawa S, Ugurbil K (1993) Functional imaging of human motor cortex at high magnetic field. J Neurophysiol 69:297–302

207. Rao SM, Binder JR, Hammeke TA, Lisk LM, Bandettini PA, Yetkin FZ, Morris GL, Meuller WM, Antuono PG, Wong EC, Haughton VM, Hyde JS (1993) Somatotopic mapping of the primary motor cortex with functional magnetic resonance imaging. In: Proceedings of the SMRM, 12th annual meeting, New York, p 1397

208. Rao SM, Binder JR, Hammeke TA, Bandettini PA, Bobholz J, Frost JA, Myklebust BM, Jacobson RD, Hyde JS (1995) Somatotopic mapping of the human primary motor cortex with functional magnetic resonance imaging. Neurology 45:919–924

209. DeYoe EA, Carman GJ, Bandettini PA, Glickman S, Weiser J, Cox R, Miller D, Neitz J, Mapping Striate and extrastriate areas in human cerebral Cortex. PNAS (1996) 93:2382–2386

210. DeYoe EA, Neitz J, Miller D, Wieser J (1993) Functional magnetic resonance imaging (FMRI) of visual cortex in human subjects using a unique video graphics stimulator. In: Proceedings of the SMRM, 12th annual meeting, New York, p 1394

211. Bandettini PA, Rao SM, Binder JR, Hammeke TA, Jesmanowicz A, Yetkin FZ, Bates S, Estkowski LD, Wong EC, Haughton VM, Hinks RS, Hyde JS (1993) Magnetic resonance functional neuroimaging of the entire brain during performance and mental rehearsal of complex finger movement tasks. In: Proceedings of the SMRM, 12th annual meeting, New York, p 1396

212. DeLaPaz RL, Hirsch J, Relkin N, Victor J, Bartoshuk L, Norgren R, Prichard T (1994) Human gustatory cortex localization with functional MRI. In: Proceedings of the SMR, 2nd annual meeting, San Francisco, p 335

213. Kim S-G, Ashe J, Hendrich K, Ellerman JM, Merkle H, Ugurbil K, Georgopoulos AP (1993) Functional magnetic resonance imaging of motor cortex: hemispheric asymmetry and handedness. Science 261:615–616

214. Jezzard P, Karni A, Meyer G, Adams M, Prinster A, Ungerleider L, Turner R (1994) Practice makes perfect: a functional MRI study of long term motor cortex plasticity. In: Proceedings of the SMR, 2nd annual meeting, San Francisco, p 330

215. Ellerman JM, Flament D, Kim S-G, Merkle H, Andersen P, Ebner T, Ugurbil K (1994) Cerebellar activation due to error detection/correction in a visuo-motor learning task: a functional magnetic resonance imaging study. In: Proceedings of the SMR, 2nd annual meeting, San Francisco, p 331

216. Rao SM, Binder JR, Hammeke TA, Harrington DL, Haaland KY, Bobholz JA, Frost JA, Myklebust BM, Jacobson RD, Bandettini PA, Hyde JS (1994) Functional magnetic resonance imaging correlates of cognitive motor learning: preliminary findings. In: Proceedings of the SMR, 2nd annual meeting, San Francisco, p 329

217. McCarthy G, Blamire AM, Rothman DL, Gruetter R, Shulman RG (1993) Echo-planar magnetic resonance imaging studies of frontal cortex activation during word generation in humans. Proc Natl Acad Sci USA 90:4952–4956

218. Hinke RM, Hu X, Stillman AE, Kim S-G, Merkle H, Salmi R, Ugurbil K (1993) Functional magnetic resonance imaging of Broca's area during internal speech. Neuroreport 4:675–678

219. Rueckert L, Appollonio I, Grafman J, Jezzard P, Johnson R, Jr, LeBihan D, Turner R (1994) Magnetic resonance imaging functional activation of left frontal cortex during covert word production. J Neuroimaging 4:67–70

220. Menon R, Ogawa S, Tank DW, Ellermann JM, Merkle H (1993) Visual mental imagery by functional brain MRI. In: Proceedings of the SMRM, 12th annual meeting, New York, p 1381

221. Ogawa S, Tank DW, Menon R, Ellermann JM, Merkle H, Ugurbil K (1993) Functional brain MRI of cortical areas activated by visual mental imagery. In: Book of abstracts, Society for Neuroscience, 23rd annual meeting, Washington DC, p 976

222. Rao SM, Binder JR, Bandettini PA, Hammeke TA, Yetkin FZ, Jesmanowicz A, Lisk LM, Morris GL, Mueller WM, Estkowski LD, Wong EC, Haughton VM, Hyde JS (1993) Functional magnetic resonance imaging of complex human movements. Neurology 43:2311–2318

223. Tyszka JM, Grafton ST, Chew W, Woods RP, Colletti PM (1994) Parceling of mesial frontal motor areas during movement using functional magnetic resonance imaging at 1.5 tesla. Ann Neurol 35:746–749

224. Binder JR, Rao SM, Hammeke TA, Yetkin FZ, Wong EC, Mueller WM, Morris GL, Hyde JS (1993) Functional magnetic resonance imaging (FMRI) of auditory semantic processing. Neurology 43 [Suppl 2]:189 (abstract)

225. Binder JR, Rao SM, Hammeke TA, Frost JA, Bandettini PA, Jesmanowicz A, Hyde JS (1995) Lateralized human brain language systems demonstrated by task subtraction functional magnetic resonance imaging. Arch Neurol 52:593–601

226. Cohen JD, Perlstein WM, Braver TS, Nystrom LE, Noll DC, Jonides J, Smith EE, (1997) Nature 386 (6625):604–608

227. Cohen JD, Forman SD, Casey BJ, Noll DC (1993) Spiral-scan imaging of dorsolateral pre-frontal cortex during a working memory task. In: Proceedings of the SMRM, 12th annual meeting, New York, p 1405
228. Blamire AM, McCarthy G, Nobre AC, Puce A, Hyder F, Bloch G, Phelps E, Rothman DL, Goldman-Rakie P, Shulman RG (1993) Functional magnetic resonance imaging of human pre-frontal cortex during a spatial memory task. In: Proceedings of the SMRM, 12th annual meeting, New York, p 1413
229. LeBihan D, Turner R, Zeffiro T, Cuenod CA, Jezzard P, Bonnerot V (1993) Activation of human primary visual cortex during visual recall: a magnetic resonance imaging study. Proc Natl Acad Sci USA 90:11802–11805
230. Tootell RBH, Kwong KK, Belliveau JW, Baker JR, Stern CE, Savoy RL, Breiter H, Born R, Benson R, Brady TJ, Rosen BR (1993) Functional MRI (fMRI) evidence for MT/V5 and associated visual cortical areas in man. In: Book of abstracts, Society for Neuroscience, 23rd annual meeting, Washington DC, p 1500
231. Karni A, Ungerleider L, Haxby J, Jezzard P, Cuenod CA, Turner R, LeBihan D (1993) Stimulus dependent MRI signals evoked by oriented line-element textures in human visual cortex. In: Book of abstracts, Society for Neuroscience 23rd annual meeting, Washington DC, p 1501
232. Sorensen AG, Caramia F, Wray SH, Kwong K, Belliveau J, Stern C, Baker J, Gazit I, Breiter H, Rosen B (1993) Extrastriate activation in patients with visual field defects. In: Proceedings of the SMRM, 12th annual meeting, New York, p 62
233. Tootell RBH, Reppas JB, Dale AD, Look RB, Malach R, Brady TJ, Rosen BR (1996) Visual motion aftereffect in human cortical area MT/V5 revealed by functional magnetic resonance imaging. Nature 375:139–141
234. Sereno MI, Dale AM, Kwong KK, Belliveau JW, Brady TJ, Rosen BR, Tootell RBH (1995) Functional MRI reveals borders of multiple visual areas in humans. Science 268:889–893
235. Hedera P, Lai S, Haacke EM, Lerner AJ, Hopkins AL, Lewin JS, Friedland RP (1994) Abnormal connectivity of the visual pathways in human albinos demonstrated by susceptibility-sensitized MRI. Neurology 44:1921–1926
236. Cao Y, Vikingstad EM, Huttenlocher PR, Towle VL, Levin DN (1994) Functional magnetic resonance studies of the reorganization of the human hand sensorimotor area after unilateral brain injury in the perinatal period. Proc Natl Acad Sci USA 91:9612–9616
237. Renshaw PF, Yurgelun-Todd DA, Cohen BM (1994) Greater hemodynamic response to photic stimulation in schizophrenic patients: an echo planar MRI study. Am J Psychiatry 151:1493–1495
238. Jackson GD, Connelley A, Cross JH, Gordon I, Gadian DG (1994) Functional magnetic resonance imaging of focal seizures. Neurology 44:850–856
239. Wenz F, Schad LR, Baudendistel K, Flomer F, Schroder J, Knopp MV (1993) Effects of neuroleptic drugs on signal intensity during motor cortex stimulation: functional MR-imaging performed with a standard 1.5 T clinical scanner. In: Proceedings of the SMRM, 12th annual meeting, New York, p 1419
240. Breiter HC, Kwong KK, Baker JR, Stern CE, Belliveau JW, Davis TL, Baer L, O'Sullivan RM, Rauch SL, Savage CR, Cohen MS, Weisskoff RM, Brady TJ, Jenike MA, Rosen BR (1993) Functional magnetic resonance imaging of symptom provocation in obsessive-compulsive disorder. In: Proceedings of the SMRM, 12th annual meeting, New York, p 58
241. Breiter HC, Rauch SL, Kwong KK, Baker JR, Weisskoff RM, Kennedy DN, Kendrick AD, Davis TL, Jiang A, Cohen MS, Stern CE, Belliveau JW, Baer L, O'Sullivan RL, Savage CR, Jenike MA, Rosen BR (1996) Functional magnetic resonance imaging of symptom provocation in obsessive compulsive disorder. Arch Gen Psychiatry 53:595–605
242. Cao Y, Towle VL, Levin DN, Grzeszczuk R, Mullian JF (1993) Conventional 1.5 T functional MRI localization of human hand senserimotor cortex with intraoperative electrophysiologic validation. In: Proceedings of the SMRM, 12th annual meeting, New York, p 1417
243. Morris GL, Mueller WM, Yetkin FZ, Haughton VM, Hammeke TA, Swanson S, Rao SM, Jesmanowicz A, Estkowski LD, Bandettini PA, Wong EC, Hyde JS (1994) Functional magnetic resonance imaging in partial epilepsy. Epilepsia 35:1194–1198
244. Turner R, Jezzard P (1994) Magnetic resonance studies of brain functional activation using echo-planar imaging. In: Thatcher RW, Hallett M, Zeffiro T, John ER, Huerta M (eds) Functional neuroimaging. Technical foundations. Academic, San Diego, pp 69–78
245. Schulman RG, Blamire AM, Rothman DL, McCarthy G (1993) Nuclear magnetic resonance imaging and spectroscopy of human brain function. Proc Natl Acad Sci USA 90:3127–3133
246. Prichard JW, Rosen BR (1994) Functional study of the brain by NMR. J Cereb Blood Flow Metab 14:365–372

247. Cohen ME, Bookheimer SY (1994) Localization of brain function using magnetic resonance imaging. Trends Neurosci 17:1994
248. Bandettini PA, Binder JR, DeYoe EA, Hyde JS (1996) Sensory activation-induced hemo-dynamic changes observed in the human brain with echo planar MRI. In: Grant DM, Harris RK (eds) Encyclopedia of nuclear magnetic resonance imaging. Wiley & Sons Ltd, Chichester (1996) pp 1051–1056

CHAPTER 16

Research Issues Using Echo-Planar Imaging for Functional Brain Imaging

K. Kwong

Introduction

Functional magnetic resonance imaging (fMRI), a technique that images intrinsic blood signal change with magnetic resonance (MR) imagers, has in the past 3 years become one of the most successful tools used to study blood flow and perfusion in the brain. Since changes in neuronal activity are accompanied by focal changes in cerebral blood flow (CBF), blood volume (CBV), blood oxygenation, and metabolism, these physiological changes can be used to produce functional maps of mental operations.

There are two basic but completely different techniques used in fMRI to measure cerebral blood flow. The first is a classical steady-state perfusion technique first proposed by Detre et al. [1], who suggested the use of saturation or inversion of incoming blood T1-weighted signal to quantify absolute blood flow [1–5]. By focusing on T1 signal *change*, and hence blood flow *change*, and not just steady-state blood flow, Kwong et al. were successful in imaging brain visual functions associated with quantitative perfusion change [6]. There are many advantages in studying blood flow change alone, as many common baseline artifacts (magnetization transfer, imperfect cancellation of signals from static tissue, etc.) associated with MR absolute flow techniques can be subtracted out when we are only interested in changes. In addition, one obtains adequate information in most functional neuroimaging studies with information on flow change alone.

The second technique also looks at change of a blood parameter – blood oxygenation *change* and its associated T2* change during neuronal activity. The utility of the change of T2* change was strongly evident in Turner's work [7] with cats with induced hypoxia. Turner found that with hypoxia the MRI signal from the cats' brains decreases as the level of deoxyhemoglobin increases, a result which was an extension of Ogawa's earlier study [8, 9] of the effect of deoxyhemoglobin on MR signals in animal's veins. Turner's new observation was that when oxygen is restored, the cats' brain signal climbs to *above* its baseline level. This suggested that the vascular system overcompensates, bringing more oxygen, and that with more oxygen in the blood the MR signal rises beyond the baseline.

Based on Turner's observation and the perfusion method suggested by Detre et al., movies of human visual cortex activation utilizing both the perfusion and blood oxygenation techniques were successfully acquired in May 1991 (Fig. 1) at the Massachusetts General Hospital with a specially equipped super-

Fig. 1. Functional MR image demonstrating activation (colored region) of the primary visual cortex (V1). Image acquired on 9 May 1991 with a blood oxygenation sensitive MR GE technique

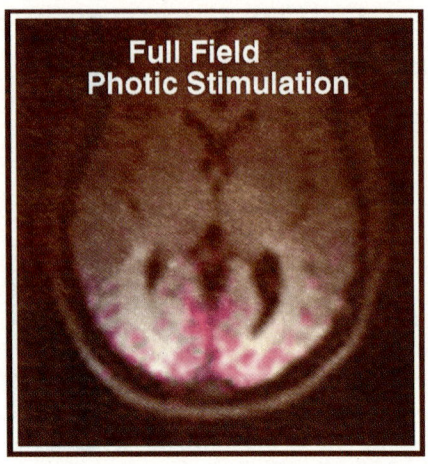

Full Field Photic Stimulation

fast 1.5-T system known as an echo-planar imaging (EPI) MR system [10]. fMRI results using intrinsic blood contrast were first presented in public at the Tenth Annual Meeting of the Society of Magnetic Resonance in Medicine in August 1991 [6, 11]. The research into visual cortex activation was carried out with flickering goggles, a photic stimulation protocol earlier employed by Belliveau et al. [12] to perform MR functional imaging of the visual cortex with the injection of the contrast agent Gd-DTPA. The use of external contrast agent allows the study of change in blood volume. The intrinsic blood contrast technique, sensitive to blood flow and blood oxygenation, uses no external contrast. Early model calculation showed that signal due to blood perfusion change is only around 1 % above baseline, and that the signal due to blood oxygenation change is also quite small. It was quite a pleasant surprise that fMRI results prove to be so robust and easily detectable.

EPI and fMRI is a "marriage made in heaven." It is impractical to collect hundreds of T1-weighted inversion recovery images with a conventional scanner whereas it is quite simple to collect T1-weighted, perfusion-indexed images with EPI. The normally unwanted susceptibility sensitivity of EPI is an additional bonus for T2* imaging in fMRI. The motion-freezing image acquisition speed of EPI makes the notorious motion artifacts of fMRI manageable. Moreover, the routinely long TR (2 s or longer) used to acquire EPI images proves to be extremely beneficial in suppressing MR signals from large vessel inflow. If we add the better signal to noise of EPI for images acquired in the same amount of time as conventional scanner and the multi-slice whole-head EPI imaging capability every 2 or 3 s, the major weakness of EPI – low spatial resolution – is an acceptable tradeoff under most conditions.

The blood oxygenation sensitive MR signal change, termed blood oxygenation level dependent (BOLD) by Ogawa [8, 9, 13], is in general much larger than the MR perfusion signal change during brain activation. Since most centers performing fMRI today are equipped only with conventional MR systems, the explosive growth of MR functional neuroimaging [14–33] in the past 3 years relies mainly on the measurement of blood oxygenation change. Both high-speed EPI and conventional MR have now been successfully employed for functional imaging in MRI systems with magnet field strength ranging from 1.5 to 4.0 T.

Advances in Functional Brain Mapping

The popularity of fMRI is based on many factors. It is safe and totally noninvasive. It can be acquired in single subjects for a scanning duration of several minutes, and it can be repeated on the same subjects as many times as necessary. The implementation of the blood oxygenation sensitive MR technique is universally available. Early neuroimaging work focused on time-resolved MR topographic mapping of human primary visual (V1; Figs. 2, 3), motor (M1), somatosensory (S1), and auditory (A1) cortices during task activation. Today, with the BOLD technique combined with EPI, one can acquire 20 or more contiguous brain slices covering the whole head (3×3 mm in plane and 5-mm slice thickness) every 3 s for a total duration of several minutes. The benefit of whole-head imaging are many. Not only can researchers identify and test their hypotheses on known brain activation centers, but they can also search for previous unknown or unsuspected sites. EPI resolution can reach 1.5×1.5 mm in plane and a slice thickness of 3 mm. Higher spatial resolution has been reported in conventional 1.5-T MR systems [34].

Of note in Fig. 3 is that with blood oxygenation sensitive MR technique one observes an undershoot [6, 15, 35] in signal in V1 when the light stimulus is

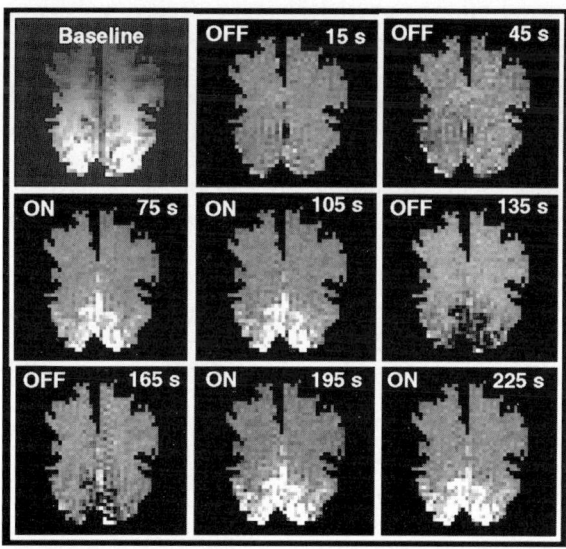

Fig. 2. Movie of fMRI mapping of primary visual cortex (V1) activation during visual stimulation. Images are obliquely aligned along the calcarine fissures with the occipital pole at the bottom. Images were acquired at 3-s intervals using a blood oxygenation sensitive MR sequence (80 images total). A baseline image acquired during darkness (*upper left*) was subtracted from subsequent images. Eight of these subtraction images are displayed, chosen when the image intensities reached a steady-state signal level, during darkness (*OFF*) and during 8-Hz photic stimulation (*ON*). During stimulation local increases in signal intensity are detected in the medial-posterior regions of the occipital lobes along the calcarine fissures

Fig. 3. Signal intensity changes for a region of interest (~60 mm^2) within the visual cortex during darkness and during 8-Hz photic stimulation. Results using oxygenation-sensitive (*above*) and flow-sensitive (*below*) techniques are shown. The flow sensitive data were collected once every 3.5 s, and the oxygenation sensitive data were collected once every 3 s. Upon termination of photic stimulation an undershoot in the oxygenation sensitive signal intensity is observed

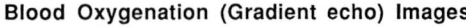

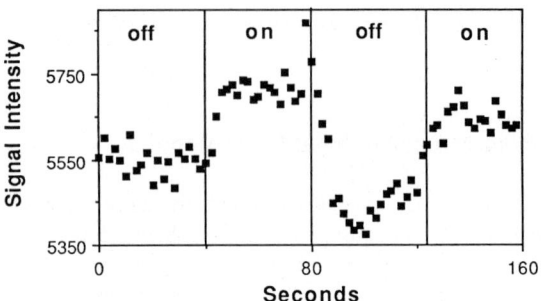

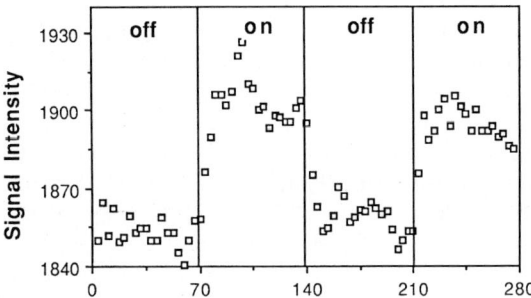

turned off. The physiological mechanism underlying the undershoot is still not well understood.

The data collected in the past 3 years have demonstrated that fMRI maps of the visual cortex are well correlated with known retinotopic organization [24, 36]. Higher visual regions such as V5/MT [37] and motor cortex organization [6, 14, 27, 38] have been successfully explored. Presurgical planning (Fig. 4) using motor stimulation [21, 39, 40] has helped neurosurgeons to preserve primary areas from tumors to be resected. For higher cognitive functions several fMRI language studies have already demonstrated known language-associated regions [25, 26, 41, 42] (Fig. 5). More detailed modeling has been carried out on the mechanism of functional brain mapping by blood oxygenation change [43–46]. Postprocessing techniques that would help to alleviate the serious problem of motion/displacement artifacts are available [47].

Fig. 4. Functional MRI mapping of motor cortex for presurgical planning. This three-dimensional rendering of the brain represents fusion of functional and structural anatomy. Brain is viewed from the top. A tumor is shown (*yellow*) in the left hemisphere, near the midline. The other colors depict sites of functional activation during movement of the right hand (*blue*), right foot (*red*), and left foot (*green*). The right foot cortical representation is displaced by tumor mass effect from its usual location. (Photo courtesy of Dr. Brad Buchbinder)

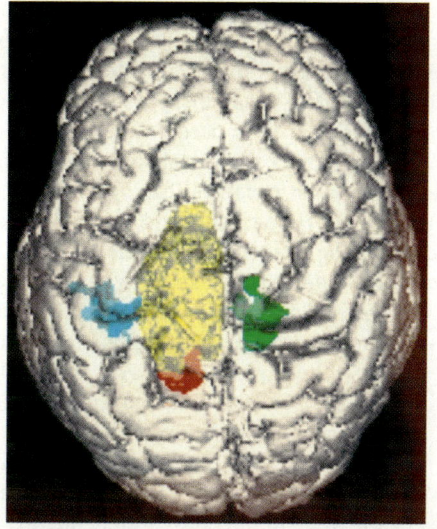

Fig. 5. Left hemisphere surface rendering of functional data (EPI, GE, 10 oblique coronal slices extending to posterior sylvian fissure) and high-resolution anatomical image obtained on a subject (age 33 years) during performance of a same-different (visual matching) task of pairs of words or nonwords (false font strings). Foci of greatest activation for this study are depicted in color and are located in dominant perisylvian cortex, i.e., inferior frontal gyrus (Broca's area),

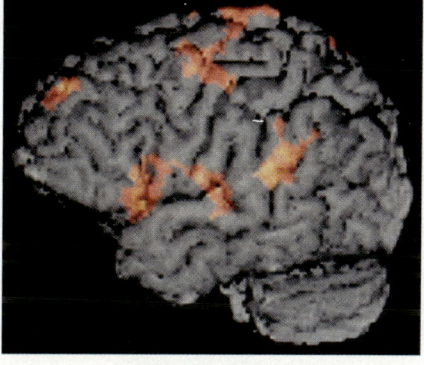

superior temporal gyrus (Wernicke's area), and inferior parietal lobule (angular gyrus). Also active in this task are sensorimotor cortex and prefrontal cortex. The perisylvian sites of activation are known to be key nodes in a left hemisphere language network. Prefrontal cortex probably plays a more general, modulatory role on attentional aspects of the task. Sensorimotor activation is observed in most language studies despite the absence of overt vocalization. (Photo courtesy of Dr. Randall Benson)

Mechanism

Flow-sensitive images show increased perfusion with stimulation, while blood oxygenation sensitive images demonstrate changes consistent with an increase in venous blood oxygenation. Although the precise biophysical mechanisms responsible for the signal changes have yet to be determined, good hypotheses exist to account for our observations.

Two fundamental MR relaxation rates, T1 and T2*, are used to describe the fMRI signal. T1 is the rate at which the nuclei approach thermal equilibrium, and perfusion change can be considered as an additional T1 change. T2* represents the rate of the decay of MR signal due to magnetic field inhomogeneities, and the change in T2* is used to measure blood oxygenation change (Fig. 6).

T2* changes reflect the interplay between changes in CBF, CBV, and oxygenation. As hemoglobin becomes deoxygenated, it becomes more paramagnetic than the surrounding tissue [48] and thus creates a magnetically inhomogeneous environment. The observed *increased* signal on T2*-weighted images during activation reflects a decrease in deoxyhemoglobin content, i.e., an increase in venous blood oxygenation. Oxygen delivery, CBF, and CBV all increase with neuronal activation. Because CBF (and hence oxygen delivery) changes exceed CBV changes by two to four times [49], while blood oxygen extraction increases only slightly [50, 51], the total paramagnetic blood deoxyhemoglobin content within brain tissue voxels decreases with brain activation The resulting decrease in the tissue-blood magnetic susceptibility difference leads to less intravoxel dephasing within brain tissue voxels and hence *increased* signal on T2*-weighted images [6, 14–16]. These results independently confirm observations obtained by positron emission tomography that activation-induced changes in blood flow and volume are accompanied by little or no increase in tissue oxygen consumption [50–52].

Since the effect of volume susceptibility difference $\Delta\chi$ is more pronounced at high field strength [53], higher field imaging magnets [16] increase the observed T2* changes.

Signal changes can also be observed on T1-weighted MR images. The relationship between T1 and regional blood flow has been characterized by Detre et al. [1]:

$$\frac{dM}{dt} = \frac{M_0 - M}{T_1} + fM_b - \frac{f}{\lambda} M \tag{1}$$

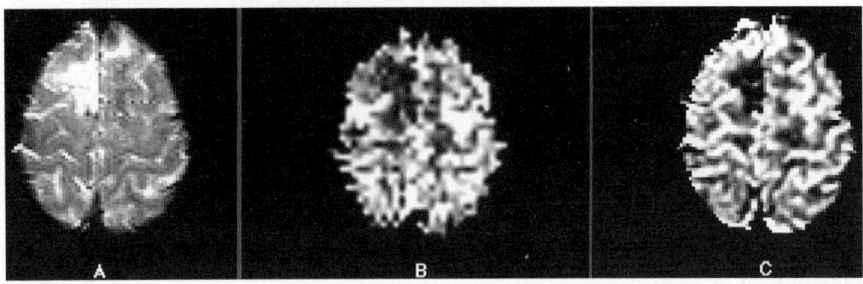

Fig. 6. Flow-related image (**B**) of a low-flow tumor obtained by subtracting a flow-nonsensitive (nonselective inversion) image from a flow-sensitive (selective inversion) image. CBV map (**C**) of the same tumor region obtained by fitting the time course of the injection of a bolus of MR contrast agent Gd-DTPA. The CBV map is a completely different and established method to measure hemodynamics with MR. T2-weighted anatomic image (**A**) of the same brain slice shows the tumor region filled with edema, bright because of its long T2 and long T1. The low-flow brain tumor (**B**; *dark region left of midline*) matches well with the CBV image (**C**). Gray-white matter differentiation is also similar between **B** and **C**

where M is tissue magnetization, and M_b is incoming blood signal. M_o is proton density, f is the flow (in milliliters per gram per unit of time), and λ is the brain-blood partition coefficient of water ($\sim$0.95 ml/g). From this equation, the brain tissue magnetization relaxes with an apparent time constant given by:

$$\frac{f}{\lambda} = \frac{1}{T_{1app}} - \frac{1}{T_1} \qquad (2)$$

where the $T1_{app}$ is the observed (apparent) longitudinal relaxation time with flow effects included. T1 is the true tissue longitudinal relaxation time in the absence of flow. If we assume that the true tissue T1 remains constant with stimulation, a change in blood flow Δf leads to a change in the observed $T1_{app}$:

$$\Delta T_{1app} = \Delta \frac{f}{\lambda} \qquad (3)$$

Thus, the MR signal change can be used to estimate the change in blood flow.

There are a number of ways to estimate baseline absolute blood flow instead of flow change. From Eq. 1, if the magnetization of blood and tissue always undergoes a similar T1 relaxation, the flow effect would be minimized. This is a condition that can be approximated by using a nonselective inversion T1 technique inverting *all* the blood coming into the imaged slice of interest. A flow-sensitive T1 sequence would be a slice-selective inversion pulse applied to the imaged slice. The flow-nonsensitive sequence can be subtracted from the flow-sensitive sequence to provide an index of CBF without the need of external stimulation [54, 55]. Initial results in tumor patients show that such flow mapping techniques are useful for mapping out blood flow of tumor regions [55] (Fig. 6).

Other flow techniques under investigation include the continuous inversion of incoming blood at the carotid level [1] and the use of a single-inversion pulse at the carotid level (EPI signal targeting with alternating radiofrequency, EPI STAR*) inverting the incoming blood [56, 57].

From our T_1 perfusion model and Eq. 2 one can derive expressions for the subtraction of signal intensity for all the baseline flow techniques mentioned above [55]. For a flow nonsensitive image subtracted from a flow-sensitive image, the MR signal becomes:

$$M_{sel} - M_{non} \approx 2M_o \cdot TI \cdot \frac{f}{\lambda} \cdot e^{\frac{-TI}{T_1}} \qquad (4)$$

where M_{sel} and M_{non} are magnetizations of the selective inversion (flow sensitive) pulse and the nonselective inversion (flow nonsensitive) pulse, respectively. M_o is proton density. TI and f are the usual TI and flow terms. One can see that the signal differences would be zero if there is no flow. With flow, the subtracted images are weighted by flow and proton density as well as by TI and T_1 terms.

The M_o in these equations is the M_o of brain matter alone, and not the M_o of mixed brain matter and CSF present at the same voxel. The CSF component has been subtracted out. It is interesting to note that Eq. 4 is merely a γ function commonly used to fit the kinetics of contrast agents entering and leaving the brain. This "coincidence" is not accidental. A slab of blood inverted at the carotid (e.g., EPI STAR*) is, in the context of the T_1 model, merely a version of the selective-nonselective inversion method. The kinetics of a slab of inverted blood can here be described as an inverted γ function.

For continuous inversion at the neck level and assuming no relaxation of the inverted blood traveling to the imaged slice, the expression of signal intensity in the steady state has already been derived as Eq. 1:

$$M_{control} - M_{inver} \approx 2M_o \cdot T_{1app} \cdot \frac{f}{\lambda} \tag{5}$$

In comparing Eqs. 4 and 5 it is interesting to note that at $TI = T_1$, which is the peak of the selective-nonselective difference, the continuous inversion technique has a theoretical advantage over the selective-nonselective inversion technique by a factor of e, if one is interested only in the subtraction of signal intensity [55]. Unfortunately, the continuous inversion technique has also a significant problem of magnetization transfer [1] which contaminates the flow signal with a magnetization transfer signal, which is several times larger.

Within the context of the T_1 model, a single-shot inversion of blood at the carotid level (EPI STAR*) would basically be the same as the nonselective-selective method [55] except with possible loss from relaxation of the inverted blood traveling to the imaged slice. The subtracted signal becomes smaller by a factor of $e^{\frac{TI}{T_1}}$

$$M_{control} - M_{tagged} \approx 2M_o \cdot (TI - TX) \cdot \frac{f}{\lambda} \cdot e^{\frac{-(TI - TX)}{T_1}} \cdot e^{\frac{-TX}{T_1}} \tag{6}$$

where TX is the time it takes blood to travel from the tagged site to the imaged slice of interest.

Baseline CBF is useful for many clinical situations such as studies of active tumor sites or epileptic centers. For most brain mapping and neurological studies the more sensitive flow change techniques are more appropriate.

Problem and Artifacts in fMRI:
The Brain-Vein Problem? The Brain-inflow Problem?

The artifacts arising from large vessels pose serious problems to the interpretation of fMRI data. It is generally believed that microvascular changes are specific to the underlying region of neuronal activation. However, MR gradient echo (GE) is sensitive to vessels of all dimensions [46, 58], and there is concern that macrovascular changes distal to the site of neuronal activity can be induced [20]. This is known as the brain-vein problem. For laboratories not equipped with EPI, GE sensitive to variations in T2* and magnetic susceptibility are the only realistic sequences available for fMRI acquisition; therefore the problem is particularly acute.

In addition, there is a non-deoxyhemoglobin-related problem which is especially acute in conventional MR. This is the inflow problem of fresh blood that can be time-locked to stimulation [28, 29, 59]. Such nonparenchymal and macrovascular responses can introduce error in the estimate of activated volumes.

Techniques To Reduce the Large Vessel Problems

In dealing with the inflow problems EPI has special advantages over conventional scanners. The use of long repetition times (2–3 s) in EPI significantly reduces the brain-inflow problem. Conventional GE sequences with very short TR must rely on smaller flip angle to reduce inflow effect [59]. Based on inflow modeling [60], one observes that at an angle smaller than the Ernst angle (Fig. 7) the inflow effect drops much more rapidly than the tissue signal response to activation [61]. One can therefore effectively remove the inflow artifacts with small flip-angle techniques.

Another simple method to suppress large vessel signals is the asymmetric spin-echo (ASE) method, which offsets the 180° by a time interval [62]. ASE maintains a high contrast-to-noise ratio in fMRI. The success of ASE is most likely due to the time-of-flight effect of its spin-echo component.

An exciting new possibility is to add small additional velocity dephasing gradients to suppress slow in-plane vessel flow ([61, 63]; W. Song, P. Bandettini, E. Wong, J. Hyde 1994, personal communication). Basically, moving spins lose signals while stationary spins are unaffected. The addition of these velocity-dephasing gradients decreases the overall MR signal (Fig. 8). The hypothesis that large vessel signals are suppressed while tissue signals remain intact is a subject of ongoing research.

Another advantage with EPI is the additional availability of another oxygenation-sensitive method such as the EPI T2-weighted spin echo (SE). T2-weighted SE methods are sensitive to the MR parameter T2, which is affected by microscopic susceptibility and hence blood oxygenation. Theoretically, T2-weighted SE methods are far less sensitive to large vessel signals [46, 58]. For conventional scanners T2-weighted SE methods take too long to perform and are therefore not practical options.

Fig. 7. Changes in inflow and tissue signal with activation (at short TR) vs. tip angle. Simulated curves show that at different velocities of (10, 20, 40 mm/s) of arterial flow (assuming laminar flow), MR signals due to inflow drop as a function of flip angle of the radiofrequency pulse. The inflow signal is compared to a simulated tissue response of 5 % signal change. MR parameters are TR = 60 ms, TE = 40 ms, with a simulated tissue T1 = 1 s. This demonstrates vividly that for a flip angle smaller than that of the Ernst angle inflow signal decreases much more rapidly than tissue signal drop

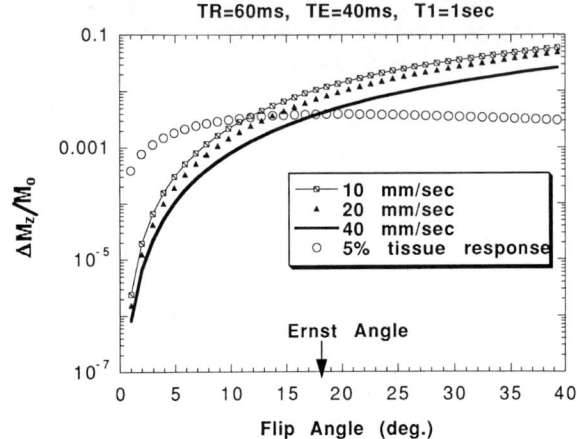

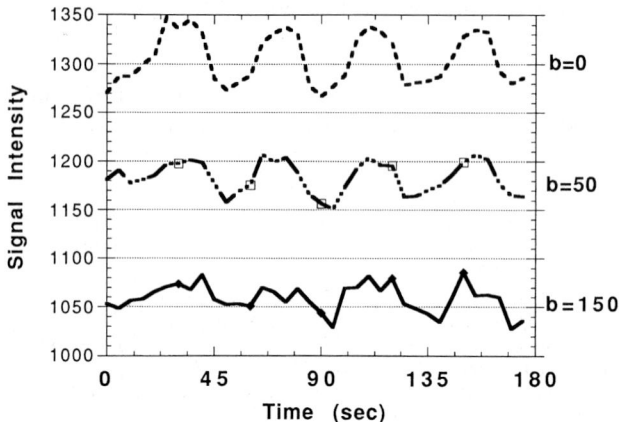

Fig. 8. fMRI (V1 stimulation) with diffusion gradients on. The curves represent time courses of MR response to photic stimulation (off-on-off-on...) with different levels of velocity dephasing gradients turned on to remove MR signals coming from the flowing blood of large vessels. *Top curve* had no velocity-dephasing gradients turned on; *bottom curve* was obtained with such strong velocity-dephasing gradients turned on that all large vessel signals were supposed to have been eliminated; *middle curve* represents a moderate amount of velocity-dephasing gradients, a tradeoff between removing large vessel signals and retaining a reasonable of MR signal to noise. b values (*right*) indicate the equivalent diffusion sensitivity for the velocity-dephasing gradients

The flow model (Eq. 1) based on T1-weighted sequences and independent of deoxyhemoglobin is also not so prone to larger vessel artifacts, as the T_1 model is a model of perfusion at the tissue level.

A study of volunteers has shown the average percentage change in T2*-weighted GE signal at V1 to be 2.5 % ±0.8 %. The average percentage change in oxygenation-weighted T2-weighted SE signal was 0.7 % ±0.3 % and the average percentage change in perfusion-weighted and T1-weighted MR signal 1.5 % ±0.5 %. These results demonstrate that T2-weighted SE and T1 methods, in spite of their ability to suppress large vessels, are not competitive with T2* effect at 1.5 T. However, since the microscopic effect detected by T2-weighted SE scales up with field strength [64], we expect the T2-weighted SE to be a useful sequence at high field strength such at 3 or 4 T. Advancing field strength should also benefit T1 studies due to the better signal-to-noise ratio and to the fact that T1 lengthens at higher field strength.

While GE sequence has a certain ambiguity when it comes to tissue versus vessels, its sensitivity at current clinical field strength makes it an extremely attractive technique to identify activation sites. By using careful paradigms that rule out possible links between the primary activation site and secondary sites one can circumvent many of the worries of "signal from the primary site draining down to secondary sites." A good example is as follows. Photic stimulation activates both the primary visual cortex and extrastriate cortex. To show that the extrastriate areas are not merely a drainage from the primary cortex, one can utilize paradigms that activate the primary visual cortex but not the extrastriate and vice versa. There are many permutations of this [37, 65]. It allows study of the higher order functions unambiguously even when one is using GE sequences.

The continuous advance of MRI mapping techniques utilizing intrinsic blood-tissue contrast promises the development of a functional human neuroanatomy of unprecedented spatial and temporal resolution.

References

1. Detre J, Leigh J, Williams D, Koretsky A (1992) Perfusion imaging. Magn Reson Med 23:37–45
2. Williams DS, Detre JA, Leigh JS, Koretsky AP (1992) Magnetic resonance imaging of perfusion using spin-inversion of arterial water. Proc Natl Acad Sci USA 89:212–216
3. Zhang W, Williams DS, Detre JA, Koretsky AP (1992) Measurement of brain perfusion by volume-localized NMR spectroscopy using inversion of arterial spins: accounting for transit time and cross relaxation. Magn Reson Med 25:362
4. Zhang W, Williams DS, Koretsky AP (1993) Measurement of rat brain perfusion by NMR using spin labeling of arterial water: in vivo determination of the degree of spin labeling. Magn Reson Med 29:416
5. Dixon WT, Du LN, Faul D, Grado M, Rosnick S (1986) Projection angiograms of blood labelled by adiabatic fast passage. Magn Reson Med 3:454
6. Kwong KK, Belliveau JW, Chesler DA, Goldberg IE, Weisskoff RM, Poncelet BP, Kennedy DN, Hoppel BE, Cohen MS, Turner R et al (1992) Dynamic magnetic resonance imaging of human brain activity during primary sensory stimulation. Proc Natl Acad Sci USA 89:5675–5679
7. Turner R, Le Bihan D, Moonen CT, Despres D, Frank J (1991) Echo-planar time course MRI of cat brain oxygenation changes. Magn Reson Med 22:159–166
8. Ogawa S, Lee T-M (1990) Magnetic resonance imaging of blood vessels at high fields: in vivo and in vitro measurements and image simulation. Magn Reson Med 16:9–18
9. Ogawa S, Lee T-M, Kay AR, Tank DW (1990) Brain magnetic resonance imaging with contrast dependent on blood oxygenation. Proc Natl Acad Sci USA 87:9868–9872
10. Cohen MS, Weisskoff RM (1991) Ultra-fast imaging. Magn Reson Imaging 9:1
11. Brady TJ (1991) Future prospects for MR imaging, vol 2. In: Proceedings Society of Magnetic Resonance in Medicine, San Francisco
12. Belliveau JW, Kennedy DN Jr, McKinstry RC, Buchbinder BR, Weisskoff RM, Cohen MS, Vevea JM, Brady TJ, Rosen BR (1991) Functional mapping of the human visual cortex by magnetic resonance imaging. Science 254:716–719
13. Ogawa S, Lee TM, Nayak AS, Glynn P (1990) Oxygenation-sensitive contrast in magnetic resonance image of rodent brain at high magnetic fields. Magn Reson Med 14:68–78
14. Bandettini PA, Wong EC, Hinks RS, Tikofsky RS, Hyde JS (1992) Time course EPI of human brain function during task activation. Magn Reson Med 25:390–397
15. Ogawa S, Tank DW, Menon R, Ellermann JM, Kim SG, Merkle H, Ugurbil K (1992) Intrinsic signal changes accompanying sensory stimulation: functional brain mapping with magnetic resonance imaging. Proc Natl Acad Sci USA 89:5951–5955
16. Turner R, Jezzard P, Wen H, Kwong K, Le Bihan D, Balaban R (1992) Functional mapping of the human visual cortex at 4 tesla using deoxygenation contrast EPI. In: Proceedings Society of Magnetic Resonance in Medicine, 11th annual meeting, Berlin, p 304
17. Frahm J, Bruhn H, Merboldt K, Hanicke W (1992) Dynamic MR imaging of human brain oxygenation during rest and photic stimulation. J Magn Reson Imaging 2:501–505
18. Blamire A, Ogawa S, Ugurbil K, Rothman D, McCarthy G, Ellermann J, Hyder F, Rattner Z, Shulman R (1992) Dynamic mapping of the human visual cortex by high-speed magnetic resonance imaging. Proc Natl Acad Sci USA 89:11069–11073
19. Menon R, Ogawa S, Tank D, Ugurbil K (1993) 4 Tesla gradient recalled echo characteristics of photic stimulation-induced signal changes in the human primary visual cortex. Magn Reson Med 30:380–386
20. Lai S, Hopkins A, Haacke E, Li D, Wasserman B, Buckley P, Friedman L, Meltzer H, Hedera P, Friedland R (1993) Identification of vascular structures as a major source of signal contrast in high resolution 2D and 3D functional activation imaging of the motor cortex at 1.5 T: preliminary results. Magn Reson Med 30:387–392

21. Cao Y, Towle VL, Levin DN, Grzeszczuk R, Mullan JF (1993) Conventional 1.5 T functional MRI localization of human hand sensorimotor cortex with intraoperative electrophysiologic validation. In: Proceedings Society of Magnetic Resonance in Medicine, 12th Annual Meeting, New York, p 1417
22. Connelly A, Jackson GD, Frackowiak RSJ, Belliveau JW, Vargha-Khadem F (1993) Functional mapping of activated human primary cortex with a clinical MR imaging system, Gadian. Radiology 188:125–130
23. Kim SG, Ashe J, Georgopouplos AP, Merkle H, Ellemann JM, Menon RS, Ogawa S, Ugurbil K (1993) Functional imaging of human motor cortex at high magnetic field. J Neurophysiol 69:297–302
24. Schneider W, Noll DC, Cohen JD (1993) Functional topographic mapping of the cortical ribbon in human vision with conventional MRI scanners. Nature 365:150–153
25. Hinke RM, Hu X, Stillman AE et al (1993) Functional magnetic resonance imaging of Broca's area during internal speech. Neuro Report 4:675–678
26. Binder JR, Rao SM, Hammeke TA, Yetkin FZ, Wong EC, Mueller WM, Morris GL, Hyde JS (1993) Functional magnetic resonance imaging (FMRI) of auditory semantic processing. Neurology [Suppl] 2:189
27. Rao SM, Binder JR, Bandettini PA, Hammeke TA, Yetkin FZ, Jesmanowica A, Lisk L, Morris GL, Mueller WM, Estowski LD, Wong EC, Haughton VM, Hyde JS (1993) Functional magnetic resonance imaging of complex human movements. Neurology 43:2311–2318
28. Gomiscek G, Beisteiner R, Hittmair K, Mueller E, Moser E, (1993) A possible role of in-flow effects in functional MR-imaging. MAGMA 1:109–113
29. Duyn J, Moonen C, de Boer R, van Yperen G, Luyten P (1994) Inflow versus deoxyhemoglobin effects in BOLD functional MRI using gradient-echoes at 1.5 T. NMR Biomed 7:83–88
30. Hajnal JV, Collins AG, White SJ, Pennock JM, Oatridge A, Baudoin CJ, Young IR, Bydder GM (1993) Imaging of human brain activity at 0.15 T using fluid attenuated inversion recovery (FLAIR) pulse sequences. Magn Reson Med 30:650
31. Hennig J, Ernst T, Speck O, Deuschl G, Feiffel E (1994) Detection of brain activation using oxygenation sensitive functional spectroscopy. Magn Reson Med 31:85
32. Constable RT, Kennan RP, Puce A, McCarthy G, Gore JC, (1994) Functional NMR imaging using fast spin echo at 1.5 T. Magn Res Med 31:686
33. Binder JR, Rao SM, Hammeke TA, Yetkin FA, Wong EC, Mueller WM, Morris GL, Hyde JS (1994) Functional magnetic resonance imaging of human auditory cortex. Ann Neurol 35:662–672
34. Frahm J, Merboldt K, Hänicke W (1993) Functional MRI of human brain activation at high spatial resolution. Magn Reson Med 29:139–144
35. Stern CE, Kwong KK, Belliveau JW, Baker JR, Rosen BR (1992) MR tracking of physiological mechanisms underlying brain activity. In: Proceedings Society of Magnetic Resonance in Medicine, annual meeting, Berlin, p 1821
36. Belliveau JW, Kwong KK, Baker JR, Stern CE, Benson R, Goldberg IE, Cohen MS, Kennedy DN, Brady TJ, Rosen BR (1992) MRI mapping of human visual cortex: retinotopic organization and frequency response of V1. In: Proceedings Society of Magnetic Resonance in Medicine, Annual Meeting, Berlin, p 310
37. Tootell RBH, Kwong KK, Belliveau JW, Baker JR, Stern CE, Hockfield SJ, Breiter HC, Born R, Benson R, Brady TJ, Rosen BR (1995) Functional analysis of human MT and related visual cortical areas using magnetic resonance imaging. J Neurosci 15:3215–3230
38. Kim S-G, Ashe J, Hendrich K et al (1993) Functional magnetic resonance imaging of motor cortex: hemispheric asymmetry and handedness. Science 261:615
39. Buchbinder BR, Jiang HJ, Cosgrove GR, Stern CE, Kwong KK, Baker JR, Alpert NM, Ogilvy CS, Fischman AJ, Rosen BR (1994) Functional mapping of sensorimotor cortex: correlation between functional MRI, O-15 PET, and intraoperative cortical stimulation in individual subjects. ASNR 162.
40. Jack CR, Thompson RM, Butts RK, Sharbrough FW, Kelly PJ, Hanson DP, Riederer SJ, Ehman RL, Hangiandreou NJ, Cascino GD (1994) Sensory motor cortex: correlation of presurgical mapping with functional MR imaging and invasive cortical mapping. Radiology 190:8592
41. Benson RR, Kwong KK, Belliveau JW, Baker JR, Cohen MS, Stern CE, Hildebrandt N, Rosen BR (1993) Magnetic resonance imaging studies of visual word recognition: words versus false font string. Society of Neuroscience 740:10
42. Benson RR, Kwong KK, Buchbinder BR, Jiang HJ, Belliveau JW, Cohen MS, Bookheimer S, Rosen BR, Brady TJ (1994) Noninvasive evaluation of language dominance using functional MRI. In: Proceedings Society of Magnetic Resonance, San Francisco, p 684

43. Ogawa S, Menon R, Tank D, Kim S, Merkle H, Ellermann J, Ugurbil K (1993) Functional brain mapping by blood oxygenation level- dependent contrast magnetic resonance imaging: a comparison of signal characteristics with a biophysical model. Biophys J 64:803–812
44. Ogawa S, Lee TM, Barrere B (1993) The sensitivity of magnetic resonance image signals of a rat brain to changes in the cerebral venous blood oxygenation. Magn Reson Med 29:205–210
45. Kennan RP, Zhong J, Gore JC (1994) Intravascular susceptibility contrast mechanisms in tissues. Magn Reson Med 31:9–21
46. Weisskoff RM, Zuo CS, Boxerman JL, Rosen BR (1994) Microscopic susceptibility variation and transverse relaxation: theory and experiment. Magn Reson Med 31:601–610
47. Bandettini PA, Jesmanowicz A, Wong EC, Hyde JS (1993) Processing strategies for time-course data sets in functional MRI of the human brain. Magn Reson Med 30:161–173
48. Thulborn KR, Waterton JC, Matthews PM, Radda GK (1982) Oxygenation dependence of the transverse relaxation time of water protons n Biochim Biophys Acta 714:265–270
49. Grubb RL, Raichle ME, Eichling JO, Ter-Pogossian MM (1974) The effects of changes in PaCo2 on cerebral blood volume, blood flow, and vascular mean transit time. Stroke 5:630–639
50. Fox PT, Raichle ME (1986) Focal physiological uncoupling of cerebral blood flow and oxidative metabolism during somatosensory stimulation in human subjects. Proc Natl Acad Sci USA 83:1140–1144
51. Fox PT, Raichle ME, Mintun MA, Dence C (1988) Nonoxidative glucose consumption during focal physiologic neural activity. Science 241:462
52. Prichard J, Rothman D, Novotny E, Petroff O, Kuwabara T, Avison M, Howseman A, Hanstock C, Shulman R (1991) Lactate rise detected by 1H NMR in human visual cortex during physiologic stimulation. Proc Natl Acad Sci USA 88:5829–5831
53. Brooks RA, Di Chiro G (1987) Magnetic resonance imaging of stationary blood: a review. Med Phys 14:903–913
54. Kwong K, Chesler D, Zuo C, Boxerman J, Baker J, Chen Y, Stern C, Weisskoff R, Rosen B (1993) Spin echo (T1, T2) studies for functional MRI. In: Proceedings Society of Magnetic Resonance in Medicine, 12th Annual Meeting, New York, p 172
55. Kwong KK, Chesler DA, Weisskoff RM, Rosen BR (1994) Perfusion MR imaging. In: Proceedings Society of Magnetic Resonance, San Francisco
56. Edelman R, Sievert B, Wielopolski P, Pearlman J, Warach S (1994) Noninvasive mapping of cerebral perfusion by using EPISTAR MR angiography. J MRI 4(P):68
57. Warach S, Sievert B, Darby D, Thangaraj V, Edelman R (1994) EPISTAR perfusion echo-planar imaging of human brain tumors. J Magn Reson Imaging 4(P):S8
58. Fisel CR, Ackerman JL, Buxton RB, Garrido L, Belliveau JW, Rosen BR, Brady TJ (1991) MR contrast due to microscopically heterogeneous magnetic susceptibility: numerical simulations and applications to cerebral physiology. Magn Reson Med 17:336–347
59. Frahm J, Merboldt K, Hanicke W (1993) Tissue vs vascular effects and changes of flow vs deoxyhemoglobin? Problems revealed by functional brain imaging high spatial resolution. In: Proceedings Society of Magnetic Resonance in Medicine, 12th annual meeting, New York, p 1427
60. Poncelet B, Weisskoff R, Wedeen V, Brady T, Kantor H (1993) Time of flight quantification of coronary flow with echo-planar MRI. Magn Reson Med 30:447
61. Kwong KK, Chesler DA, Boxerman JL, Davis TL, Weisskoff RM, Rosen BR (1994) Strategies to reduce macrovascular effects in fMRI. In: Proceedings Society of Magnetic Resonance, San Francisco, p 650
62. Baker JR, Hoppel BE, Stern CE, Kwong KK, Weisskoff RM, Rosen BR (1993) Dynamic functional imaging of the complete human cortex using gradient echo and asymmetric spin echo echo-planar magnetic resonance imaging. In: Proceedings Society of Magnetic Resonance in Medicine, New York, p 1400
63. Boxerman JL, Weisskoff RM, Kwong KK, Davis TL, Rosen BR (1994) The intravascular contribution to fMRI signal change. Modeling and diffusion-weighted in vivo studies. In: Proceedings Society of Magnetic Resonance, San Francisco, p 619
64. Zuo C, Boxerman J, Weisskoff R (1992) Compartment size determines T2 relaxivity in susceptibility contrast agents: theory and experiment. In: Proceedings Society of Magnetic Resonance in Medicine, 11th annual meeting, Berlin, p 866
65. Tootell RBH, Reppas JB, Kwong KK, Malach R, Belliveau JW, Brady TJ, Rosen BR (1995) Visual motion aftereffect in human cortical area MT revealed by functional magnetic resonance imaging. Nature 375:139–141

CHAPTER 17

Echo-Planar Imaging on Small-Bore Systems

A. J. S. de Crespigny

Introduction

While echo-planar imaging (EPI) has only recently become popular on clinical imaging systems as a result of improved hardware and the added stimulus of the new field of functional magnetic resonance imaging (MRI), the capability has existed on small-bore experimental systems for several years. High-performance gradient hardware is needed to achieve good spatial resolution for the small-scale structures imaged on these systems, and this same performance is also required for EPI. The two most important uses of small-bore MRI systems are in the oil exploration industry for analyzing potentially oil bearing rock samples, and in the biomedical field for studying laboratory animals. While submillimeter spatial resolution is needed in both of these fields, biomedical MRI has the additional need for efficient data collection, and in many cases motion insensitivity which can be met through the use of echo-planar imaging techniques.

Problems and Advantages of EPI on Small Bore Systems

SNR and Resolution

The greatest challenge of all MRI experiments on small systems is the tremendous loss in sensitivity that comes with the reduction in scale. From imaging the brain of a human (approx. 18 cm) to imaging the brain of a rat (approx. 1 cm) is a decrease in linear dimension of a factor of about 18, which corresponds to a reduction of about 1000 in voxel size to resolve comparable brain structures (factors of 18×18 in plane and 3 in the slice direction). This factor of 1000 less signal is partially offset by the higher field strengths of 2 and 4.7 T typically used on experimental systems along with the application of more sensitive volume and localized RF coils. Nevertheless there remains a significant penalty in terms of the signal-to-noise ratio (SNR) for animal imaging which must be addressed with careful experiment design and use of efficient data collection techniques.

On the positive side, the reduction in scale significantly reduces the inductance and increases the "magnetic-field-per-amp" of the gradient windings. These small, often self-shielded, high-efficiency gradients yield switching times of a few hundred microseconds or less, with maximum gradient strengths ranging from 7 G/cm (22 cm diameter), 20 G/cm (15 cm diameter) to 150 G/cm

(7.5 cm diameter). This is compared to 1 G/cm (60 cm diameter) on typical clinical systems. The maximum gradient strength, together with the SNR achievable with the radiofrequency (RF) coil, generally sets a limit on the spatial resolution that can be obtained on small bore systems, although on microscopy systems with gradient strengths in excess of 100 G/cm the ultimate limit on spatial resolution is set by diffusion of the spins through applied and internal magnetic field gradients [2].

A source of image degradation which is a particular problem for EPI is the effect of eddy currents induced in the magnet cryostat by the rapidly changing field gradients. This is a limiting factor for both clinical and experimental systems but can be alleviated by using self-shielded gradients. In many cases, however, there are residual effects resulting from imperfect shielding or eddy current compensation, and some form of phase correction of the EPI data is needed to remove these effects. The small size of gradients in experimental systems often means that the gradient windings are further away from the magnet cryostat and therefore induce less eddy currents: the combination of active shielding and the rapid fall off of the B field with distance means that the magnetic field penetrating into the cryostat is very small.

Magnetic Susceptibility Distortions

Geometrical distortions blurring and signal dropout in EPI images are problems common to the technique regardless of the scale of the imaging system and are often caused by magnetic susceptibility effects. Disruption of the main magnetic field (B_0) occurs close to boundaries between two regions of differing magnetic susceptibility (e.g., air-tissue) within the object of interest and often extend some distance from the boundary, depending on the shape and orientation of the object. EPI is particularly sensitive to magnetic susceptibility distortions because of the small image bandwidth in the phase-encode direction. While the readout bandwidth (receiver bandwidth) of the image is often 100 kHz or more, the phase-encode bandwidth can be a few tens of Hertz. This is comparable to the B_0 distortions caused by magnetic susceptibility differences, so that pixels can be shifted and dephased significantly in the phase-encode direction. Magnetic susceptibility effects are generally local and cannot be completely removed by shimming. The only effective solution is a reduction in the phase-encode bandwidth by more rapid sampling of the data (shortening the readout train, requiring even higher gradients) or interleaving the acquisition (multi-shot EPI).

In human brain imaging the air-tissue interface in the sinuses generally limits EPI of lower brain sections, while in the abdomen air in the lungs and intestines can compromise EPI of those regions. In animal imaging, however, magnetic susceptibility effects can be devastating. Since the field change caused by magnetic susceptibility difference scales with field strength, at 4.7 T the air-tissue interface in the sinus of a rat, for instance, can cause signal loss over the whole of the posterior part of the brain. Figure 1 compares EPI image quality in rat brain at two different field strengths and two different gradient strengths. Geometric distortion due to magnetic field inhomogeneities is particularly

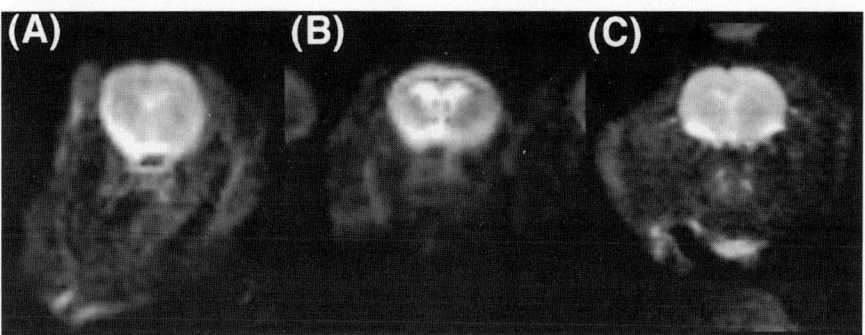

Fig. 1A–C. Single-shot EPI images of rat brain acquired on three small-bore MR systems with different field strengths and gradient coils but otherwise identical hardware, showing varying magnetic susceptibility effects (blurring, distortions). **A** 4.7 T, 80 kHz bandwidth, 64×64 (max. gradient ±7G/cm). **B** 2 T, 80 kHz bandwidth, 64×64 (max. gradient ±7G/cm). **C** 2 T, 200 kHz bandwidth, 128×128 (max. gradient ±20 G/cm). Note that the lower strength gradients limit the maximum bandwidth that can be used

noticeable at 4.7 T (Fig. 1A) however the greatest advantage is achieved by increasing the bandwidth (i.e., reducing the readout time) which is possible using stronger gradients.

EPI Pulse Sequences on Small Bore Systems

For the most part, the pulse sequences used on small-bore systems are the same as on the larger human imaging machines. However, one useful modification is the addition of 180° RF pulses to the EPI echo train to refocus dephasing caused by magnetic susceptibility variations. This can be done using a 180° pulse for every echo, as in rapid acquisition relaxation enhancement (RARE) [10], or for groups of echoes, as in gradient and spin echo [7].

Another way to circumvent the susceptibility problem (for the images at least) is the use of an EPI spectroscopic imaging sequence [15]. Here a rapid gradient echo (GRE) train is used without phase-encoding blips to encode the readout spatial dimension and the chemical shift dimension, while traditional phase encoding is performed in a multi-shot sequence to acquire the second spatial dimension. This is a very time efficient way to acquire a spectroscopic image with high spatial resolution. Figure 2 shows the simple pulse sequence (A) and spectroscopic image of rat brain (B) used here to show spatial variations in the water resonance frequency due to susceptibility and chemical shift. After Fourier transformation in all three dimensions the spectra at each pixel were fitted to a single Lorentzian lineshape function and the fit parameters displayed as images. With the addition of a water suppression pulse the sequence could be used for metabolite mapping in the brain.

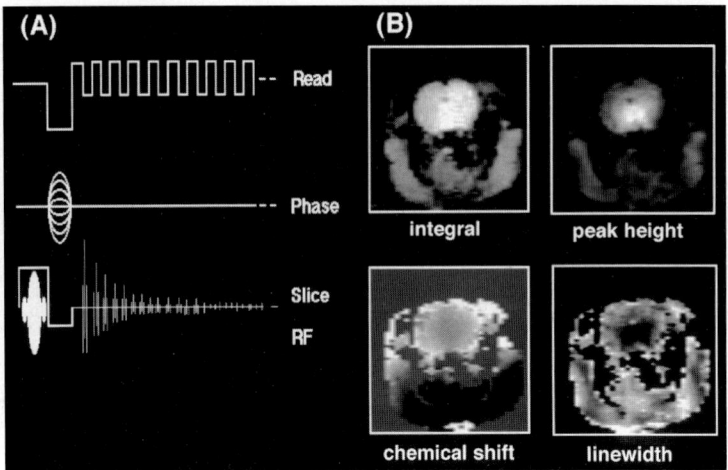

Fig. 2. Pulse sequence for spectroscopic EPI (**A**) and spectroscopic images of the water resonance across a coronal section of an in vivo rat head at 4.7 T (**B**). Parameters were 128×64 spatial×128 spectral dimensions. The maps of resonance frequency and linewidth in particular demonstrate the susceptibility induced magnetic field changes around the head

Applications: Animal Studies

Brain Imaging: Cerebral Ischemia

Uses of EPI to study animal models of various human disease states have focused largely on snapshot measurement of perfusion and diffusion, with application to experimental ischemia. The discovery of the decrease in apparent diffusion coefficient (ADC) with acute cerebral ischemia was first made on an animal imaging system [18] using a conventional spin-echo (SE) technique. In spite of the fact that the animals are anesthetized and the head mechanically immobilized, there are often significant motion-ghosting artifacts (resulting from respiratory motion) when using the large diffusion weighting gradients. These can be moderated by acquiring multiple averages but at the expense of long imaging times. Therefore, as soon as EPI became available on these small systems [29], the pulse sequence immediately found application in diffusion imaging of acute stroke [18]. Here the high speed imaging modality allows multiple, motion free, diffusion-weighted images with increasing b values to be acquired in a short time, thus allowing temporal mapping of regional ADC changes after the onset of ischemia. Figure 3 shows EPI diffusion-weighted images of a coronal slice through the brain of a cat, approximately 60 min after the onset of focal ischemia caused by inflation of a balloon occluder around the middle cerebral artery (MCA) [25]. Images were acquired on a GE chemical shift imaging (CSI) Omega system, equipped with ±20 G/cm Acustar shielded gradients. ADC maps produced from these data using a linear least-squares fitting program (Fig. 3B) clearly define the ischemic tissue as the region of significantly lower ADC than normal brain.

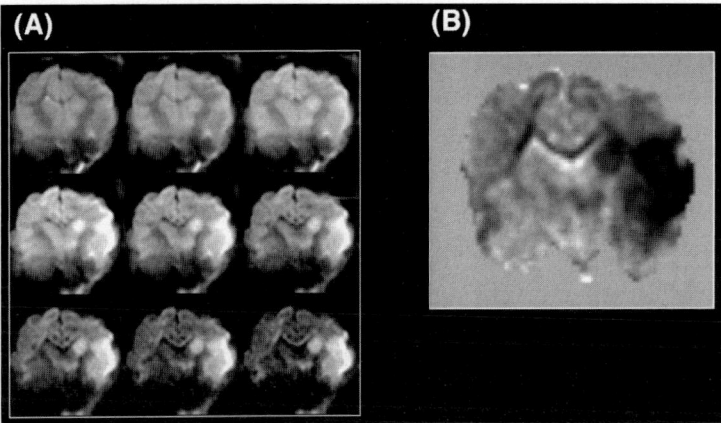

Fig. 3. A EPI diffusion-weighted images of ischemic cat brain at 2.0 T. Imaging parameters: 128×128 matrix, 70 mm FOV, 3 mm slice, TR 4 s, TE 80 ms, b values increased in equal steps from 10 to 1200 s/mm^2. Images are scaled individually to enhance the contrast between normal and ischemic tissue. The area of ischemia is clearly visible as the bright region in the left hemisphere. B ADC image calculated from the diffusion weighted data; pixel values are in units of 10^{-3} cm^2 s^{-1}, and give values of ~0.4 in the ischemic hemisphere and ~0.85 for the contralateral normal brain tissue

A vital counterpart to the diffusion data in stroke is information about relative cerebral blood flow patterns after an ischemic insult. Such information can be obtained by tracking a bolus injection of paramagnetic contrast agent with some high-speed imaging technique. EPI is of course well suited to this task and can easily follow the time course of a bolus transit, even with the relatively fast transit times found in animals [13, 16] and give perfusion information over multiple slices at once [5]. Figure 4 shows an example of high speed bolus tracking using a SE-EPI sequence to follow an injection of DyDTPA into ischemic cat brain (60 min post-MCA occlusion). The imaging parameters in this case were identical to those used for diffusion imaging shown in Fig. 3 (except that the diffusion gradients were turned off) allowing areas of tissue on both the diffusion and perfusion scans to be directly correlated. Figure 4A shows SE-EPI (TE 80 ms) images acquired with 2-s time resolution, clearly showing signal loss in the normal hemisphere due to T2 and T2* shortening as the paramagnetic agent passes through the microvasculature, with signal intensity largely recovering as the bolus washes out. Note the lack of signal change in the nonperfused brain. This is highlighted on the relative blood volume (rCBV) maps calculated by integrating the $\Delta R2$ transit curves for each pixel [$\Delta R2 = -\ln(S(t)/S(0))/TE$] shown in Fig. 4B. Here the dark area on the right of the image corresponds to the region of perfusion deficit.

While such rCBV maps do not give absolute blood flow or volume information, they are very valuable in distinguishing regions of normal and compromised perfusion, and particularly for following changes in blood flow during ischemia formation and subsequent therapy. A good example of this is the treatment of cerebral embolism using anticoagulant/thrombolytic agents. If successful

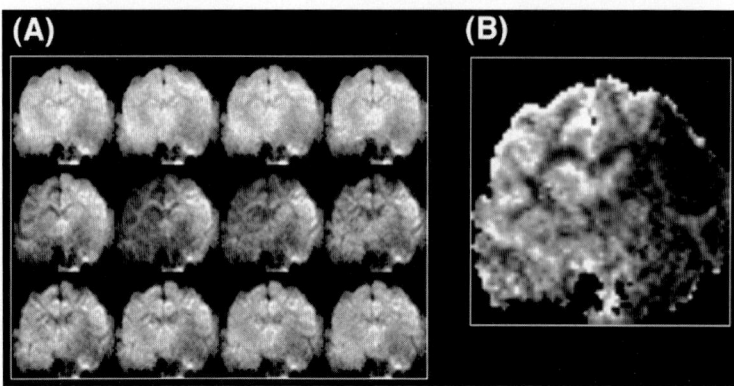

Fig. 4. A EPI T2-weighted images acquired with 2-s time resolution during the first pass transit of a bolus injection of paramagnetic contrast agent in focally ischemic cat brain at 2.0 T. The images are scaled identically to show the signal change as the agent passes through normally perfused brain tissue, while in ischemic brain there is no signal decrease. **B** The rCBV calculated from these images; ischemic brain is again visible as the region of severely reduced blood volume compared to the normally perfused tissue

blood clot lysis occurs following a thromboembolic stroke, blood supply may be returned to the ischemic tissue and resulting brain damage reduced or eliminated. Work performed in a rat model has shown the feasibility of using rCBV mapping to follow ischemia formation due to thromboembolic stroke, and treatment using streptokinase [5]. In this model, focal ischemia is induced by injection of a blood clot into the internal carotid artery. This model more closely mimics the corresponding human disease than most other models of experimental stroke in animals. However, due to clot fragmentation it produces regions of ischemia which are variable in position and extent throughout the brain, so that a 3D or multi-slice imaging approach is needed to fully characterize the injury.

Using multi-slice SE EPI on a 4.7 T GE CSI system to track a bolus injection of contrast agent, relative perfusion can be mapped over four sections through rat brain following embolic stroke. At this field strength magnetic susceptibility distortions can severely degrade echo-planar image quality, particularly near air-tissue interfaces in the sinuses. For this reason the most posterior slices of the rat brain could not be imaged, and careful shimming had to be performed on a slab containing the slices of interest. Linewidths of 60–80 Hz were typically obtained from a 12-mm thick slab. To further reduce susceptibility artifacts a SE-EPI sequence was used, rather than a GRE sequence, to track the first pass of a bolus injection of T2* shortening contrast agent. The spin echo refocuses much of the spin dephasing due to static field distortions while retaining sensitivity to the effects of the contrast agent via diffusion driven motion of water protons through microsusceptibility gradients around the capillaries and small veins of the cerebral microvasculature.

The EPI sequence used a 64×64 matrix size, 40-mm FOV, 74-kHz bandwidth, and 60-ms echo time. A 2-s repetition time was used in which four adjacent 3-mm-thick slices were acquired. Relative blood volume maps were generated as described above, and are shown in Fig. 5A for timepoints before and after stroke by clot injection and subsequent treatment with streptokinase. A large hemispheric region of perfusion deficit (dark area in images) is clearly seen after embolization (second set of images) compared to the uniform perfusion apparent in normal brain. Two injections of streptokinase were given shortly before image sets 3 and 4 to dissolve the blood clot, and a reduction in the region of perfusion deficit is clearly seen as time goes on. The same data are presented in Fig. 5B as a graph of the volume of deficit, calculated from the four imaged slices, showing the return of blood flow to the brain as a result of clot dissolution, compared to another animal which received no treatment.

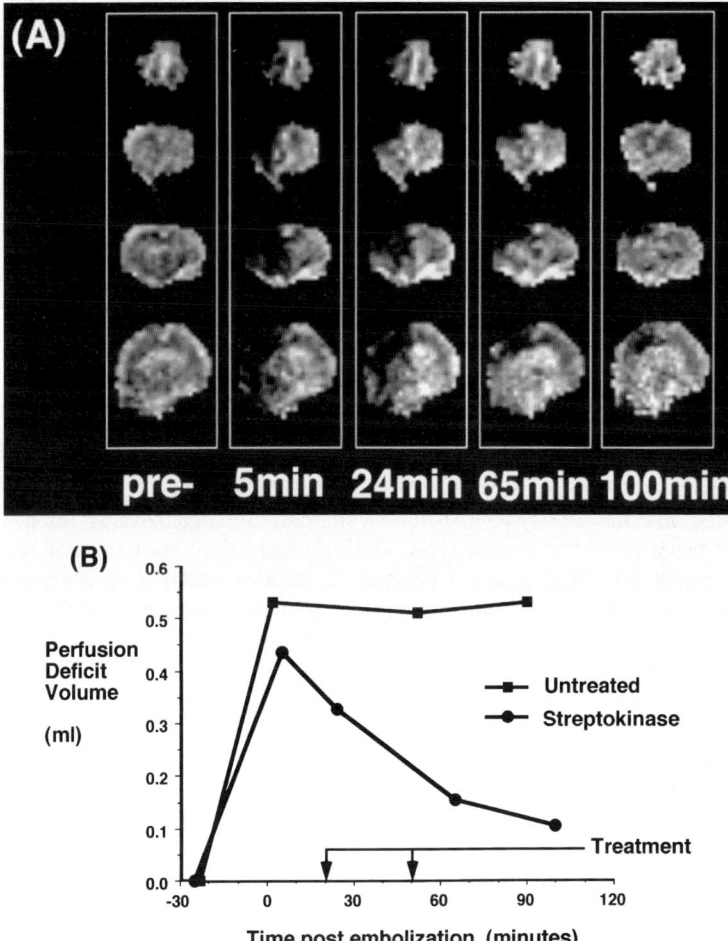

Fig. 5. A Maps of relative cerebral blood volume in four slices of rat brain before and at intervals after stroke by carotid embolization, and subsequent treatment with streptokinase. **B** Plots of volume of perfusion deficit calculated from the four slice rCBV maps for an animal receiving streptokinase compared to an untreated animal

Brain Imaging: Spreading Depression

The phenomenon of cortical spreading depression (SD) is a transient depression of cortical electrical activity, starting from the "initiation point" and spreading outwards as a wave at about 3 mm per minute. A change in the cells' ionic distributions also occurs, resulting in transient cellular swelling. SD may occur in such human conditions as stroke, migraine, and head trauma and is also believed to cause a local, temporary, increase in blood flow. Spreading depression has been observed in a rat model using conventional GRE MRI [8], where a transient 10 % signal increase was observed after cortical stimulation, which may be attributable to the blood oxygenation level dependent (BOLD) effect. The cellular swelling that occurs with SD might be expected to reduce the observed diffusion coefficient of the brain tissue, exactly as occurs in stroke following cerebral ischemia, except that in the case of SD blood flow is increased.

Diffusion imaging of SD presents a considerable challenge since multiple diffusion-weighting b values must be acquired repeatedly at high speed in order to map the transient diffusion changes occurring in this highly dynamic effect, and EPI is probably the only technique available for this task. EPI diffusion imaging of SD in rat brain has been carried out [14] using a 45-cm bore 2-T imaging system (GE CSI) equipped with ±20 G/cm shielded gradients. In this work SD was initiated by direct application of 40 μl KCl solution to the surface of the brain via a small burr hole. Diffusion weighted EPI (TR 1 s, TE 90 ms, 2 NEX) was carried out *continuously* for 6.5 min to monitor ADC changes over a single slice of brain as a function of time after SD initiation. Six b-values were used in order to generate ADC maps; however, since the SD effect changes quite rapidly over time, a "sliding window" method was used to combine the various b values into an ADC map with high temporal resolution. Rather than simply acquiring images with an increasing b-value sequence, (i.e., b~1, 2, 3, 4, 5, 6), b-values were acquired in an interleaved manner (b~1, 5, 3, 6, 2, 4) so that the high b-value images were acquired more evenly over time. The "sliding window" of six images used therefore generates ADC images at 2-s timepoints, each of which is an average over a 12-s time window. Figure 6 shows the result of such an experiment; the horizontal axis is time in seconds after SD initiation. The dark area of reduced ADC appears about 1 min after KCl administration and can clearly be seen moving down the cortex, disappearing after about 3 min, when brain ADC values return to normal. No such effect is seen in a control series of images after saline administration.

Using the same EPI techniques, SD has also been observed immediately following the onset of cerebral ischemia [26, 27]. After remotely occluding the middle cerebral artery of a rat inside the magnet a transient wave of ADC decrease was seen to travel bidirectionally away from the edge of the ischemic lesion into the peri-infarct tissue at a rate of about 3 mm/min.

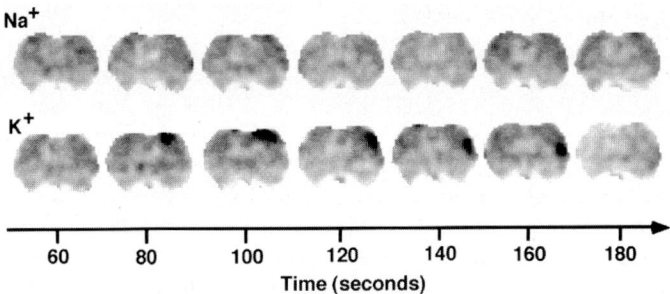

Fig. 6. Time-resolved ADC maps (12-s temporal resolution) of rat brain during an episode of cortical spreading depression initiated by application of KCl to the brain surface, compared to a control series using NaCl. *Black patch* (KCl series), a region of tissue with ADC values transiently reduced by 35% compared to normal, indicating temporary cell membrane depolarization. This patch of cellular "depression" propagates at a rate of ~3.3 mm/min. The ADC images were calculated from six diffusion-weighted EPI images using a "sliding window" method. (Data courtesy of Dr. L. Latour, Worcester Polytechnic Institute, Mass.)

Brain Imaging: Blood Oxygenation Level Dependent Contrast

Forming the basis for the new field of functional MRI, BOLD image contrast was first observed on a high-field small-bore system [22], where the paramagnetic effect of deoxyhemoglobin is most significant. Studies in animals at 2 T have shown that reversible "stresses" that alter cerebral blood flow and oxygenation, such as anoxia and apnea [32] result in observable signal changes in T2*-weighted EPI images. A decrease in blood oxygenation, as in apnea, causes signal loss due to the build up of paramagnetic deoxyhemoglobin in the blood. Conversely, an increase in cerebral blood flow, as occurs after the end of an anoxic or apneic challenge, can result in a transient increase in blood oxygenation in the brain and hence an increase in T2*-weighted image intensity.

The same effect can be used to observe the very earliest effects of cerebral ischemia, namely the deoxygenation of static blood in the brain as the arterial supply is cut off. In a global animal model of cerebral ischemia [31] signal decrease in T2*-weighted images was observed within the first few seconds. Figure 7 shows images from a similar experiment in which transient focal ischemia in cat brain was effected by inflating and deflating a balloon occluder surgically positioned around the middle cerebral artery (MCA) [4]. In this work GRE EPI images were acquired (GE CSI 2 T system, 64×64 matrix, 70 mm field of view (FOV), TE 24 ms, TR 2 s, 4 NEX) with 8-s time resolution during variable length periods of focal ischemia.

Figure 7 shows subtraction images to highlight signal changes, which occur predominantly in gray matter. The balloon occluder was inflated at point "A," and within 16 s this results in image intensity decrease, which plateaus out at about 8% after 20–30 s as the (now static) blood in the region of the brain supplied by the MCA becomes deoxygenated. After reperfusion, by deflating the occluder, signal intensity immediately returns to normal and transiently overshoots by 5% before returning to baseline. This overshoot is attributed to a tem-

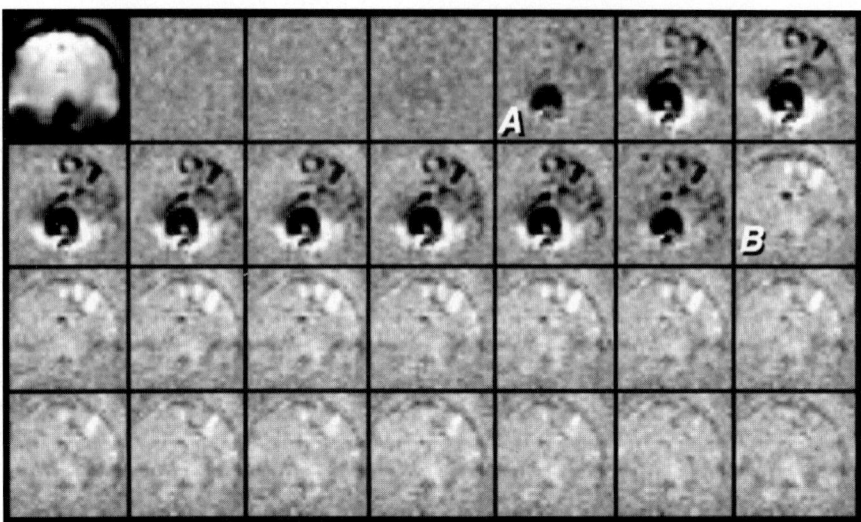

Fig. 7. GRE EPI baseline (*top left*) and time-resolved subtraction images during a 2.5-min episode of transient focal ischemia, acquired at 2 T. In the data shown, the time from one image to the next is 16 s. The MCA was occluded at *A* and released at *B*. Immediate signal loss due to the buildup of deoxyhemoglobin is observed in the MCA territory, with a transient overshoot in intensity after reperfusion, suggestive of a reactive hyperemia effect. *Circular black region* (at the base of the brain during ischemia), is a susceptibility artifact caused by the balloon occluder

porary increase in blood flow (hyperemia) to the region, and consequent overoxygenation, which leads to a reduction in deoxyhemoglobin, and T2* increase. The arteries and arterioles become maximally dilated during ischemia, resulting in increased CBF after reperfusion, and they subsequently constrict back to normal size after flow is resumed (causing the signal overshoot to return to normal). The length of the overshoot was found to increase with the length of ischemia.

The length and size of overshoot in signal intensity after transient ischemia may be an indication of the reactivity of the cerebral microvasculature, i.e., its ability to increase or decrease flow as a result of various metabolic conditions. As the vessels become damaged by prolonged ischemia, they are less able to respond to these changes and their reactivity is compromised. Tests of the reactivity of the cerebral microvasculature are performed clinically using an intravenous vasodilator agent, such as acetazolamide, combined typically with Xenon computed tomography to monitor the blood flow changes. A similar reactivity test is possible by functional MRI, using T2*-weighted GRE EPI to monitor changes in deoxyhemoglobin levels as a result of blood flow and volume changes following acetazolamide injection [34].

Figure 8A shows serial GRE EPI subtraction images of cat brain acquired during and after acetazolamide injection (100 mg/kg i.v., imaging parameters as in preceding subsection). The images were acquired 120 min after the onset of focal ischemia caused by MCA occlusion, as indicated by the area of hyperintensity in the diffusion-weighted image (Fig. 8B). The initial transient darkening in the

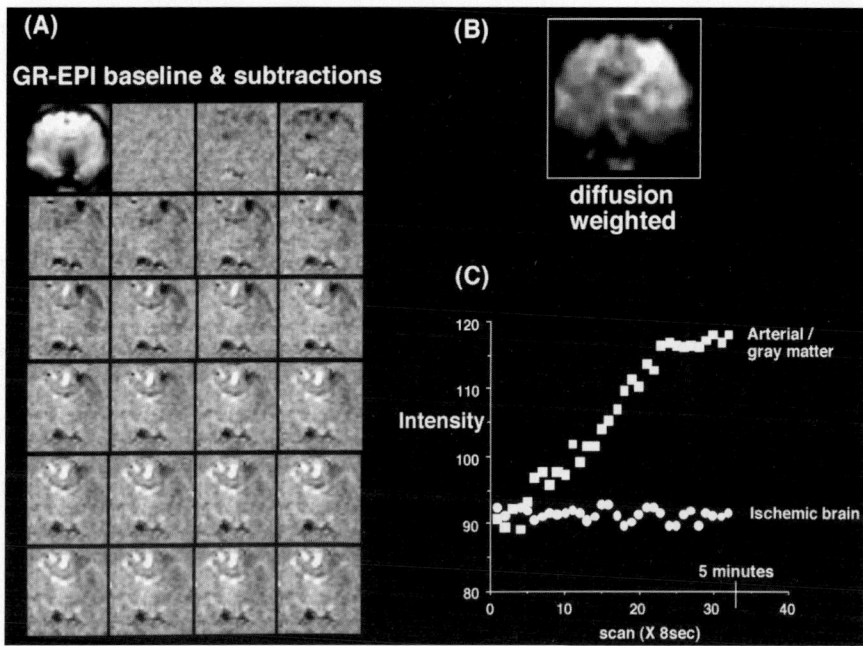

Fig. 8. Serial GRE EPI subtraction images (**A**) during acetazolamide injection (i.v.) in focally ischemic cat brain. The diffusion-weighted image (**B**) indicates the area of injury. For the data shown, the time between one image and the next is 8 s. Signal changes are observed only in normally perfused brain, while the ischemic tissue does not respond (**C**). *Bright areas* (later images), the result on T2* lengthening due to a reduction in deoxyhemoglobin concentration, which in turn is the result of the continuing increase in CBF in normal brain

images is most likely due to a drop in blood flow caused by a blood pressure decrease following injection. Signal intensity in perfused brain subsequently continues to increase for the rest of the imaging time, while ischemic brain shows no response. Figure 8C plots signal changes from regions of normal and ischemic cortical gray matter. Assuming that tissue oxygen usage does not significantly change, the signal increase observed may be directly attributable to an increase in blood flow to the normally perfused brain tissue. Thus functional MRI is able to monitor, though qualitatively, the ability of the microvasculature to respond to this "stress test" injection of vasodilator, and also distinguishes normal from unresponsive, ischemic tissue. As in the preceding subsection, the use of EPI allows imaging speed to be combined with high SNR per unit time to observe small (a small percentage) transient changes in T2*.

Cardiac EPI

EPI of the hearts of small laboratory animals presents a special challenge to the MR scanner hardware; not only is good spatial resolution necessary to resolve this (~10-mm-sized) organ but short echo times and readout times are required to avoid motion blurring since RR intervals are typically only 200–300 ms. Nevertheless, such scans have been performed on an in vitro preparation [1] and also in vivo on rat hearts [36] in a study of contrast-enhanced perfusion imaging of myocardial ischemia. For contrast bolus tracking the single-shot approach is necessary, and cardiac gating is used only to synchronize image acquisition to a particular point in the cardiac cycle.

Figure 9 shows a set of 64 single-shot GRE EPI images of a rat heart in an open-chest experimental myocardial ischemia preparation. The images were gated to every R wave for 64 consecutive beats, so that TR~350 ms. The TE was 10 ms, with asymmetric echo acquisition to minimize spin dephasing due to motion. Other imaging parameters were: GE 2 T CSI system, ±20 G/cm gradients, 50 mm FOV, 2 mm slice, 64×64 matrix, and 32 ms total image acquisition time. T2*-shortening contrast agent (Gd-DTPA) was injected after the second image of the series; signal loss can be seen as the bolus passes through the myo-

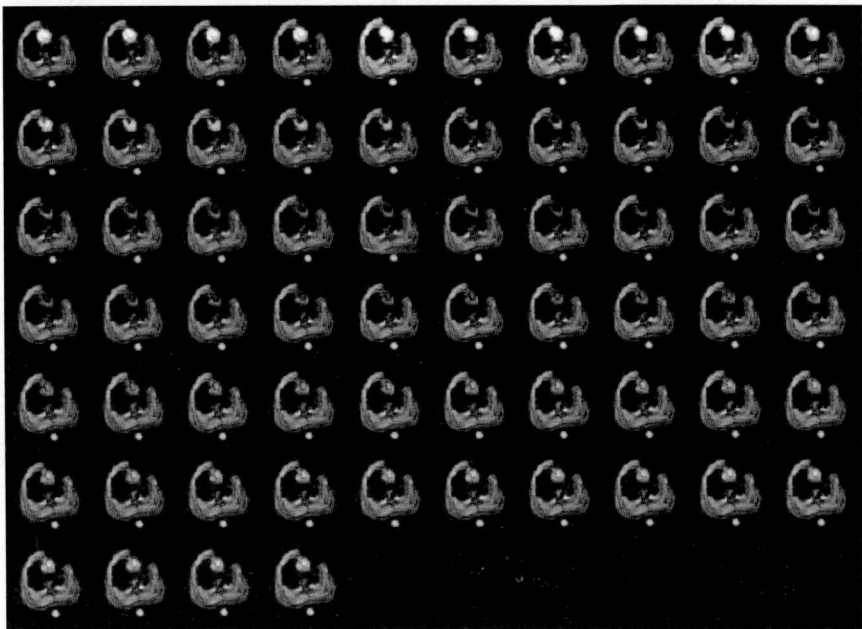

Fig. 9. Single-shot GRE EPI images of ischemic rat heart in vivo, gated to every heart beat for 64 consecutive beats (total imaging time 22 s). Echo time is 10 ms, 50 mm FOV, 64×64 matrix, 32 ms acquisition time. A bolus of Gd-DTPA was injected after the second image in the series and can be seen to cause darkening in perfused heart wall and in the chamber blood as the first pass goes through. (Images courtesy of Dr. M.F. Wendland, University of California, San Francisco)

cardium and ventricular chambers. Image intensity returns to normal after the end of the first pass. In this model of coronary artery occlusion part of the myo-cardium is ischemic and does not darken as the contrast is injected. In a similar experiment the use of endogenous deoxyhemoglobin contrast also indicated regions of perfusion deficit during episodes of apnea [35].

Cardiac imaging in an open-chest rat model is at the very limit of the 2-T small-bore scanner's hardware capability. Great care was required in positioning of the animal within the probe, shimming on the imaging slice and ensuring that adequate ventilation was maintained in order to keep the heart at the correct position within the chest cavity. Failure to take these precautions would result in image degradation due to susceptibility artifacts. In plane spatial resolution in the images in Fig. 9 was approximately 780 µm, although blurring due to motion and asymmetric echo sampling reduces this somewhat. Although this resolution is sufficient to resolve the heart wall, it gives only three to five pixels over this important piece of tissue. Further increases in resolution would require a larger matrix size, leading to longer readout time and greater chances of blur-ring due to motion. Another option is the use of echo-planar "zoom" imaging whereby a reduced region-of-interest (ROI) in the imaging slice is selectively excited (to remove image aliasing artifacts) and then imaged with a small FOV [30]. In this case, due to the problem of motion, a preferable option is to leave spins inside the ROI undisturbed and saturate everything outside [3]. Figure 10 shows an example of this approach in the rat heart. Figure 10A shows the full 50-mm FOV image, from which a circular region is chosen by saturating magnetization from surrounding tissue (Fig. 10B). Doubling the read-out and phase-blipped gradients then halves the FOV without any artifacts from signal folding back from outside the FOV shown in Fig. 10C. The subsequent

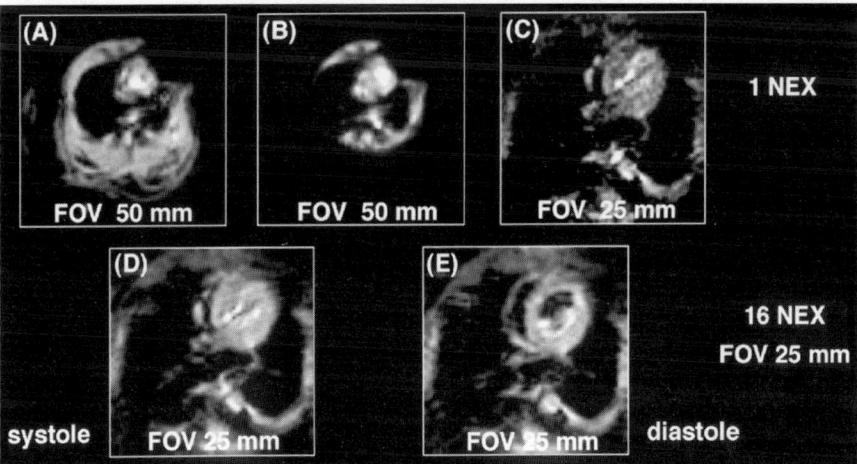

Fig. 10. Image (A) shows the full FOV section of an in vivo rat heart, from which a circular ROI is chosen by selective saturation (B). Reducing the FOV to 25 mm then yields ~400 µm resolution with no aliasing artifacts. The original image SNR may be obtained by signal averaging (D, E)

reduction in SNR due to the smaller voxel size may be recovered by signal averaging if required, as in Fig. 10D,E.

EPI of Liver Perfusion

As with clinical abdominal MRI in humans, the major concern is controlling the effects of respiratory motion on image quality, and snapshot imaging techniques are highly advantageous. In animals the higher respiratory rate requires still faster imaging, although in many experimental models the use of mechanical ventilation allows MRI image acquisition to be quite accurately gated. Nevertheless, dynamic imaging is required to follow rapid changes such as contrast bolus transit in perfusion imaging or blood oxygenation changes in functional fMRI experiments. Bolus tracking experiments in the liver have been carried out in a canine model [24] using iron oxide particles as a T2* contrast agent [23]. Such intravascular contrast agents are useful in liver perfusion experiments as they do not immediately leak into the surrounding tissue and can thus maintain a good first pass bolus concentration-time profile.

Gadolinium agents such as Gd-DTPA can also be used if they are attached to some large molecule to keep them from leaking out of the intravascular space. An example of this is the use of polylysine-Gd-DTPA in bolus tracking experiments in the rat liver [33]. Figure 11 shows a series of single-shot EPI images during a bolus injection of polylysine-Gd-DTPA. Selected images are displayed from a series acquired with 1.5-s time resolution during the injection (2.0 T, GRE EPI, TE 20 ms, TR 1.5 s, FOV 50 mm, 64×64, 1 NEX). The T2*-shortening effect of the contrast agent produced up to 40 % signal loss in the liver tissue, which clearly highlights the implanted tumor (shown by the arrow in Fig. 11) as a region of perfusion deficit.

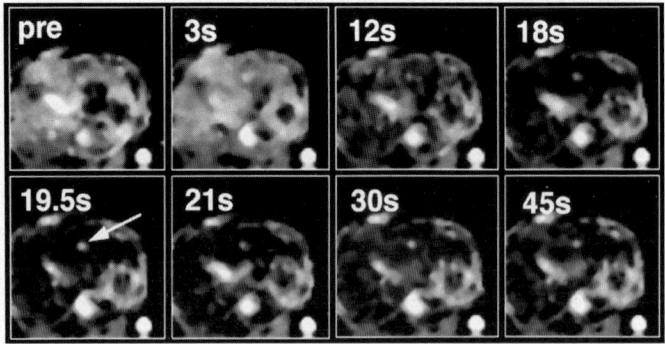

Fig. 11. GRE EPI images selected from a bolus tracking series acquired during injection of polylysine-Gd-DTPA in a rat liver with implanted tumor (*arrow*). The tumor is highlighted as a region of reduced blood flow, and hence reduced signal loss during the contrast passage. (Images reproduced courtesy of Dr. V. Vexler, University of California, San Francisco)

Kidney Perfusion/Function

Regional tissue perfusion can also be obtained using a functional MRI approach, relying on changes in blood deoxyhemoglobin concentration during some paradigm or "stress test." Such an experiment in the kidneys might be expected to yield a large BOLD contrast effect compared to the brain because of the relatively large blood volume in this organ. Figure 12 shows an example of such a functional MRI paradigm carried out as part of an experiment on focal renal ischemia [33]. The images are single-shot GRE EPI coronal slices through rat kidneys at 2 T, acquired using the "zoomed EPI" technique described above. A circular 30-mm-diameter region including both kidneys was isolated by selective saturation, and automatic shimming performed on this ROI. Blood deoxygenation was effected by 60-s apneic episodes (by ceasing mechanical ventilation) which caused up to 40% signal loss in the parenchyma of nonischemic kidneys (Fig. 12A).

In this model focal ischemia was caused by i.v. injection of glycerol, which is known to cause a vasoconstrictive decrease in renal perfusion, predominantly in the inner cortex. An identical apnea experiment carried out 2 hours after the onset of ischemia (Fig. 12B) again shows significant decrease in parenchymal signal after 60 s, but now a bright band is visible in the inner cortex which

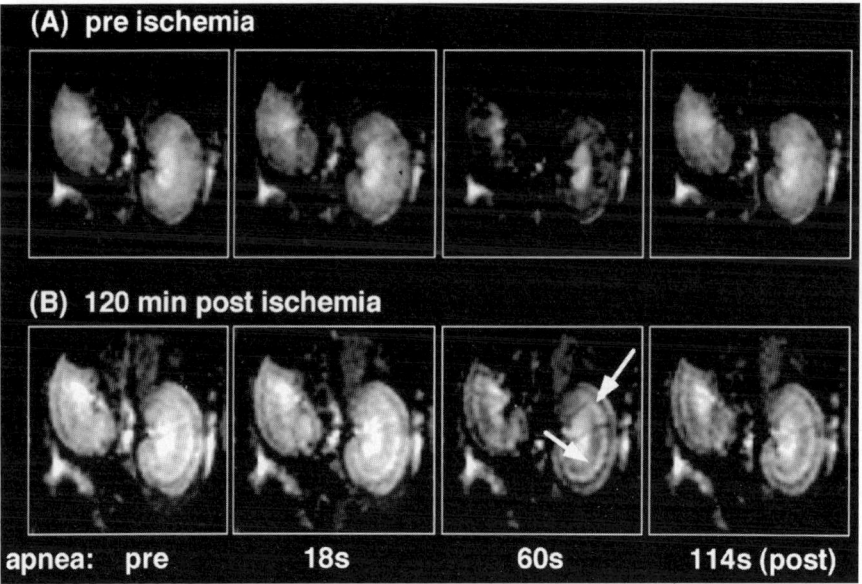

Fig. 12. Single-shot zoomed GRE EPI images of rat kidneys selected from a series acquired during 60-s episodes of apnea before (**A**) and after (**B**) focal renal ischemia by glycerol administration. Image FOV is 35 mm with 64×64 matrix, TE 20 ms, TR 6 s. BOLD signal loss is observed in normal kidney parenchyma, but this signal change is markedly reduced in the inner cortex (*arrows*) after glycerol injection. (Images reproduced courtesy of Dr. V. Vexler, University of California, San Francisco)

does not darken with global blood deoxygenation due to the reduction in blood flow to this region. The location of this area of renal perfusion deficit was later confirmed by contrast bolus tracking, and postcontrast T1-weighted MRI. Thus changes in renal perfusion are clearly observable using only endogenous BOLD contrast.

Applications: Human Studies

The high-performance of small-bore MRI systems may be used to image human peripheral organs such as arms and legs. Once again, measurement of in vivo diffusion coefficients benefits from the motion insensitivity of EPI in organs that are harder to immobilize than the brain. Rapid, motion artifact free imaging is essential to measure T2 and ADC changes before, during, and after exercise in human arm muscle. The problems of motion in such a study are obvious; however, high-speed scanning is also required as the buildup and washout of water in the muscle is expected to be relatively fast. Figure 13 shows the results of such a study [17, 19] using a 2-T small-bore animal system with 16-cm inner diameter shielded gradients. The magnet design is asymmetric, so that the isocenter of the B_0 field is nearer one end than the other, enabling the forearm of a volunteer sitting beside the magnet to be easily positioned inside the RF probe at the center of the field. EPI images acquired in real time during exercise show up to 80 % signal increases in the active muscle groups (TE = 46 ms, TR = 3 s). The EPI sequence used a 64×64 matrix, 5-mm slice, 80-mm FOV and an inversion pulse was used for fat suppression (TI = 170–190 ms). Measure-

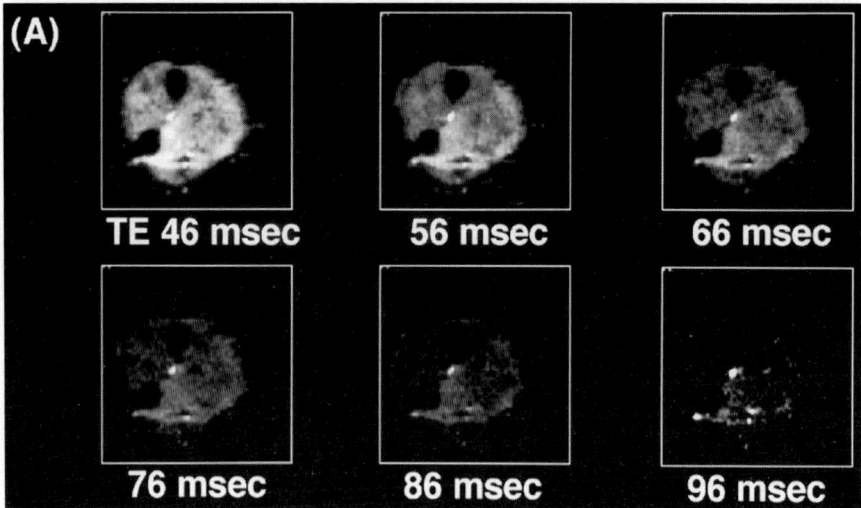

Fig. 13. A Single-shot SE EPI images of human forearm after exercise acquired with increasing echo time (*TE*) and long repeat time TR = 15 s; total acquisition time 2.5 min. *Brighter regions*, exercised muscle with T2 value of 40 ms, compared to 30 ms in the resting state.

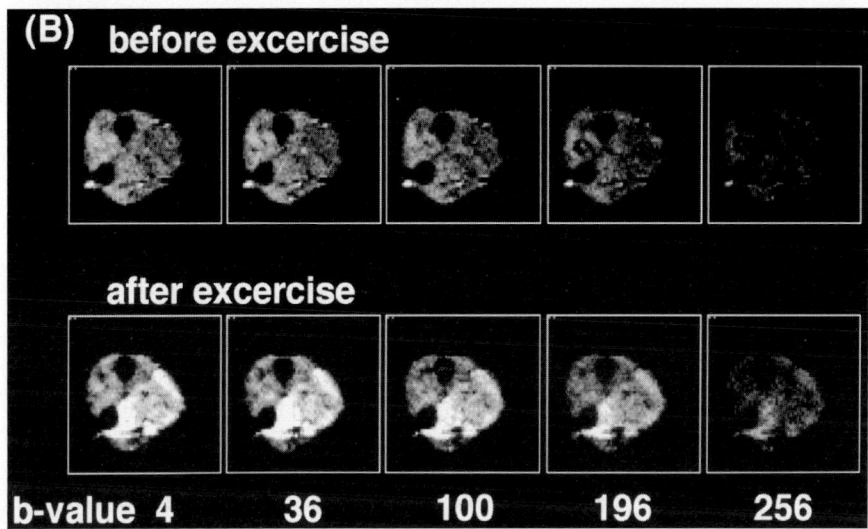

Fig. 13. B Diffusion-weighted EPI images (TE 46 ms, TR 15 s) with increasing b value before and after exercise: total acquisition time 2.5 min. ADC values increased by 6%–8% in exercised muscle, and also 5%–8% in resting muscle. (Images courtesy of Dr. M. Moseley, Stanford University, California)

ments of T2 were made after exercise using multiple acquisitions with increasing echo time (TE 46–96 ms, TR 15 s; Fig. 13A) and yielded values of 40 ± 5 ms for exercised muscle groups and 30 ± 4 ms for relaxed groups. The increased T2 is probably due to increased water content.

The same pulse sequence was used with diffusion gradients added to measure ADC values before and after exercise. Measurements of diffusion anisotropy before exercise gave relative diffusivity values (ADC/ADC_{H2O}) of 0.63, 0.61, 0.89 for the X, Y, and Z directions, where Z is oriented along the arm, consistent with a picture of faster diffusion in directions parallel with the muscle fibers. ADC_z was measured before and after exercise, as shown in Fig. 13B. ADC values increased by 6%–8% in exercised muscle, but also by 5%–8% in nonexercised muscle groups, suggesting that this observed change may be due mostly to a temperature increase of the arm.

Applications: EPI Microscopy

As we move to yet higher fields, into the realm of NMR microscopy, the demands on gradient hardware continue to increase. Fortunately, magnet bore sizes tend to decrease in these systems, and therefore it is quite possible to design self-shielded gradients that can produce ±40 G/cm or more over a FOV of a few centimeters without drawing excessive currents into the necessarily small coil windings. At first sight, EPI might seem an unlikely pulse sequence to use for micro-

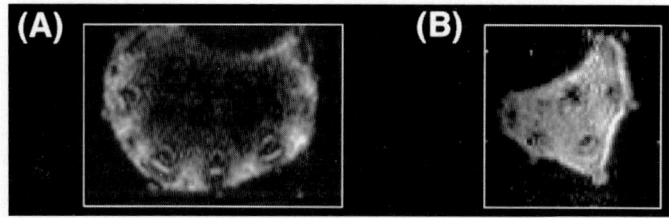

Fig. 14A,B. Microscopic single-shot EPI sections through a celery stem acquired at 9.4 T. In plane resolution 94 µm (**A**) and 53 µm (**B**). (Images courtesy of Dr. S. Sukumar, Bruker Instruments Inc.)

scopic imaging at high magnetic fields, where magnetic susceptibility effects are large and high spatial resolution is required. However, the efficient data sampling of the EPI sequence makes the best possible use of available NMR signal and can provide optimum SNR in the small voxel sizes. The sequence can also be interleaved to increase the maximum imaging matrix size, while the addition of 180° refocusing pulses overcomes some of the magnetic susceptibility effects.

For microscopic MRI of living organisms or other biological systems problems of small sample size are compounded by the problem of sample motion and stability over long imaging times. For cellular organisms suspended in fluid only a snapshot imaging approach can hope to be successful, without moving to some form of sample immobilization such as use of a gel matrix, which may adversely affect the organisms themselves. A demonstration of the kind of spatial resolution possible at high fields with the availability of high gradients is shown in Fig. 14. In this example a 9.4-T vertical bore GE CSI system, equipped with 150 G/cm self-shielded gradients [28], was used to image two sections through a celery stem. Both images were acquired with a single-shot SE EPI sequence. The first image (Fig. 14A) has an in-plane resolution of 94 µm (128×128 matrix, 12 mm FOV, 2 mm slice thickness, 100 kHz bandwidth) and clearly shows the structure present within the vascular bundles around the edge of the stem. The second image (Fig. 14B) shows a thinner portion of the same stem with 53 µm in-plane resolution (128×128 matrix, 6.8 mm FOV, 2 mm slice thickness, 100 kHz bandwidth).

Applications: EPI of Flow

The use of EPI as a rapid acquisition technique opens the possibility of performing multidimensional MRI experiments in much reduced times. In this section, rapid three-dimensional MR anemometry by motion sensitive phase-encoded echo-planar MRI is demonstrated to visualize all three components of the velocity. Conventionally the acquisition of such data would require an extremely long experimental time. EPI is therefore a key technology in the practical development of these techniques.

Measurement of fluid flow patterns has been performed using EPI [9] in humans and on small-bore systems [11, 12]. Recent measurements in three dimensions [6] were carried out using an experimental baffled duct flow system which generates a number of interesting flow features in a single system. A motion-encoding scheme employing pulsed field gradients (PFGs) with a stimulated echo was implemented as a magnetization preparation module in front of each EPI acquisition. Motion encoding was performed using encoding gradients with duration, $\delta = 3$ ms and a displacement evolution interval, $\Delta = 109$ ms. The use of longitudinal storage of the magnetization allows much longer evolution intervals to be employed with this sequence than inclusion of the PFGs in the imaging sequence. Seventeen motion-encoded images were obtained for each of the three Cartesian components of the motion with a constant 3510 Hz/cm increment between successive images. The approximate volumar flow rate of the fluid, measured at the point of runoff, was 14 ml per minute. A 100-ms z storage period was allowed between motion encoding and imaging. A slab selected, phase-encoded MBEST sequence was used to acquire 64^3 voxel images with TE = 47 ms, TR 2 s, readout time 40 ms, $4.5 \times 4.5 \times 5.5$ cm FOV, four averages. Experiments performed at 2 T using 10 cm inner diameter ± 30 G/cm unshielded gradients.

Each complex motion encoded image took approximately 17 min to acquire. For each of the three Cartesian components of the velocity, 17 three-dimensional images were generated; one for each increment of the displacement encoding

Fig. 15. Images from a six dimensional EPI velocity dataset of a cylindrical fluid flow phantom containing two flat baffles. Three-dimensional rendered images are shown for each of the three Cartesian components of velocity (*a–c*) together with the speed, v , image (*d*). (Images courtesy of Dr. J.A. Derbyshire, Herschel Smith Laboratory, Cambridge University, UK)

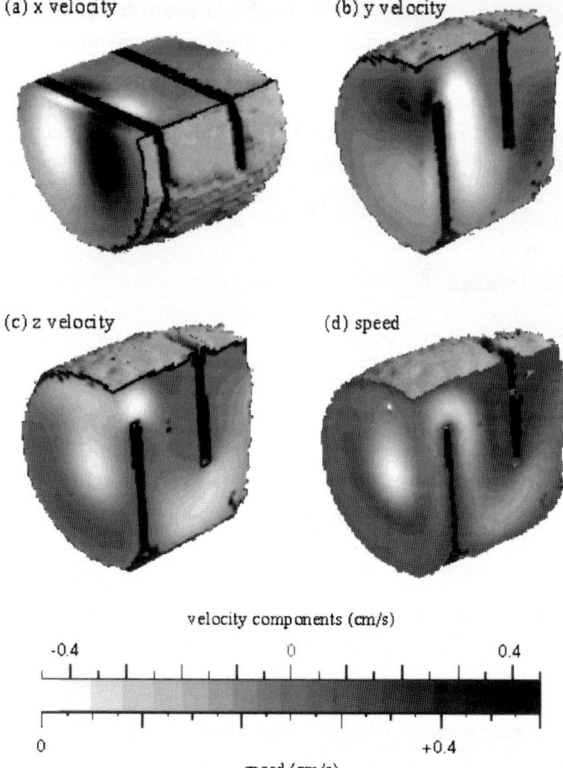

(a) x velocity

(b) y velocity

(c) z velocity

(d) speed

velocity components (cm/s)

-0.4   0   0.4

0   +0.4

speed (cm/s)

number, q. The individual pictures were processed using a three-dimensional image rendering software to obtain a two-dimensional view of the baffle phantom data by ray casting. This software allows the external structure to be cut away to reveal the internal features of the dataset.

Frequency analysis of the motion encoded data sets can be performed using an interpolated Fourier transform of the q space signal at each voxel followed by identification of the modal frequency (velocity). The modal values of the velocity components were then used to construct velocity component maps of the data, shown in Fig. 15 which clearly shows the pattern of fluid flow around the flat baffle obstructions in the tube.

Rapid imaging protocols such as the EPI method minimize the data acquisition time required for each image in the sequence, but a completely time-efficient protocol must also minimize the number of images to be acquired. The use of motion encoded, three-dimensional EPI in combination with nonuniform q-space sampling represents a powerful experimental technique.

Conclusions

In spite of the technical difficulties of imaging small objects, EPI has proved useful in a wide variety of imaging applications in which speed and motion insensitivity are required. Physiological motion in animals is significantly faster than in humans; nevertheless with sufficient optimization EPI can capture images of a rapidly beating animal heart, while the efficient data sampling allows the collection of six dimensional images (three spatial + three flow). With further advances in small diameter and local gradient coil design and magnet homogeneity the use of the EPI technique in biomedical and nonmedical imaging on small bore systems is only likely to increase.

References

1. Blackband SJ, Chatham JC, O'Dell W, Day S (1990) Echo planar imaging of isolated perfused rat hearts at 4.7 T: a comparison of Langendorff and working heart preparations. Magn Reson Med 15(2):240–245
2. Callaghan PT, Eccles CD (1988) Diffusion-limited resolution in nuclear Magn Reson microscopy. J Magn Reson 78:1–8
3. de Crespigny A, Carpenter T, Hall L (1990) Zoom imaging using noise pulses. J Magn Reson 88:406–416
4. de Crespigny AJ, Wendland MF, Derugin N, Kozniewska E, Moseley ME (1992) Real-time observation of transient focal ischemia and hyperemia in cat brain. Magn Reson Med 27(2):391–397
5. de Crespigny AJ, Tsuura M, Moseley ME, Kucharczyk J (1993) Perfusion and diffusion MR imaging of thromboembolic stroke. J Magn Reson Imaging 3(5):746–754
6. Derbyshire J, Gibbs S, Carpenter T, Hall L (1994) Rapid three-dimensional velocimetry by nuclear Magn Reson Imaging Am Inst Chem Engineering J 40(8):1404–1407
7. Feinberg DA, Oshio K (1991) GRASE (gradient- and spin-echo) MR imaging: a new fast clinical imaging technique. Radiology 181(2):597–602
8. Gardner-Medwin AR, van Bruggen N, Williams SR, Ahier RG (1994) Magnetic resonance imaging of propagating waves of spreading depression in the anaesthetised rat. J Cereb Blood Flow Metab 14(1):7–11

9. Guilfoyle D, Gibbs P, Ordidge R, Mansfield P (1991) Real-time flow measurement using echo-planar Imaging Magn Reson Med 18(1):1–8
10. Hennig J, Nauerth A, Friedburg H (1986) RARE imaging: a fast imaging method for clinical MR. Magn Reson Med 3:823–833
11. Kose K (1991) One-shot velocity mapping using multiple spin-echo EPI and its application to turbulent flow. J Magn Reson 92(3):631–635
12. Kose K (1992) Visualization of turbulent motion using echo-planar imaging with a spatial tagging sequence. J Magn Reson 98(3):599–603
13. Kucharczyk J, Vexler ZS, Roberts TP, Asgari HS, Mintorovitch J, Derugin N, Watson AD, Moseley ME (1993) Echo-planar perfusion-sensitive MR imaging of acute cerebral ischemia. Radiology 188(3):711–717
14. Latour L, Hasegawa Y, Formato J, Fisher M, Sotak C (1994) Spreading waves of decreased diffusion coefficient after cortical stimulation in the rat brain. Magn Reson Med 32(2):189–198
15. Mansfield P (1984) Spatial mapping of the chemical shift in NMR. Magn Reson Med 1(3):370–386
16. McKinstry RC, Weiskoff RM, Belliveau JW, Vevea JM, Moore JB, Kwong KW, Halpern EF, Rosen BR (1992) Ultrafast MR imaging of water mobility: animal models of altered cerebral perfusion. J Magn Reson Imaging 2:377–384
17. Moseley M, Wendland M (1991) Acute effects of exercise on echo-planar T2- and diffusion-weighted MRI of skeletal muscle in volunteers. Tenth Annual Meeting of the Society of Magnetic Resonance in Medicine, San Francisco, p 108
18. Moseley ME, Kucharczyk J, Mintorovitch J, Cohen Y, Kurhanewicz J, Derugin N, Asgari H, Norman D (1990) Diffusion-weighted MR imaging of acute stroke: correlation with T2-weighted and magnetic susceptibility-enhanced MR imaging in cats. AJNR 11:423–429
19. Moseley M, Wendland M, Asgari H (1991) High speed MRI of human forearm muscle, applications note. GE NMR Instruments
20. Moseley ME, Sevick R, Wendland MF, White DL, Mintorovitch J, Asgari HS, Kucharczyk J (1991) Ultrafast magnetic resonance imaging: diffusion and perfusion. Can Assoc Radiol J 42(1):31–38
21. Moseley ME, Wendland MF, Kucharczyk J (1991) Magnetic resonance imaging of diffusion and perfusion. Topics Magn Reson Imaging 3:50–75
22. Ogawa S, Lee T-M, Nayak A, Glynn P (1990) Oxygenation-sensitive contrast in magnetic resonance image of rodent brain at high magnetic fields. Magn Reson Med 14:69–78
23. Reimer P, Kwong KK, Weisskoff R, Cohen MS, Brady TJ, Weissleder R (1992) Dynamic signal intensity changes in liver with superparamagnetic MR contrast agents. J Magn Reson Imaging 2(2):177–181
24. Reimer P, Weissleder R, Nickeleit V, Brady T (1992) Animal models for magnetic resonance imaging research of the liver. Invest Radiol 27(5):390–393
25. Roberts TP, Vexler Z, Derugin N, Moseley ME, Kucharczyk J (1993) High-speed MR imaging of ischemic brain injury following stenosis of the middle cerebral artery. J Cereb Blood Flow Metab 13(6):940–946
26. Röther J, de Crespigny A, D'Arceuil H, Yoshikawa J, Iwai K, Seri S, ME M (1995) MRI detection of cortical spreading depression after focal ischemia. Society of Magnetic Resonance, Third Annual Meeting, Nice, p 27
27. Röther J, de Crespigny A, D'Arceuil H, Moseley M (1996) MRI detection of cortical spreading depression immediately following focal ischemia in rat. J. Cereb Blood Flow Metab 16:214–220
28. Sukumar S (1990) High field echo planar imaging relaxation times. GE NMR Instruments 7(2):7–8
29. Turner R, LeBihan D (1990) Single-shot diffusion imaging at 2.0 tesla. J Magn Reson 86:445–448
30. Turner R, von KM, Moonen CT, Van Zijl PC (1990) Single-shot localized echo-planar imaging (STEAM-EPI) at 4.7 tesla. Magn Reson Med 14(2):401–408
31. Turner R, Bizzi A, Despres D, Alger J, Di Chiro G (1991) Dynamic gradient-echo echo-planar imaging of deoxygenation in reversible global ischemia of cat brain. Society of Magnetic Resonance in Medicine, Tenth Annual Scientific Meeting and Exhibition, San Francisco, p 1032
32. Turner R, Le Bihan D, Moonen CTW, Frank J (1991) Echo-planar imaging of deoxygenation episodes in cat brain at 2 T. J Magn Reson Imaging 1 (2):227–230

33. Vexler VS, de Crespigny AJ, Wendland MF, Kuwatsuru R, Muhler A, Brasch RC, Moseley ME (1993) MR imaging of blood oxygenation-dependent changes in focal renal ischemia and transplanted liver tumor in rat. J Magn Reson Imaging 3(3):483–490
34. Wendland M, de Crespigny A, Vexler Z, Derugin N, Moseley M (1992) Inherent contrast enhancement of focal cerebral ischemia on GRE EPI by vascular challenge. Eleventh Annual Meeting, Society of Magnetic Resonance in Medicine, Berlin, p 916
35. Wendland MF, Saeed M, Lauerma K, de Crespigny A, Moseley ME, Higgins CB (1993) Endogenous susceptibility contrast in myocardium during apnea measured using gradient recalled echo planar imaging. Magn Reson Med 29(2):273–276
36. Wendland MF, Saeed M, Masui T, Derugin N, Moseley ME, Higgins CB (1993) Echo-planar MR imaging of normal and ischemic myocardium with gadodiamide injection. Radiology 186(2):535–542

CHAPTER 18

Single Shot RARE

J. Hennig

Introduction

In his original paper on echo-planar imaging (EPI) Mansfield foresaw the using of a train of RF pulses to create multiple signals that could phase encoded to produce a magnetic resonance (MR) image [15]. Despite several attempts to produce a practical pulse sequence according to this concept it took several years before such a sequence could be demonstrated [5]. Even after the first successful demonstration of such a system in 1984 on a clinical scanner it took another 7 years before the method found widespread acceptance [18]. Segmented acquisition, which uses more than one excitation of the spin system to generate all phase-encoding steps for image reconstruction, is currently installed on all state-of-the-art MR systems under various terms (fast spin echo, turbo-spin echo) and plays an important role in clinical diagnosis [1, 12, 13, 16, 17, 19, 20, 22, 26–29, 33]. The single-scan rapid spin echo (RARE) technique has as yet been installed only on a limited number of systems despite its useful clinical applications [3, 6, 7, 8, 14, 24, 25, 30, 31]. This chapter discusses the problems in generating a long echo train under the conditions of a clinical MR system and presents an overview of the clinical use of the technique.

Method

The crucial difficulty in generating a long echo train on a clinical MR system is the treatment of the numerous echoes, which arise whenever the flip angle of the refocusing pulse is not exactly 180°. In this case the behavior of magnetization can be described as a splitting of the phase graph of transverse magnetization into four different trajectories. One describes magnetization that passes through the pulse as though the pulse had not occurred (Fig. 1B, a), one corresponds to refocused magnetization (Fig. 1B, b), and two have trajectories corresponding to z-magnetization (Fig. 1B, c and d). The latter two are created from magnetization that behaves as thought the refocusing pulse had flip angles of 90° and –90°, respectively. The actual phase of the transverse magnetization is stored in the amplitude of the z magnetization. Any subsequent RF pulse retrieves some of this z magnetization and creates a stimulated echo.

The possibility of describing the behavior of magnetization as a superposition of these four states rather than the usual terms of pure M_x, M_y, and M_z magnetization can be derived straightforwardly from the papers of Hahn [4] and

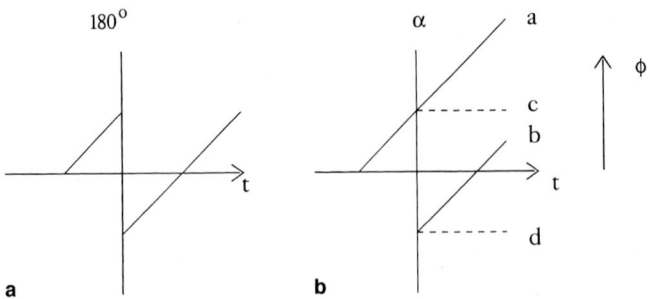

Fig. 1a,b. a Phase graph for refocusing by a refocusing pulse with 180° flip angle under a constant gradient. The phase Φ evolves linearly before the pulse, is negated by the pulse, and evolves linearly after the pulse. The time of zero crossing with the baselines gives the echo time. **b** The behavior of magnetization under a refocusing pulse α can be described as a separation of the refocusing pathway into four parts: one in which magnetization behaves as though no pulse had occurred (*a*), one which corresponds to the case of ideal refocusing (*b*) as shown in **a**, and two pathways (*c*) and (*d*) which store the phase at the time of the pulse for later retrieval as a stimulated and virtual stimulated echo

Woessner [32]. The use of this description to calculate the signal behavior in multi-pulse sequences was presented in 1988 [9]. The transition matrix formalism described there not only allows a simple calculation of the amplitude of all signals generated by an arbitrary number of refocusing pulses. It also lends itself to an pictorial illustration of the various magnetization pathways contributing to a given signal [11]. For a Carr-Purcell-Meiboom-Gill sequence with equally spaced refocusing pulses the number of possible pathways leading to a given echo increases very rapidly with the echo number. Without additional gradients all possible magnetization pathways lead, however, to a coherent superposition of signals such that a single train of echoes is produced (Fig. 2).

Fig. 2. Magnetization pathways in a multi-pulse sequence with a switched read gradient G_{Read}. Although multiple refocusing pathways contribute to signal formation, all echoes interfere coherently and therefore produce artifact-free signals

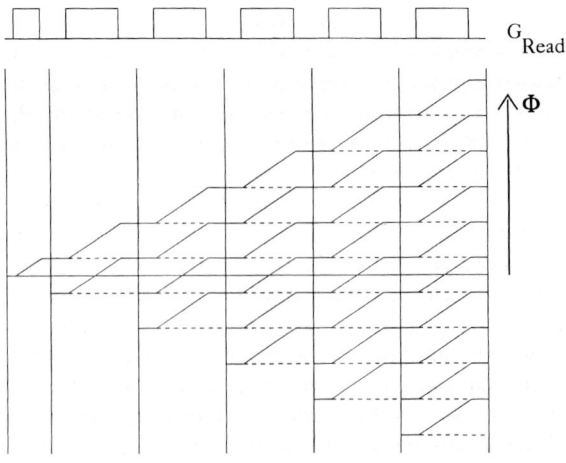

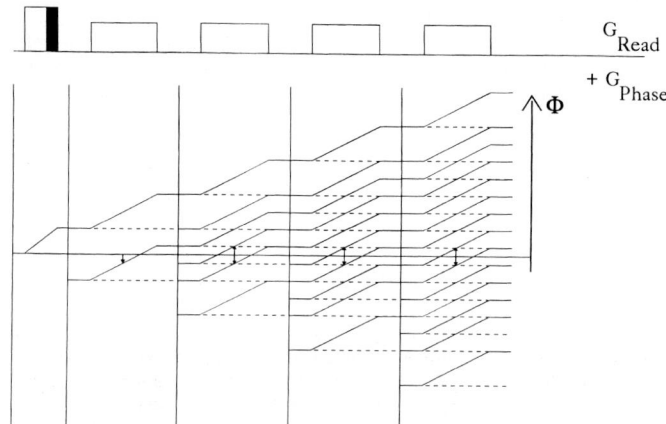

Fig. 3. Magnetization pathways for the same experiment as in Fig. 2 but with an additional phase-encoding gradient G_{Phase}, which is applied only once between the excitation and first refocusing pulse (*black box*). Magnetization is divided into two groups, leading to the formation of two signals with opposite phase encoding

The situation changes, however, when a phase-encoding gradient is introduced into the sequence. Even a single phase-encoding gradient introduced between the excitation pulse and the first refocusing pulse leads to a splitting of the resulting refocusing pathways into two groups with opposite phase encoding (Fig. 3). Images produced with such a sequence therefore show a pronounced mirror artifact. Schemes which have been proposed to produce a single-shot imaging sequence with straightforward incrementing phase-encoding gradients create a superposition of multiple signals with different phase encoding with the result of disastrous image artifacts.

The benign and self-correcting behavior of the Carr-Purcell-Meiboom-Gill sequence can be maintained in imaging only if the phase-encoding gradient is applied prior to the echo acquisition and "rewound" before the next refocusing pulse. The resulting sequence is shown in Fig. 4. In addition to providing images free of ghosting artifacts, the coherent superposition of echoes offers the advantage that the flip angle of the refocusing pulses can be reduced without serious effect on signal amplitude [9]. This can be important if the sequence is applied at high fields or with very short echo spacing, where the radiofrequency (RF) power may be limiting if 180° pulses are being used. A 60° refocusing pulse with only 1/9th of the RF power of a 180° pulse generates 50% of the maximum echo amplitude.

An additional benefit of rewinding the phase-encoding gradient is the possibility of freely varying the sequence of phase-encoding steps. The signal attenuation due to the relaxation time, T2, of the tissues under observation serves as a weighing function of the respective phase-encoding steps and thus affects the point spread function of the imaging sequence, and a continuous sweep of k space is therefore advisable to minimize image artifacts. This can be achieved either by a continuous trajectory [5] or by centric phase encoding [18].

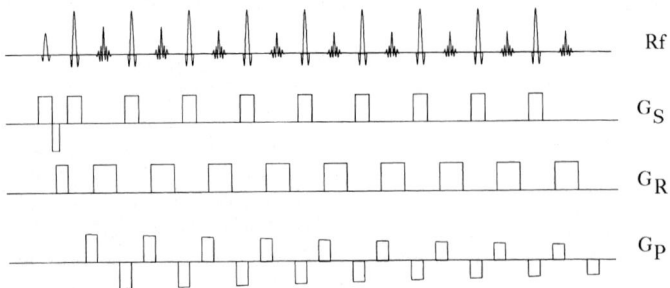

Fig. 4. Scheme of the RARE sequence. *Rf*, Radiofrequency pulses and signals; G_S, slice selection gradient; G_R, read gradient; G_P, phase-encoding gradient. By rewinding the effect of the phase-encoding gradient to zero before each refocusing pulse all later signal contributions interfere coherently, as shown in Fig. 2

The image contrast is generally given by the signal amplitude of the projection carrying the zero phase-encoding step [5, 16, 18]. For single-shot RARE performed on a conventional scanner with 15-ms echo interval and a phase-encoding zero point placed in the 64th of 256 phase-encoding steps, this leads to a signal attenuation of brain tissue (T2 = 80 ms) of 0.0006 % of the spin density value, whereas liquid water (T2 = 3 s) retains more than 70 % of its available magnetization. This extreme contrast selection for fluids has led to such clinical applications of this sequence as MR RARE myelography, MR RARE urography, and most recently MR RARE cholangiography, which are discussed in Chap. 10.

The set of images shown in Fig. 5 demonstrates that the total suppression of soft-tissue signals allows acquisition without slice selection. The resulting projection mode images are especially useful for examining fluid-filled structures such as the spinal canal and the ureters, which tend to go in and out of the slice in a slice-selective measurement and thus can lead to serious partial volume effects.

Pushing the phase-encoding zero point into early echoes to generate images with soft-tissue signals does not produce satisfactory results when performed with echo intervals of more than 10 ms. The T2 decay then acts as a low pass filter, with considerable blurring of the respective tissues (Fig. 5c). The creation of high-quality soft-tissue images requires fast gradients resulting in echo intervals significantly below 10 ms. Figure 6a shows one such image acquired on a 2-T whole body system (S 200 F, Bruker); Fig. 6b shows a similar result acquired on a 1-T system (Magnetom Impact, Siemens) with a sequence using half-Fourier acquisition single-shot turbo-spin echo imaging.

Although the images display satisfying detail and a lack of susceptibility artifacts and the problems of chemical shift misregistration common to EPI images, the clarity and detail of resolution is currently not competitive with multi-shot RARE images. Their role in standard clinical diagnosis, where the reduction in imaging time from a few seconds to below 1 s is not significant, is therefore somewhat doubtful. A very useful application, however, appears to be the combination of single-shot RARE with pulse schemes for manipulation of the image contrast. One such approach uses a 180° pulse to introduce T1 contrast via an

Fig. 5a–c. a Sagittal single-shot RARE image acquired with 30-ms echo interval and phase-encoding zero in the 64th of 128 echoes (0.23 T, Bruker R23) with 8-mm slice thickness. The long readout time of the projection with zero phase-encoding suppresses all tissue and displays CSF only. **b** Same experimental conditions as in **a** but without slice selection. This yields a projection view of the total ventricular spaces. Note that the eyes also appear bright. **c** Same experimental conditions as in **a** but with zero phase encoding in the 8th echo. The signal of soft tissues yield signal which is, however, smeared due to the T$_2$ filtering in the phase-encoding direction

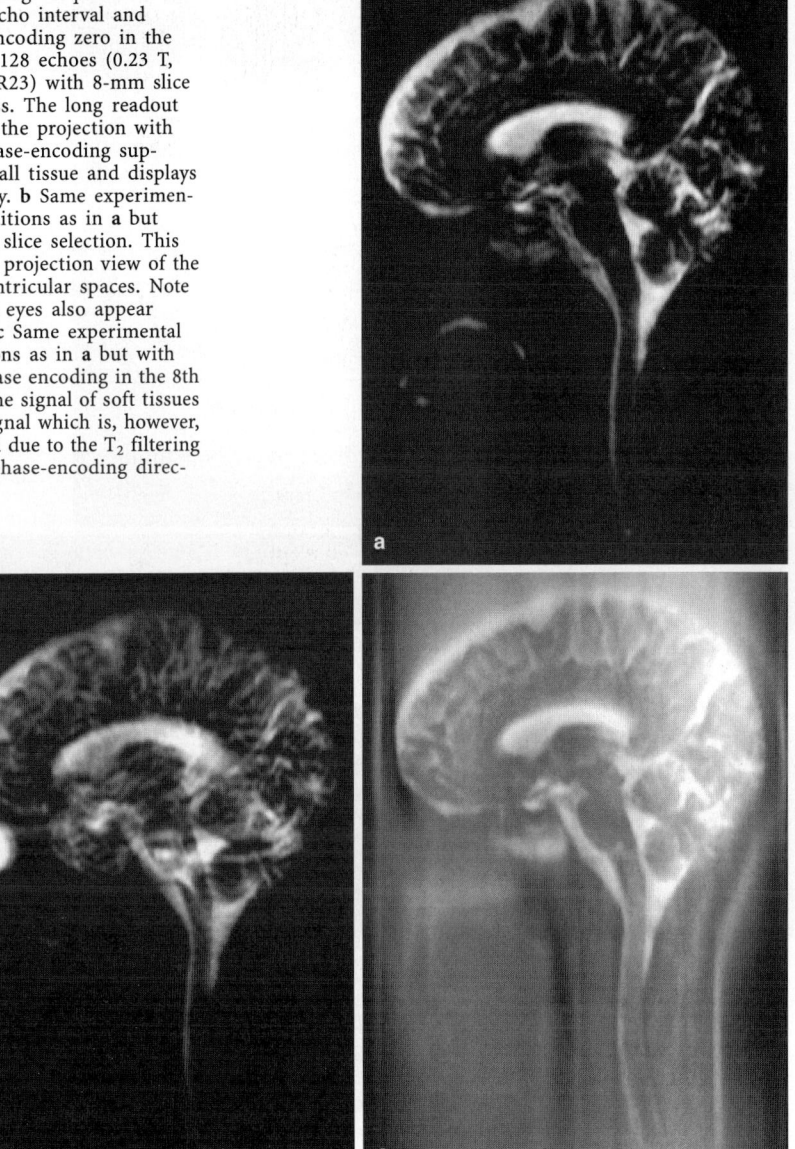

Fig. 6a–b. Single-shot RARE
images. **a** With 7-ms echo
interval acquired at 2 T
(Bruker S 200F). **b** With 5-ms
echo interval acquired at 1 T
(Siemens Magnetom Impact,
courtesy of B. Kiefer, Siemens,
Erlangen) demonstrating good
image quality for soft tissues
with reduced echo interval

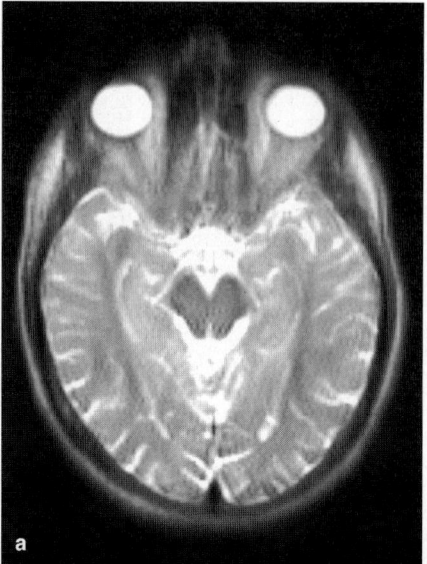

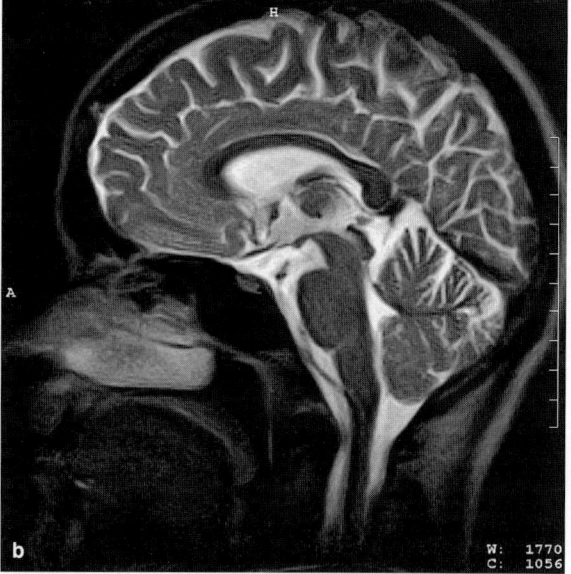

inversion recovery scheme (Fig. 7). Especially with a timing set to nullify signal
from CSF according to the fluid-attenuated inversion recovery sequence introduced by Bydder [2], this is a very useful experiment for detecting lesions
close to the inner or outer ventricular spaces [23].

A different approach to manipulate the contrast of RARE images uses the time
between the excitation pulse and the first refocusing pulse as a magnetization
preparation period. If the time is simply prolonged with respect to the refocusing

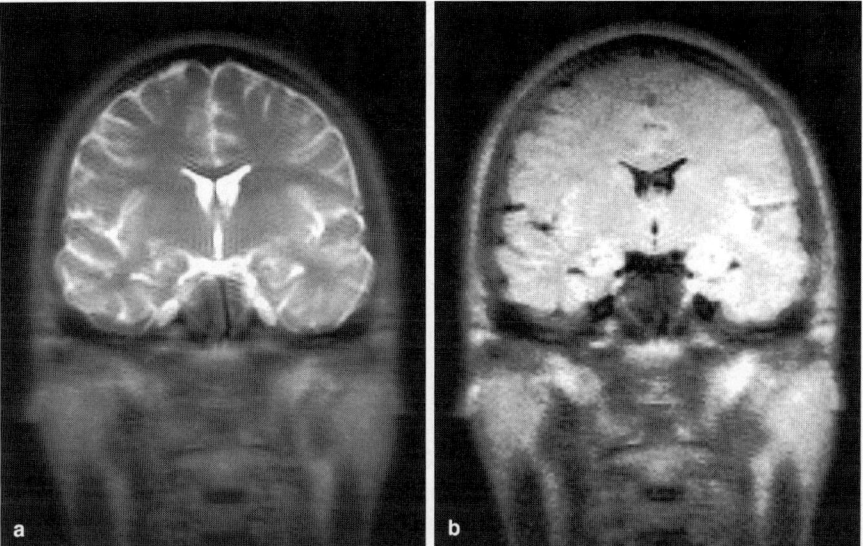

Fig. 7. a Single-shot half-Fourier acquisition single-shot turbo-spin echo (HASTE) image. **b** Inversion recovery-HASTE image (1-T Siemens Magnetom Impact). The echo interval was 8 ms with phase-encoding zero in the 8th echo and half Fourier image reconstruction for both images. The inversion time in **b** was set to 2000 ms, where signal from CSF is nulled

interval, the signal behaves with respect to magnetic field inhomogeneities exactly as described in Fig. 3. Susceptibility-dependent phase shifts thus lead to a reduction in the signal amplitude via incoherent superposition of the two groups of echoes with opposing susceptibility-dependent phase. This leads to susceptibility-dependent variation in the signal amplitude.

A second useful variant is to produce a spin echo with long echo time and additional motion-sensitive gradients prior to the multi-echo train. This leads to a diffusion weighting of the resulting image if a sufficient b value is used. The original intravoxel incoherent motion sequence, which uses diffusion weighting with conventional spin echoes, produces considerable motion problems as a consequence of small and irreproducible phase shifts due to motion from one acquisition to the next. The single-shot RARE experiment avoids these problems and thus combines the extremely stable and robust multi-echo readout sequence with diffusion encoding.

Other preparation procedures such as generating a stimulated echo and introducing flow-encoding gradients can be used to add a broad range of additional information to single-shot RARE in addition to its native T2 contrast.

A final variant of the sequence has been used to visualize and quantitate extremely slow flow [10]. The double phase-encoding sequence uses phase-encoding rewind gradients which differ by a fixed amount from the preceding phase-encoding gradient loops. This leads to a division of the echo train into two groups, which appear time shifted with respect to each other. Fourier transformation then produces an interferographic image, which is sensitive to very slow flow in the range below 0.5 mm/s. This sequence has found useful applications in the examination of CSF dynamics.

Clinical Applications

MR Myelography

Single-shot RARE with an echo interval of 15–25 ms and phase-encoding zero in the 64th–128th of 256 echoes generates images that display fluid only [6]. It is thus an ideal screening technique either for fluid-filled lesions or for lesions surrounded by CSF [3, 6, 8, 31]. Typical examples that show positive contrast in images of the head are hydrocephalus, the cystic portion of Hippel-Lindau and other tumors, and subarachnoidal cysts. The advantage of the technique compared to conventional examinations is – apart from the short acquisition time of 2–8 s – the possibility of choosing arbitrarily thick slices and thus establishing the extent of a lesion in a single projection scan. Indications for head examinations with dark lesion contrast are the assessment of compression of the ventricular system by a space-occupying lesion and the distinction of (bright) cystic tumor portions from (dark) edema, especially in lesions with complex topography such as primary neuroectodermal tumors.

For applications to examinations of the spinal chord, a single-shot RARE experiment in coronal view without slice selection is extremely useful as a localizer image. The exact location and orientation of the spinal canal is thus established unambiguously for subsequent scans in sagittal or transverse orientation. Indications for further use of the sequence for diagnosis include ependymoma, hemangioblastoma, periventricular cysts, and syringomyelia, which all appear in bright contrast. Useful applications for dark contrast lesions are the search for small tumors and metastasis in the spinal canal such as neurinoma and drop metastasis as well as compression of the spinal canal due to disc prolapse or rheumatoid arthritis. The compression status of nerve roots can be easily established by projection images in two or three different orientations.

In all spinal canal examinations the possibility of performing the examination in projection mode is especially beneficial. Ambiguous assessments due to partial volume effects, which are common in slice-selective conventional examinations can thus be ruled out. An additional sagittal scan with soft-tissue contrast (T1-weighted spin echo or segmented RARE) is normally performed to establish the location of a lesion with respect to the spinal column.

Figure 8 presents an example of single-shot RARE used in the diagnosis of a stenosis of the cervical spine. A similar example in the thoracic spine is demonstrated in Fig. 9. In both cases the complex contrast behavior of the different tissues around the spinal canal makes it difficult to establish the diagnosis with the conventional scans. Figure 10 shows sagittal and coronal RARE myelograms of a patient with two small neurinoma. The final example in Fig. 11 of a patient with the accidental diagnosis of a small nerve root cyst in the lumbar spine was chosen to demonstrate the high spatial resolution of the method and its ability to visualize the nerve roots.

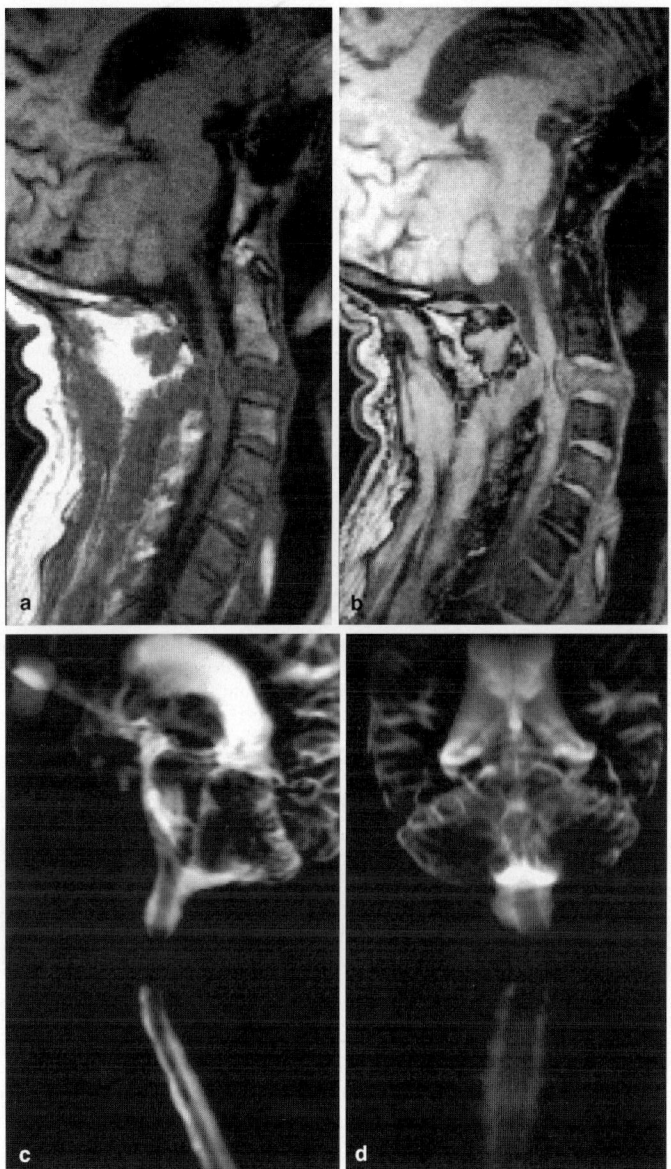

Fig. 8. a Slice-selective images of a patient with bone metastasis in the cervical spine demonstrated with a spin-echo sequence (TE = 16 ms, TR = 500 ms). **b** Gradient echo sequence (TE = 8 ms, TR = 100 ms, 45° flip angle). Full stenosis of the spinal canal is established with the RARE myelogram in sagittal (**c**) and coronal (**d**) views

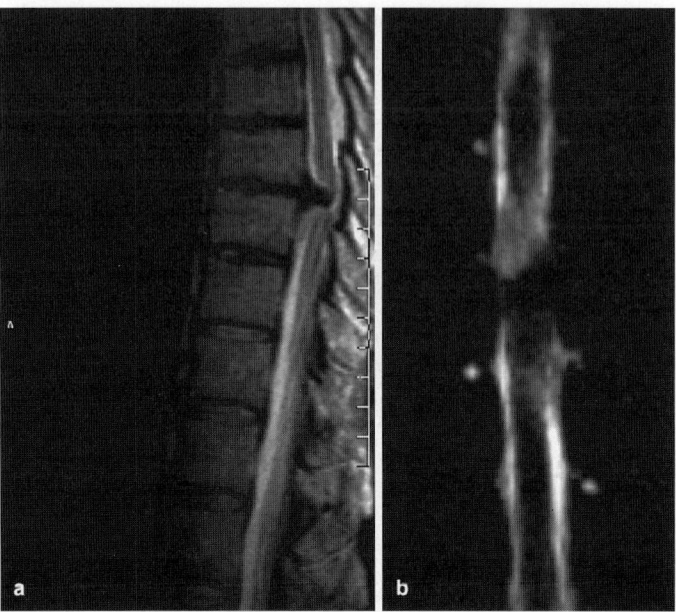

Fig. 9a,b. Assessment of stenosis of the spinal canal in a patient with severe spinal compression due to hyperostosis. **a** The T2-weighted segmented RARE (turbo-spin echo) image an does not allow a conclusive diagnosis due to signal contributions from tissues surrounding the subarachnoidal space. **b** The RARE myelogram demonstrates total stenosis of the CSF-filled spaces. Experimental conditions as in Fig. 8. (0.28-T Bruker R 28, courtesy of M. Mueri, Spectrospin, Zurich)

Fig. 10. Single-shot RARE of two neurinomas located in the thoracic spine in coronal (*left*) and sagittal (*right*) projection (echo interval 15 ms, phase-encoding zero at 640 ms, 1-T Siemens Magnetom Impact)

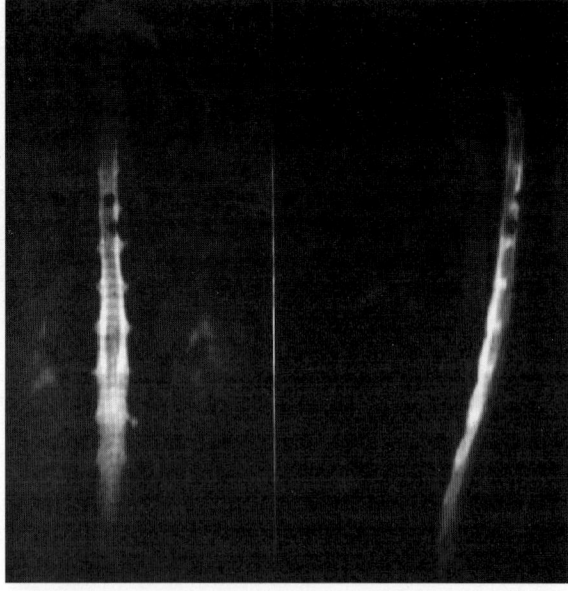

Fig. 11. Accidental finding of a small nerve root cyst in the lumbar spine demonstrated at two different projection angles. Note the clear demonstration of the nerve roots. Experimental conditions as in Fig. 10 (1-T Siemens Magnetom Impact)

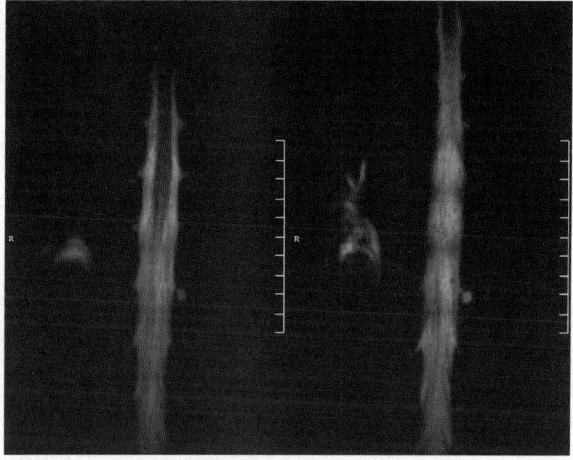

MR Urography

Single-shot RARE offers the possibility to examine the urinary system. Kidney cysts, hydronephrosis, duplicate kidneys, and calicectasis are readily displayed [24, 25]. The advantages of MR compared to ultrasound are the lack of interference with bowel gas, display of the entire excretion system including the renal pelvis, ureters, and bladder in a single projection mode image, and the user independence of the images, which allow follow-up studies on an objective basis. The greater availability and the reduced cost of ultrasound make this modality the primary screening tool for kidney cysts. MR is indicated in cases with complex renal pathology and in the search for small cystic lesions.

The morphology of dilated ureters is readily displayed with RARE urography. An example is shown in Fig. 12, which demonstrates images from a patient with a large bladder tumor. Slice-selective images do not allow assessment of the total stenosis of the ureter (Fig. 12a), whereas RARE images yield full information about the urinary system in a single scan (Fig. 12b).

In patients with pelviuretric obstruction, renal duplication, megaureter, and hydronephrosis the MR examination in corroboration with ultrasound, vesiculography, and renal scintigraphy diagnosis can be reached without resorting to the invasive and radiative X-ray excretion urography. This appears to be especially important for examinations of children.

Fig. 12. a Sagittal segmented RARE (turbo-spin echo) of a patient with a large bladder tumor. The slice-selective images do not allow assessment of whether the ureter (bright structure at the center of the image) is totally blocked or merely leaves the image plane. **b** The sagittal single-shot RARE image demonstrates the total stenosis, the enlarged ureter and the enlarged renal pelvis (bright lemon-shaped structure in the center of the image). Note that the liquid-filled stomach (above the kidney) and the spinal canal are also shown in this projection image. Conditions as in Fig. 10

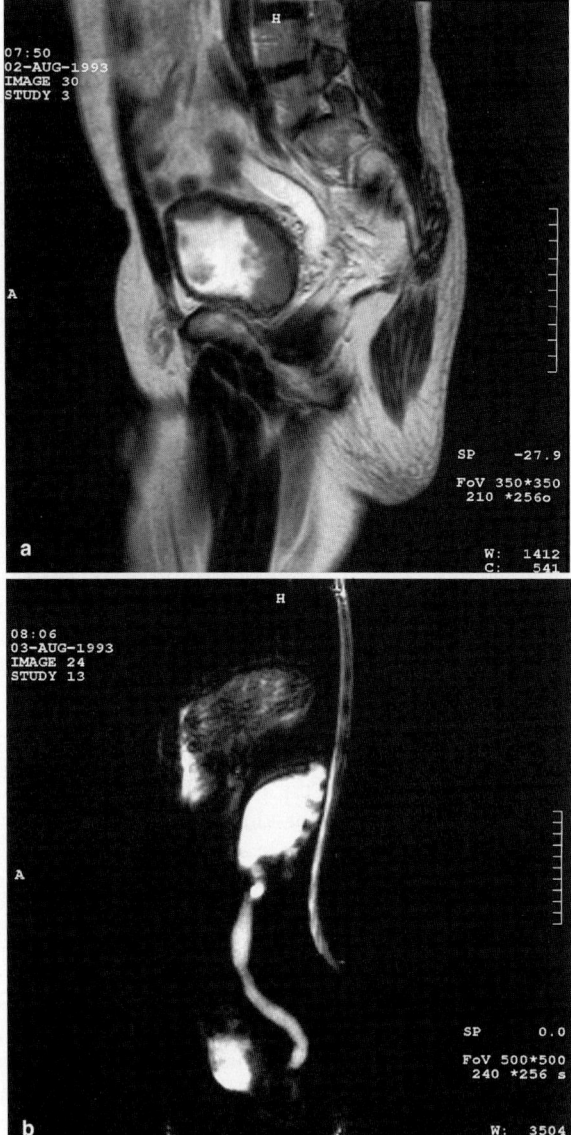

MR Cholangiography

The application of single-shot RARE for the examination of the hepatobiliary system has only recently been introduced [14]. Single-shot RARE allows projection images of the biliary ducts as well as the pancreatic duct. For suppression of the signal from the spinal canal a slice thickness of 80–100 mm is normally chosen to provide overlap-free images. The short acquisition time for a single image allows time-resolved studies of the common bile duct and the papilla of Vater. The excretion of bile into the duodenum can be demonstrated (Fig. 13).

   The conventional diagnosis of stenosis of the common bile duct and the pancreatic duct requires X-ray observation with endoscopic intervention. This is an onerous examination for the patients. The fast and noninvasive MR method is therefore a significant improvement in terms of patient care despite its somewhat reduced spatial resolution. The preliminary data demonstrate that the MR method is sufficient for diagnosis, and that ERCP should be reserved for patients in whom the diagnosis is accompanied by immediate endoscopic intervention.

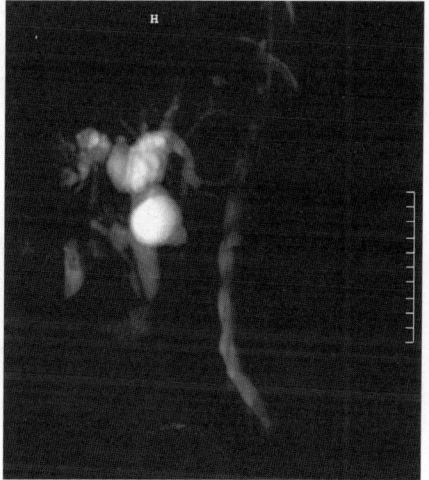

Fig. 13. Sagittal RARE cholangiogram of a patient with benign stricture of the papilla of Vater with subsequent dilation of the bile ducts. The dilated biliary system is shown at the center of the image. The diffuse bright signal originating at the comma-shaped papilla of Vater originates from bile, which is excreted into the duodenum. Note the liquid-filled bowel (*halfmoon-shaped area, left*) and the demonstration of several small liver cysts (*top right*). The elongated structure on the right of the image corresponds to the spinal canal. Conditions as in Fig. 10 except 80-mm slice thickness

Other Applications

Single-shot RARE is also useful as an additional examination for cystic lesions outside of the main indications discussed above [30]. The speed of the single-shot RARE technique allows its use for three-dimensional data acquisition (Fig. 14). The resulting images can be used for highly exact, quantitative determination of the CSF volume. Potential practical applications include the assessment and follow-up of hydrocephalus and brain atrophy; however, no clinical data have yet been published based on this technique. This is also true for three-dimensional urograms, which may be helpful in planning surgical intervention.

Fig. 14. Surface reconstruction of the outer ventricular spaces of a normal volunteer. A cut-off plane at the right of the image allows visualization of the ventricular system. (0.23-T, Bruker R 23)

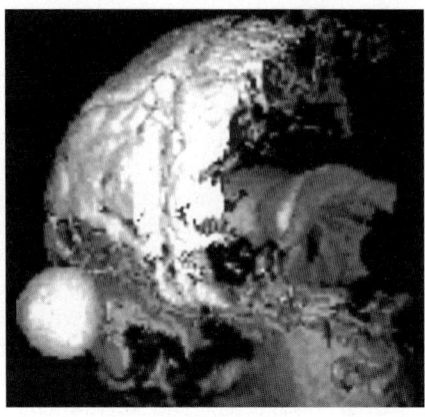

Conclusions

The lack of widespread availability of the single-shot RARE technique has restricted its use for clinical diagnosis to a few centers. With the introduction of the next generation of MR scanners with considerably enhanced soft- and hardware features, this situation is likely to change in the near future. At our institute, where the technique has been available since 1986, single-shot RARE is used for all indications discussed above, at least as an accompanying examination. For a few indications, such as RARE urography in newborn children, single-shot RARE is the only examination performed if the image is diagnostic.

Since efficient gradient systems that allow single-shot RARE with soft-tissue contrast have been available for only a few months, there are not yet sufficient clinical data to assess the clinical usefulness of this technique.

The production of signals by gradient reversal is intrinsically faster than RF refocusing due to the reduced number of gradient switching steps required. Therefore EPI and gradient and spin echo imaging [21] are faster than single-shot RARE. The disadvantage of the high speed of these sequences is their sensitivity to a wide range of factors such as magnetic field inhomogeneity (macroscopic susceptibility), chemical shift, and motion. Because of its much more stable and predictable signal behavior single-shot RARE can be expected to find its place along with EPI and segmented RARE for applications in which speed is less important than reliable and predictable image contrast.

References

1. Chien D, Mulkern RV (1992) Fast spin-echo studies of contrast and small-lesion definition in a liver metastasis phantom. J Magn Reson Imaging 2:483
2. De Coene B, Hajnal JV, Gatehouse P et al (1992) MR of the brain using fluid-attenuated inversion recovery (FLAIR) pulse sequences. AJNR 13:1555–1564
3. Friedburg HG, Hennig J (1986) RARE myelography: clinical experience in 128 Cases. Proceedings of the 5th annual meeting, Society of Magnetic Resonance in Medicine, Montreal, p 818
4. Hahn EL (1950) Spin echoes. Phys Rev 80:580–594
5. Hennig J, Nauerth A, Friedburg H (1986) RARE imaging: a fast imaging method for clinical MR. Magn Reson Med 3:823–833
6. Hennig J, Friedburg H, Stroebel B (1986) Rapid nontomographic approach to MR myelography. J Comput Assist Tomogr 10:375–378
7. Hennig J, Friedburg H, Ott D (1987) Fast three-dimensional imaging of cerebrospinal fluid. Magn Reson Med 5:380–383
8. Hennig J, Friedburg H (1988) Clinical applications and methodological developments of the RARE technique. Magn Reson Imaging 6:391–395
9. Hennig J (1988) Multiecho imaging sequences with low refocusing flip angles. J Magn Reson 78:397–407
10. Hennig J, Ott D, Adam T, Friedburg H (1990) Measurement of CSF Flow using an interferographic MR technique based on the RARE-fast imaging sequence. Magn Res Imaging 8:543–556
11. Hennig J (1991) Echoes – how to generate, recognize, use or avoid them in MR imaging sequences. I. Fundamental and not so fundamental properties of spin echoes. Concepts in Magn Res 3:125–143; II. Echoes in imaging sequences. Concepts in Magn Res 3:179–192
12. Jolesz FA, Jones KM (1993) Fast spin-echo imaging of the brain. Top Magn Reson Imaging 5:1–13
13. Jones KM, Mulkern RV, Mantello MT, Melki PS, Ahn SS, Barnes PD, Jolesz FA (1993) Brain hemorrhage: evaluation with fast spin-echo and conventional dual spin-echo images. Radiology 182:53–58
14. Laubenberger J, Büchert M, Schneider B, Blum U, Hennig J, Langer M (1995) Breath-hold projection magnetic resonance–cholangio-pancreaticography (MRCP): a new method for the examination of the bile and pancreatic ducts. Magn Reson Med 33:18–23
15. Mansfield P (1977) Multi-planar image formation using NMR spin echoes. J Phys C Solid State Phys 10:L55–58
16. Melki PS, Mulkern RV, Panych LP, Jolesz FA (1991) Comparing the FAISE method with conventional dual-echo sequences. J Magn Res Imaging 1:319–326
17. Melki PS, Jolesz FA, Mulkern RV (1992) Partial RF echo planar imaging with the FAISE method. I. Experimental and theoretical assessment of artifact. Magn Reson Med 26:328–341; II. Contrast equivalence with spin-echo sequences. Magn Reson Med 26:342–354
18. Mulkern RV, Wong STS, Winalski C, Jolesz FA (1990) Contrast manipulation and artifact assessment of 2D and 3D RARE sequences. Magn Reson Imag 8:557–566
19. Norbash AM, Glover GH, Enzmann DR (1993) Intracerebral lesion contrast with spin-echo and fast spin-echo pulse sequences. Radiology 185:661–665
20. Oshio K, Jolesz FA, Melki PS et al (1991) T2-weighted thin-section imaging with the multi-slab three-dimensional RARE-technique. J Magn Res Imaging 1:695
21. Oshio K, Feinberg DA (1991) GRASE (gradient- and spin-echo) imaging: a novel fast MRI technique. Magn Reson Med 20:344–349
22. Oshio K, Mulkern RV (1992) Rapid fat/water assessment in knee bone marrow with inner-volume RARE-spectroscopic imaging. J Magn Res Imaging 2:601
23. Panush D, Fulbright R, Sze G, Smith RC, Constable RT (1993) Inversion-recovery fast spin-echo MR imaging: efficacy in the evaluation of head and neck lesions. Radiology 187:421–426
24. Sigmund G, Stoever B, Zimmerhackl LB et al (1991) RARE-MR-urography in the diagnosis of upper urinary tract abnormalities in children. Pediatr Radiol 21:416–420
25. Sigmund G, Stoever B, Zimmerhackl LB et al (1991) Cystic diseases of the kidney in children: MRI, including RARE-MR-urography. Eur Radiol 1:27–32
26. Smith RC, Reinhold C, Lange RC, McCauley TR, Kier R, McCarthy S (1993) Fast spin-echo MR imaging of the female pelvis. I. Use of a whole-volume coil. Radiology 184:665–669
27. Sze G, Merriam M, Oshio K, Jolesz FA (1992) Fast spin-echo imaging in the evaluation of intradural disease of the spine. AJNR 13:1383–1392

28. Tice HM, Jones KM, Mulkern RV, Schwartz RB, Kalina P, Ahn S, Barnes P, Jolesz FIN (1993) Fast spin-echo imaging of intracranial neoplasms. J Comp Assist Tomogr 17:425–431
29. Tien RD, Felsberg GJ, MacFall J (1992) Practical choices of fast spin echo pulse sequence parameters: clinically useful proton density and T2-weighted contrasts. Neuroradiology 35:38–41
30. Vinee P, Stoever B, Sigmund G, Laubenberger J, Hauenstein KH, Weyrich G, Hennig J (1992) MR Imaging of the Pericardial Cyst. J Magn Res Imaging 2:593–596
31. Wakhloo AK, van Velthoven V, Schumacher M, Krauss J (1991) Evaluation of MR imaging, digital subtraction angiography and CT cisternography in diagnosing CSF fistula. Acta Neurochir (Wien) 111:119–127
32. Woessner DE (1961) Effects of diffusion in nuclear magnetic resonance spin-echo experiments. J Chem Phys 34:2057–2061
33. Zoarski GH, Mackey JK, Anzai Y, Hanafee WN, Melki PS, Mulkern RV, Jolesz FA, Lufkin RB (1993) Head and neck: initial clinical experience with fast spin-echo MR imaging. Radiology 188:323–327

CHAPTER 19

Turbo Spin-Echo Imaging

B. Kiefer

Introduction

Turbo spin-echo imaging (TSE; also known as Rapid Acquisition with Relaxation Enhancement, Fast Spin Echo, and Fast Acquisition Interleaved Spin Echo) can also be described as radiofrequency (RF) refocused echo-planar imaging (EPI) [25]. After a single RF excitation multiple RF refocusing pulses are applied, thus refocusing multiple spin echoes, which are progressively phase encoded. In the extreme all echoes required to form an image are recorded after the initial RF excitation. This sequence was first implemented successfully by Hennig in 1986 under the term RARE [11]. In most TSE sequences the raw data needed for image formation are acquired in several consecutive passes instead of one. This segmentation has several advantages: shorter effective echo time, lower bandwidth, less T2 decay, and fewer artifacts.

Since its conception and clinical implementation TSE imaging has become a standard imaging technique on clinical magnetic resonance (MR) systems because it provides tissue contrast closely resembling the contrast of conventional spin echo imaging (SE) at significantly shorter acquisition times [11, 27]. With the currently implemented "single contrast" and "dual contrast" sequences T1-, proton density- (PD), and T2-weighted images can be obtained, with time-saving factors between 3 and 240 with regard to SE. TSE sequences with an inversion recovery (IR) prepulse, i.e., short inversion time IR (STIR) [21, 33, 37] or fluid-attenuated IR (FLAIR) [3, 46], can be used to increase lesion conspicuity without the disadvantage of unacceptably long acquisition times of IR SE sequences. While SE is limited to two-dimensional (2D) acquisition because of its relatively long acquisition times, with TSE three-dimensional (3D) volume imaging with multi-slab acquisition can be performed within reasonable acquisition times [12, 32].

Method

Principle

What are the main differences between TSE and SE? In a conventional spin echo sequence with multiple echoes the echoes are phase encoded equally, so that one line in k space is acquired per RF excitation. From scan to scan the phase encode gradient is incremented to acquire the next line. To obtain, say, a 128×128 matrix, 128 scans with a repetition time TR must be performed, resulting in a total acquisition time of 128×TR. The number of echoes of the multi-echo pulse train determines the number of reconstructed images, each image with different T2 weighting.

In contrast to this, each echo in a multi-echo pulse train can be phase encoded individually, so that all *number of echoes* k space lines required for generating the image can be acquired after only one RF excitation pulse. The resulting time saved with regard to SE is then *number of echoes*. This sequence type was first implemented successfully by Hennig in 1986 [11]. A disadvantage of this technique is that the images are heavily T2 weighted [11], which limits the application of this technique to MR myelography, urography, and cholangiography.

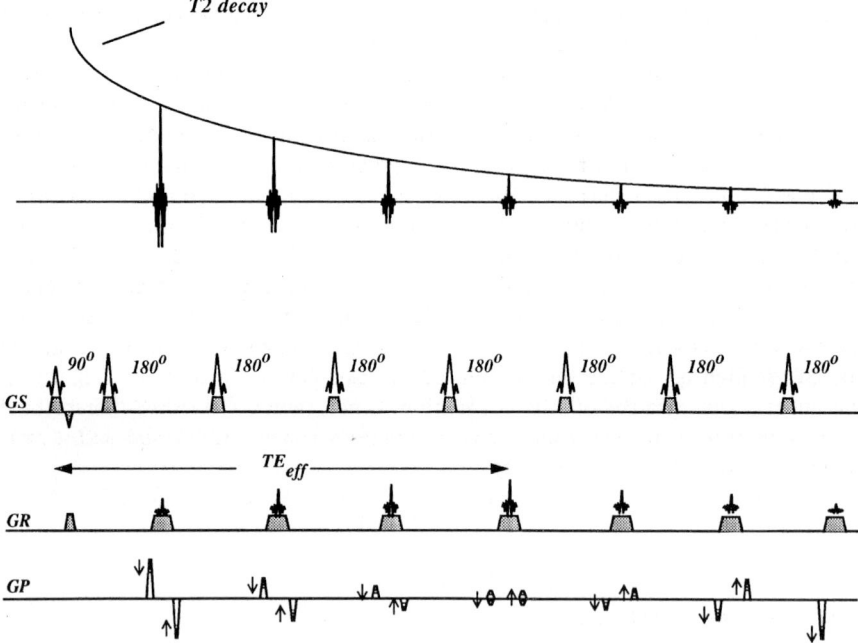

Fig. 1. Sequence diagram for a multi-excitation TSE sequence with seven echoes. The scans are repeated with different phase encoding until all lines in k space are acquired. Image contrast and SNR are determined basically by the effective echo time (TE_{eff}). Note that with a higher number of echoes per scan the acquisition time can be reduced, but, on the other hand, the pulse train length is increased, so that for a given TR fewer slices can be acquired

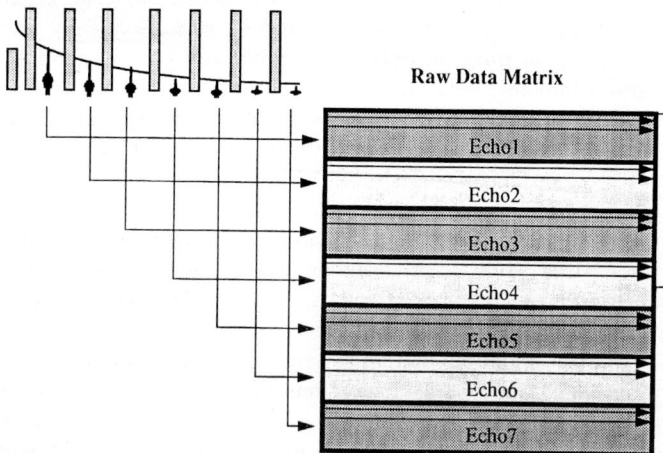

Fig. 2. Ordering scheme in k space for a 7 echo TSE sequence to obtain T2 contrast. Image contrast is determined mainly by the fourth echo. The echoes located in the outer part of k space determine the spatial resolution

TSE was derived from RARE with the goal of increasing the range of possible clinical applications. Introducing multi-excitation sequences with different raw data ordering schemes allows one to cover the full spectrum of contrast variations as known from SE. Figure 1 shows the sequence diagram of a seven-echo train single-contrast TSE sequence together with a T2 decay curve. In analogy to SE all echoes are RF refocused as so-called spin echoes, so that the relaxation curve reflects true T2 decay. The echo signals, each with different T2 weighting, are phase encoded individually and then collected in one raw data set (Fig. 2). To prevent ringing artifacts in the final image the phase encode order must be such that abrupt amplitude discontinuities in k space are minimized when going from echo group to echo group. This restriction limits the flexibility in sequence design. The signal to noise ratio (SNR) and the contrast of the image is determined essentially by the temporal position of the echo for which the phase encode gradient has the smallest amplitudes, that is, the echo with the weakest spin dephasing in phase encode direction and therefore with the highest signal intensity. The temporal distance between the excitation pulse and the echo is called the effective echo time (TE_{eff}) and determines the T2 contrast of the TSE image.

Stimulated Echo Contribution

An important difference between SE and TSE is the treatment of stimulated echoes. Stimulated echoes are generated after a previously excited free induction decay, if more than one RF pulse is applied with a flip angle not exactly 180° [9]. Flip angles which are not equal to 180° always occur at the flanks of the necessarily imperfect slice-selective RF refocusing pulses (see also Chap. 2). The maximum number of distinct echo paths generated by N subsequently applied RF pulses is 3^N [13]. In SE imaging only the regular spin echo contributes to the echo signal and stimulated echoes, which evolve along different magnetization pathways, are dephased during the data sampling period by additional spoiler gradients. In long echo train sequences with multiple RF pulses a dephasing of the various "unwanted" echo signals by additional gradients is not possible. Therefore the TSE sequence is designed such that the stimulated echoes contribute to the total signal by interfering coherently with the regular spin echoes. This, however, causes some restrictions in sequence design and makes such sequences more sensitive to eddy current contributions. Figure 3 shows the magnetization pathways of the regular spin echo and the first stimulated echo for a modified Carr-Purcell-Meiboom-Gill pulse sequence [2, 26]. The magnetization is brought into the x-y plane by a 90° excitation pulse; after the time τ a refocusing pulse is applied, so that after 2τ a spin echo is refocused. This is repeated to refocus the second and third echoes and so forth. The signal amplitude of the recorded echoes decays with T2. In the case of imperfect RF refocusing pulses a second pathway is possible, where after RF excitation the spins "see" only a 90° pulse instead of the 180° refocusing pulse. The effect is that between the second and third RF pulse the magnetization is stored in the z direction. During this time period the magnetization decays with T1 only. After the third RF pulse a stimulated echo is refocused, which is equal in phase to the spin echo

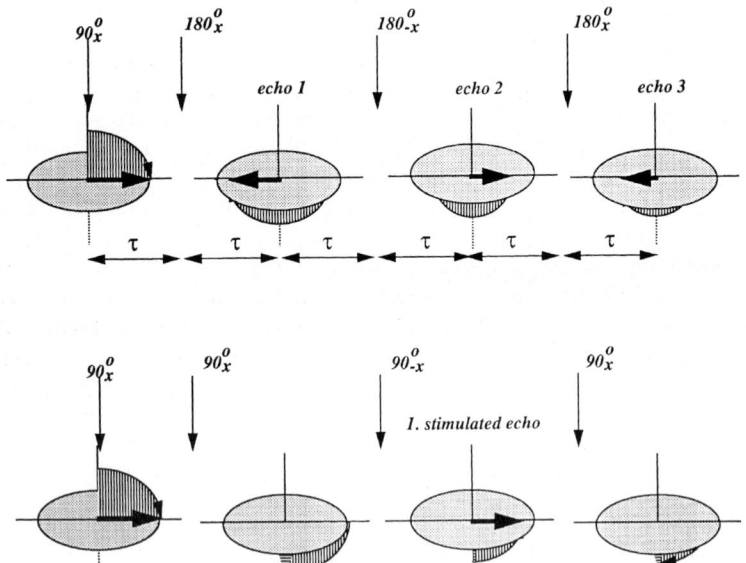

Fig. 3. Stimulated echo contribution to the total signal amplitude in TSE. Shown is the magnetization pathway for the regular spin echo (*above*) and for a stimulated echo in the presence of imperfect RF refocusing pulses (*below*)

but has a different weighting. This T1 contribution might have an effect on the contrast of the final image.

The following considers in detail a number of important issues in the design of TSE sequences caused by the stimulated echo contribution:

- Let us assume the time between the RF excitation pulse and the first RF refocusing pulse to be τ, the RF refocusing pulses must be precisely equally spaced with the time 2τ.

  Reason: A static or dynamic magnetic field contribution (e.g., a gradient offset, magnetic susceptibility, or eddy current) causes a phase evolution of the spins between the first and second RF refocusing pulse as shown in the example in Fig. 3. For the stimulated echo the magnetization is stored in the z direction during this time and is not affected by a gradient field. If the time between RF excitation pulse and first RF refocusing pulse is τ, and the time between first and second RF refocusing pulse is $\tau+\tau_1$, the stimulated echo is refocused after the time τ, the spin echo after the time τ_1 after the second refocusing pulse. Superposition of these echoes results in image artifacts, for example, signal drop down and shading, if τ is unequal to τ_1.

- The phase encode gradient must be applied between each RF refocusing pulse and data acquisition interval and must be rewound after each data acquisition interval and before the next RF pulse (see Fig. 1).

  Reason: A phase encode gradient applied during the time when the magnetization for one echo pathway is stored in z direction is "invisible" for this echo. As a result echoes with different phase encoding would be superimposed if the phase encode gradient is not rewound before each RF refocusing pulse.

- The gradient scheme for flow compensation must be designed so that it works for all acquired echoes.

  Reason: For SE sequences the flow compensation is calculated that the gradient moments are nulled at the echo center. To have an effective flow compensation for all magnetization pathways in TSE the gradient moments must be nulled at the center of the RF pulses *and* at the center of the echoes [15]. The disadvantage of this method is that only one axis can be flow compensated, in either read or slice-select direction. Additional gradients along the second axis are necessary to dephase the free induction decay generated by each imperfect RF refocusing pulse during the data sampling interval.

Image Contrast

The most striking difference in contrast between SE and TSE images is the increased signal intensity of fat [27], which is observed even in strongly T2-weighted images (Fig. 4). The reasons which account for this effect are:

- Magnetization transfer saturation (MT): In TSE a large number of RF refocusing pulses is applied. In single-slice TSE the RF pulses are all on-resonance, and in this case a MT effect is not observable. In multi-slice TSE RF refocusing pulses are also applied for adjacent slices and therefore act as off-resonance pulses. The MT effect in multi-slice TSE causes a loss in contrast between

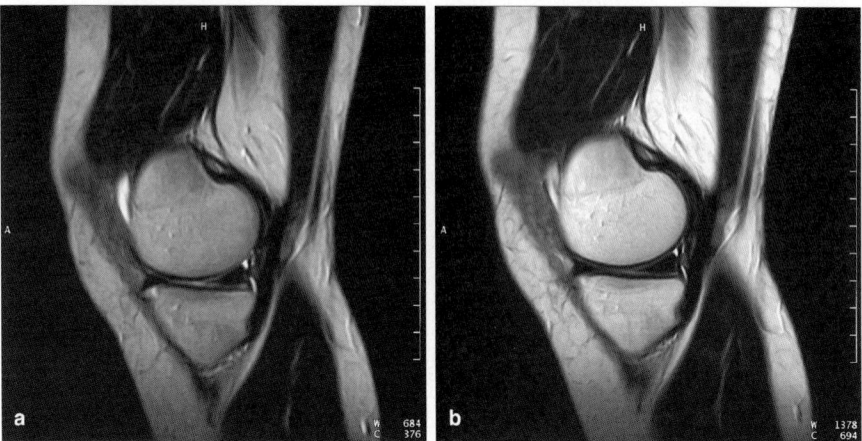

Fig. 4a,b. Sagittal knee images obtained with the CP extremity coil on the 1.5-T Magnetom Vision. a With SE, TA = 10:15 min; TR/TE = 2200 ms/120 ms, in plane resolution = 0.94×0.70 mm; Sl = 3 mm. b With 15-echo TSE, bandwidth = 130 Hz/pixel; echo spacing = 15 ms; TA = 5:11 min; TR/TE = 4400 ms/120 ms; in plane resolution = 0.67 mm×0.51 mm; Sl = 3 mm. Especially with a short echo spacing, fat appears brighter in the TSE image

white and gray matter of the brain and a signal attenuation of white and gray matter compared to fat tissue [28]. The relative decrease in brain signal compared to the unattenuated fat makes fat appear relatively brighter (Fig. 5)

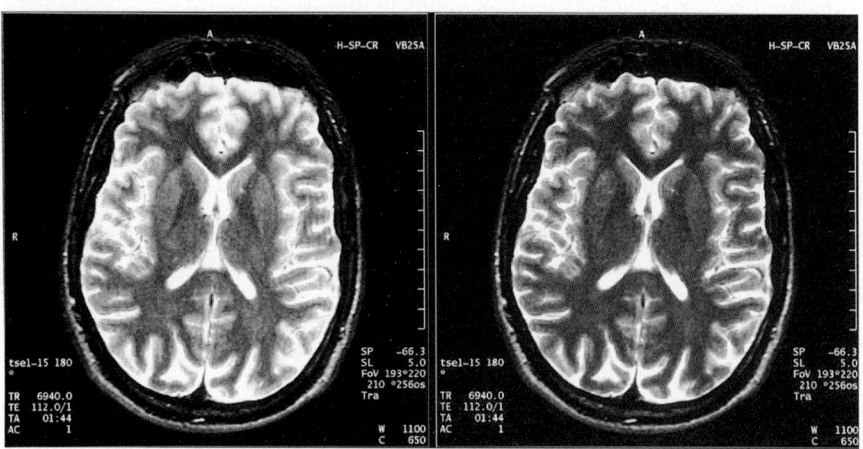

Fig. 5. Multi-slice TSE images display additional magnetization transfer contrast due to the large number of off-resonant 180° pulses from neighboring slices. White and gray matter signal appears significantly darker on the multi-slice TSE image out of a study with 19 slices (*right*) than on the single slice image (*left*). Signal from CSF and fat remains unaffected. Therefore the magnetization transfer saturation contributes to the "bright fat" effect. Images were obtained on the 1.5-T Magnetom Vision with a 15-echo TSE sequence

- Spin-spin coupling of fat protons: Lipids and fat actually show multiple resonances with different chemical shifts and with multiple resonances from spin-spin coupling. In these complex coupled systems the apparent relaxation times are strongly dependent on the pulse rate of the RF refocusing pulses [4, 10]. With increasing pulse rate, i.e., the closer the RF-RF pulse distance in TSE, the brighter fat appears.
- Stimulated echoes: As mentioned in the above section, stimulated echoes contribute to the total echo signal. During their magnetization paths the spins are stored for a certain time period in the z direction. During this time the magnetization decays with T1 instead of T2, which could cause a noticeable contrast difference [4].

Less sensitivity to magnetic susceptibility is observed with TSE than with SE, which is due to the multi-echo refocusing train [27]. This effect might be desirable for example, for imaging of the sella region, but, on the other hand, it may reduce the conspicuity of hemorrhagic lesions [18, 31].

Image Resolution

The ordering of the spin echoes in k space affects the spatial resolution of TSE images [5, 11]. To obtain T2 contrast early echoes are phase encoded such that they form the outer lines in k space (Fig. 2), thus defining the spatial resolution. Late echoes, on the other hand, are phase encoded such that they are located at the center of k space, thus defining mainly the image contrast. The early echoes have the weakest T2 decay and therefore the highest signal amplitude, in contrast to later echoes which are attenuated by T2. This T2 filter can cause an edge enhancement on tissue boundaries, so that images appear well resolved.

The behavior is different for T1- and for PD-weighted TSE. For this type of sequences the early echoes, i.e., the echoes with the highest signal amplitude, are located in the central lines of k space; the late echoes in this case define the spatial resolution. This T2 filter can cause a loss of resolution in the phase encode direction, which is most severe for tissues with short T2. To compensate for this the TSE echo train must be short and the echo-echo distance as short as possible. As a consequence the number of echoes that can be acquired per scan, defining the time saving factor of TSE, is limited.

Dual Contrast TSE

The dual-contrast TSE sequence was developed as a counterpart to the double-echo SE sequence, with a time-saving factor between 3 and 9 versus double echo SE in the current implementations. In dual-contrast TSE in its simplest form the data for the PD image are acquired in the first part of the echo train and the data for the T2-weighted image in the second part. A more effective method is the so-called shared-echo technique (Fig. 6). With this technique the echoes, located in the outer part of the k space, are recorded only once

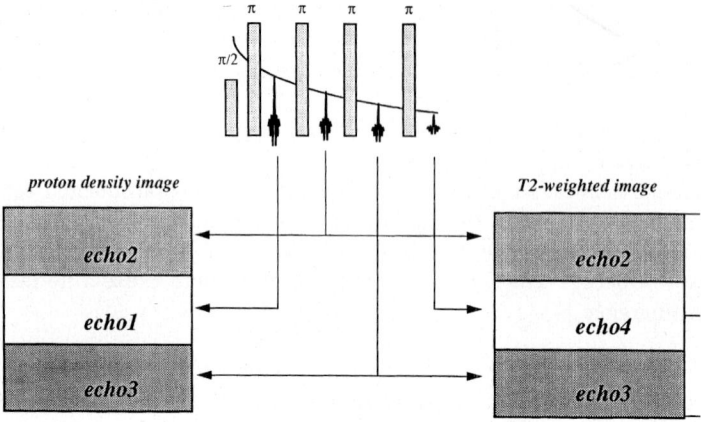

Fig. 6. Shared-echo technique used in dual-contrast TSE. Only the central echoes for the PD- and T2-weighted image are acquired individually; the outer echoes are shared. The advantage of this technique is that the pulse train can be kept shorter. Consequently more slices can be measured for a given TR, and the RF power deposition is reduced

and are shared for the PD and T2 raw data set; the echoes located in the central part of k space, and therefore defining the contrast of the final image, are acquired for each raw data set individually [14]. The advantage is that the echo train length can be shortened so that for a given TR more slices can be obtained and the RF power deposition is reduced.

To obtain PD-weighted TSE images with a contrast similar to that known from SE a TR not longer than 3 s should be used (Fig. 7). The reason is that in double-echo SE imaging a TR of about 2 s is usually employed to stay within an acceptable imaging time. With this "short" TR substances with long T1 such as CSF cannot completely relax. Therefore CSF appears dark in the PD image, which is important in clinical imaging to differentiate CSF-filled spaces from lesions. With dual-contrast TSE one is tempted to increase TR to longer than 3 s, especially in the case of long echo trains which limit the available number of slices for a given TR. A long TR, however, reduces the T1 weighting, thus resulting in a contrast closer to the "true" PD contrast with which CSF appears bright.

TSE with Prepulse for Spin Preparation

Techniques for spin preparation are well known from SE sequences and can also be applied in TSE. Because of the relatively long preparation periods of some of these techniques the performance of SE is low. This drawback can be overcome with TSE. Spin preparation techniques are commonly used in TSE to obtain fat [7, 19, 21, 33, 37] and fluid suppression [3, 46].

Fat suppression can be obtained by using a frequency selective prepulse. For this technique a good field homogeneity is necessary to achieve a homogeneous fat suppression. A drawback of this method is that it is sensitive to magnetic

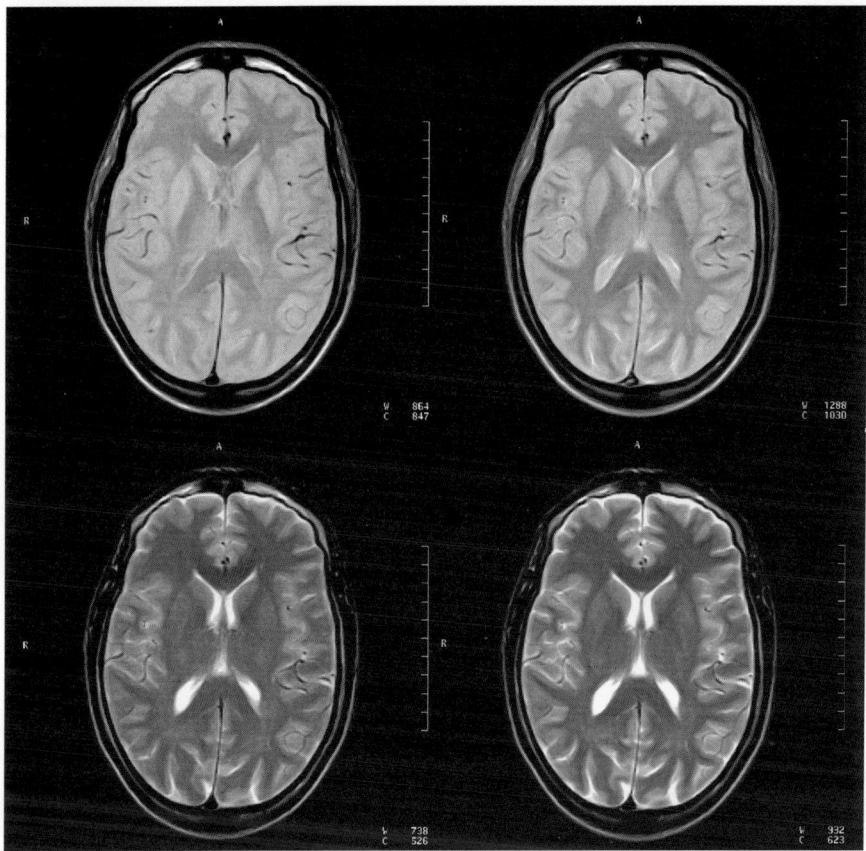

Fig. 7. Axial head images obtained with dual-contrast TSE at two different TRs on the 1.5-T Mag-netom Vision. Dual contrast TSE sequence: shared-echo technique; 5 echoes per raw data set; TE = 16 ms, 98 ms; in plane resolution = 0.91×0.90 mm; Sl = 4 mm; 42 images. *Left,* PD- and T2-weighted image, obtained with a "short" TR of 2700 ms, TA = 1:49 min; *right,* PD- and T2-weighted image, obtained with a "long" TR of 5000 ms, TA = 3:16 min. Result: With a "short" TR CSF is dark in the PD image, as is desired in clinical imaging; with the long TR CSF is bright in the PD image

susceptibility. This can cause incomplete fat suppression and/or even water sup-pression for example, in the paranasal sinuses, at the skull base, and in the region of the neck where the air filled trachea and the overall geometry accounts for magnetic susceptibility changes.

A more robust method for fat suppression is the STIR technique (Fig. 8). Spins are inverted by a 180° prepulse. The inversion time TI is selected so that the lon-gitudinal magnetization of the fat is zero at the time when the excitation pulse of the TSE sequence is applied. In STIR TSE not only is fat suppressed, but the tis-sue contrast in general is affected. STIR TSE sequences with short TE_{eff} produce an "inverted" T1 contrast. This means that tissues with long T1 values, for exam-

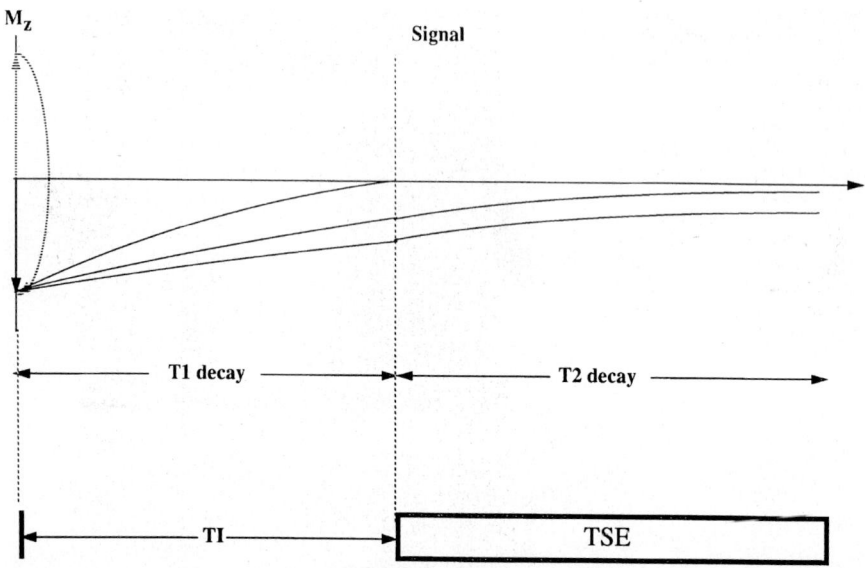

Fig. 8. TSE with inversion prepulse for spin preparation. To obtain fat suppression (STIR) or fluid suppression (FLAIR) the inversion time TI is adjusted so that after spin inversion the magnetization of the tissue to be suppressed is just at zero crossing point when the 90° excitation pulse is applied. Note that fat suppression with STIR gives the image an additional "inverted" T1 contrast

ple, gray matter, appear brighter than tissues with short T1 values, for example, white matter. With a long TE_{eff}, the "inverted" T1 contrast enhances the T2 contrast, creating the appearance of a very heavy T2 weighting [21] (Fig. 9). This contrast enhancement can increase lesion conspicuity, as has been reported, for example, in abdominal imaging [37]. A drawback is the reduction of the SNR of STIR TSE especially for tissues with short T1.

When increasing the T1 to values of 300–600 ms the image contrast is very heavily T1 weighted. After real-part reconstruction substances with a long T1 are displayed with negative sign corresponding to the direction of the longitudinal component of the magnetization vector at the time when the RF excitation pulse is applied; tissues with short T1 are displayed with positive sign (Fig. 10). This heavily T1-weighted contrast may become clinically important for diagnosis, for example, in pediatric imaging.

In dark fluid TSE the inversion prepulse is used to null the fluid signal, for example, the CSF. For this a TI of about 2 s is necessary because of the long T1 of fluid. With both a long TE_{eff} and a long TR "long T2" lesions can be made visible which are normally obscured by the bright CSF (Fig. 11). One problem of dark fluid TSE with a selective inversion prepulse is the fact that during the long spin preparation period inflow effects of unsaturated CSF can occur, resulting in white areas such as in the ventricles.

In cardiac imaging flow compensated SE sequences have been used to image congenital heart disease. With these sequences slowly flowing blood appears

Fig. 9a,b. Axial head images obtained with 11-echo TSE (TA = 6:35 min, TR = 5000 ms, in plane resolution = 0.78×0.58 mm, Sl = 4 mm) on the 1.5-T Magnetom Vision.
a With frequency selective prepulse for fat suppression, TE = 99 ms.
b With STIR prepulse; TE/TI = 60/150 ms. The STIR prepulse produces an additional "inverted" T1 contrast, so that the resulting image looks very heavily T2 weighted

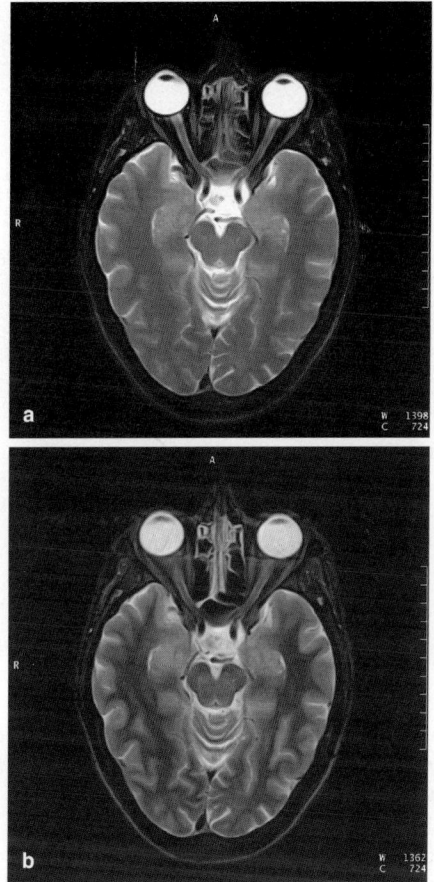

Fig. 10. Coronal head image with a nice T1 contrast, obtained with 11-echo TSE and inversion prepulse (TR/TE/TI = 5800/60/350 ms, TA = 6:40 min, in plane resolution = 0.61×0.45 mm, Sl = 5 mm) on the 1.5-T Magnetom Vision. Because of the real-part reconstruction substances with long T1 are displayed with negative sign corresponding to the direction of the longitudinal component of the magnetization vector at the time when the RF excitation pulse is applied; tissues with short T1 are displayed with positive sign

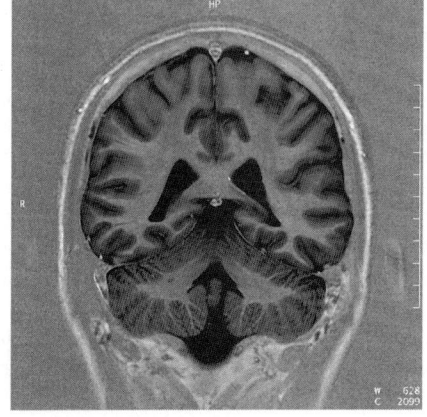

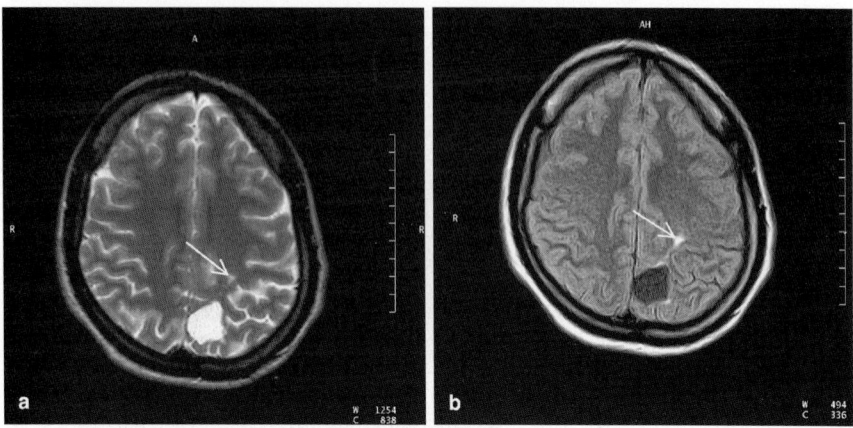

Fig. 11a,b. Head images of a patient after glioma operation obtained on the 1.0-T Magnetom Impact. a T2-weighted TSE image: TA = 3:15 min; TR/TE = 5000/90 ms. b Dark fluid image obtained with a 15-echo TSE sequence with Inversion prepulse. TA = 2:33 min; TR/TE/TI = 9000/150/2500 ms; in plane resolution = 0.96×0.89 mm; 11 images. The lesion is detectable only with the dark fluid (FLAIR) sequence

bright, thus reducing the ability to obtain morphological information. This problem is avoided by using a "black blood" spin preparation [6] to null the vascular signal without reducing the signal intensities of stationary tissue. A nonselective inversion prepulse is first applied to invert the signal of blood and tissue followed immediately by a slice selective "reversion" pulse. By appropriate selection of the inversion time TI of about 700 ms the blood appears black. Combination of the "black blood" spin preparation with TSE makes this technique fast enough for breath-hold ECG-triggered T2-weighted imaging of the heart with few or no motion artifacts [42] (Fig. 12). The blood and fat signal can be nulled simultaneously by applying a slice selective STIR prepulse during the inversion time of the "black blood" spin preparation.

3D Fourier Transform TSE

The majority of 3D Fourier transform (FT) sequences which are implemented on currently available scanners are based upon gradient echo techniques. The combination of 3D FT acquisition with SE would result in unacceptably long acquisition times. TSE, however, makes it possible to acquire images in a 3D acquisition mode in reasonable times [12, 32]. Most interesting is the application to obtain T2 contrast with 3D TSE because this is not possible with the commonly used gradient echo sequences. With 3D TSE T1 and PD contrast can also be obtained.

In a 3D experiment one or multiple slabs are excited similarly to slices in a multi-slice 2D SE experiment during the TR interval, but are further divided into thin partitions using a second phase encode gradient in slice select direction. A possible implementation of 3D TSE is to perform the segmentation of

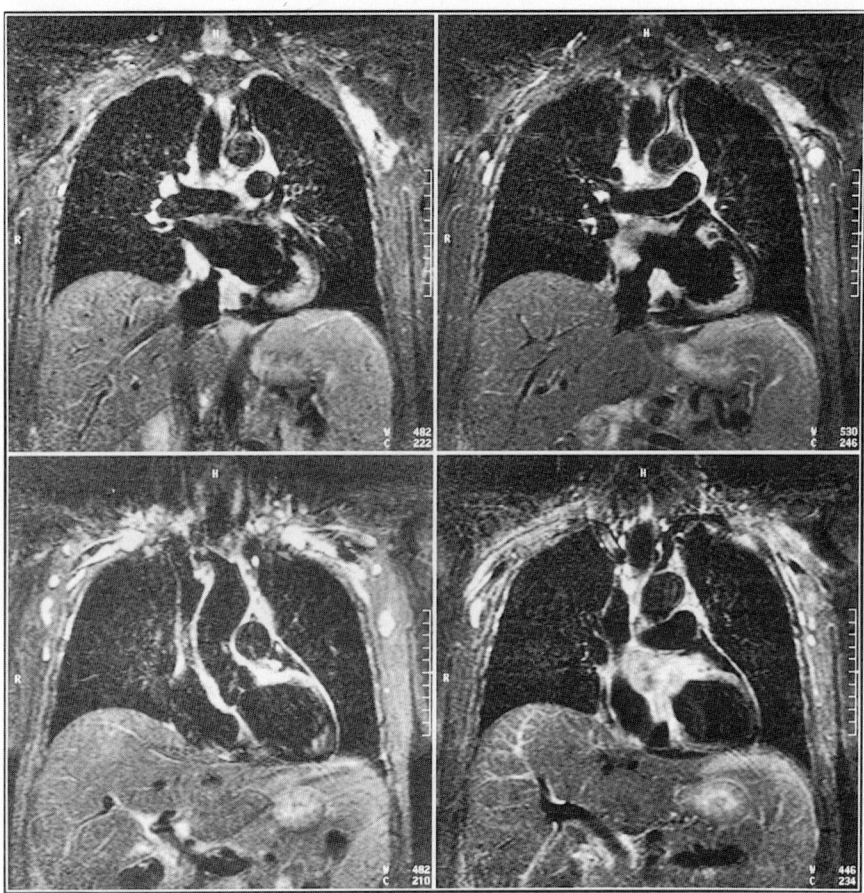

Fig. 12. Single-slice breath-hold ECG-triggered "black blood" STIR TSE image of the heart in a patient with recurrent angiosarcoma of the right atrium and ventricle. Due to the fat and blood signal nulling and the T2 weighting of this sequence type the increased T2 of the tumor can be beautifully differentiated as high signal from normal cardiac structures. Images were obtained on the 1.5-T Magnetom Vision with the CP body phased array coil. (Courtesy of the Grosshadern Clinic, Munich)

the gradient table in the phase encode direction, as shown in Fig. 1. In addition, gradient tables are introduced in the slice select direction, located directly before the data sampling period. A rewinder table is located directly after the data sampling period. The 3D phase encode tables are equal in amplitude during a scan, and change their amplitude for the next scan.

The acquisition time is longer with a 3D than with a 2D data set by the number of partitions per slab. In spite of the time saving of TSE the number of partitions obtainable in reasonable scan times is limited. To obtain T2-weighted images with a 27-echo TSE sequence, TR of 3 s, matrix of 216×256, 8 partitions per slab, the acquisition time is 216/27×8×3 [s] = 3 min. Depending on the

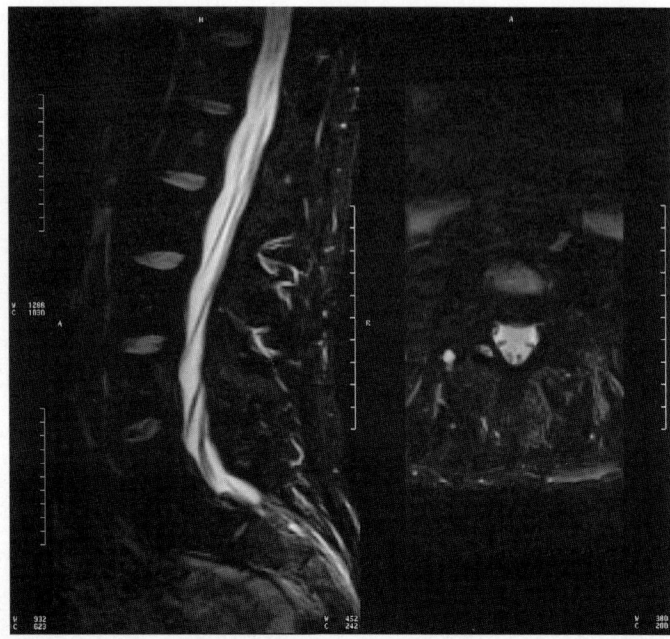

Fig. 13. Lumbar spine images obtained in 9:39 min with 23-echo 3D TSE with fat suppression and long TE = 149 ms on the 1.5-T Magnetom Vision. *Left,* one sagittal image out of the original data set with 1.1-mm partition thickness. The reformatted axial image reconstructed out of this data set shows a good visualization of the nerve roots without disturbing flow artifacts. The original data set is also well suited to obtaining myelograms by using a maximum intensity projection program. Parameters are: TR/TE = 3600/149 ms; resolution = 1.1×1.1×1.1 mm

pulse train length multiple slabs can be excited within one TR. If, for example, 10 slabs are excited with 8 partitions per slab, the total number of partitions that can be acquired in about 3 min is 80. A drawback of multi-slab acquisition is that between adjacent slabs crosstalk can occur, as known from 2D multi-slice imaging, which can cause image quality degradation of the partitions located at the edges of the slabs. This problem can be solved by performing two sequence runs, the first to acquire slabs with an interslab gap of one slab and the second to fill the gaps. The total acquisition time is then increased to about 6 min in the example above. The obtained 3D data sets are suitable for multi-planar reconstruction so that the original dataset can be reformatted into images with different obliquity (Fig. 13)

HASTE

To provide a complete overview of TSE-type sequences we mention the single-shot variant of half-Fourier acquisition single-shot turbo-spin echo (HASTE). Single-shot sequences are described in more detail in Chap. 9. HASTE is derived from single-shot RARE with the goal of increasing the range of possible clinical applications [22]. The phase encode order is chosen in a way that the central Fourier lines are acquired early in the pulse train so that images with moderate T2 weighting can be obtained with acquisition times of less than 1 s per image (Fig. 14). Because of the infinite TR, however, fluid appears very bright. HASTE can be combined with prepulses for fat or fluid suppression to increase lesion conspicuity [23]. Applications of this technique include imaging of noncooperative patients (Fig. 15), functional joint imaging, and fast screening for pathology in the abdomen [41, 45]. Because of the bright fluid signal together with RARE this technique is also increasingly applied for noninvasive MR myelography, urography, and cholangiography [24, 34, 35, 40]. A drawback of HASTE is the strong T2 decay during the long data acquisition period. This T2 filter causes loss of spatial resolution in phase encode direction especially for tissues with short T2 (see "Image Resolution"). The T2 filter effect is reduced with double-shot HASTE, a double-segment version of this technique, because of the shorter data acquisition period per shot. With this sequence the liver can be scanned in a single breath-hold (Fig. 16).

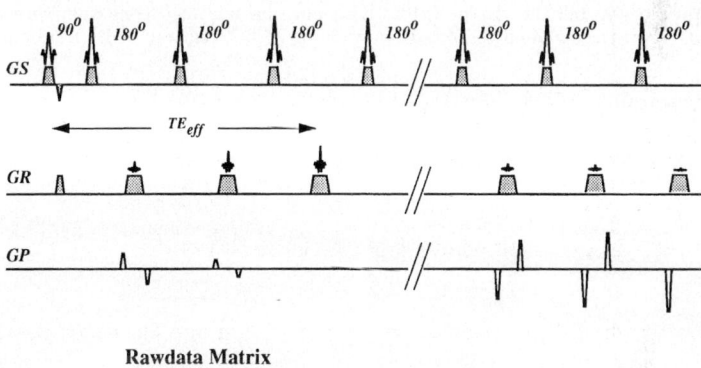

Rawdata Matrix

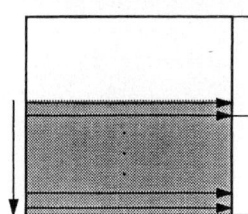

Fig. 14. Sequence diagram and k space ordering scheme for a HASTE sequence. All lines in k space are acquired after only one excitation pulse, so that the full magnetization is available. To have a short TE_{eff} the central Fourier line is acquired early in the pulse train. Images are obtained after half Fourier reconstruction

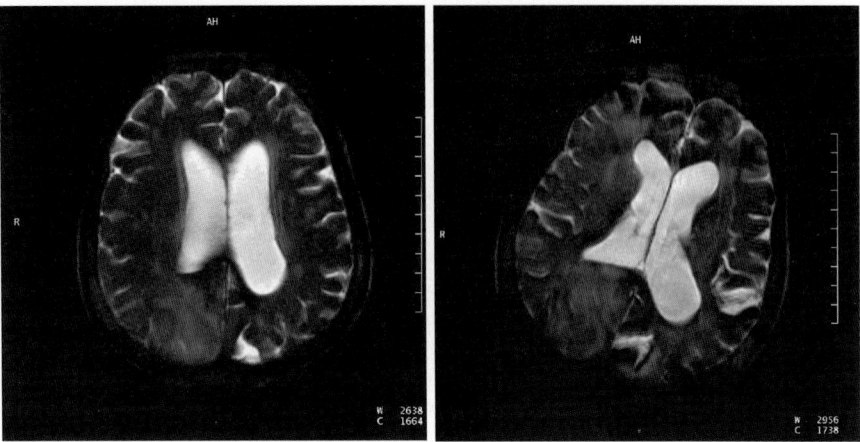

Fig. 15. Two images from a sequential multi-slice study obtained with HASTE on the 1.0-T Magnetom Impact. The patient is an infant with hydrocephalus who moved his head during the examination. Because of the fast acquisition time per image of 1.2 s no motion artifacts are visible in the images, but the change in the head position was registered from slice to slice. TE = 87 ms, in plane resolution = 1.0×0.94 mm; Sl = 5 mm. (Courtesy of Dr. Friedburg, Freiburg)

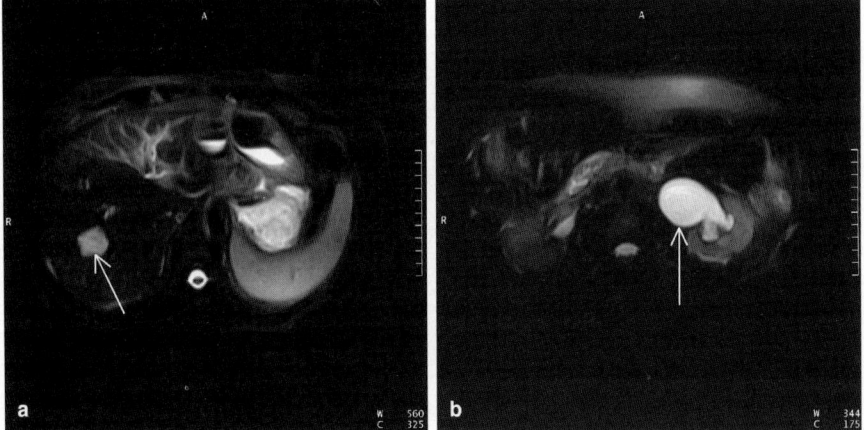

Fig. 16a,b. Two images from a breath-hold study with double-shot HASTE combined with STIR prepulse to increase lesion conspicuity. Two lesions are detected in this study. A hemangioma (a) and a hydronephrosis of the left kidney (b). Images are obtained with a CP body phased array coil on the 1.5-T Magnetom Vision. This sequence can be used as a fast screening technique for pathology. TA = 16 s, TR/TE/TI = 8000/66/140 ms; in plane resolution = 2.0×1.4 mm; Sl = 8 mm; 17 images per breath-hold. (Courtesy of Grosshadern Clinic, Munich)

Clinical Applications of TSE

Brain and Spine

TSE is now well established for neurological applications [1, 8, 17, 38, 44]. Dual-contrast TSE studies with a good coverage of the brain can be obtained in about 2 min (Fig. 7). Flow artifacts in head and spine can be largely suppressed with flow compensated TSE sequences. However, because of the stimulated echo contribution (see "Stimulated Echo Contribution") some residual flow artifacts can remain, visible for example, in spine imaging.

TSE with fat suppression [33] (Fig. 9) and dark fluid TSE [3, 46] (Fig. 11) are used to increase lesion conspicuity.

HASTE allows the examination of noncooperative patients because of its short acquisition time and its sequential slice capability [22, 23] (Fig. 15). T2-weighted high resolution imaging of small neural structures in scan times between 3 and 9 min is possible with 2D and 3D single-contrast TSE sequences. Sagittal spine images with 1-mm partition thickness can be obtained with 3D TSE and can be reformatted in all planes without loss of resolution [16, 32] (Fig. 13). The major drawback of TSE in the brain is its reduced sensitivity to hemorrhagic lesions [18, 31].

Abdomen and Pelvis

The substantially reduced imaging time combined with strong T2-weighted contrast makes TSE an interesting technique for abdominal imaging [20, 29, 36, 41, 45]. TSE images acquired with multiple acquisitions to reduce motion artifacts are superior to SE images obtained with typically 2 acquisitions. Alternatively the time saving can be used to increase the spatial resolution. (Fig. 17a). In combination with fat suppression techniques artifacts from breathing can be reduced, which improves the conspicuity of pathological structures. Especially STIR TSE was found to be best for lesion detection [37].

With the introduction of body phased array coils and the resulting strongly increased SNR TSE sequences optimized for breath-hold imaging are expected to replace conventional T2-weighted TSE sequences in the abdomen (Figs. 16, 17b). Breath-hold sequences minimize motion-related artifacts and can therefore depict lesions not seen with other sequences.

In pelvic imaging the time saving of TSE can be translated into a larger matrix for high resolution. TSE imaging, especially when combined with fat suppression, can depict subtle architectural details of the prostate and uterus [7, 30, 43] (Fig. 18).

Most recently single-shot RARE and multi-slice HASTE sequences have provided MR cholangiograms of outstanding quality. Although still under evaluation, MR cholangiography has become an important adjunct and in some cases an alternative for the evaluation of biliary pathology. Whereas RARE provides a projection image of the biliary system in about 3-s acquisition time [24, 34] (Fig. 19a) and thus an overview of the anatomy and major pathology, the

Fig. 17. a High-resolution T2-weighted liver image on a patient with multiple metastases obtained with the body coil on the 1.0-T Magnetom Impact. The time saving of TSE is used to increase the spatial resolution. 11-echo TSE sequence with flow compensation in read: TA = 5:41 min; TR/TE = 4660/112ms; 2 acquisitions; in plane resolution = 1.0×0.76 mm; Sl = 8 mm. **b** Breath-hold liver study of a patient with a pancreatic tumor obtained with the CP body phased array coil on the 1.5-T Magnetom Vision. 29-echo TSE sequence; TA = 19 s; TR/TE = 2200/132ms; in plane resolution = 2.5×1.5 mm; 9 images. (Courtesy of the Grosshadern Clinic, Munich)

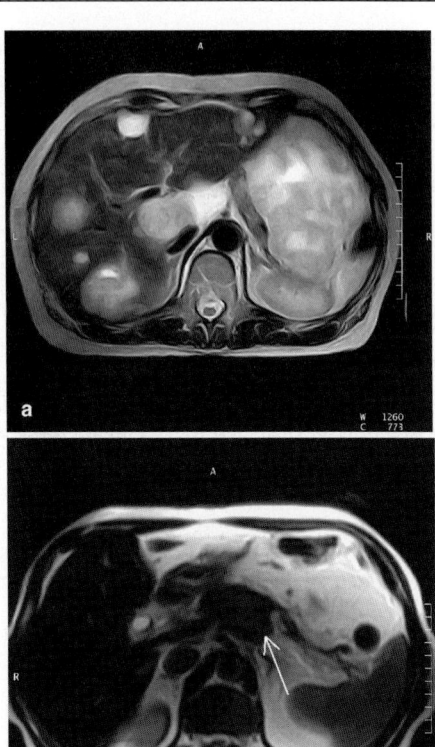

Fig. 18. Imaging of the pelvis with the CP body phased array coil on the 1.5-T Magnetom Vision. 7-echo TSE sequence: TA = 9:06 min; TR/TE = 5000/96ms; in plane resolution = 0.89×0.78 mm; Sl = 3 mm. Prostate carcinoma stage C: hypointense capsule (*arrow 1*) on the left side of the organ, tumor nodule in the hypointense peripheral zone (*arrow 2*). (Courtesy of K. Engelhard, Martha Maria Hospital Nuremberg)

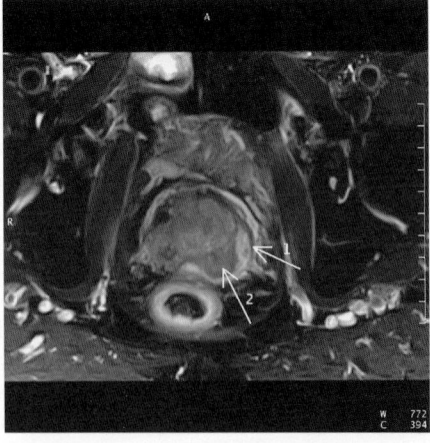

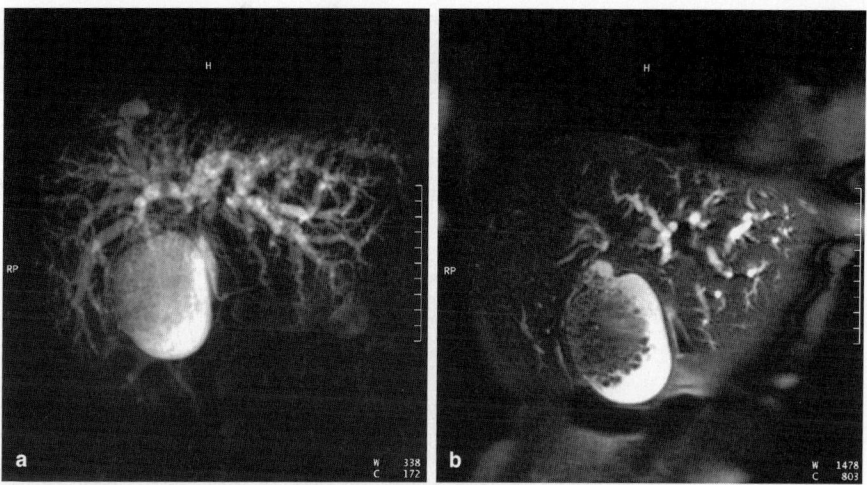

Fig. 19. a Projectional RARE cholangiogram obtained in 3 s on the 1.0-T Magnetom Expert with the CP body phased array coil provides an overview over the biliary anatomy in this patient with stones in the gallbladder. 240-echo single shot TSE sequence; TE = 1100 ms; in plane resolution = 1.17×1.09 mm; Sl = 70 mm. **b** Multi-slice HASTE images obtained in a 16 s breath-hold provide more detail of the individual anatomic structures and show also signal from the surrounding tissue. A maximum intensity projection can be applied. TE = 87 ms; in plane resolution = 1.17×1.09 mm; Sl = 5 mm, 8 images

stack of 3- to 5-mm- thin HASTE images (Fig. 19b) provides exquisite detail of structures within a breath-hold [40].

RARE and HASTE are also increasingly used for noninvasive urography.

Heart

Both breath-hold TSE and HASTE sequences have recently provided reliably artifact-free T2-weighted images of the heart. Particularly when combined with "black blood" and STIR spin preparation, suppression of the blood pool signal and fat improves the depiction of cardiac structures and enhances the conspicuity of pathological processes (Fig. 12). The enhanced T2 weighting provided by STIR prepulses facilitates the depiction of ischemic myocardium, cardiac, and mediastinal tumors involving the heart and of inflammatory conditions.

Ultrafast single-shot HASTE images, obtained in 330 ms, have been shown to provide images of great detail of the heart (Fig. 20). In contrast to gradient echo EPI sequences, they are free of magnetic susceptibility artifacts. Within a single breath-hold it is possible to depict the heart along its major axis with a stack of 5-mm-thick HASTE images.

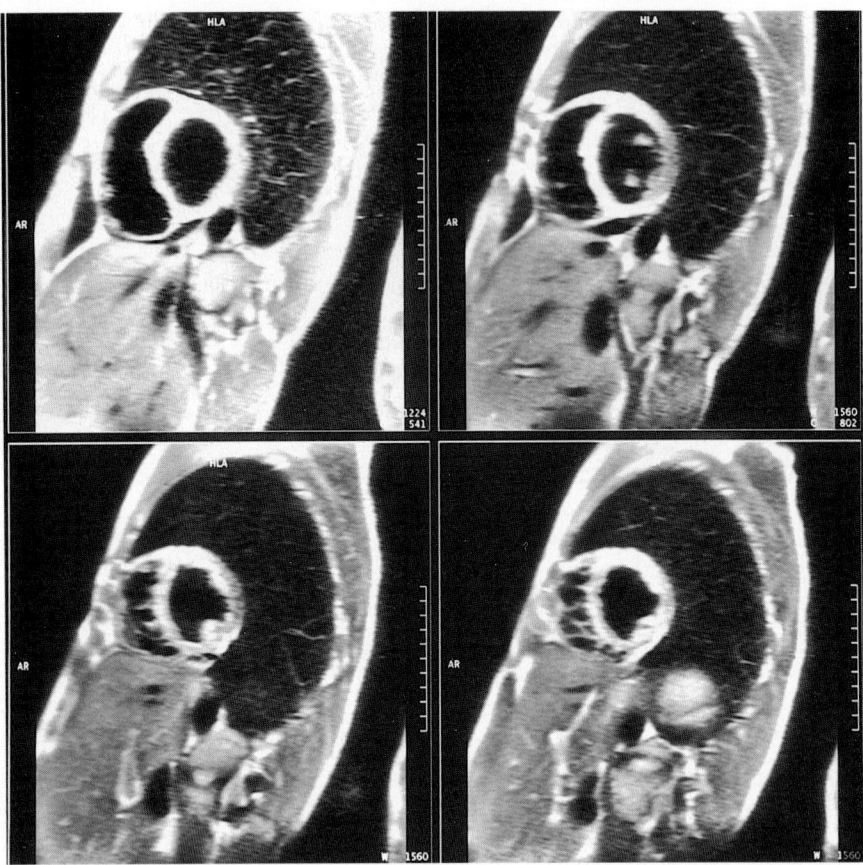

Fig. 20. HASTE images obtained in 330 ms on the 1.5-T Magnetom Vision with the CP body phased array coil provide complete coverage of the heart along one of its major axis in a stack of 5-mm-thick sections in a single breath-hold. A "black blood" prepulse provides reliable suppression of blood signal

Orthopedics

TSE has not yet found full acceptance in orthopedic imaging. TSE is considered to be less sensitive to bone disease due to the bright fat signal. TSE with fat suppression, however, should solve this problem [19]. It has also been reported that rotator cuff tears and meniscal tears can be missed or mimicked [39]. These problems are controversial at the moment and might be solved by shorter echo trains, shorter echo-echo spacing, and modified k space ordering schemes. The short imaging time of TSE makes it possible to obtain PD- and T2-weighted images with high resolution (up to 1024 matrix), as it is needed to differentiate joint spaces, ligaments, and their pathologies (Figs. 4, 21).

Fig. 21. High-resolution shoulder study of a patient with a cyst obtained with a CP flexible coil on the 1.5-T Magnetom Vision. 7-echo TSE sequence: TA = 4:26 min, TR/TE = 5000/96ms; in plane resolution = 0.55×0.39 mm; Sl = 3 mm. (Courtesy of Grosshadern Clinic, Munich)

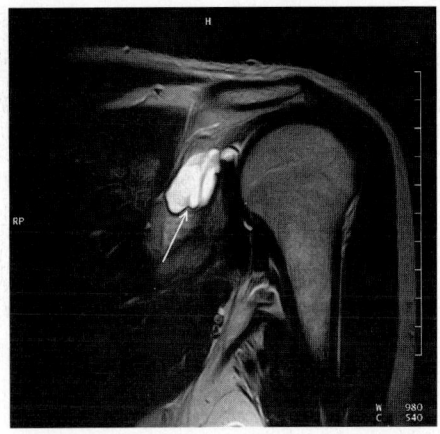

References

1. Atlas SW, Hackney DB, Listerud J (1993) Fast spin-echo imaging of the brain and spine. Magn Reson Q 9:61–83
2. Carr HY, Purcell EM (1954) Effects of diffusion on free precision in nuclear magnetic resonance experiments. Phys Rev 94:630–638
3. Coene BD, Hajnal JV et al (1992) MR of the brain using fluid-attenuated inversion recovery (FLAIR) pulse sequences. AJNR 13:155–1564
4. Constable RT, Anderson AW et al (1992) Factors influencing contrast in fast spin-echo MR imaging. Magn Reson Imaging 10:497–511
5. Constable RT, Gore JC (1992) The loss of small objects in variable TE imaging: implications for FSE, RARE, and EPI. Magn Reson Med 28:9–24
6. Edelman RR, Chien D, Kim D (1991) Fast selective black blood MR imaging. Radiology 181:655–660
7. Engelhard K, Hollenbach HP et al (1994) Anwendung neuer Turbo-Spin-Echo-Pulssequenzen mit und ohne Fettunterdrückung bei der Diagnostik und Stadieneinteilung des Prostatakarzinoms. Fortschr Rontgenstr 160(1):59–65
8. Fellner F, Schmitt R et al (1993) Wertigkeit schneller Spinecho-(Turbo-Spinecho)- Sequenzen in der MR-Routinediagnostik des Zerebrums bei 1.0 Tesla. Klin Neuroradiol 3:111–117
9. Hahn EL (1950) Spin echoes. Phys Rev 80:580–594
10. Henkelman RM, Hardy PA et al (1992) Why fat is bright in RARE and fast spin-echo imaging. JMRI 2:533–540
11. Hennig J, Nauerth A, Friedburg H (1986) RARE imaging: a fast imaging method for clinical MR. Magn Reson Med 3:823–833
12. Hennig J, Friedburg H, Ott D (1987) Fast three-dimensional imaging of cerebrospinal fluid. Magn Reson Med 5:380–383
13. Hennig J (1991) Echoes – how to generate, recognize, use or avoid them in MR-imaging sequences I. Concepts Magn Reson 3:125–143
14. Hinks RS, Einstein S (1991) Shared data dual echo in fast spin echo imaging. SMRM 10:1011
15. Hinks RS, Constable RT (1992) Flow compensation in fast spin echo imaging. SMRM 11:891
16. Holland GA, Mitchell J (1994) Optimization and initial experience with high resolution 3D fast spin-echo imaging of the cervical spine. JMRI 4(P):112
17. Jones KM, Mulkern RV et al (1992) Fast spin-echo MR imaging of the brain and spine: current concepts. AJR 158:1313–1320
18. Jones KM, Mulkern RV et al (1992) Brain hemorrhage: evaluation with fast spin-echo and conventional spin-echo images. Radiology 182:53–58
19. Kapelov SR, Teresi LM et al (1993) Bone contusions of the knee: increased lesion detection with fast spin-echo MR imaging with spectroscopic fat saturation. Radiology 189:901–904
20. Kreft B, Layer G et al (1994) Evaluation of turbo spin echo sequence for MRI of focal liver lesions at 0.5T. Eur Radiol 4:106–113

21. Kiefer B, Hollenbach HP et al (1992) Fat suppression with turboSE using an inversion or frequency selective prepulse. SMRM 11:4523
22. Kiefer B, Hausmann R (1993) Fast imaging with single-shot MR imaging techniques based on turboSE and turboGSE. Radiology 189(P):289
23. Kiefer B, Grässner J, Hausmann R (1994) Image acquisition in a second with half-Fourier acquisition single-shot turbo spin echo. JMRI 4(P):86
24. Laubenberger J, Büchert M et al (1995) Breath-hold projection magnetic resonance-cholangio-pancreaticography (MRCP): a new method for the examination of the bile and pancreatic ducts. Magn Reson Med 33:18–23
25. Mansfield P (1977) Multi planar image formation using NMR spin-echoes. J Phys C (Solid St Phys) 10:L55–L58
26. Meiboom S, Gill D (1958) Modified spin echo method for measuring nuclear relaxation times. Rev Sci Instr 29:688–691
27. Melki PS, Mulkern RV et al (1991) Comparing the FAISE method with conventional dual-echo sequences. JMRI 1:319–326
28. Melki PS, Mulkern RV (1992) Magnetization transfer effects in multislice RARE sequences. Magn Reson Med 24:189–195
29. Mitchell DG (1993) Hepatic imaging: techniques and unique applications of magnetic resonance imaging. Magn Reson Q 9:84–112
30. Nghiem HV, Herfkens RJ et al (1992) The pelvis: T2-weighted fast spin-echo MR imaging. Radiology 185:213–217
31. Norbash AM, Glover GH, Enzmann DR (1992) Intracerebral lesion contrast with spin-echo and fast spin-echo pulse sequences. Radiology 185:661–665
32. Oshio K, Jolesz FA et al (1991) T2-weighted thin-section imaging with the multislab three-dimensional RARE technique. JMRI 1:695–700
33. Panush D, Fulbright R et al (1993) Inversion-recovery fat spin-echo MR imaging: efficacy in the evaluation of head and neck lesions. Radiology 187:421–426
34. Reuther G, Tuchmann B, Kiefer B (1996) Cholangiography before bile surgery: single shot MR cholangiography versus intravenous X-ray cholangiography. Radiology 198:561–566
35. Reuther G, Kiefer B (1995) 2D-MR-myelography (2D-MRM) in single-shot technique versus 3D-MR-myelography with fat suppression (3D-MRM) as an adjunct to MR-tomography of lumbar disc herniations. Eur Radiol 5 [Suppl]:S141
36. Rijcken TH, Davidoff A et al (1994) Optimized tissue characterization with fast spin-echo imaging at 1.5T. JMRI 4(P):43
37. Rofsky NM, Weinreb JC et al (1994) Comparison of fat-suppression techniques for hepatic MR imaging: turbo-SE, breath-hold turbo-SE, GRASE and turbo STIR. JMRI 4(P):66
38. Ross JS, Ruggieri P et al (1993) Lumbar degenerative disk disease: prospective comparison of conventional T2-weighted spin-echo imaging and T2-weighted rapid acquisition relaxation-enhanced imaging. AJNR 14:1215–1223
39. Rubin DA, Underberg-Davis SJ (1992) Fast-SE imaging of meniscal pathology in the knee: comparison with SE imaging. Radiology 185(P):308
40. Sananes JC, Secesne R et al (1995) MR Cholangiography (MRC) using a breath hold fast spin echo sequence. Eur Radiol 5 [Suppl]:S4
41. Semelka RC, Kelekis NL et al (1996) HASTE MR Imaging: Description of Technique and Preliminary Results in the Abdomen. J MRI 6:698–699
42. Simonetti OP, Laub G, Finn JP (1994) Breath-hold T2-weighted Imaging of the Heart with TurboSE. SMR 2:1499
43. Smith RC, Reinhold C et al (1992) Fast spin-echo MR imaging of the female pelvis: part I. use of the whole-volume coil. Radiology 184:665–669
44. Sze G, Kawamura Y et al (1993) Fast spin-echo MR imaging of the cervical spine: influence of echo train length and echo spacing on image contrast and quality. AJNR 14:1203–1213
45. Van Hoe L, Bosmans H et al (1996) Focal Liver Lesions: Fast T2-weighted MR Imaging with Half-Fourier Rapid Acquisition with Relaxation Enhancement. Radiology 201:817–823
46. White SJ, Hajnal JV et al (1992) Use of fluid-attenuated inversion-recovery pulse sequences for imaging the spinal cord. Magn Reson Med 28:153–162

CHAPTER 20

Gradient and Spin-Echo (GRASE) Imaging

D. A. Feinberg

Introduction

Magnetic resonance (MR) imaging pulse sequences are developed through an evolutionary process rather than by entirely de nova invention. Useful new imaging sequences evolve by combining new and existing methodology. For example, spin warp phase encoding was incorporated into selective line scan imaging to produce contemporary 2D FT gradient echo imaging (4). The incorporation of a 180° RF refocusing pulse into 2D FT gradient echo imaging yielded spin echo imaging (1). Spin echo images and gradient echo images differ considerably in their static field inhomogeneity and susceptibility artifacts, tissue contrast and the effects of blood flow. Elimination of field inhomogeneity artifacts allowed for much later echo times, increasing T2 contrast in spin echo images, which is extremely useful for tissue characterization in medical diagnosis. Development of pulse sequences may in retrospect appear straightforward. In reality, there are often major difficulties in removing unanticipated image artifacts in new imaging sequences for which solutions often require more creativity than do the original sequence. Imaging with multiple spin echoes was hypothetically suggested as a simple variant of gradient refocused echo-planar imaging (EPI) but without consideration of artifacts from stimulated echo magnetization. It took years and contributions from several scientists [19, 31] to overcome stimulated echo artifacts for successful implementation of spin-echo train imaging.

The gradient- and spin-echo (GRASE) pulse sequence generates a train of echoes by means of multiple gradient reversals between multiple RF pulses in the Carr-Purcell-Meiboom-Gill (CPMG) sequence. The GRASE sequence has unique complexity due to modulated signal phase errors occurring through the echo train in addition to signal amplitude decay. Severe ghosting artifact arising from phase modulation (PM) and amplitude modulation (AM) are eliminated using k space trajectories and echo time shift (ETS) methodology described below.

The GRASE sequences incorporates methodologies used in EPI [23, 24] and rapid spin-echo (RARE) imaging [19, 20]. The use of switched gradients to refocus signals is derived from EPI and contributes to the high rate of signal refocusing in GRASE. The CPMG sequence in GRASE gives T2 decay in the echo train rather than the shorter T2* decay of echo-planar sequences (Fig. 1). Consequently, single-shot GRASE produces more signals than EPI (Fig. 2) and can achieve higher spatial resolution in single-shot imaging. A second improvement over EPI is that the GRASE technique eliminates image artifacts, distortions, and

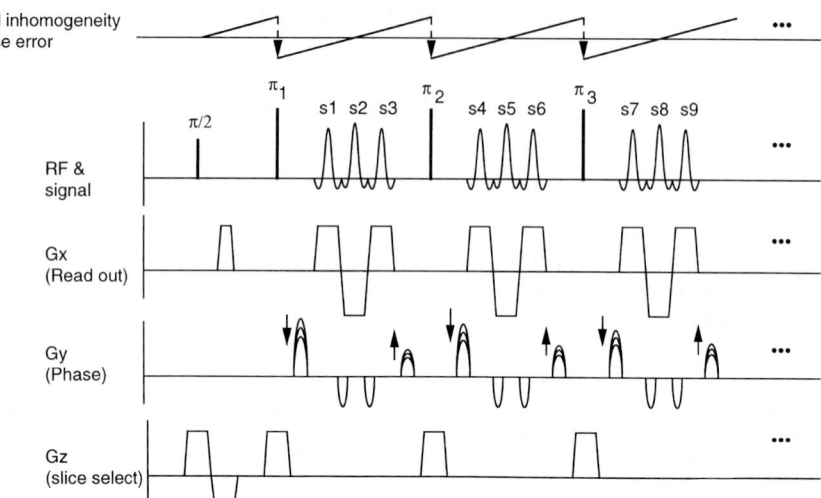

Fig. 1. GRASE pulse sequence. The phase errors in the echo train are refocused by each 180° RF pulse. (From [9])

signal loss which have plagued EPI. The CPMG sequence reduces the accumulated field inhomogeneity and susceptibility errors in the echo train (Fig. 3). In GRASE the off-resonance errors from magnetic field inhomogeneity are maintained at a low level and can be adjusted by the gradient-echo train lengths and RF pulse spacing. Furthermore, the requirement of high-performance gradients in EPI to rapidly refocus signals during their short T2* decay is not so strict a requirement for GRASE.

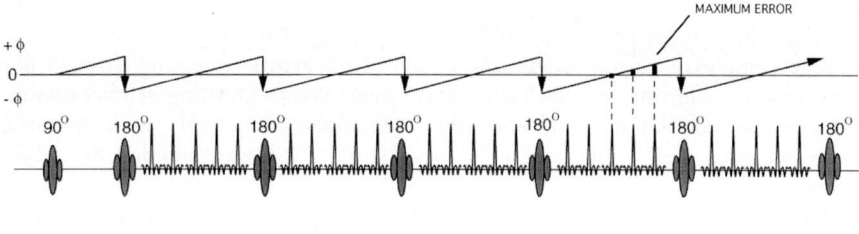

a   GRASE

Fig. 2a,b. Comparison of phase errors from static magnetic field inhomogeneity in GRASE versus SE EPI. The GRASE sequence can be extended over a longer time than EPI which more than offset its lower signal refocusing rate. **a** In GRASE the multiple 180° pulses of create a periodic phase error function with identical errors in each spin-echo envelope. The phase errors increase with distance from the Hahn SE position in each group of echoes, but phase errors do not accumulate in the total echo train. The modulated phase error function is removed in the computer data matrix (k space) by interleaving groups of signals taken from the same echo train

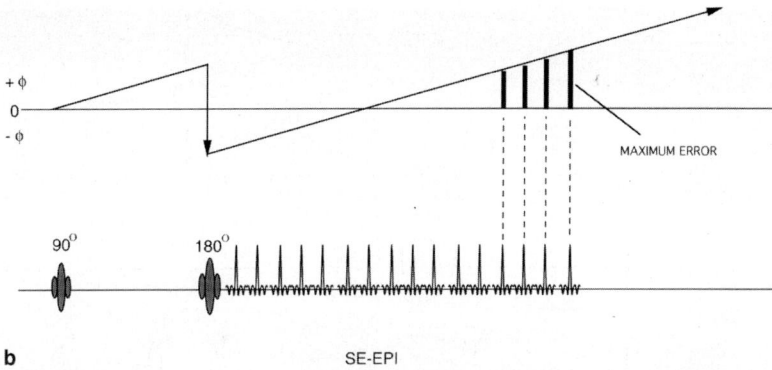

b

SE-EPI

Fig. 2a,b. b SE EPI, gradient-echo train follows the 180° RF pulse. Signals accumulate field inhomogeneity phase errors with time, maximum error at the two ends of the echo train. Field inhomogeneity limits total echo train time, but there is no modulation of the phase error function. There is a larger τ period of dead time between the 90° and 180° RF pulses in SE EPI than in GRASE

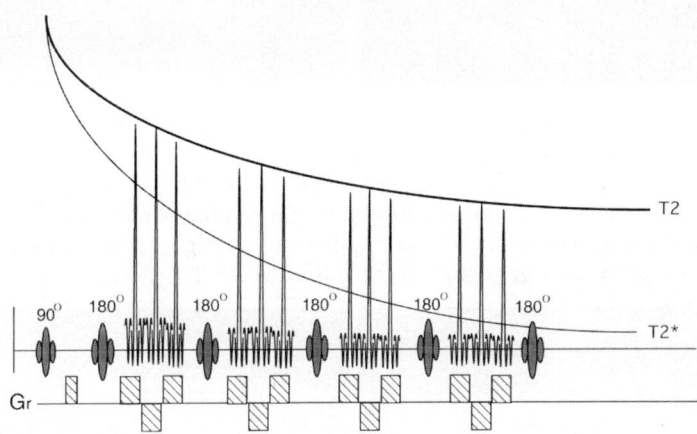

Fig. 3. Echo train refocusing in GRASE. A group of gradient refocused signals is centered on each spin-echo time. These signals are distinctly different from a conventional gradient-echo acquired in absence of an RF refocusing pulses. Field inhomogeneity errors accumulate with time from the Hahn echo in each spin-echo envelope but do not accumulate between spin-echo times. This elimination of accumulated errors in effect eliminates T2* decay in the echo train which instead has T2 decay

The image contrast in GRASE [9] has features of both conventional SE and RARE (Figs. 4–6). The signal from fat is of similar intensity in GRASE and SE and not bright as in RARE. Cystic fluid structures which have long T2 are brighter in both GRASE and RARE than in SE images. Similar to EPI, GRASE has chemical shift on the image's phase-encoded axis. As discussed below, the image contrast in GRASE is affected by its magnetization pathway, stimulated echo magnetization, RF pulse spacing, and k space trajectories.

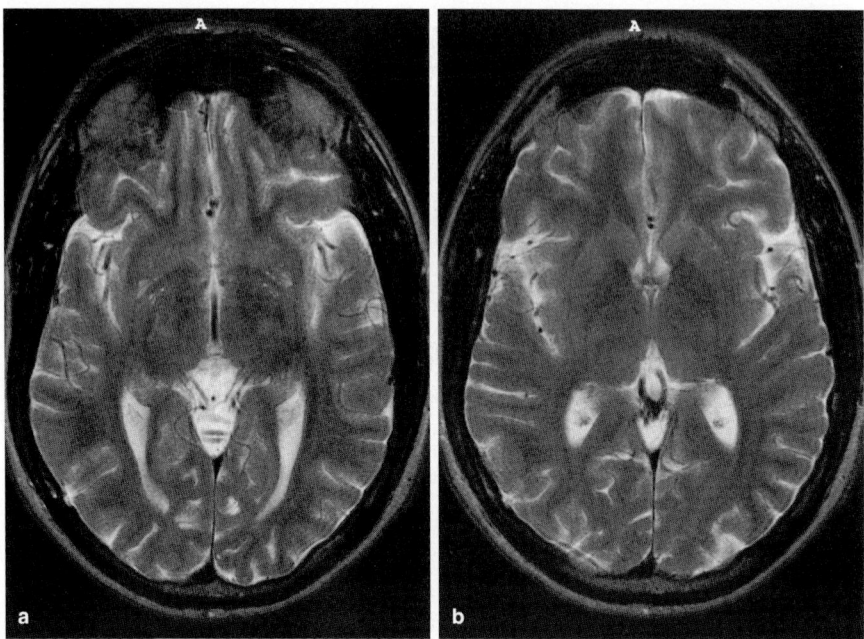

Fig. 4a,b. T2-weighted axial GRASE images of normal brain TR/TE/3500/108 ms acquired in 512×512 matrix with 22-cm field of view, acquisition time 3:40 min, at 1.0 T with 15 mT/m gradients

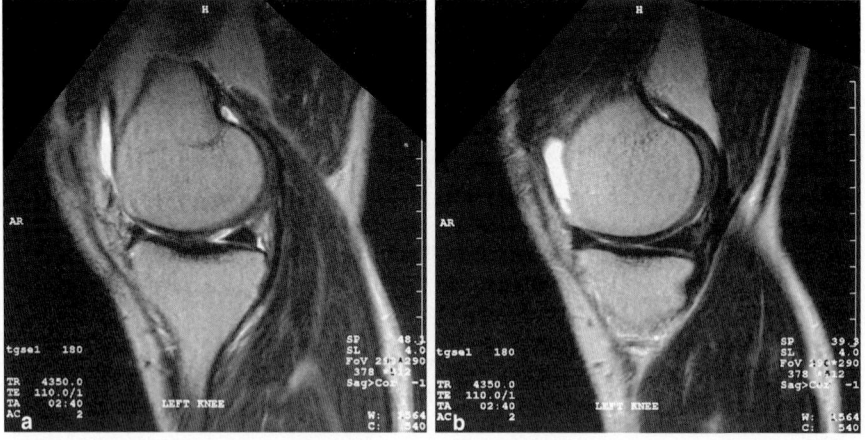

Fig. 5a,b. T2-weighted sagittal GRASE images of knee shows bright synovial fluid and lower signal intensity from fat. The GRASE technique does not produce bright fat signal as do several variants of the RARE technique (fast SE) so that clinical misinterpretations of edema for fat in the bone marrow and soft tissues is avoidable

Fig. 6. GRASE imaging study of patient with metastatic carcinoid tumor in liver. 17 sections acquired in 18 s, TR 3500 ms, TE 105 ms, 192×256 matrix at 1.0-T with 15 mT/m gradients

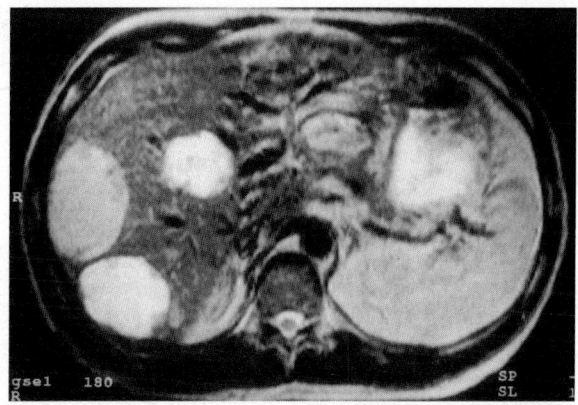

Background and Evolution of GRASE

Hahn first demonstrated how stimulated echoes and spin echoes are components of the same magnetization when applying multiple RF pulses. In the presence of pulsed field gradients the stimulated echoes and spin echoes have different phase pathways, which becomes problematic in MR imaging sequences. The CPMG pulse sequence gave accurate T2 measurements in spin-echo trains but was problematic for image spatial phase encoding. Perhaps for these reasons the earliest echo train images (EPI) utilized gradient refocusing techniques and not RF-refocused spin echoes. The earliest "RF-refocused" EPI method proposed by Mansfield and Pykett [24] utilized a phase-encoding scheme derived from gradient-refocused EPI whereby the signals accumulate phase shifts from prior spin echoes. The proposed method alternates the polarity of a constant phase-encode gradient after each RF pulse but certainly creates considerable image artifact from improperly phase-encoded stimulated echoes. Magnetization stored on the longitudinal axis does not experience the alternating polarity phase-encoding gradients. The stimulated echoes and spin echoes therefore would accumulate different net phase shifts through the echo train sequence.

Strobel and Ratzel [31] overcame the artifacts from stimulated echo magnetization in spin-echo train sequences using a brilliant design approach to phase encoding. They developed the concept of "new phase rewind" to maintain a constant phase in each π-π pulse time interval (Fig. 7). Each phase-rewind pulse has equal area but opposite polarity as the preceding phase-encode pulse and effectively nulls the accumulated phase from one π-π pulse time interval to the next. This eliminated the problem encountered in RF-refocused EPI caused by the different accumulated phase history of stimulated echoes and spin echoes. The RARE sequence developed by Hennig [19, 20] overcame the problems of stimulated echoes in RF-refocused EPI sequence by incorporating this phase-rewind methodology.

The "blipped" phase-encoding scheme for EPI developed by Edelstein [3, 21] is a very important element in the GRASE sequence. As originally conceived, this

Fig. 7. a Phase encoding using rewind pulses in the CPMG sequence (redrawn from [31]). The phase-rewind pulse has opposite polarity and identical amplitude as the phase-encoding pulse, in presence of constant read gradient (*dashed line*). *Below*, the phase of the magnetization. **b** GRASE phase-rewind pulse accomplishes nulling of several phase-encode gradient pulses. The net accumulated phase shift of the gradient pulses is zero in each 180°–180° time interval. Note that GRASE requires a phase-rewind pulse of the same polarity and different magnitude than the first gradient pulse because the encoded k space trajectories of the three signals covers both halves of k space rather than consecutive spatial frequency lines

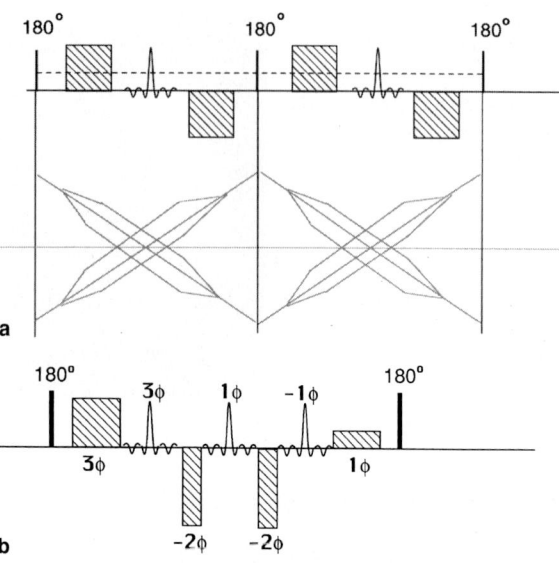

method gives an orthogonal k space trajectory in EPI for two-dimensional FT by independent time of read and phase-encode gradients. GRASE incorporates blipped phase encoding using a discontinuous phase-encode order necessary for k space interleaving. The spin-warp phase-encoding methodology, yet another invention of Edelstein [4], is incorporated into multi-shot GRASE, similar to multi-shot RARE. Free induction decay spoiler gradient pulses are used to remove free induction decay artifacts in GRASE, similarly to most other optimized SE sequences. Gradient moment nulling [32] to reduce flow-related artifacts can be incorporated into read gradients of the GRASE sequence.

Some differences between the physical limitations on GRASE, EPI, and RARE are worth mentioning. GRASE was developed to increase the speed of signal refocusing by using switched gradients within the CPMG sequence. Therefore GRASE sequence has two independent refocusing parameters, RF refocusing and gradient refocusing, which can be adjusted independently. Image artifacts due to field inhomogeneity, susceptibility, and chemical shift can be maintained at an acceptably low level [13, 17]. Much of the magnetization in the later portion of the GRASE echo train is contributed by stimulated magnetization. This is different from SE EPI where the two ends of the echo train decay with T2* and ultimately limit the echo train length. RARE and GRASE differ in their susceptibility contrast, which depends on differences in RF pulse spacing and on the number of gradient refocusings. Differences between RARE and GRASE images are apparent as RARE has bright lipid signal intensity, whereas GRASE does not.

RARE has a one-to-one dependence of echo refocusing rate on the number of RF pulses, thus a direct dependence of echo train length or imaging speed on RF heating. The biological hazard of RF heating (specific absorption rate) can be overcome in the RARE technique by using a reduced number of slices or reduced RF refocusing rate. As diagrammed in Fig. 8, specific absorption rate is less of a

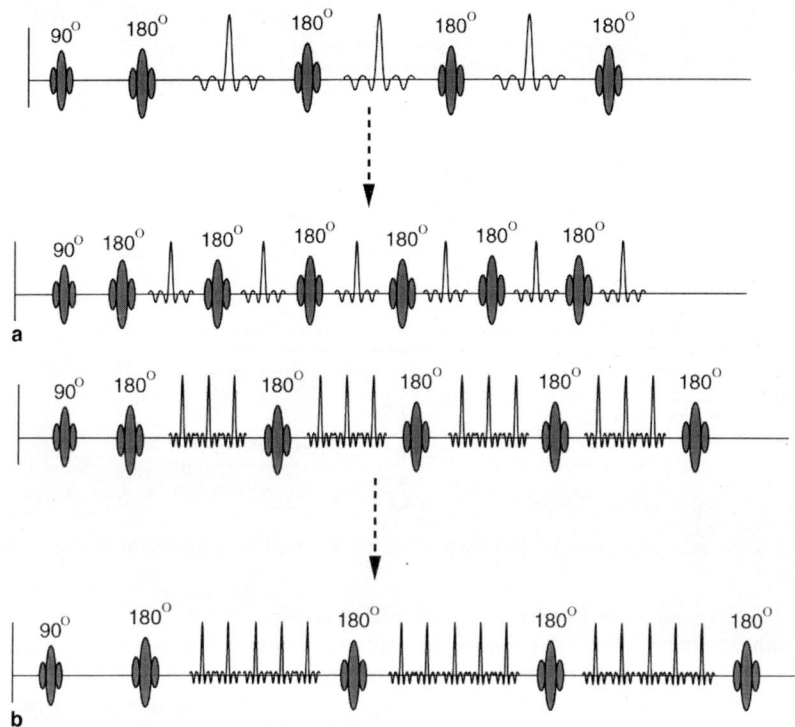

Fig. 8a,b. Use of the CPMG sequence particularly at higher field strengths increases the heating of biological tissue. **a** RARE generates one signal per π pulse and to increase the number of signals in the echo train the number of π pulses must be increased by closer spacing. Increased tissue heating occurs with decreased RF pulse spacing for faster imaging. **b** In GRASE the RF power deposition and tissue heating is dependent on RF refocusing rate but independent of signal refocusing rate. Increased RF pulse spacing decreases RF power and allows additional gradient refocusings, increasing signal refocusing rate

problem in GRASE due to the wider spacing of the RF pulses given the multiple intervening gradient refocusing pulses.

Phase Error Modulation

A unique problem encountered in the development of the GRASE sequences is that phase errors from field inhomogeneity, susceptibility, and frequency differences between lipid and water tissues are all modulated in the echo train (Fig. 2). Phase modulation (PM) gives severe image ghosting if not properly dealt with. The PM artifacts are not present in EPI or RARE where gradient refocusing or RF refocusing is performed separately. In GRASE the periodic π pulse refocusing of field inhomogeneity, susceptibility, and other off-resonance effects result in a modulated phase errors function through the echo train. In k space the modu-

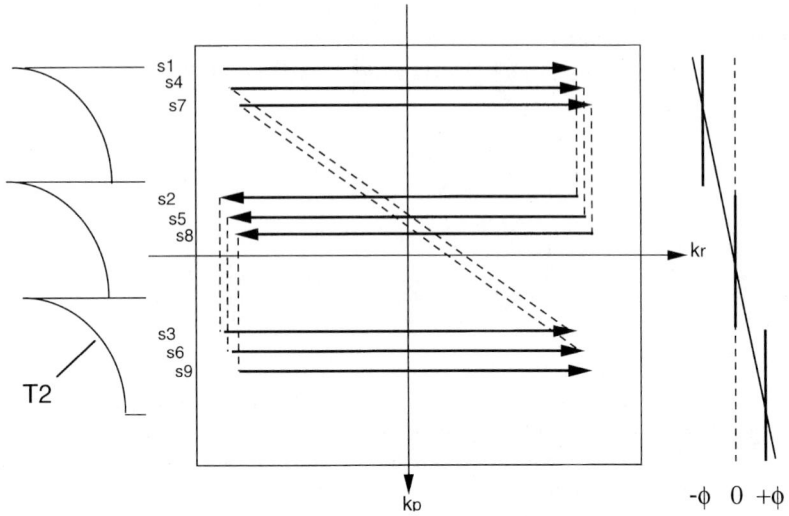

Fig. 9. K space diagram of GRASE showing the T2 error function and phase error function on the k_p axis

lated phase error function is convolved with the spatial frequency data and gives severe ghosting artifact in the image domain.

Methodology to demodulate the phase error function is needed for successful imaging, regardless of the RF pulse timing. The CPMG sequence creates groups of echoes centered at Hahn spin-echo times. Each group of echoes are thus created within the spin-echo time envelope and each group has an identical phase error function imposing an exact periodicity to the modulated phase error function. These groups of signals can be interleaved in k-space so that signals of identical phase error and phase polarity are regrouped together and placed adjacent to each other in k-space data matrix. To accomplish the interleaving in k space the phase-encoding ordering in the echo train is not a monotonically increasing order as in EPI or RARE (Fig. 9). With interleaving, the PMs are transformed into a single long-stepped phase error function across the phase axis of k space. As described below, a specific timing in gradient refocusing known as ETS, is additionally incorporated to the pulse sequence to further remove phase discontinuities in k space.

Echo Formation in GRASE

The MR signals can be described in terms of magnetization M(r), magnetic field gradients G(t), and spatial position r-as:

$$S(t) = M(r)\exp[-j(k(t)\ r+\gamma E(r)t)]d\ r \tag{1}$$

$$k(t) = \gamma \int_D^t G(t')dt' \tag{2}$$

where $E(r)$ is the field component due to static magnetic field inhomogeneities, susceptibility, and chemical shift. In two-dimensional Fourier imaging Eq. 1 can be rewritten in terms of ϕ_1, y-phase encoding, and ϕ_2, phase error:

$$S(t) = M(r)\exp[-j(k_x x + \phi_1 + \phi_2)]dr$$
$$\phi_1 = k_y(i)y \tag{3}$$
$$i = 1, 2, N$$

$$\phi_2 = \gamma E(x, y) n - \frac{G_{GE} + 1}{2} T_{GE} \tag{4}$$
$$n = 1, 2, ..., G_{GE}$$

where i is the y-encoding index, n is the gradient-echo index, and T_{GR} the gradient-echo time interval and N is the total number of y-encodings.

The magnetization pathway of the GRASE sequence differs considerably from both gradient-echo trains and spin-echo train as it passes through multiple phase error null points corresponding to the Hahn echo time of each gradient-echo train segment of the total echo train. Each gradient-echo train can be considered to occur in a "spin-echo envelope." Phase errors increase with echo position from the center of the envelope but without increasing from one spin-echo envelope to the next. Therefore the phase errors recur identically in each of the multiple SE envelopes resulting in a modulated phase error function.

The total number of echoes per echo train is the product of the number of RF refocused spin echoes using switched read gradients, N_{RF}, and the number of gradient refocused echoes, N_{GR}, in each spin-echo time period; thus $N_{signals} = N_{RF} \times N_{GR}$. Using N_{RF} as an additional 1 degree of freedom, field inhomogeneity errors are not directly dependent on echo train length as in EPI. By increasing N_{RF} and decreasing N_{GE} the off-resonance errors can be adjusted to an acceptable level to eliminate artifacts in a particular clinical or biological application.

Phase-Encoding Methodology

Phase encoding in GRASE is designed to accomplish a specific interleaved reordering of signals to remove PMs in k space [9, 27]. In exchange this interleaving process transforms the monotonic T2 decay across k space into a modulated T2 magnitude error function (Fig. 9). In effect the periodic phase error function is replaced by a periodic magnitude error function consisting of multiple T2 decays on the k_p axis which eliminates the severe ghost artifacts from the GRASE image.

Phase encoding is performed in a periodic manner using each spin echo as a temporal reference frame. Signals of identical phase error occurring in identical relative positions in the SE envelopes are grouped together in k space. The phase-encoding value, k_y, in the *l*th excitation, *m*th RF refocused spin-echo envelope, and *n*th gradient refocused echo of each spin-echo envelope is expressed as:

$$k_y (l, m, n) = l + N_{EX} (m-1) + N_{EX} N_{RF} (n-1) \tag{5}$$

where N_{EX} is the total number of excitations and N_{RF} is as defined above. The signals from each SE envelope are then assigned in the computer to a k space position which corresponds to an interleaving process.

The time required for the blipped phase-encoding pulse must be sufficient to allow for traversal of a larger segment of k space. The larger phase-encoding step in GRASE is more of a time-limiting step than in EPI, where in the latter the blipped phase gradient traverses only one k space line. By increasing the number of gradient refocusings per spin echo in GRASE the number of k space lines traversed by each blipped gradient becomes smaller, as do the time requirements.

Any constant phase shifts due to slight timing errors between the odd and even gradient echoes, or DC offsets, can be removed by post acquisition phase correction. A template set of correction data can be obtained in an echo train without phase encoding and used to normalize unwanted phase shifts in the image data. The zero phase-encoded correction data can be obtained from the first excitation in multi-shot imaging or from a spin-echo envelope period in single-shot imaging.

Following the teachings of Strobel and Ratzel [31], the stimulated echo magnetization is phase encoded identically with the spin-echo magnetization. The net accumulated phase in each π-π interval is zero as a result of the "phase-rewind pulses." In the CPMG spin-echo train [31] and in the RARE sequence [19] the phase-encode and phase-rewind pulses are identical in size and shape but of opposite polarity (Fig. 7). In GRASE the phase-rewind pulse must cancel the accumulated phase of several phase-encoding pulses in each π-π interval and therefore is of unequal size. The phase-rewind methodology also serves to readily allow an interleaved k space trajectory.

Echo Time Shifting

A sequence design feature known as ETS [10, 11, 14] removes artifacts resulting from discontinuities in the k space phase error function in GRASE. ETS has also been used to improve image quality of multi-shot EPI [25, 29]. ETS incrementally changes the timing (temporal position) of gradient refocused signals relative to Hahn spin-echo times in the CPMG sequence. The resulting phase error function has reduced and redistributed phase discontinuities so as not to produce a low level ghosting otherwise present in multi-shot EPI or GRASE images.

In single-shot EPI the phase error function results from the temporal accumulation of field inhomogeneity errors. This phase of the error function incrementally increases with time and is mapped onto consecutive k space point, creating a smooth continuous function on the phase axis of k space. The phase error function in GRASE data is dissimilar due to the interleaving process which groups data from N_{RF} gradient-echo trains, each with identical phase error functions. This regrouping or interleaving creates a discrete jump in the net phase error function which appear as a bidirectional tilted stairstep function on the phase axis of the data (Fig. 10a). In segmented, multi-shot EPI interleaved gradient-echo train data create the same stairstep phase error function and not the

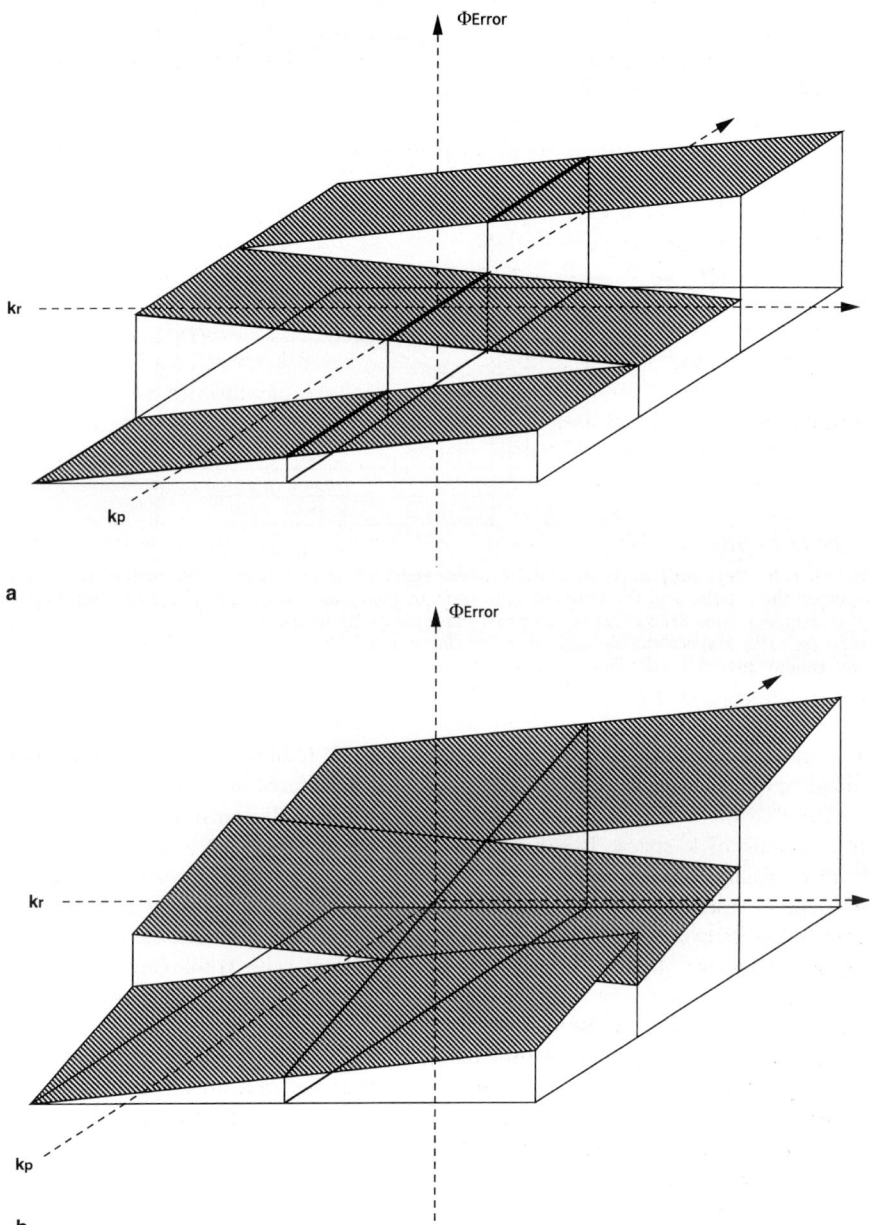

Fig. 10a,b. Diagram of phase error function in GRASE and in interleaved multi-shot EPI using three gradient-recalled echoes. An echo train of three echoes is diagrammed with time reversal of the middle echo. **a** Without ETS. **b** With ETS the phase discontinuities are reduced and moved to the outer regions of k space. This removes ghosting from images. Increased time between echoes as caused by longer read periods causes larger phase error discontinuities in the higher spatial frequencies of the k_r axis. The longer gradient-echo trains of EPI increases the net phase error across the k_p axis. In GRASE the RF refocusing time interval of the CPMG sequence sets the maximal phase error on the phase axis. (From [14])

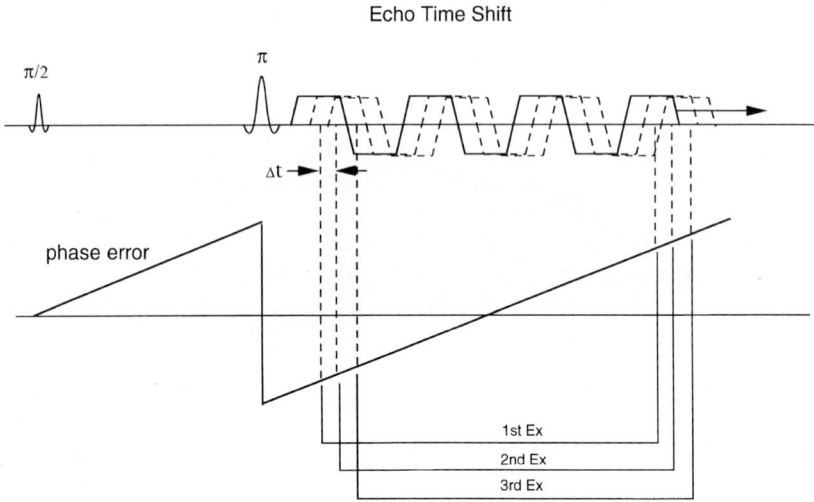

Fig. 11. Echo time shift in multi-shot EPI pulse sequence incorporates a differential time delay between the π pulse and the gradient-echo train in each excitation cycle. The echo train occurs at incremental time delays (*Δt*) on the phase error curve. By interleaving echoes from consecutive echo trains in k space causes signals on the phase axis to become sequentially ordered in time and equally spaced by the time shift increment

smooth or continuous phase steps in single-shot EPI. This error function creates image artifacts often visible at fat-water tissue interfaces and as ghosting.

The ETS method reduces artifacts caused by phase discontinuities in the central regions of k space. It can be used in both multi-shot EPI and GRASE to remove discontinuities in the phase error function present in the central regions of k space, resulting from the interleaving process. By incorporating a differential time delay between each π pulse and the subsequent gradient-echo train the phase errors are slightly different in each gradient-echo train (Fig. 11). With appropriate choice of the ETS the interleaved data have continuous incremental phase steps identical to the smooth function of single-shot EPI.

In general, the increment of time delay in ETS always equals the gradient-echo spacing divided by the number of interleaves (number of π pulses and excitation cycles). With multi-shot (segmented) EPI the delay increment equals T_{GE}, the read gradient A/D time, and switching time, divided by N_{EX} the number of excitation cycles (shots or segmentations):

$$Dt = (1-1)\frac{T_{GE}}{N_{EX}} - \frac{T_{GE}}{2} \tag{6}$$

As shown in Fig. 12, the short gradient-echo trains are shifted in time around the Hahn time of each spin-echo envelope. Since the phase error functions of EPI and GRASE are monotonic on the k_p axis, ETS can effectively be applied to both techniques. The magnitude of the off-resonance phase errors differs between EPI and GRASE. Though SE EPI utilizes a 180° RF pulse to halve the magnitude of phase errors, the errors remain proportional to the total echo train time. Reduction of the maximal phase error in GRASE can be made independent of total echo train time by changing the number and spacing of 180° RF pulses in the CPMG sequence. Consequently the maximum phase error of GRASE is typically five to ten times smaller than that of SE EPI.

Certain generalizations can be made about the phase error discontinuities as shown in the phase error plots of Fig. 10. Longer read periods or increased echo time interval creates larger phase tilt on the k_r axis, causing larger phase error discontinuities in the higher spatial frequency data of ETS. Secondly, longer echo train times increase the phase error tilt on the k_p axis but do not affect the k_r axis phase tilt. Longer signal read periods for higher spatial resolution or for lower bandwidth increase the phase discontinuity (net tilt) on k_r axis.

It is noted that ETS slightly increases the TE of the image. In using ETS in EPI an additional time of half an echo time interval, $T_{GE}/2$, is required before the π pulse, increasing the minimal obtainable TE of SE EPI by one echo time interval and increasing the TE of gradient-echo EPI by $T_{GE}/2$. Also there is an increase in

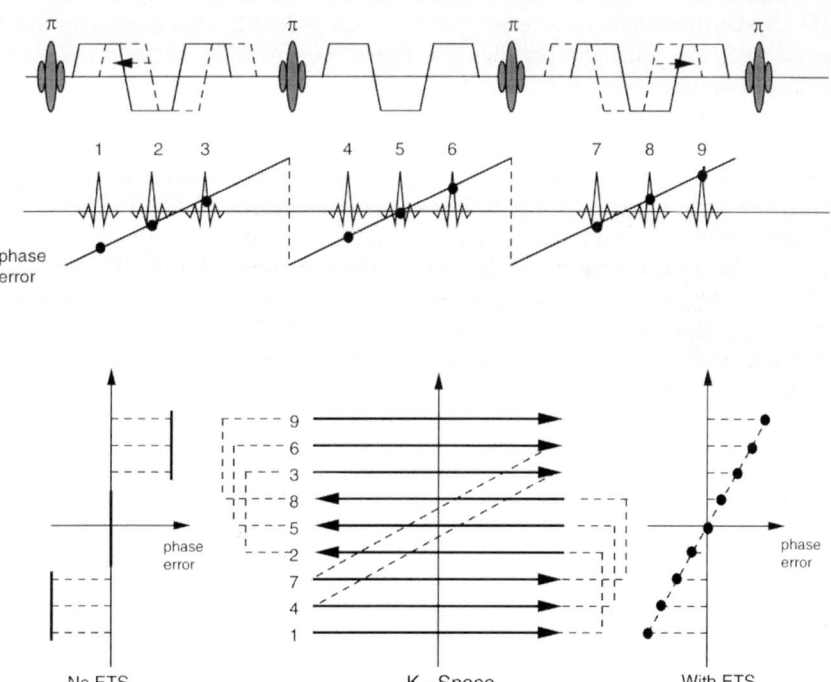

Fig. 12. Echo time shift in GRASE. Without ETS (*broken lines*) the read gradients are symmetrically positioned about each Hahn echo time. With ETS (*solid lines*) a linear variation of phase error is present on the phase axis so that there are no phase error discontinuities in the lowest spatial frequencies, the center of each signals (*black dots*). In effect, the phase discontinuities are moved from the central of k space to the higher spatial frequency in the outer regions of k space. (From [11])

the maximal phase error due to this net longer sampling time of the phase error function. In SE EPI and GRASE the phase error function is zero in the middle of k space (Fig. 10). In gradient-echo EPI the phase error function does not pass through a null point which would occur at the 90° RF pulse time.

The implementation of ETS can be problematic since it removes redundancy in sequence code in excitation cycles and within the a single gradient-spin-echo pulse sequence. Limitations of certain pulse sequence control computer programs have been revealed in attempts to implement ETS. This is different from most imaging pulse sequences, which can simply reload gradient table values in each cycle. Echo time shifting requires either the reloading of time tables not available on all sequence control software. Alternatively, the entire pulse sequence with unique code for each cycle must be downloaded into the sequencer memory, and this may be possible only for single-shot imaging.

Dual-Contrast Imaging

The CPMG sequence necessitates equal time spacing between 180° RF pulses. This results in a constraint on the duration of the read period which must be held constant throughout the echo train, as used in RARE. This constraint differs considerably when using more than one signal refocusing in each π-π time interval (Fig. 13). Here the net time of the multiple read periods instead of one read period is constrained by the constant RF pulse spacing. A mixed number of read periods of different duration can be interchanged during any particular π-π interval as long as the equal time spacing of the CPMG sequence is maintained. This additional degree of freedom has not previously been studied in echo train imaging [16].

In the T2-weighted image signals are obtained at a later time in the echo train and have considerably lower signal amplitude than signals used for the proton density (PD) weighted image. Longer read periods can be used for the T2-weighted image than for the PD-weighted image to produce narrower bandwidth signals for lower noise, which is desirable to compensate for the relatively low signal amplitudes. Such balancing the SNR of the PD- and T2-weighted images can avoid signal averaging corresponding to longer data acquisition times to compensate for this deficient SNR in T2-weighted images. Several variants of mixed signal bandwidth when acquiring dual-contrast (PD- and T2-weighted) images can be implemented.

Single-Shot GRASE Imaging

One promising use of GRASE is as a T2-weighted single-shot imaging technique [7, 18, 28]. Paradoxically, the incorporation of the CPMG sequence in GRASE permits greater utilization of the available magnetization than with EPI given the removal of constraints on signal acquisition time. At present it appears that single-shot GRASE provides several advantages over SE EPI, most notably higher spatial resolution, improved image quality, and ability to image in regions of

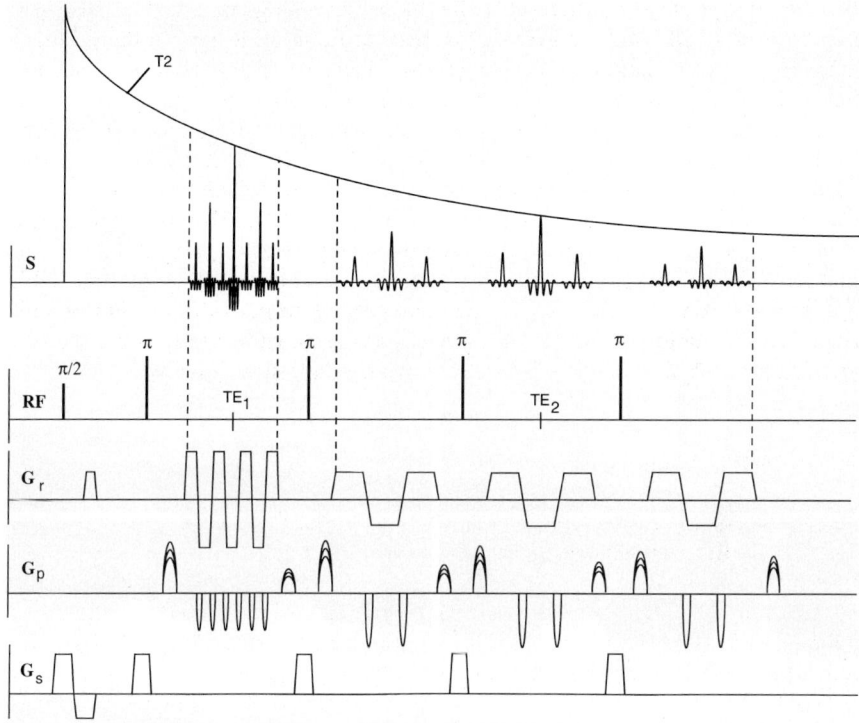

Fig. 13. Pulse sequence timing diagram for creating mixed double echo imaging, proton density weighted (*PDW*) and T2-weighted (*T2 W*). A different number of gradient-recalled echoes with a corresponding difference in signal bandwidth is used for the two images. Seven signals of relatively high bandwidth are used for the PD-weighted image. The last nine signals incorporated into the T2-weighted image have a lower signal bandwidth than those of the PD-weighted image. This difference in image bandwidth compensates for signal amplitude differences and more closely equilibrate the SNR of the two image. (From [16])

high susceptibility; i.e. at air and bone interfaces of the brain near the paranasal sinuses (Fig. 14).

Acquiring an image from a single echo train using only one excitation RF pulse has generally been assumed to require extremely fast signal refocusing rates, necessitating special EPI hardware including fast gradient rise times and static field uniformity beyond that used for conventional clinical MR systems. In the earliest single-shot GRASE imaging experiments [7] we assumed that the slower signal refocusing rate due to additional RF pulses would limit the image spatial resolution. Higher resolution was obtained using inner-volume "zooming" of a subsection region of the body.

In single-shot imaging sequences both the field of view and spatial resolution are determined by the net area of the read gradient and phase-encoding gradient pulses and by the number of echoes acquired in the echo train. The product of the signal refocusing rate and echo train time determines the echo train length and the obtainable spatial resolution on the phase axis. The interdependence of

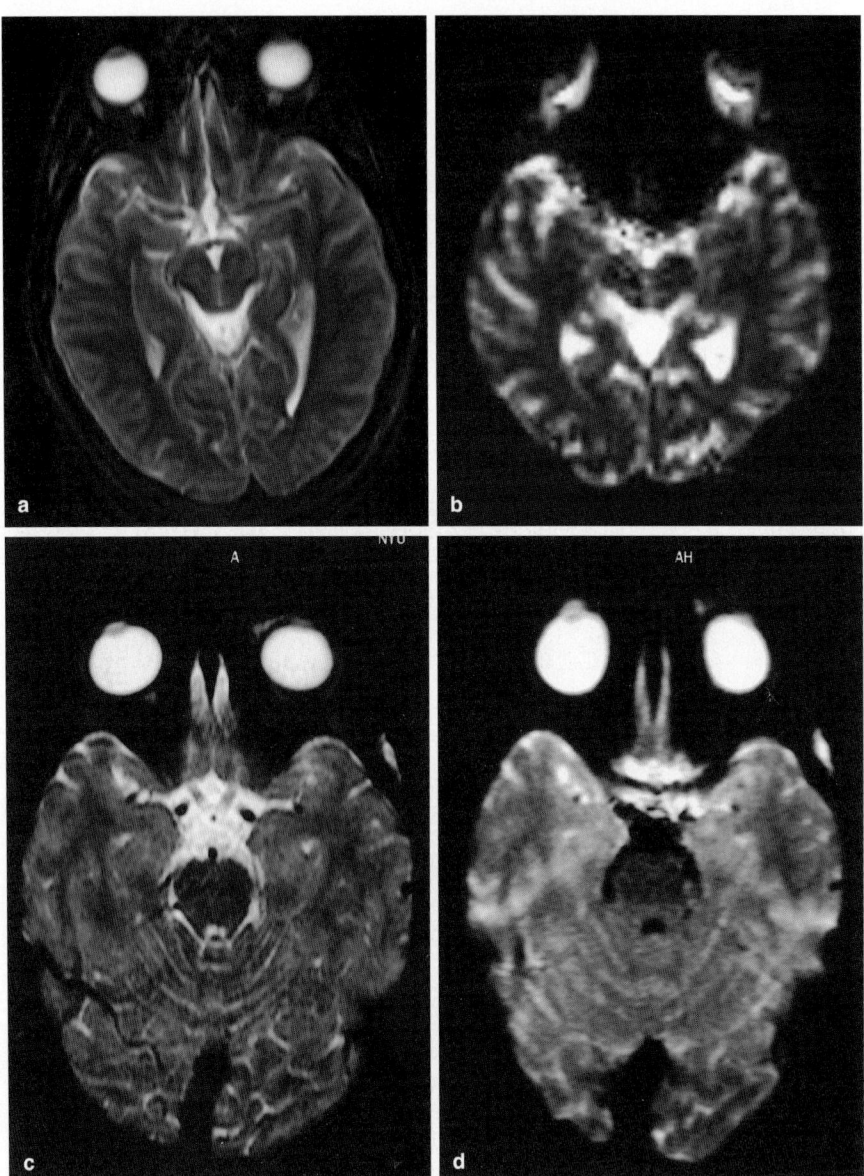

Fig. 14a–f. Comparison of single-shot GRASE and SE EPI using conventional gradients and high performance gradients. All images are 5 mm thickness. **a,b** Acquired with conventional gradients with 600-μs rise time to maximum 25 mT/m (see [33]). **a** Single-shot GRASE image acquired in 330 ms, TE_{eff}: 160 ms. **b** SE EPI image in 150 ms, TE_{eff}: 86 ms having signal loss from susceptibility errors near the paranasal sinus. **c–f** Acquired with high performance gradients with 300-μs rise time to maximum 25 mT/m. **c,e** Single-shot kbGRASE images acquired in 380 ms TE_{eff}: 75 ms, field of view: 20 cm, 144×256 matrix (full Fourier data sampling). K space banded phase encoding was used to obtain an earlier effective TE. **d,f** SE EPI images acquired in 180 ms with TE_{eff}: 96 ms, field of view: 21 cm, 128×200 matrix (partial Fourier sampling)

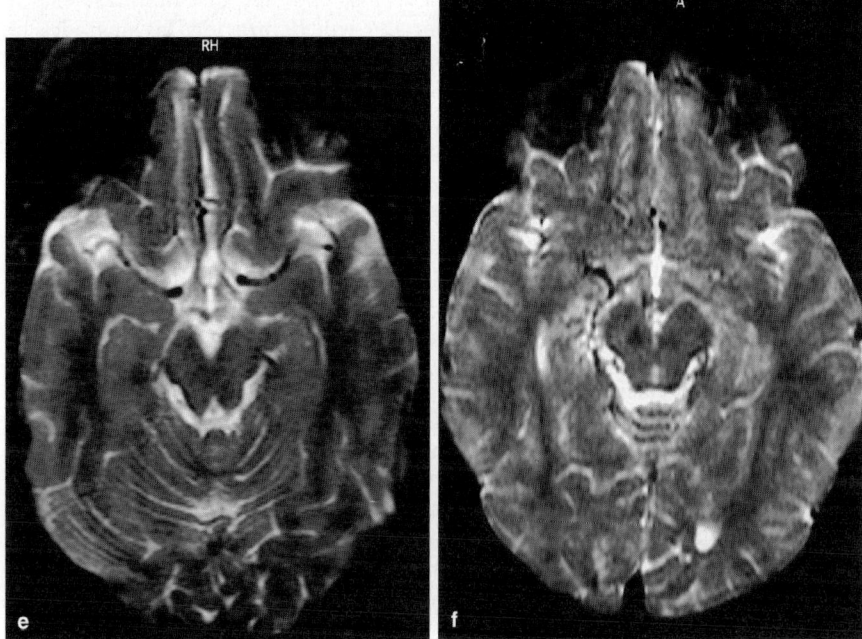

echo time and the acceptable levels of field inhomogeneity and susceptibility errors has always limited the echo train time of EPI, so that higher spatial resolution is reached through improved gradient hardware performance to increase the echo refocusing rate.

Single-shot GRASE differs most significantly from EPI sequences in that field inhomogeneity errors are not coupled to the echo train time, as the echo train decays with T2 not T2*. It is important to note that field inhomogeneity and susceptibility errors do not accumulate in the echo train of GRASE whereas they do accumulate in EPI and SE EPI. Nor do they accumulate in RARE imaging; however, the signal refocusing rate is entirely dependent on RF pulses, which can have RF heating limitations and are much slower than gradient switching used in GRASE and EPI. Therefore single-shot GRASE images can be obtained with long echo train times of 200–400 ms, depending on the tissue T2. Using SE EPI for T2-weighted imaging, even in the best of circumstances, the gradient-echo train typically does not exceed 100 ms. With this difference in echo train time EPI has a disadvantage in obtaining the same spatial resolution as GRASE, when using the same gradient hardware. The faster refocusing rate of EPI is a definite advantage when there are time constraints on the echo train time. When biological motion limits imaging time, i.e., cardiac imaging requiring 50-ms echo trains, single-shot GRASE is more limited in spatial resolution than EPI.

As the signal refocusing rate of single-shot GRASE imaging is highly dependent on gradient switching speed, similarly to EPI, it also obtains higher spatial resolution with faster and stronger gradient. It is expected that improvements in gradient hardware originally designed for EPI will be provided as upgrades on clinical imaging machines and will permit improved performance of single-shot GRASE as well as of multi-shot GRASE.

Figure 14 compares single-shot GRASE images performed with 25 mT/M with moderate gradient rise time of 800 ms and faster 300 ms. The spatial resolution is increased by faster gradient switching obtainable with EPI gradient hardware, as calculated in Table 3. Image distortions due to field inhomogeneity and signal loss in regions of large variations in susceptibility are absent in single-shot GRASE performed on either gradient system.

Theoretical Comparison of EPI, RARE, and GRASE

Experimental comparison of different echo train imaging sequences is intrinsically affected by the hardware constraints and MR system design. Both static field inhomogeneity and gradient hardware parameters (gradient switching time and maximum gradient strength), as discussed above, are critical determinants in echo train imaging performance. As one particular MR system design may be more favorable for a certain echo train sequence, there may be an intrinsic bias when comparing the imaging performance of different techniques.

One approach is to compare the performance of different echo train sequences by defining identical sequence parameters in which hardware design constraints can be freely varied. EPI, RARE, and GRASE share common elements of sequence design which can be rearranged to create each of the imaging sequences (Fig. 15). This makes possible their comparison using a variable parameter pulse sequence timing diagram. In such a sequence the gradient pulse sequence variables of number of gradient refocusings and RF refocusings can be freely varied in

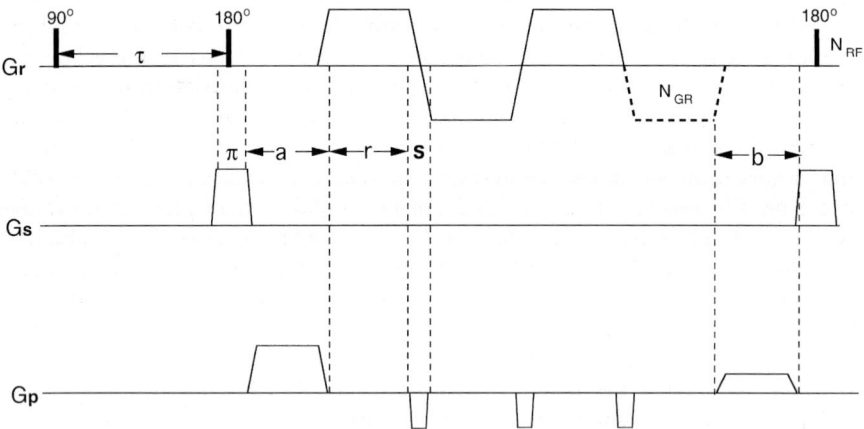

Fig. 15. Generic pulse sequence timing diagram for EPI, SE EPI, RARE, and GRASE. The timing parameters are defined as follows: τ, by convention defined as time between the 90° and 180° RF pulses; π, the time of the 180° RF pulse, a, delay time used for spoiler gradients and phase-encode gradient, r, read gradient time, s, read gradient switching time, b, delay time used for phase-rewind pulse (typically $a = b$), N_{RF}, number of π pulses, N_{GR}, number of read gradients per π pulse

their order and number to create the different echo train sequences. Identical sequence parameters are therefore used to create different echo train sequence, making possible a direct comparison of the affect of changing either hardware parameters or pulse sequence timing parameters. For each of several different echo train sequences a common sequence diagram can be used to calculate the efficiency and speed of signal refocusing, and the number of echoes so generated. Such imaging parameters can be expressed in equation form and derived from common hardware constraints.

In the following analysis echo train sequences are parameterized identically using the sequence timing diagram of Fig. 15. The timing parameters are defined as: π time of section-selective 180° RF pulse; s, read gradient switching time; r, read period of signal (A/D sampling time); a, delay time between RF pulse and read period; b, delay time between read period and subsequent RF pulse; τ, time from 90° RF spin excitation pulse to first π pulse; 2τ, π pulse spacing in the CPMG sequence; N_{RF}, number of refocusing π pulses; and N_{GR}, number of read gradient refocusing pulses used between each pair of π pulse.

The RARE sequence is generated using N_{GR} equal to 1 and N_{RF} equal to the number of spin echoes. The GRASE sequence is generated using N_{RF} equal to 2 or greater and N_{GR} equal to an odd number 3, 5 or greater. In current practice with GRASE, N_{GR} equals an odd number to position the lowest spatial frequencies (k_o) in the middle of the π-π interval at the Hahn spin-echo position where the phase errors are minimal.

The EPI sequence is generated in two ways, with a π pulse prior to the gradient-echo train ($N_{RF} = 1$) often denoted as SE EPI [26] and generated without the use of a π pulse, simply denoted as EPI. Both EPI and SE EPI use one gradient-echo train, where N_{GR} equals to the number of signals. In SE EPI a time delay between the 90° and 180° RF pulses is useful to create T2-weighted EPI images and also serves to reduce off-resonance errors by centering low spatial frequency signals (k_o) on the spin-echo time. With k_o positioned at the Hahn SE time there is a factor of 2 reduction in off-resonance errors, T2* errors, in SE EPI compared to conventional EPI permitting longer echo trains typically 70–100 ms long.

The generic pulse sequence is shown in Fig. 15 with the timing parameters defined in the legend. In this sequence the signal is refocused by N_{RF} π pulses and N_{GR} gradient reversals between each π pulse. The RARE sequence is generated from the generic sequence by using N_{GR} equal to 1 and N_{RF} equal to the total number of phase-encoding steps. The GRASE sequence is generated using N_{GR} equal to a number greater than 1 and N_{RF} adjusted to generate the desired number of phase-encoding steps. Normally N_{GR} is odd so as to position the lowest spatial frequencies (k_o) in the middle of the π-π interval at the Hahn echo time where the phase errors are minimal. The EPI sequence uses N_{GR} echoes, and the SE EPI sequence is similar but uses a single π pulse ($N_{RF} = 1$).

The derived parameters of the generic pulse sequence are: t, half the time between the π pulses; R, the average echo refocusing rate (echoes/ms); N_E, number of echoes per train; and E, an efficiency factor which is the fraction of time of signal sampling in the echo train. Table 1 gives the expressions for each of these parameters for each sequence. The echo train time, T_{AQ}, is longer for RARE and GRASE, which decay with T2 and are even further prolonged by sti-

Table 1. Expressions used to calculate derived sequence parameters for RARE, GRASE, SE EPI, and EPI sequences using the timing parameters defined in the pulse sequence timing diagram in Fig. 15

	RARE	GRASE	SE EPI		EPI
τ (ms)	$(\pi+a+r+b)/2$	$[(N_{GR}(s+r))+(\pi+a+b)-s]/2$	$N_{GR}(s+r)/2$		0
T_{AQ} (ms)	$2N_{RF}\times\tau$	$2N_{RF}\times\tau$	$N_{GR}(s+r)$		$N_{GR}(s+r)$
R (ms/echo)	$(T_{AQ}+\tau)/N_{RF}$	$(T_{AQ}+\tau)/N_{RF}\times N_{GR}$	$(T_{AQ}+\tau)/N_{GR}$		T_{AQ}/N_{GR}
E	r/R	r/R	r/R		r/R
N_E	$(T_{MX}-\tau)/2\tau$	$N_{GR}\times(T_{MX}-\tau)/2\tau$	$(T_{MX}-\tau)/(s+r)$		$T_{MX}/(s+r)$

τ, Half the time between consecutive π pulses; T_{AQ}, acquisition time (the time between the first and last echoes); S, average echo separation; E, efficiency expressed as the fraction of the total acquisition time during which the signal is actually being sampled; N_E, echo train length (number of signals per excitation) when the last echo occurs at T_{MX}.

mulated echo magnetization. EPI and SE EPI decay by T2*. In human head imaging experiments with GRASE and RARE the useful T_{AQ} was 330 ms and this value was used in the calculations. The signal acquisition time for EPI and SE EPI was taken from the longest T_{AQ} published, 70 ms for EPI, and 140 ms for SE EPI.

Calculation of the above expressions is presented in Table 2 for our current clinical imager (Siemens Vision) – 25 mT/m gradients with 1-ms rise times and in Table 3 for a similar system with specialized echo-planar hardware – gradient strength of 32.5 mT/m with 300 ms gradient rise time. Experiments with

Table 2. Comparison of EPI, RARE and GRASE performance with gradient hardware typical of a current commercial MR system: 24 mT/m gradients with 625-μs rise times

	RARE	GRASE	SE EPI	EPI
τ (ms)	2.8	7.0	70	0
T_{MX} (ms)	330	330	210	70
R (ms/echo)	5.69	2.87	3.18	2.12
E	0.23	0.45	0.41	0.61
N_E	58	115	66	33

Timing parameters are p = 1.3 ms, a = 1.5 ms, b = 1.5 ms, r = 1.3 ms, s = 0.8 ms. For GRASE: $N_{GR} = 5$, $N_{RF} = 23$. See Table 1 and Fig. 15 for corresponding expressions and definitions.

Table 3. Comparison of EPI, RARE, and GRASE performance with gradient hardware typical of an EPI MR system: 32.5 mT/m gradients with 150-μs rise times

	RARE	GRASE	SE EPI	EPI
τ (ms)	2.0	8.5	70	0
T_{MX} (ms)	330	330	210	70
R (ms/echo)	4.02	1.59	1.96	1.32
E	0.25	0.63	0.51	0.76
N_E	82	208	107	53

Timing parameters are p = 1 ms, a = 1 ms, b = 1 ms, r = 1 ms, s = 0.3 ms. (This value of r gives the same spatial resolution with these gradients as that obtained with the values in Table 2.) For GRASE, $N_{GR} = 11$ was used. The Hahn echo time is placed asymmetrically in the SE EPI train to reduce dead time. Other values are the same as those in Table 2. See Table 1 and Fig. 15 for corresponding expressions and definitions.

single-shot GRASE imaging of the brain (Fig. 14) used parameters similar to those of Table 2.

Differences in R, N_E, and E in these sequences result from several factors. The initial τ time between the $\pi/2$ and π RF pulses and the τ delay is in general a loss of signal acquisition time which reduces sequence efficiency. The τ delay in GRASE or RARE is smaller than that in SE EPI due to the closer spaced $\pi/2$ and π pulses of the CPMG sequence. The EPI gradient-echo train accumulates phase errors throughout the echo train which reduces image quality; however, its lack of π pulses gives it the highest signal refocusing rate. As shown in the generic sequence, the lower efficiency and lower echo refocusing rate of RARE is due to the time requirement of the phase-encode–rewind methodology. The use of blipped phase encoding in GRASE accumulates the phase shifts of several gradient pulses of relatively short duration, and proportionately fewer rewind pulses are required.

As described above, in GRASE the field inhomogeneity errors can be adjusted independently of N_E. This control of phase error in GRASE is possible given the two independent refocusing techniques of gradient and RF refocusing, parameters N_{RF} and N_{GR}, respectively. This is different from the spin-echo variant of EPI, SE EPI, which has one Hahn echo time Fig. 2b, but where the temporal accumulation of field inhomogeneity errors still occurs with echo train position. In SE EPI the field inhomogeneity errors are proportional to $N_E/2$, and in effect T2* decay remains coupled to the total echo train time.

K Space Banded Phase Encoding

Sequential signal ordering, used typically in EPI and RARE, is not used in GRASE due to the phase error modulation in GRASE echo trains. An interleaved or discontinuous signal ordering eliminates PM in GRASE k space but introduces AM which also causes artifacts when significant T2 decay occurs in the echo train. The frequency of AM is much slower than that of phase error modulation, and therefore the artifacts fall much closer to the true image and can appear as ringing (under- and over-shoot at edges). The standard GRASE phase-encoding order has two further disadvantages. First, the "effective TE" (TE_{eff}, i.e., the echo time of the zero phase-encoding echo) is half the total echo train time. Second, partial Fourier sampling cannot be implemented easily in the phase-encoding direction so that imaging times cannot be reduced by using half Fourier techniques [6, 7].

A more flexible phase-encoding scheme for GRASE has been developed to allow a minimization of AM and PM artifacts. The scheme encodes different k space bands in different time segments of the echo train. Within each band echoes are reordered in an interleaved manner similar to standard GRASE to remove PMs in k space. This approach to phase encoding in GRASE is intermediate between sequential signal ordering found in EPI or RARE and interleaved order of standard GRASE. This phase-encode order reintroduces moderate modulations of phase error to reduce the size of T2 AM. In addition to artifact reduction, the method allows an earlier effective TE for higher image SNR and allows for implementation of partial Fourier imaging.

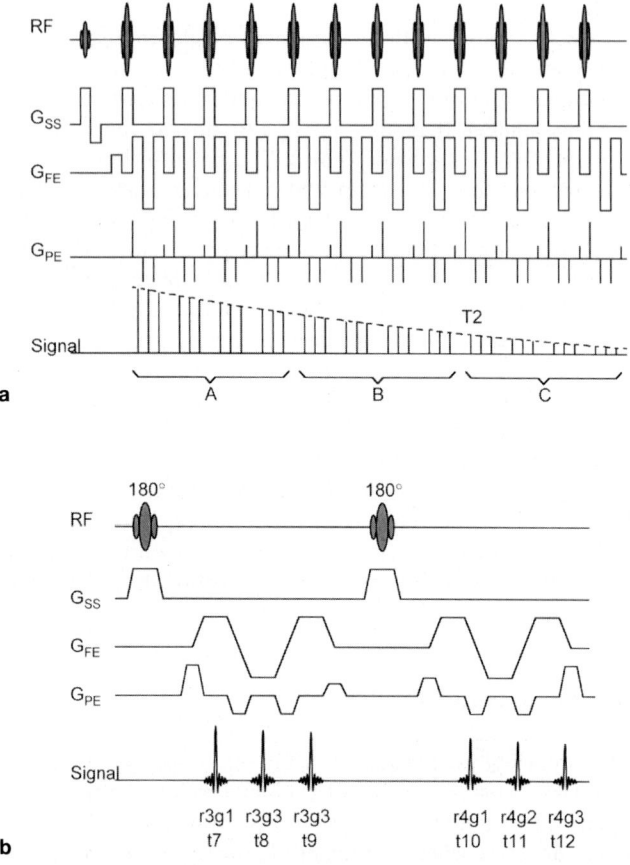

Fig. 16a,b. The k space banded GRASE pulse sequence. **a** Complete sequence with a typical k banding arrangement with equal width segments, A, B, and C. **b** Expansion of a section of the sequence after the third RF refocusing pulse. The echoes are labeled with RF, gradient, and echo number. (From [34])

Different time segments of the echo train are encoded with different bands of spatial frequency in k space (hence "k banding"). Figure 16 shows a typical instance with three equal time segments labeled A, B, and C. Figure 17b shows the corresponding positions of the echoes in k space. Segment A is encoded with the central k space band, segment B with one of the outer bands, and segment C is encoded by the final band. Within each band the echoes are grouped as in the standard GRASE order with echoes with equal g values together. With this ordering the lowest amplitude echoes are encoded with high spatial frequencies, thus avoiding the gaps in the central regions of k space that can occur in standard GRASE with long echo trains.

The original motivation behind k space banded (kb) GRASE was to reduce artifacts; however, the k space trajectory has two further advantages over stan-

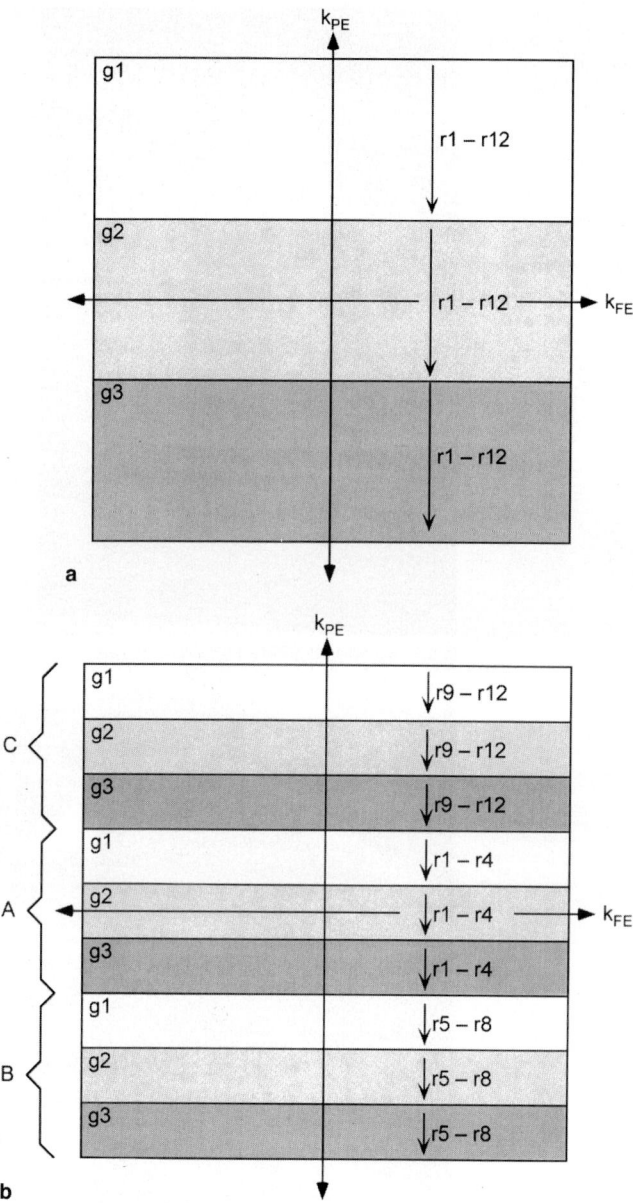

Fig. 17a,b. The k space diagrams showing the echoes encoded with different areas in k space. **a** Standard GRASE phase-encoding order. **b** kbGRASE order with three equal bands, A, B, and C, corresponding to the three time segments of the echo train shown in Fig. 16

Fig. 18a–c. High-resolution GRASE images in 1024 matrix. **a** The head image has 0.27 mm×0.28 mm and a 4-mm slice thickness TR/ 7000 ms, TE/115 ms, 19 sections in 4.3 min acquisition time. **b,c** Magnified subsection of 1024 matrix shows details of the trigeminal nerves, cochlea, and neurovascular bundle within the internal auditory canal. (From [15])

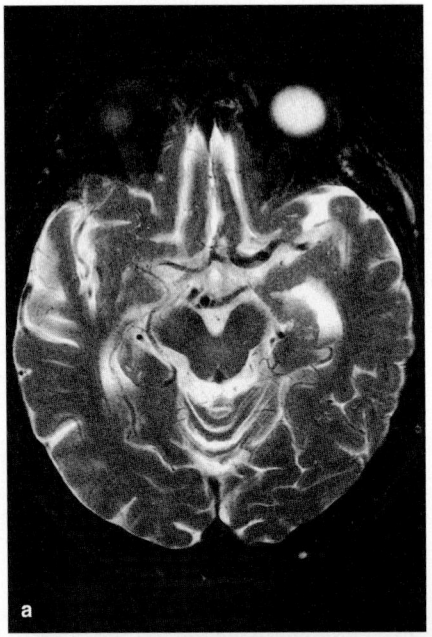
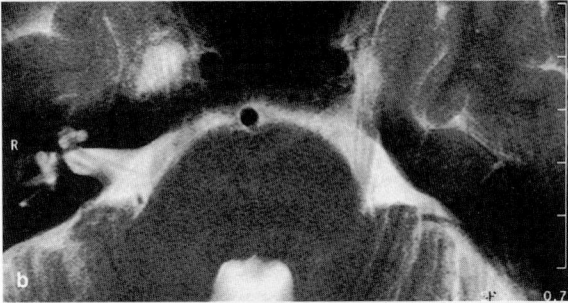
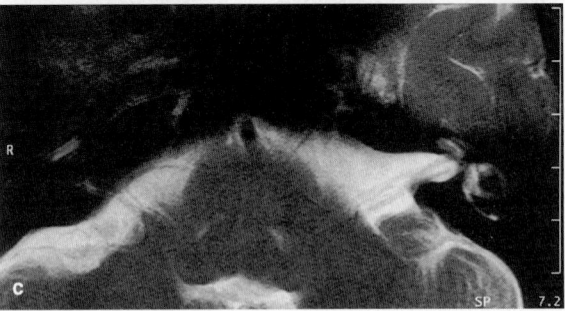

dard GRASE. First, there is more flexibility in choosing an effective echo time, TE_{eff}, reflected by the time of echoes encoding the low spatial frequencies that determines, at least superficially, contrast. In standard GRASE TE_{eff} (k_o) is positioned at half the time of the echo train. T_{eff} can be reduced in standard GRASE by shifting the position of k_o to an earlier spin-echo period [17] with zero filling the missing outermost k space lines. With kbGRASE the T_{eff} can be reduced by encoding the low spatial frequency band into early echoes (or, conversely, increased by encoding low spatial frequencies into late echoes). Examples of kbGRASE are given for single-shot imaging in Fig. 14 and for high-resolution imaging in Fig. 18. A second advantage of kbGRASE is that asymmetric Fourier sampling can be implemented very simply by dropping one or more bands in the negative half of k space. Asymmetric sampling can be achieved with standard GRASE by encoding the origin of k space with an echo that does not occur at the Hahn echo time, but this could cause problems in reconstructing the accurate phase information required for conjugate synthesis.

Future Directions for GRASE Imaging

GRASE is a versatile imaging sequence and can be performed with various system hardware and magnetic field strengths. As a fast imaging technique GRASE can be used to overcome artifacts from respiration, peristalsis, and cardiovascular sources of body motion. The high data acquisition rate of GRASE can substantially reduce the time three-dimensional FT imaging [15] which has additional advantage in removing modulation artifacts. Reduction of modulation artifacts with new k space trajectories such as k space banding continues to be an active area of GRASE development. GRASE gives markedly improved image quality over EPI, as seen in high-resolution 1024 matrix images and in single-shot images. The spin-echo contrast mechanisms in GRASE images make it desirable for routine clinical studies. Development of k space trajectories for shorter effective TE will be useful for higher SNR and for high-resolution single-shot diffusion imaging and velocity imaging, currently under investigation.

GRASE imaging will likely be useful for brain activation imaging (fMRI) for two reasons. At higher magnetic field strength (3–4 T) GRASE gives better control field inhomogeneity artifacts than EPI while obtaining susceptibility sensitivity useful for activation studies. Preparatory pulses and changes in the RF pulse spacing can be used to adjust susceptibility and field inhomogeneity affects in GRASE sequences. A second possibility is to use GRASE to directly image blood contrast in brain tissue. The possibility of very high spatial resolution single-shot GRASE images may also improve spatial localization. The RF power deposition of the CPMG sequence will not be problematic at high magnetic field strengths as the number of gradient refocusing to RF refocusing can be adjusted for fewer RF pulses in GRASE, and low flip angle RF pulses can be used.

Single-shot GRASE imaging obtains high spatial resolution and distortion-free anatomical detail which has useful applications for several patient groups, i.e., for children to avoid sedation, for rapid screening of noncompliant patients, and for those who have limited tolerance for the MR magnet environment. High-performance gradients which are required for EPI also increase the spatial resolution of single-shot GRASE images. The cost of gradient hardware upgrades for existing clinical imaging systems may be better justified when it benefits several different fast imaging techniques. The clinical niche of different fast imaging sequences will undoubtably vary.

References

1. Crooks LE, Arakawa M, Hoenninger J, Watts J, McRee R, Kaufman L, Davis PL, Margulis AR, DeGroot J (1982) Nuclear magnetic resonance whole-body imager operating at 3.5 K Gauss. Radiology 143:169–174
2. Crooks LE, Watts J, Hoenninger J, Arakawa M, Kaufman L, Guenther H, Feinberg DA (1985) Thin section definition in magnetic resonance imaging: technical concepts and their implementation. Radiology 154:463–467
3. Edelstein WA, Hutchison JM, Johnson G, Redpath TW, Mallard JR (1980) UK Patent no GB2,079,463A, methods of producing image information from objects (priority date: 3/14/1980)
4. Edelstein WA, Hutchison JM, Johnson G, Redpath TW, Mallard JR (1980) Spin warp imaging and applications to whole body imaging. Phys Med Biol 25:751–756
5. Feinberg DA, Mills CM, Posin JP, Ortendahl DA et al (1985) Multiple spin-echo magnetic resonance imaging. Radiology 155:437–442
6. Feinberg DA, Hale JD, Watts JC, Kaufman L, Mark A (1986) Halving MR imaging time by conjugation: demonstration at 3.5 kG. Radiology 161:527–531
7. Feinberg DA, Hale JD (1986) Inner-volume echo planar imaging in book of abstracts. Proceedings of 5th annual meeting, Society of Magnetic Resonance in Medicine, p 950
8. Feinberg DA, Oshio K (1991) US Patent no 5,270,654 Ultra-fast multi-section MRI using gradient and spin echo (GRASE) imaging (priority date: 7/6/1991)
9. Feinberg DA, Oshio K (1991) GRASE (gradient and spin echo) MR imaging: a new fast clinical imaging technique. Radiology 181:597
10. Feinberg DA, Oshio K (1991) Gradient-echo time shifting in fast imaging. In: Book of abstracts (works in progress), 10th annual meeting, Society of Magnetic Resonance in Medicine, San Francisco, p 1239
11. Feinberg DA, Oshio K (1992) Gradient-echo shifting in fast MRI techniques (GRASE) for correction of field inhomogeneity errors and chemical shift (communication). J Magn Reson 97:177–183
12. Feinberg DA, Turner R, Jakab PD, von Kienlin M (1990) Echo-planar imaging with asymmetric gradient modulation and inner-volume excitation. Magn Res Med 13:162–169
13. Feinberg DA (1993) GRASE imaging provides image quality and speed, Diagnostic Imaging. Miller Freeman, 2: p 71–78
14. Feinberg DA, Oshio K (1994) Phase errors In multi-shot echo planar imaging with echo time shift. Magn Res Med 32:535–539
15. Feinberg DA Kiefer B, Litt AW (1995) High resolution GRASE MRI of the brain and spine: 512 and 1024 matrix imaging. J Comput Assist Tomogr 19(1):1–7
16. Feinberg DA Kiefer B, Litt AW (1994) Dual contrast GRASE (gradient-spin echo) imaging using mixed bandwidth. Magn Res Med 31:461–464
17. Feinberg DA, Kiefer B (1994) High resolution imaging of the brain with GRASE (TGSE). First meeting of the Society of Magnetic Resonance in Medicine. J Magn Res Imaging 4(P):48
18. Feinberg DA, Kiefer B (1994) High speed T2-weighted imaging of the liver with single-shot GRASE (TGSE). First meeting of the Society of Magnetic Resonance in Medicine. J Magn Reson Imaging 4(P):48
19. Hennig J, Friedburg H, Strobel B (1986) Rapid nontomographic approach to MR myelography without contrast agent. J Comput Assist Tomogr 10:375–380
20. Hennig J, Neurith A, Friedburg H (1986) RARE imaging: a fast imaging method for clinical MR. Magn Reson Med 3:823–833
21. Johnson G, Hutchison JMS, Redpath TW, Eastwood LM (1983) Improvements in performance time for simultaneous three-dimensional imaging. J Magn Res 54:374–378

22. Kiefer B, Hollenbach HP, Feinberg DA (1994) T2-weighted imaging with long echo train 3D turbo gradient spin-echo for neurological applications with high resolution. Second meeting of the Society of Magnetic Resonance in Medicine, San Francisco, 1994
23. Mansfield P (1977) J Phys C 10:L55
24. Mansfield P, Pykett IL (1978) Biological and medical imaging by NMR. J Magn Reson 29:355–373
25. McKinnon GC (1993) Ultrafast interleaved gradient-echo-planar imaging on a standard scanner. Magn Res Med 30:609–616
26. Ordidge JR Howseman A, Coxon R et al (1989) Snapshot imaging at 0.5T using echo-planar technique. Magn Reson Med 10:227
27. Oshio K, Feinberg DA (1991) GRASE (gradient- and spin-echo) imaging: a novel fast MRI Technique. Magn Res Med 20:344–349
28. Oshio K, Feinberg DA (1992) Single-shot GRASE imaging without fast gradients. Magn Res Med 26:355–360
29. Oshio K, Jolesz F (1994) Fast T1-weighted imaging with multiexcitation EPI. Proceedings from the 1st meeting of the Society of Magnetic Resonance, p 37
30. Rofsky NM, Weinreb JC, Safir J, Mercado C, Goldman JP, Megibow AJ (1994) Comparison of fat suppression techniques for hepatic MR imaging: turbo-SE, breath-hold turbo-SE, GRASE, and turbo STIR. First meeting of the Society of Magnetic Resonance in Medicine. J Magn Reson Imaging 4(P):66
31. Strobel B, Ratzel D (1984) US Patent no 4,697,148. Process for the excitation of a sample for NMR tomography (priority date: 4/18/84)
32. Xiang QS Nalcioglu O (1987) A formalism of generating multiparametric encoding gradients in NMR tomography. IEEE Trans Med Imaging 6:14–20
33. Feinberg DA, Kiefer B, Johnson G (1995) GRASE improves spatial resolution in single shot imaging. Magn Reson Med 33:529–533
34. Feinberg DA, Kiefer B, Johnson G (1995) GRASE increased flexibility in GRASE imaging by k-space-banded phase encoding. Magn Reson Med 34:149–155

CHAPTER 21

Spiral Echo-Planar Imaging

C. H. Meyer

Introduction

This chapter departs somewhat from the others in this volume. Echo-planar imaging (EPI) typically refers to a scan that covers k-space in a nearly rectilinear fashion, with an oscillating gradient on one axis. Here we discuss scanning k-space in a spiral fashion, with two oscillating gradients. Of course there are many similarities between EPI and spiral k-space scanning. In fact the first research group to implement spiral scanning [1] called it spiral EPI, because it involves collecting a large portion of k-space with time-varying gradients after a single excitation, much as in Mansfield's original experiment. For clarity, however, in this chapter the term "EPI" refers to *rectilinear* EPI and its variants, and "*spiral scanning*" refers to covering k-space in a spiral fashion. This chapter is an overview of spiral scanning rather than a systematic comparison of spiral scanning with EPI. However, we try to point out the ways in which spiral scanning differs from EPI.

What difference does it make whether one scans k-space in a rectilinear fashion or a spiral fashion? What does one need to know to implement a spiral scanning system? What does one need to know to use spiral scanning? What are some applications of spiral scanning? Have any lessons been learned from research in spiral scanning that might apply to "regular" EPI? Finally, given a choice, should one purchase an EPI system or a spiral scanning system? These are the sorts of questions that this chapter addresses. (As a preview, the answer to the last question is "both.")

Spiral scanning is a newer technique than EPI, and thus fewer researchers and physicians have experience with it. The first paper to suggest spiral scanning was published by Ljunggren in 1983 [2], although it had been independently suggested in an earlier patent by Likes [3]. Spiral scanning was not implemented until the middle of the 1980s, first by Ahn et al. [1] and then by the present author's group at Stanford University [4–8]. In the 1990s a number of groups implemented spiral scanning, and by the middle of the 1990s spiral scanning had been implemented on scanners from all of the major manufacturers. This chapter does not attempt to present a comprehensive survey of all spiral scanning research to date because such a survey is beyond the scope of this chapter and would very quickly become out of date. Of course, the author refers to such research whenever appropriate. The particular spiral scanning implementation described is that developed at Stanford by the author and his colleagues. Similarly, many of the applications described are those studied by the author and

Fig. 1. Spiral design in the Forbidden City in Beijing, China

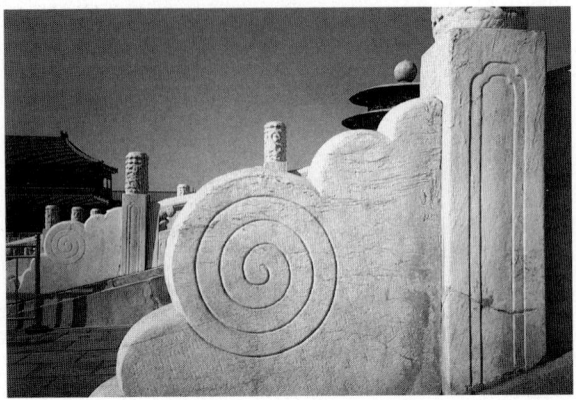

others at Stanford. The reason for this is simply that the author is most familiar with the work described there; much interesting work in spiral scanning, however, has also been performed at other institutions.

Figure 1 illustrates an archimedean spiral, in which the cumulative angle traced by the spiral starting from the origin is proportional to the radius of the trajectory at that point. One consequence of this is that the distance between successive turns of the spiral is constant along any particular spoke from the origin. Thus, when a spiral is used for scanning k-space, the k-space sampling is uniform along each spoke.

Fig. 2. Single k-space spiral

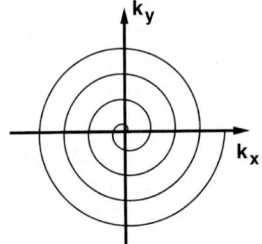

With proper hardware, single-shot spiral scanning is possible, and for some applications it is appropriate. Figure 2 illustrates a single-shot spiral k-space trajectory. In most situations, however, it makes more sense to interleave the spiral scans. Figure 3 illustrates interleaved spiral k-space trajectories. Each interleaf differs from the others by a simple rotation, which can easily be implemented by rotating the x and y gradients. Interleaving decreases the hardware requirements for a given spatial resolution and increases the signal-to-noise ratio (SNR). To be specific, with N interleaves the gradient power is reduced by about $1/N^2$, the receiver bandwidth is reduced by $1/N$, and the SNR is increased by $\sqrt{N}$.

The philosophy that has guided much interleaved spiral scanning research is this: a scan should be as fast as necessary, but not faster. How fast a scan must be is determined by the physiology of the area to be imaged. For example,

Fig. 3. Four interleaved spiral k-space trajectories. The gradients are rotated by 0°, 90°, 180°, and 270° on successive excitations to produce the four interleaved spirals in k-space

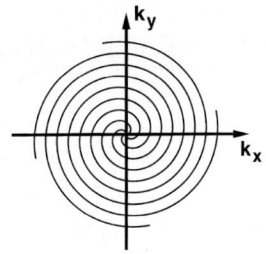

in scanning the head a scan that takes a few minutes is often fast enough. In this case many interleaves can be used. For scans of the abdomen, on the other hand, it is often desirable to complete the scan in a breath-hold, which requires faster scanning and fewer interleaves. In the case of heart studies it may be necessary to complete the cardiac-gated scan in a breath-hold, which puts additional constraints on the scan in order to freeze both cardiac and respiratory motion. Finally, in tracking dynamic events, for example, imaging the heart without gating, it is necessary to use very few interleaves to achieve temporal resolution of well under 1 s.

The rest of this chapter is organized as follows. First, there is a section on the properties of spiral scanning, which includes some discussion of how these properties differ from those of EPI. This section covers the advantages and disadvantages of spiral scanning, as well as the sort of artifacts that may appear in a spiral scan image. The next section is an overview of the implementation of spiral scanning, including such issues as gradient waveform design and image reconstruction. The final section surveys a number of the applications of spiral scanning.

Figure 4 can be thought of as a preview of the rest of the chapter. It is a breath-held interleaved spiral scan of the proximal left coronary artery system

Fig. 4. High-resolution spiral coronary angiogram. Breath-held 2D spiral image with 0.57-mm spatial resolution showing the left anterior descending artery and its first-order branches in an LAO-caudal view

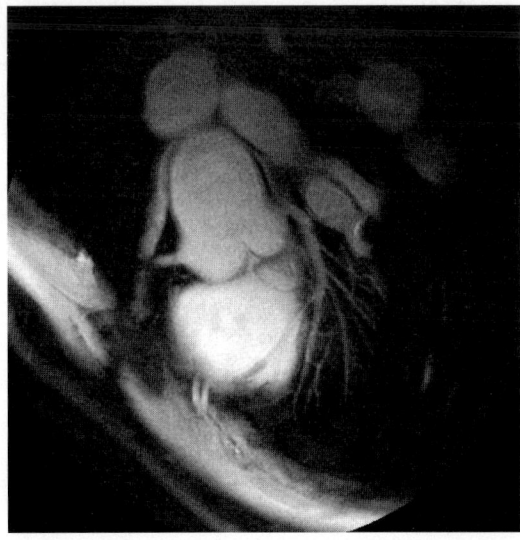

of a normal volunteer. Several coronary arteries are well visualized, including the left main coronary artery, the left anterior descending coronary artery (LAD), and several diagonal arteries. Note that the flowing blood in the heart is well visualized with minimal flow artifacts in this spiral scan. This good performance in the presence of moving material is one of the main advantages of spiral scanning, and this is discussed further in the section on properties of spiral scans. Because the data for this spiral scan were not collected on a two-dimensional (2D) grid, a technique called gridding was needed to reconstruct the image; this technique is discussed further in the implementation section. Magnetic resonance (MR) coronary angiography is one of the major applications of spiral scanning, and it is discussed in more detail in the section on applications.

Properties

Because many of the properties of spiral scans stem from the basic geometry of spiral scanning, we first consider this, and then specific properties.

Geometry of Spiral Scanning

Whereas EPI treats the two readout directions differently, spiral scanning treats them essentially in the same manner. This circular symmetry is the source of many of the properties of spiral scanning.

The circular symmetry of spiral scans can be seen simply by observing the k-space trajectory of Fig. 2. There is no essential difference between the k_x and k_y axes other than the slight difference at the origin resulting from the choice of initial trajectory angle. Even this slight asymmetry is largely eliminated by interleaving as in Fig. 3. It is easy to see that such circular symmetry in k-space translates to similar symmetry in image space. One can also see this by thinking about a spiral scan in object space. During a 2D spiral scan, both x and y gradients are applied in a time-varying manner. However, at any given time during the scan there is a single effective gradient, oriented along the vector sum of the x and y gradients. During a spiral scan the direction of this gradient continually rotates. As this gradient rotates, linear phase develops across the object in a direction orthogonal to the gradient itself at any given time, and thus this linear phase rotates as well.

Figure 5 illustrates the effect of this rotation in object space. The signal produced in an MR imaging scan at a given time is a space integral of the magnetization multiplied by a spatially varying complex exponential weighting factor. Depicted in Fig. 5 is the real part of this complex exponential weighting factor at three sequential times during a spiral scan. As the scan proceeds, note that the direction of the weighting rotates. Also note that spatial frequency of the weighting factor increases as the scan proceeds, so that finer details are encoded later in the scan. Of course this merely restates familiar k-space ideas from an object-space viewpoint.

Fig. 5. The k-space position and the real part of the complex spatial weighting factor at three different times during a spiral readout. Note that as the scan proceeds, the encoded direction rotates and the spatial frequency of the weighting factor increases

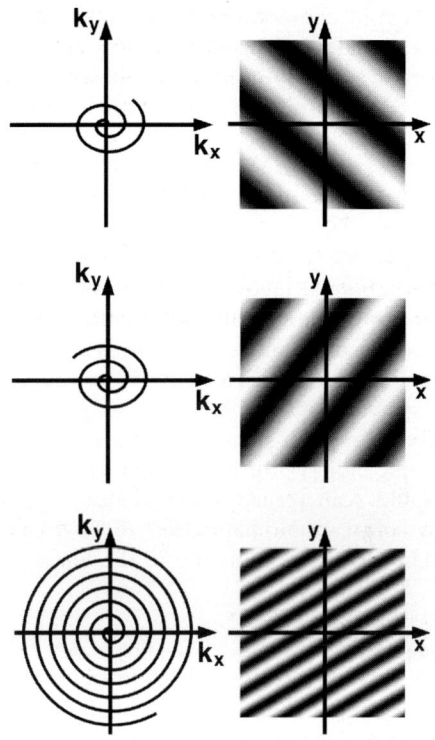

How does this rotating gradient make a spiral scan different from an EPI scan? The basic idea is that there is no difference between the x and y axes in the image. Thus many familiar ideas from spin-warp imaging and EPI do not apply. For example, there is no "phase-encoding direction," nor is there a "frequency-encoding direction." The idea of a series of evenly spaced echoes from EPI does not really apply either. An important benefit of this is that spiral scanning does not suffer from the broad range of "odd-even" artifacts from which EPI sometimes suffers.

The circular symmetry of spirals leads to other positive imaging characteristics, such as isotropic response to T2 decay and flow. However, it also leads to some negative imaging properties, most notably in the isotropic response that spirals have to main field inhomogeneity, which leads to image blurring. Issues such as these are discussed in the following sections.

Contrast

The contrast of interleaved spiral scans is similar to that of spin-warp scans. Traditional T1-weighted, T2-weighted, and density-weighted scans can be performed with spiral readouts, although spiral scans are typically shorter than spin-warp scans. Both gradient-echo and spin-echo scans can be performed.

Although by convention we refer to spiral gradient-echo scans, a spiral readout does not actually call back a gradient echo because the readout starts at the k-space origin with no gradient dephaser. This means that spiral gradient scans can have very short echo times, limited only by the excitation pulse.

T2 Decay

This section refers not to T2 decay between the excitation and the readout, which affects the contrast merely in the usual way, but to T2 decay during the readout. Every imaging method suffers some impulse response distortion due to T2 decay. This effect becomes more pronounced with longer readouts, and therefore it is a somewhat greater concern with EPI or spiral scanning readouts than it is with spin-warp readouts.

T2 decay during a spiral scan of k-space leads to the relatively benign effect of an isotropic blur [1]. To understand why this occurs, consider that T2 decay during a spiral scan results in a circularly symmetric apodization of the k-space data. By contrast, the main effect of T2 decay during an EPI scan is anisotropic resolution loss, predominantly in the phase-encoding direction [9].

Inhomogeneity

Spiral scanning in the presence of main field inhomogeneity leads to a space-variant image blur unless steps are taken to compensate for this blur in the image reconstruction [5, 8, 10]. This effect is the major disadvantage of spiral scanning relative to spin-warp imaging because in spin-warp imaging inhomogeneity causes mild geometric distortion rather than blurring, which is typically a less objectionable effect. It is easy to understand why an off-resonance spin is reconstructed at a different position along the readout direction in spin-warp imaging. In spiral imaging one can see that a spatial shift becomes a blur as the spiral readout gradient is rotated during the scan. This is an example of the disadvantage due to the circular symmetry of spiral scanning.

The inhomogeneity response of EPI is somewhat similar to that of spin-warp imaging although a bit more complicated [9]. The main effect of inhomogeneity is, once again, geometric distortion, although the distortion is typically more pronounced than in spin warp because of the extended readout window. In EPI an off-resonance spin is reconstructed at a shifted position along the phase-encoding direction. There is also an effect resulting from alternating shifts along the readout direction, but it is less pronounced. Thus, while the EPI off-resonance response is worse than that of spin-warp imaging, it is typically preferable to the (uncorrected) response of spiral scanning.

Figure 6 illustrates the effect of off-resonance on a spiral image. Depicted here is an interleaved spiral scan of a phantom reconstructed both on resonance and 50 Hz off-resonance with 17.6-ms readouts. Note that the off-resonance image appears blurred. Different spiral scans have different off-resonance sensitivities; shorter readouts and more interleaves lead to less blurring for a given amount of inhomogeneity.

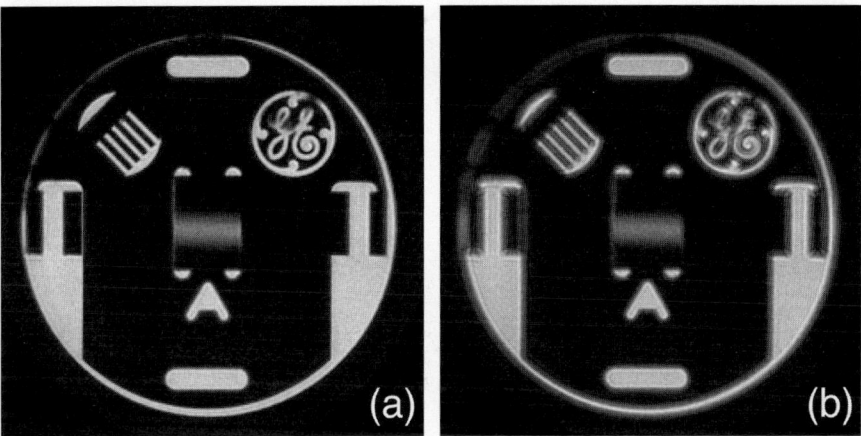

Fig. 6. a Spiral phantom image reconstructed on-resonance. **b** Spiral phantom image reconstructed 50 Hz off-resonance with a 17.6-ms readout window. Note the blurring of the image

Because of this off-resonance blurring in spiral scans it is important to take account of off-resonance when implementing spiral scans. First, it is often best to suppress fat in spiral scans, at least at 1.5 T. If fat is not suppressed, it might blur into water pixels. Second, it is very important to tune the sequence to the resonant frequency of the slice of interest, either during acquisition or in reconstruction. Otherwise, the entire image is blurred as in Fig. 6, even if the shim within the slice is quite good. For multislice studies the proper frequency offsets can be determined by collecting free induction decays (FIDs) or field maps of each slice [8]. Finally, it is often best to include some form of spatially varying inhomogeneity compensation in the image reconstruction [11–13]. Often this compensation can be performed with minimal computation [13]. A discussion of this topic follows in the section on image reconstruction.

Flow

From the earliest experiments it was apparent that spiral scanning is relatively insensitive to flow-related dropouts and ghosting, even though the readouts are relatively long. For example, the heart image in Fig. 4 has no obvious flow artifacts. This section discusses some of the theoretical reasons for the good flow performance of spiral scans.

Perhaps the most important flow-related advantage of spirals scanning is simply that the trajectory starts at the origin in k-space and moves out. This means that the center of k-space is collected at the start of the scan and thus with zero transverse moments of all orders. (The moments of gradients in MR imaging determine how sensitive a particular pulse sequence is to motion.) This factor alone reduces flow-related dropouts and ghosting due to phase variations from pulsatile flow. By contrast, full k-space EPI scans often have significant flow

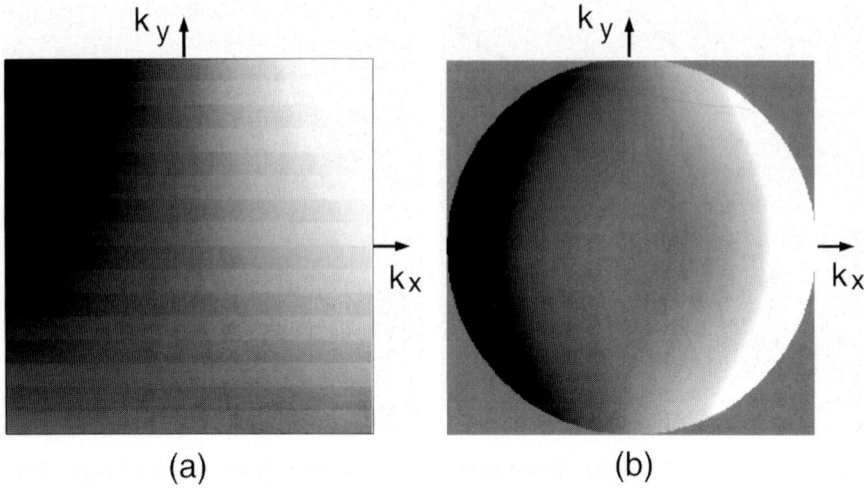

Fig. 7. Velocity k-space trajectories for interleaved spiral scan (a) and interleaved EPI scan (b). Shown here is the velocity k-space component corresponding to flow in the x direction. The EPI scan has discontinuities in the velocity k-space trajectory, which can lead to flow ghosting, whereas the trajectory of the spiral scan is smooth. (Courtesy of Dwight Nishimura)

dropouts because there are a number of gradient lobes before the center of k-space is traversed. This effect can be reduced in EPI by partial k-space scans or by flow compensation along the phase-encoding direction, but there are still more gradient moments of some order at the center of k-space than with a spiral scan.

Another spiral scanning advantage is that the moments of spiral readout gradients continue to have desirable properties as the scan spirals out from the k-space origin. One way to study the velocity sensitivity of a readout gradient is to plot the first moment in a particular direction as a function of the spatial k-space trajectory. Nishimura et al. used this velocity k-space approach to study the flow sensitivity of both spiral scanning and EPI [14].

Figure 7 (from [14]) shows an image of the first moment along the x direction as a function of k_x and k_y for two different sequences. Figure 7a shows the velocity k-space trajectory for an interleaved spiral scan, and Fig. 7b shows the equivalent plot for an interleaved EPI scan. Compare the smoothness of the plot for the spiral scan with the alternating bands in the EPI scan. These discontinuities in k-space lead to the well-known flow ghosting of (uncompensated) EPI scans. This can be seen in the simulated vessel images of Fig. 8. Figure 8a shows a simulated spiral image of vessel model with parabolic flow, and Fig. 8b shows the corresponding echo planar image. The spiral image shows no apparent flow distortion, but the echo planar image shows substantial flow ghosting.

Figure 7a also shows another desirable flow property of spiral scans. Note that the phase variation is monotonic and is oriented almost entirely along the horizontal direction – the direction of flow. This means that the main effect of flow during the scan is a shift and blurring along the direction of flow. One can intui-

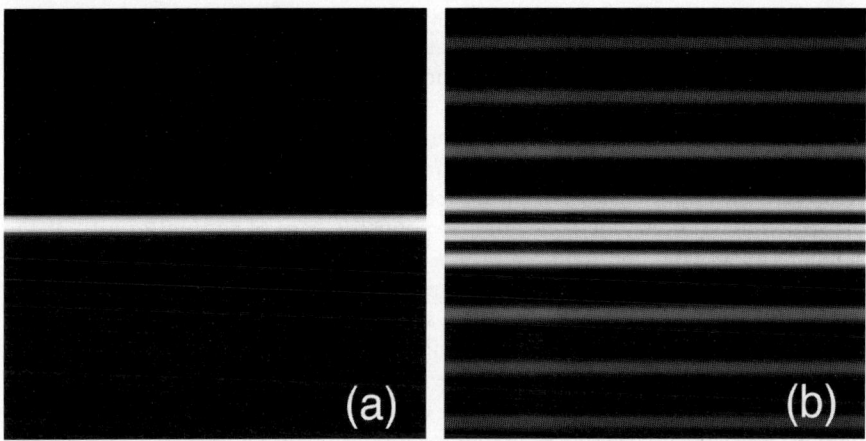

Fig. 8. Simulated vessel images for interleaved spiral scan (**a**) and interleaved EPI scan (**b**) of Fig. 7. The vessel model was a straight in-plane vessel with circular cross-section and 40 cm/s parabolic flow. (Courtesy of Dwight Nishimura)

tively think of this shift as a time-of-flight effect during the readout. This is the least objectionable effect of flow since one is typically most interested in resolving across a vessel or perpendicular to the main direction of flow. There is a small component in Fig. 7a perpendicular to the direction of flow. This produces a small shift of the vessel perpendicular to the direction of flow, but this shift is quite small for typical flow velocities.

Figures 7 and 8 illustrate the velocity k-space analysis for flow along the EPI readout direction. The EPI results would be different if the flow were oriented along the phase-encoding direction. In particular, the effect of the velocity moments during the scan would be much less, but the effect of the higher order moments might be worse. In oblique scans the effects would be intermediate. On the other hand, the symmetry of the spiral scan means that its response to flow is isotropic. Thus spiral scanning exhibits the same good flow behavior regardless of the direction of flow.

Efficiency

What does one mean when one discusses the efficiency of an imaging method? A number of possible meanings come to mind, but here we are mainly concerned with two issues: (a) SNR, the fundamental issue of how efficiently the technique collects and uses the available signal, and (b) the practical issue of how efficiently the technique uses the available hardware, in particular the gradient system.

First, how efficiently does spiral scanning use the available signal? Overall, spiral scanning, much as with traditional EPI, uses the signal quite efficiently. Some reasons for this efficiency are that the readout window is longer and the flip angle larger than in many rapid imaging methods. The main SNR difference between spiral scanning and EPI is that they have different sampling patterns. For optimal SNR (assuming no prior knowledge of the image) the sampling pattern should be uniform.

There are two elements to the sampling pattern: the k-space trajectory and the sampling along the trajectory. Both spiral and EPI trajectories sample k-space reasonably uniformly. The SNR differences result from the way in which the samples are spread along the trajectory. A good measure of the uniformity of the sampling is whether the trajectory has a constant k-space velocity, which is proportional to the readout gradient magnitude. Thus a constant gradient magnitude leads to optimal SNR, with either spiral scanning or EPI.

Practical spiral scanning and EPI sequences seldom have a constant gradient magnitude throughout the scan because of gradient hardware limitations. However, the sampling is close enough to uniform in the two sequences that the loss in SNR due to sampling nonuniformity is a minor effect. There is also some minor spatial noise coloration due to the sampling nonuniformity. Whether spiral scanning or EPI has a small advantage in SNR depends upon the details of the gradient design; the closer a sequence approaches constant gradient magnitude, the better is the SNR. As it turns out, this is also often a good measure of how efficiently a sequence uses the gradient system.

How well does spiral scanning use the available gradient system? It uses it very efficiently in most cases, leading to short scan times. It is easy to understand intuitively why this is the case. One important reason is that spiral scans cover a circular region in k-space rather than a square region, leading to a $\pi/4$ reduction in the k-space area that needs to be covered. It turns out that this acceleration comes at little or no cost because not collecting the corners of k-space leads to an isotropic impulse response, which is typically preferred to an anisotropic response. Indeed, the data from the corners of k-space are often not used in 2D Fourier transform (FT) scans for this reason. Typically EPI scans spend time collecting these corners of k-space, although there are circular EPI variants.

Not only does spiral scanning cover an efficient (i.e., circular) region of k-space, but it can cover this region rapidly under the typical hardware constraints of a maximum gradient amplitude and a maximum gradient amplifier voltage. The maximum gradient amplitude sets a limit on the maximum k-space velocity. The amplifier voltage limits how rapidly the gradient can change, which corresponds to a limit to how rapidly the k-space trajectory can speed up, slow down, or change direction. Spiral scanning is one of the most efficient ways of using this limited amplifier voltage. The trajectory is continually turning, which is accomplished by slowly changing from one gradient amplifier to the other and reduces the need for rapid changes of gradient amplifier polarity such as those needed in an EPI scan. In a properly designed spiral readout, the vector gradient amplitude increases monotonically during the scan until it reaches the amplitude limit (set by gradient or bandwidth constraints). After the amplitude limit is reached, often early in the scan, the scan proceeds with the desired constant k-space velocity. By contrast, the velocity in an EPI scan usually fluctuates because the velocity along the readout direction continually changes sign and thus traverses zero. The velocity along the phase-encoding direction is often highest around the zero crossing of the readout gradient, but typically not high enough to maintain a constant net velocity.

A simple example may help to illustrate the efficiency of spiral scanning. In this example, we will compare the scan time for a full k-space, blipped, interleaved EPI scan with the scan time for an interleaved spiral scan, assuming the same gradient hardware, the same spatial resolution, and the same readout window width. The scans cover 256×256 pixels over a 24-cm field-of-view (FOV) using a 4-µs sampling time and using gradients with 24.5 mT/m maximum amplitude and 77 mT/m slew rate. Using these parameters, an EPI scan with 32 interleaves and 8 echoes per interleaf requires a 13.6-ms readout window, not including the 1.17-ms dephasing gradient or any flow-compensating gradients. By contrast, a spiral scan with a 13.6-ms readout window achieves the same resolution in only 18 interleaves. What is the source of this scan time reduction from 32 to 18 interleaves? Roughly half of the reduction comes from the spiral scan not collecting the corners of k-space. The other half comes from the higher average k-space velocity of the spiral scan.

Of course, this is only a simple example, and the actual numbers vary somewhat depending upon the assumptions. For example, if the dephaser time is included as part of the readout window, the spiral scan requires only 16 interleaves. On the other hand, the EPI scan time is reduced if the k-space corners are rounded rather than right-angle blips. Also, EPI can reach the same pixel area more rapidly by using asymmetric resolution. However, the overall result would be the same: the spiral scan would be faster with a given readout window.

A more difficult question is whether it is fair to compare these scans based on the readout window width. An argument could be made that spiral readouts need to be shorter to avoid unacceptable blurring due to inhomogeneity. On the other hand, if flow performance is an important consideration, adding flow compensation and perhaps flyback techniques to the EPI scan would slow it. The overall conclusion is that both EPI and spiral scans are efficient, but spiral scans appear to be more efficient.

Eddy Currents

Spiral scanning is surprisingly immune to the effects of eddy currents. In standard EPI some sort of sequence-specific eddy current calibration is typically required. This sort of calibration is seldom needed for spiral scanning, especially on a commercial scanner with hardware eddy current compensation or actively shielded gradients (or both). This makes spiral scanning easier to implement than EPI with regard to gradient fidelity.

In a study of a technique for eddy current calibration, Kerr et al. studied both interleaved EPI and interleaved spiral scanning sequences [15]. Their conclusion was that calibration is necessary to avoid ghosts and other artifacts with the EPI sequence, but that the improvement in the interleaved spiral scans is less dramatic. On a well-tuned scanner, the only eddy-current correction usually needed is for the gradient group delay; none of the images presented in this chapter have additional correction. However, on systems with more severe eddy currents, additional correction may be necessary; several groups have reported improvement from measuring the actual spiral trajectory [16–20].

It is easy to see why eddy currents do not have severe effects on spiral scans. Firstly, the symmetry of spiral scans mean that there are no even-odd echo effects, as mentioned above. Ghosting due to eddy currents is one of the most obvious even-odd problems in EPI. Secondly, the spiral readout gradients oscillate with a slowly increasing amplitude, and the gradients are thus close to sinusoidal. The first-order effect of eddy currents on a sinusoid is simply a reduction in amplitude and a phase shift.

The most significant eddy currents in most systems are the linear and B_0 terms. The effect of the linear term on a spiral scan is mostly an easily corrected gradient time delay. Optimized spiral gradients are not purely sinusoidal, and a single time delay therefore leads to minor rotational misregistration between low and high spatial frequencies. The effect of the B_0 eddy current term on a spiral scan is simply a slowly varying phase shift across the image. On a typical system this phase shift causes a small subpixel shift in the reconstructed image, which typically has no effect on the utility of the image.

Maxwell Fields

Maxwell's equations dictate that it is not possible to generate a magnetic field gradient without also generating unwanted "concomitant gradients," or "Maxwell fields" [21, 22]. King et al. studied the effect of these Maxwell fields on spiral scans [23]. For nonaxial scans or axial scans away from isocenter the effect of these fields is a time-varying frequency shift, which leads to image blurring in a spiral scan. This blurring is typically not noticeable for scans with 10 mT/m gradients at 1.5 T, but can become significant at higher gradient strengths or lower field strengths. King et al. showed that it is possible to correct for this blurring using multifrequency reconstruction [11, 23].

Field of View

In spiral scanning the acquired FOV is circular rather than square. Often the region outside this circular area is blacked out for display purposes. The FOV has in fact two components: (a) the trajectory component, which is that determined by the spacing between the spirals, and (b) the filter component, which is that determined by the spacing between the samples along the spirals. The trajectory component is a function of the gradient waveforms, and the filter component is a function of the receiver filter. Both of these components must be equal to or larger than the object FOV to image without aliasing or distortion.

The trajectory component is somewhat analogous to the phase-encoding FOV in spin-warp imaging. However, because of the different sampling patterns aliasing occurs differently. In spin-warp imaging an object outside the FOV in the phase-encoding direction appears in the well-known wrap-around artifact, as

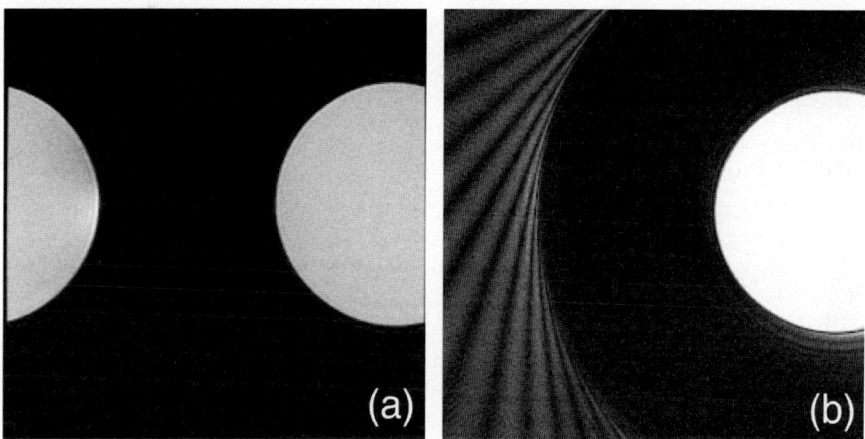

Fig. 9a,b. Images of an object placed partially outside the acquired FOV. **a** Spin-warp image. Note the coherent wrap-around artifact. **b** Spiral scan image has been windowed to accentuate the aliasing artifact. The maximum intensity of the spiral aliasing artifact is significantly lower than that in the spin-warp case

shown in Fig. 9a. In spiral scanning the aliased energy appears in somewhat of a semicircular swirl, as shown in Fig. 9b. The spin-warp aliasing artifact is typically more intense, whereas the spiral aliasing artifact is more spread out. The reduced intensity of the spiral artifact may be advantageous in some instances. Of course in most cases the FOV should be set to avoid either artifact.

The filter component is somewhat analogous to the readout FOV in spin-warp imaging. In both cases the sampling bandwidth must be set so that a spin on the edge of the FOV is within this bandwidth when the readout gradient amplitude is at its maximum. However, the effect of setting the sampling bandwidth too small is different in the two cases. In spin-warp imaging the filter can be used to restrict the FOV. However, in spiral scanning this is not the case; setting the bandwidth too small results in rotational blurring and artifacts in the periphery of the image, as shown in Fig. 10. The inability to restrict the FOV using the receiver filter is a significant disadvantage of spiral scanning relative to spin-warp imaging.

One interesting consequence of the gridding image reconstruction used in spiral scanning is that there is little or no SNR penalty for using a higher filter bandwidth than necessary because the additional data samples are effectively averaged in the reconstruction. Thus the filter bandwidth in spiral scanning should be set to be greater than or equal to the largest expected object FOV at the peak readout gradient amplitude.

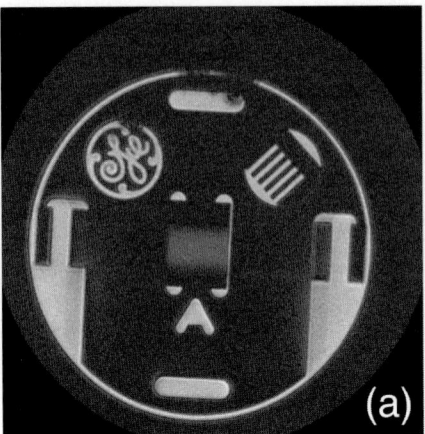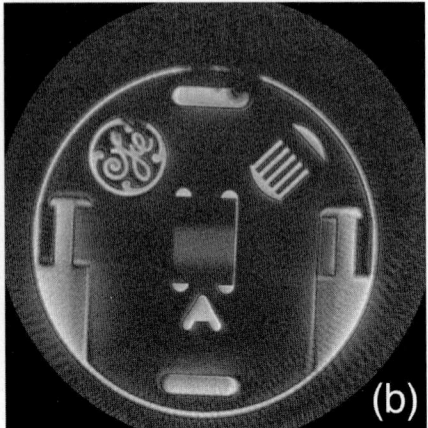

Fig. 10a,b. Illustration of the effect of receiver filter bandwidth on a spiral image. **a** Image with the receiver filter bandwidth set correctly. **b** Image with the receiver filter bandwidth set to too narrow a bandwidth. Note the blurring and artifacts near the edge of the phantom

Implementation

This section presents an overview of some of the issues involved in implementing spiral scanning. The first part discusses how to reconstruct images from data collected along spiral paths in k-space. The next part discusses how to design gradient waveforms to trace out a spiral path. The final part discusses various pulse sequences used for spiral scanning.

Image Reconstruction

Reconstructing spiral images is of course more complicated than reconstructing 2D FT images; the collected data points do not fall on a 2D grid, and therefore some operations must be performed in a addition to a fast FT (FFT). Ahn et al. reconstructed the first spiral scans using techniques from computed tomography [1], much as the very first MR images were reconstructed. However, this method of image reconstruction applies only to a spiral scan with constant angular velocity, which is slower and has lower SNR efficiency than some alternatives. Thus the author's group and others have used the gridding image reconstruction technique ("gridding") from radioastronomy to reconstruct spiral images [7, 8, 24–26].

The basic idea of gridding is to transform a set of arbitrary samples in k-space into a rectilinear array, so that they can then be rapidly transformed into an image using an FFT. What is the best way to do this transformation? At first glance it might seem that a straightforward 2D interpolation is the best way. However, there are good reasons why it is actually better to use a convolution rather than a simple interpolation. O'Sullivan provides a good discussion of some of these reasons [24]. The basic idea is that the data represent samples of the continuous FT of a finite object. However, one has no hope of reconstructing this object exactly using a finite extent of k-space data because an object and its transform cannot both be finite. Thus it is best to recognize this fact and use a convolution kernel to suppress aliasing side lobes. Another reason why it is better to use a convolution than an interpolation is that all of the data are then used in the reconstruction, which maximizes the SNR.

A basic outline of the algorithm is as follows:

- Multiply the data points by a k-space density compensation factor. This factor should weight points in oversampled regions of k-space less than those in critically sampled regions, and the effective k-space density after compensation is thus uniform. A number of density compensation factors have been proposed [27–31]; one that works well for archimedean spirals is Eq. 1 [8]; the first term of Eq. 1 compensates for the varying k-space velocity and the second term for the increased density of the spirals near the origin:

$$|g(t)| \cdot |\sin[\arg\{g(t)\} - arg\{k(t)\}]| \tag{1}$$

- Convolve the data into the 2D array. This is done by multiplying each density-compensated data point by a Kaiser-Bessel window a few grid points in width, evaluating the result at each grid point within the window, and adding the result into the array.
- Perform a complex 2D FFT.
- Divide by the transform of the Kaiser-Bessel window to remove the apodization resulting from the convolution of step 4.
- Take the magnitude of the result.

If the density compensation is performed properly, the artifacts resulting from gridding are minimal. In some cases, however, a bright object near the edge of the FOV leads to an aliasing artifact on the opposite side of the image. Such artifacts can be reduced by using a two-to-one gridding method. In this method the number of pixels in the gridding array is doubled along each dimension, leading to a finer sampling of k-space. The gridding proceeds as before, but after the FFT only the inner half of the resulting image along each dimension is preserved. The outer parts that are thrown away contain most of the artifacts resulting from the gridding procedure, and the final image is largely free of these artifacts.

The above outline of gridding omits one essential element: compensation for off-resonance effects. At a bare minimum, the effective center frequency of a spiral scan must be correct. Figure 6 shows the effect of the center frequency being grossly incorrect, but even small frequency offsets can result in detectable image blurring. Often the center frequency obtained during tuning prior to the scan is not accurate enough. This is true particularly for multislice studies in which a single center frequency is used. Thus it is best to determine the proper center frequency Δf for each image – for example, by collecting an FID or a field map of the slice – and then to demodulate the received signal to that center frequency by multiplying by $e^{i2\pi\Delta ft}$.

It most cases it is best to compensate for spatially varying inhomogeneity in addition to center frequency offsets. Noll et al. [11, 12] developed techniques for carrying out inhomogeneity compensation that involve reconstructing a series of images at different demodulation frequencies and then choosing the correct pixel value on a pixel-by-pixel basis. This can be performed using a separately acquired field map [11] or by deriving the field map automatically from the spiral data itself [12], [32]. This technique works well although it does require some additional computation. Man et al. proposed a method for reducing the computation [33], and Kadah and Hu have proposed an alternative method for correcting for inhomogeneity [34].

An inhomogeneity compensation technique that requires little additional computation involves the use of a linear approximation to the field map [13]. If the field inhomogeneity varies linearly with position across the FOV, it is the same as a constant readout gradient added to the spiral gradients. Once the value of this effective gradient is known, the k-space trajectory used for reconstruction can be changed to include the gradient, which then compensates for the inhomogeneity. The effect on the k-space trajectory is that it gradually shifts along the axis of the gradient, such that the successive turns of the spiral become closer together on one side and farther apart on the other.

Of course, inhomogeneity functions are never perfectly linear. Nevertheless, fitting a linear function to an acquired field map is often sufficient to remove the noticeable blurring from a spiral scan. Figure 11a shows an image reconstructed without linear inhomogeneity compensation, and Fig. 11b shows the same data reconstructed with inhomogeneity compensation. Note that the compensated image is significantly sharper. In this study a low-resolution field map was acquired using two single-shot spirals with different echo times, and a linear function was then fit to this field map using a χ^2 procedure. This technique is used routinely for spiral image reconstruction in the author's laboratory, sometimes in combination with the pixel-by-pixel deblurring described above.

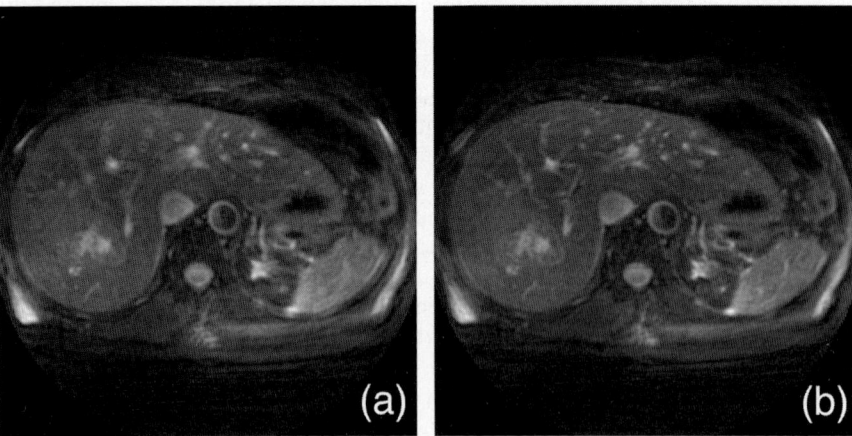

Fig. 11. a Image reconstructed with no spatially varying inhomogeneity compensation. **b** The same data as in **a**, reconstructed with linear inhomogeneity compensation. Note the decreased image blurring

Gradient Design

There are an infinite number of gradient waveforms that trace out a particular spiral k-space trajectory. The design of these gradient waveforms is an important element of spiral scanning, and a number of iterative [8, 17, 35, 36] and analytical [37, 38] approaches have been successfully applied to this problem. This section discusses an analytical, noniterative, graphical solution to this problem [39]. This approach is fast and intuitive and easily incorporates different gradient circuit models.

This design method rests on one simple discrete-time approximation, which is valid for the sampling time, T, of a typical digital gradient waveform. The algorithm checks the validity of this approximation and reduces the internal value of T in the design as necessary. Here we discuss the application of this method to one important design problem: the design of gradient waveforms that trace a given spiral trajectory in the minimum time, assuming a gradient circuit model with a given maximum slew rate and maximum gradient amplitude. We constrain the absolute value of the slew and amplitude to be no greater than the values available on one axis, so that the gradients can be rotated to generate different interleaves, and so that oblique scans pose no problems.

The desired k-space trajectory is:

$$k(\tau) = A\tau e^{i\omega\tau}, \tag{2}$$

where τ is a function of time and is designed to be as large as possible in each sampling period. The discrete-time gradient waveform is g_n and the discrete-time k-space trajectory is

$$k_n = \sum_{i=0}^{n} g_i. \tag{3}$$

The design starts with a given g_0 (typically zero) and then calculates g_n successively for increasing values of n, terminating when either a desired radius in k-space is reached or after a desired number of samples. Two gradient amplifier parameters are needed: (a) the maximum step in gradient amplitude in a given gradient sampling period (S), and (b) the maximum allowed gradient.

Figure 12 illustrates the first step in the design. Starting from a given g_n, we want to determine g_{n+1}. Because spiral gradients are continually rotating, g_{n+1} points in a slightly different direction than g_n. The first step in the design is to determine this direction, $\angle g_{n+1}$. We do this by evaluating the continuous first derivative of the expression $k(\tau)$ at the current value of τ and taking the argument of this evaluation. This step leads to the following expression:

$$L g_{n+1} = \tan^{-1}\left(\omega\frac{|k_n|}{A}\right) + \omega\frac{|k_n|}{A}. \tag{4}$$

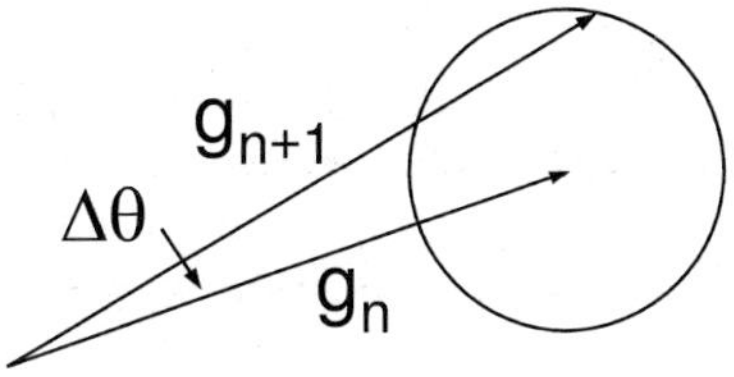

Fig. 12. First step in spiral gradient design: find $\Delta\theta$ by evaluating the continuous derivative of k at t_n

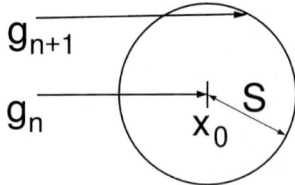

Fig. 13. Second step in spiral gradient design: determine maximum $|g_{n+1}|$ by finding intersection between line at $\Delta\theta$ and constraint circle

Figure 13 illustrates the second step in the design. (The gradient vectors have been rotated to lie along the x-axis, which does not change the problem.) Given the angle of g_{n+1}, we solve for the maximum $|g_{n+1}|$ allowable under the gradient constraints. The gradient constraints are represented by the circle, and solving for $|g_{n+1}|$ simply involves finding an intersection of the circle and the g_{n+1} line. Note that there are two intersections; we want the one corresponding to an increase in the gradient amplitude for a minimum-time design. The radius of the constraint circle is simply S, defined above. Using this circuit model the center of the circle is at the tip of g_n; with other circuit models the center of the circle shifts [39]. Solving for the intersection leads to the following expression:

$$|g_{n+1}| = Cx_0 + \sqrt{S^2 + x_0^2 (C^2 - 1)}, \tag{5}$$

where:

$$x_0 = |g_n| \tag{6}$$

and

$$C = 1/\sqrt{1 + \tan^2 \Delta\theta}. \tag{7}$$

If $|g_{n+1}|$ exceeds the maximum allowed gradient in any step, it is simply set to that value.

This spiral design approach is simple to understand and implement and leads to accurately optimized gradients. The speed of this approach makes it feasible to reoptimize spiral gradients as parameters change at scan time, which is the routine practice in the author's laboratory.

Pulse Sequences

Figure 14 illustrates a basic spiral pulse sequence. This consists of a spectral-spatial excitation pulse followed by spiral readout gradients. The readout gradients shown were optimized by the technique described in the previous section. Note that at the beginning of the scan the vector amplitude of the gradients steadily increases, with the rate of increase limited by the available gradient amplifier voltage. A few milliseconds into the readout the amplitude ceases to increase because the maximum allowed gradient amplitude is reached.

The spectral-spatial excitation pulse simultaneously selects the slice and a particular range of frequencies [40]. Typically it is used to excite only water, and thus lipids are suppressed. For most spiral scans at high field lipids must be sup-

Fig. 14. Timing diagram of a spiral pulse sequence. It consists of a spectral-spatial excitation pulse designed to excite water and suppress fat followed by optimized spiral readout gradients

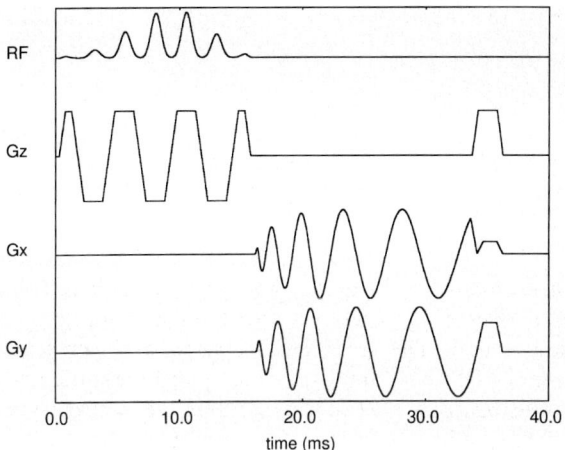

pressed so that they do not blur into the neighboring water regions. Spectral-spatial pulses provide an efficient and robust method of lipid suppression, although other methods such as lipid presaturation can be used as well.

A number of different spiral pulse sequence variations have been studied. An early spiral technique was square-spiral scanning, which permitted image reconstruction using only 1D interpolation and an FFT [4–7]. Recently other nonarchimedean spirals have been studied to match the capabilities of particular amplifier systems [31, 41]. Another variation is spiral-in/spiral-out scanning, in which the scan starts at the edge of k-space, spirals in to the center, and then spirals back out to the edge [42, 43]. This technique is best suited when a longer echo time is desired, for example, in T2-weighted spin-echo imaging. Rapid acquisition relation enhancement (RARE) spiral scanning is another variation suited to T2-weighted scanning, in which spiral annuli are acquired during the echoes of a RARE pulse train [44]. Finally, 3D variations of spiral scanning have been studied, including a (phase-encoded) cylindrical stack-of-spirals, a spherical stack-of-spirals, and a cones trajectory consisting of spirals wound onto the surfaces of various cones [45–48].

Applications

Spiral scanning has been applied to a number of different applications, and this section mentions a few of them. Some of the most successful applications have been cardiac imaging, coronary angiography, and angiography [8, 45, 48–52]. Spiral scanning in these applications takes advantage of the good flow properties of spirals. Figure 15 illustrates two frames from a spiral heart movie depicting the opening of the mitral valve. Note that there is little flow-related dephasing. Figures 4 and 16 are high-resolution 2D breath-held spiral coronary angiograms [52]. In a given breath-hold spiral coronary angiograms have higher temporal and spatial resolution and better SNR than segmented 2D FT coronary angiograms. Figure 17 is a coronary angiogram acquired using a 3D spherical stack-

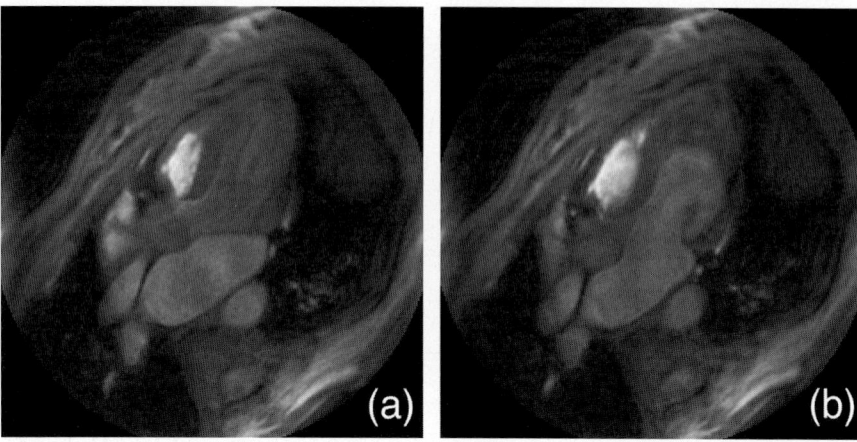

Fig. 15a,b. Two frames from a breath-held spiral heart movie. Note that the mitral valve is closed in the first image and open in the second

Fig. 16. Breath-held 2D spiral image with 0.83-mm spatial resolution showing the LAD and diagonal arteries in an LAO-caudal view. One of five slices acquired in a breath-hold

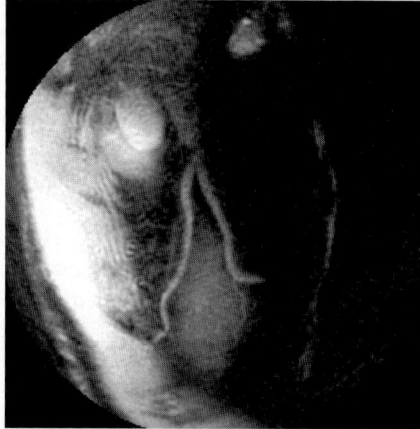

Fig. 17. 3D spiral coronary angiogram. Respiratory compensation via the diminishing variance algorithm. Reformated along a curved surface. Shown are the LAD and its first-order branches in an LAO-caudal view.
(Courtesy of Daniel Thedens)

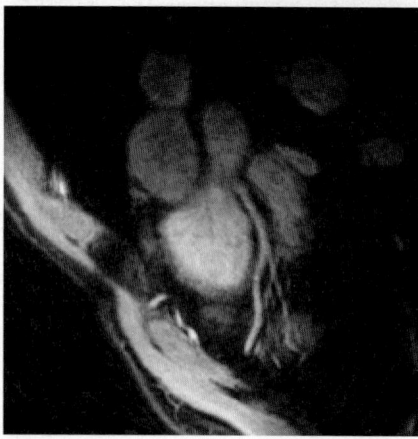

Fig. 18. 3D spiral flow-independent angiogram of the
popliteal trifurcation.
(Courtesy of Jean Brittain)

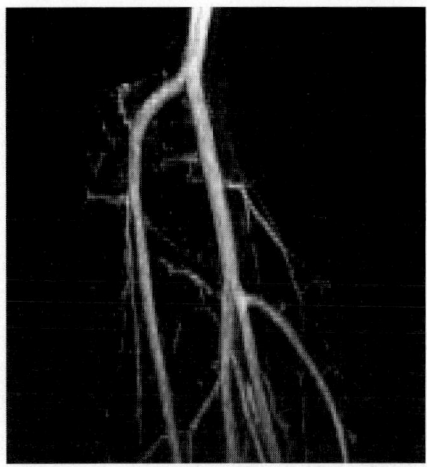

of-spirals trajectory [45, 48]. This image was acquired while the subject was breathing freely, with the diminishing variance algorithm used for respiratory compensation [53]. Figure 18 is a flow-independent peripheral angiogram also acquired using a 3D spherical stack-of-spirals trajectory [54]. Spiral scanning has also been used for phase-contrast studies of the heart [49, 50].

Abdominal tumor imaging is another application of spiral scans. For these scans the most important property of spiral scans is their efficiency. However, because susceptibility-induced inhomogeneity is significant in the abdomen, shimming and inhomogeneity compensation are important to achieve reliable results. Figure 19 compares a conventional spin-warp scan and a breath-held,

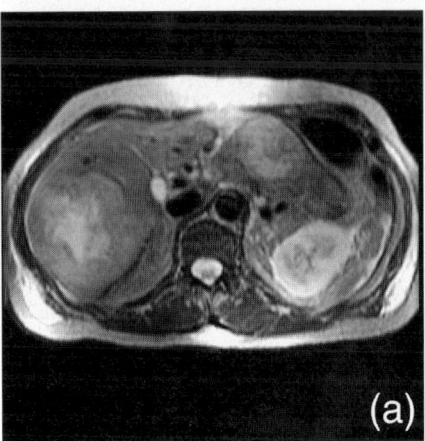
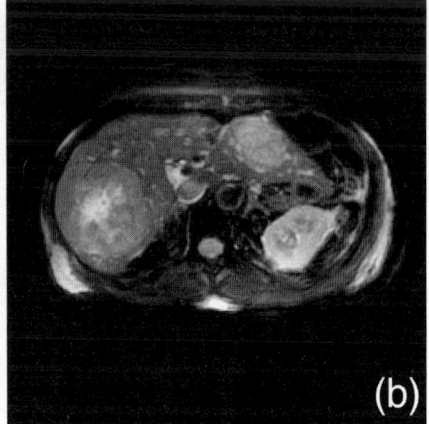

Fig. 19. a Spin-warp 2-NEX 128×256 T2-weighted multicoil image that took long than 12 min to acquire. The patient has metastatic lesions in the liver from lung carcinoma. **b** Breath-held (24-s) spiral-in/spiral-out image of the patient in **a**. The image quality is comparable to that in the spin-warp scan, in-plane and through-plane blurring due to breathing is eliminated, and the scan time is decreased 30-fold

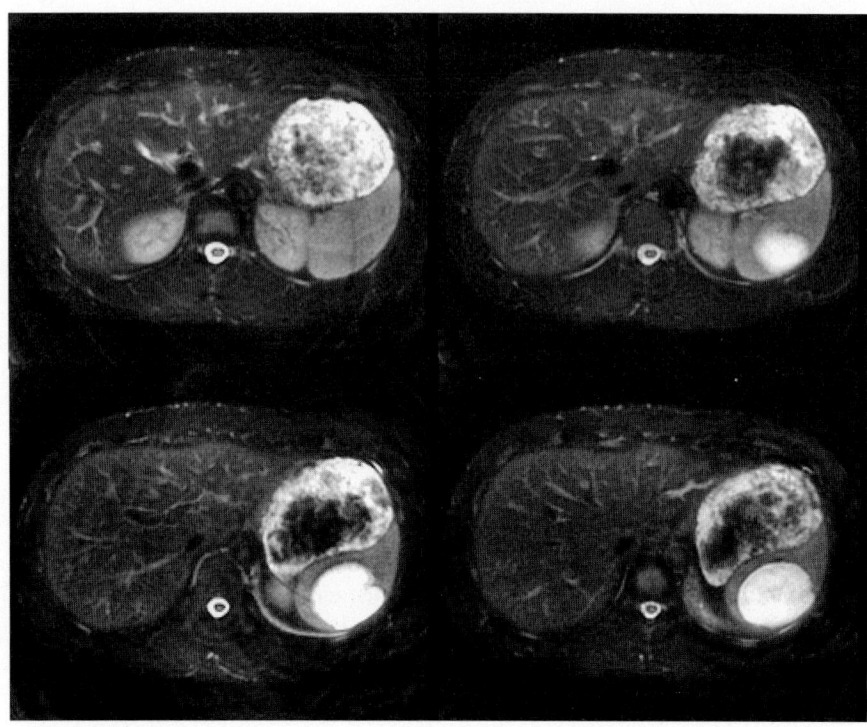

Fig. 20. RARE spiral images of a subject with a splenic cyst. TE = 80, TR = 4000, three interleaves, 1.5-mm resolution. Four of 11 slices acquired over 12 s. (Courtesy of Walter Block)

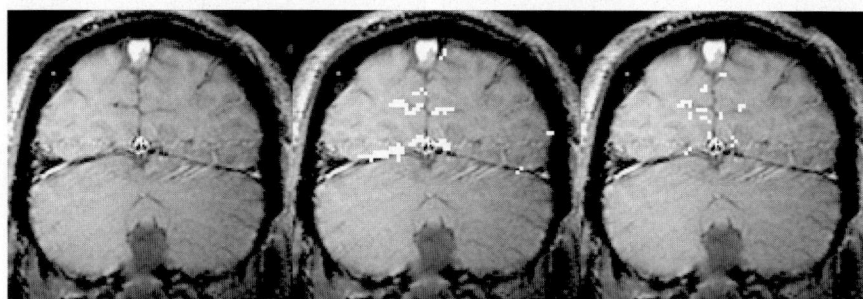

Fig. 21. High-resolution spiral 3.0-T functional MR imaging study; 8-Hz checkerboard visual stimulation; 1.5×1.5 mm in-plane resolution, 3-mm slice thickness; eight interleaves, 27-ms readouts. *Left*, T1 image; *center*, gradient echo (TE = 20 ms) functional MR image overlay; *right*, spin-echo (TE = 100 ms) functional MR image overlay. Note that the signal in the transverse sinus eliminated in the spin-echo image. (Courtesy of Douglas Noll)

T2-weighted, spiral-in/spiral-out scan of a patient with liver metastases [42, 43]. The spiral scan has reduced artifacts and a much shorter scan time. Figure 20 illustrates a breath-held, T2-weighed, RARE spiral image of a subject with a splenic cyst [44]. T2-weighted spiral-out scanning has been applied to imaging the pelvis [55].

Another major application area is functional imaging [47, 56–60]. This takes advantage of the efficiency and good motion properties of spiral scanning. Figure 21 illustrates a high-resolution spiral functional MR imaging study performed at 3.0 T at the University of Pittsburgh [56, 57]. Finally, one of the most exciting recent applications of spiral scanning is fluoroscopy, or dynamic imaging [61–65]. Kerr et al. have developed a system that allows ungated spiral images of the heart to be acquired and displayed in real time [65].

Conclusions

Spiral scanning is a promising alternative to traditional EPI. The properties of spiral scanning stem from the circularly symmetric nature of the technique. Among the attractive properties of spiral scanning are its efficiency and its good behavior in the presence of flowing material; the most unattractive property is that uncorrected inhomogeneity leads to image blurring. Spiral image reconstruction can be performed rapidly using gridding, and there are a number of techniques for compensating for inhomogeneity. There are good techniques for generating efficient spiral gradient waveforms. Among the growing number of applications of spiral scanning are cardiac imaging, angiography, abdominal tumor imaging, functional imaging, and fluoroscopy.

Spiral scanning is a promising technique, but at the present it is still not in routine clinical use. There are many theoretical reasons why spiral scanning may be advantageous for a number of clinical problems, and initial volunteer and clinical studies have yielded very promising results for a number of applications. Still, until spiral scanning is established in routine clinical use, some caution is warranted about proclaiming it to be the answer for any particular question.

Acknowledgements. The author would like to thank all of his spiral scanning colleagues for their help and discussions, especially Dr. Albert Macovski. The author would also like to thank the following researchers for graciously providing figures for this chapter: Dr. Dwight Nishimura, Dr. Daniel Thedens, Dr. Jean Brittain, Dr. Walter Block, and Dr. Douglas Noll.

References

1. Ahn CB, Kim JH, Cho ZH (1986) High Speed Spiral Scan Echo Planar Imaging. IEEE Trans Med Imaging 5(1):2–5
2. Ljunggren S (1983) A simple graphical representation of Fourier-based imaging methods. J Magn Reson 54:338–343
3. Likes RS (1981) United States patent 4,307,343
4. Macovski A, Meyer C (1986) A novel fast scanning system. From: Works in Progress, Fifth Annual Meeting of the Society of Magnetic Resonance in Medicine, pp 156–157
5. Meyer CH, Macovski A (1987) Square spiral fast imaging: interleaving and off-resonance effects. From: Proceedings, Sixth Annual Meeting of the Society of Magnetic Resonance in Medicine, pp 230
6. Meyer CH, Macovski A, Nishimura DG (1989) Square-spiral fast imaging. From: Proceedings, Eighth Annual Meeting of the Society of Magnetic Resonance in Medicine, pp 362
7. Meyer CH, Macovski A, Nishimura DG (1990) A comparison of fast spiral sequences for cardiac imaging and angiography. From: Proceedings, Ninth Annual Meeting of the Society of Magnetic Resonance in Medicine, pp 403
8. Meyer CH, Hu BS, Nishimura DG, Macovski A (1992) Fast spiral coronary artery imaging. Magn Reson Med 28 (2):202–213
9. Farzaneh F, Riederer SJ, Pelc NJ (1990) Analysis of T2 limitations and off-resonance effects on spatial resolution and artifacts in echo-planar imaging. Magn Reson Med 14:123–139
10. Yudilevich E, Stark H (1987) Spiral sampling in magnetic resonance imaging-the effect of inhomogeneities. IEEE Trans Med Imaging 6(4):337–345
11. Noll DC, Meyer CH, Pauly JM, Nishimura DG, Macovski A (1991) A homogeneity correction method for magnetic resonance imaging with time-varying gradients. IEEE Trans on Med Imaging 10 (4):629–637
12. Noll DC, Pauly JM, Meyer CH, Nishimura DG, Macovski A (1992) De-blurring for non-2D Fourier transform magnetic resonance imaging. Magn Reson Med 25 (2):319–333
13. Irarrazabal P, Meyer CH, Nishimura DG, Macovski A (1996) Inhomogeneity correction using an estimated linear field map. Magn Reson Med 35 (2):278–282
14. Nishimura DG, Irarrazabal P, Meyer CH (1995) A velocity k-space analysis of flow effects in echo-planar and spiral imaging. Magn Reson Med 33 (4):549–556
15. Kerr A, Pauly J, Nishimura D (1996) Gradient measurement and characterization for spiral and echo-planar sequences. From: Proceedings, Fourth Annual Meeting of the International Society for Magnetic Resonance in Medicine, pp 364
16. Takahashi A, Peters T (1995) Compensation of multi-dimensional selective excitation pulses using measured k-space trajectories. Magn Reson Medicine 34 (3):446–456
17. Spielman DM, Pauly JM (1995) Spiral imaging on a small-bore system at 4.7 T. Magn Reson Med 34 (4):580–585
18. Alley MT, Kerr AB, Glover GH (1996) A Fourier-transform approach for k-space trajectory measurement. From: Proceedings, Fourth Annual Meeting of the International Society for Magnetic Resonance in Medicine, pp 1406
19. Mason GF, Harshbarger T, Hetherington HP, Zhang Y, Pohost GM, Twieg DB (1997) A method to measure arbitrary k-space trajectories for rapid MR imaging. Magn Reson Med, 38 (3):492–496
20. Papadakis NG, Wilkinson AA, Carpenter TA, Hall LD (1997) A general-method for measurement of the time integral of variant magnetic-field gradients: application to 2D spiral imaging. Magn Reson Imaging 15 (5):567–578
21. Norris DG, Hutchinson JMS (1990) Concomitant magnetic field gradients and their effects on imaging at low magnetic field strengths. Magn Resonance Imaging 8:33–37
22. Weisskoff RM, Cohen MS, Rzedzian RR (1995) Nonaxial whole-body instant imaging. Magn Reson Med 29 (6):796–803
23. King K, Ganin A, Zhou X, Bernstein M (1997) Effect of Maxwell fields in spiral scans. From: Proceedings, Fifth Annual Meeting of the International Society for Magnetic Resonance in Medicine, pp 1917
24. O'Sullivan JD (1985) A fast sinc function gridding algorithm for Fourier inversion inversion in computed tomography. IEEE Trans Med Imaging 4 (4):200–207
25. Jackson JI, Meyer CH, Nishimura DG, Macovski A (1991) Selection of a convolution function for Fourier inversion using gridding. IEEE Trans Med Imaging 10:473–478
26. Schomberg H, Timmer J (1995) The gridding method for image reconstruction by Fourier transformation. IEEE Trans Med Imaging 14 (3):596–607

27. Hardy CJ, Cline HE, Bottomley PA (1990) Correcting for nonuniform k-space sampling in two-dimensional NMR selective excitation. J Magn Reson 87 (3):639–645
28. Morrel G, Macovski A (1997) 3-dimensional spectral-spatial excitation. Magn Reson Med 37 (3):378–386
29. Hoge RD, Kwan RKS, Pike GB (1997) Density compensation functions for spiral MRI. Magn Reson Med 38 (1):117–128
30. Papadakis NG, Carpenter TA, Hall LD (1997) An algorithm for numerical calculation of the k-space data weighting for polarly sampled trajectories: application to spiral imaging. Magn Reson Imaging 15 (7):785–794
31. Liao JR, Pauly JM, Pelc NJ (1997) MRI using piecewise-linear spiral trajectory. Magn Reson Med 38 (2):246–252
32. Man LC, Pauly JM, Macovski A (1997) Improved automatic off-resonance correction without a field map in spiral imaging. Magn Reson Med 37 (6):906–913
33. Man LC, Pauly JM, Macovski A (1997) A multifrequency interpolation for fast off-resonance correction. Magn Reson Med 37 (5):785–792
34. Kadah YM, Hu XP (1997) Simulated phase evolution rewinding (SPHERE): a technique for reducing B0 inhomogeneity effects in MR images. Magn Reson Med 38 (4):615–627
35. Hardy CJ, Cline HE (1989) Broadband nuclear magnetic resonance pulses with two-dimensional spatial selectivity. J Magn Reson 66 (4):1513–1516
36. King KF, Foo TKF, Crawford CR (1995) Optimized gradient waveforms for spiral scanning. Magn Reson Med 34 (2):156–160
37. Heid O (1996) Archimedian spirals with Euclidean gradient limits. From: Proceedings, Fourth Annual Meeting of the International Society for Magnetic Resonance in Medicine, pp 114
38. Salustri C, Yang Y, Duyn JH, Glover GH (1997) Comparison between analytical and numerical solutions for spiral trajectory in 2D k-space. From: Proceedings, Fifth Annual Meeting of the International Society for Magnetic Resonance in Medicine, pp 1813
39. Meyer CH, Pauly JM, Macovski A (1996) A rapid, graphical method for optimal spiral gradient design. From: Proceedings, Fourth Annual Meeting of the International Society for Magnetic Resonance in Medicine, pp 392
40. Meyer CH, Pauly JM, Macovski A, Nishimura DG (1990) Simultaneous spatial and spectral selective excitation. Magn Reson Med 15 (2):287–304
41. Pipe JG, Haj-Ali A (1996) An approximation to spiral imaging using trapezoidal waveforms and collapsing spirals. From: Proceedings, Fourth Annual Meeting of the International Society for Magnetic Resonance in Medicine, pp 391
42. Meyer CH, Li KCP, Pauly JM, Macovski A (1994) Fast spiral T2-weighted imaging. From: Proceedings, Second Annual Meeting of the Society of Magnetic Resonance, pp 467
43. Meyer CH (1997) United States patent 5,650,723
44. Block W, Pauly J, Nishimura D (1997) RARE spiral T2-weighted imaging. Magn Reson Med 37 (4):582–590
45. Irarrazabal P, Nishimura DG (1995) Fast 3-dimensional magnetic resonance imaging. Magn Reson Med 33 (5):656–662
46. Thedens DR, Gold GE, Irarrazabal P, Nishimura DG (1996) Fast 3D Imaging with a short readout short TE cones trajectory. From: Proceedings, Fourth Annual Meeting of the International Society for Magnetic Resonance in Medicine, pp 113
47. Yang YH, Glover GH, Vangelderen P, Mattay VS, Santha AKS, Sexton RH, Ramsey NF, Moonen CTW, Weinberger DR, Frank JA (1996) Fast 3D functional magnetic resonance imaging at 1.5 T with spiral acquisition. Magn Reson Med 36 (4):620–626
48. Thedens DR, Irarrazaval P, Sachs TS, Meyer CH, Nishimura DG (1997) Three-dimensional coronary angiography with spiral trajectories. From: Proceedings, Fifth Annual Meeting of the International Society for Magnetic Resonance in Medicine, pp 835
49. Gatehouse PD, Firmin DN, Collins S, Longmore DB (1994) Real time blood flow imaging by spiral scan phase velocity mapping. Magn Reson Med 31 (5):504–512
50. Pike GB, Meyer CH, Brosnan TJ, Pelc NJ (1994) Magnetic resonance velocity imaging using a fast spiral phase contrast sequence. Magn Reson Med 32 (4):476–483
51. Liao JR, Sommer FG, Herfkens RJ, Pelc NJ (1995) Cine spiral imaging. Magn Reson Med 34 (3):490–493
52. Meyer CH, Nishimura DG (1997) High-resolution multislice spiral coronary angiography with real-time interactive localization. From: Proceedings, Fifth Annual Meeting of the International Society for Magnetic Resonance in Medicine, pp 439

53. Sachs TS, Meyer CH, Irarrazabal P, Hu BS, Nishimura DG, Macovski A (1995) The diminishing variance algorithm for real-time reduction of motion artifacts in MRI. Magn Reson Med 34 (3):412–422
54. Brittain JH, Olcott EW, Szuba A, Gold GE, Wright GA, Irarrazaval P, Nishimura DG (1997) Three-dimensional flow-independent peripheral angiography. Magn Reson Med 38 (3):343–354
55. Yacoe ME, Li KCP, Cheung L, Meyer CH (1997) Spiral spin-echo magnetic-resonance-imaging of the pelvis with spectrally and spatially selective radiofrequency excitation: comparison with fat-saturated fast spin-echo imaging. Can Asso Radiol J 48 (4):247–251
56. Noll DC, Cohen JD, Meyer CH, Schneider W (1995) Spiral k-space MR imaging of cortical activation. J Magn Reson Imaging 5 (2):49–56
57. Noll DC (1995) Methodologic considerations for spiral k-space functional MRI. Int J Imaging Syst. Technology 6:175–183
58. Lee AT, Glover GH, Meyer CH (1995) Discrimination of large venous vessels in time-course spiral blood-oxygen-level-dependent magnetic-resonance functional neuroimaging. Magn Reson Med 33 (6):745–754
59. Glover GH, Lee AT (1995) Motion artifacts in fMRI: comparison of 2DFT with PR and spiral scan methods. Magn Reson Med 33 (5):624–635
60. Glover GH, Lemieux SK, Drangova M, Pauly JM (1996) Decomposition of inflow and blood oxygen level-dependent (BOLD) effects with dual-echo spiral gradient-recalled echo (GRE) fMRI. Magn Reson Med 35 (3):299–308
61. Meyer CH, Spielman D, Macovski A (1993) Spiral Fluoroscopy. From: Proceedings, Twelfth Annual Meeting of the Society of Magnetic Resonance in Medicine, pp 475
62. Holz D, Rasche V, Schomberg H (1994) Continuous imaging using spiral k-space trajectories. From: Proceedings, Second Annual Meeting of the Society for Magnetic Resonance, pp 464
63. Spielman DM, Pauly JM, Meyer CH (1995) Magnetic-resonance fluoroscopy using spirals with variable sampling densities. Magn Reson Med 34 (3):388–394
64. Meyer CH, Macovski A (1996) United States patent 5,485,086
65. Kerr AB, JM Pauly, Hu BS, Li KCP, Hardy CJ, Meyer CH, Macovski A, Nishimura DG (1997) Real-time interactive MRI on a conventional scanner. Magn Reson Med 38 (3):355–367

Subject Index